Illustrated Tips and Tricks for

Intraoperative Imaging in Fracture Surgery

Illustrated Tips and Tricks for

Intraoperative Imaging in Fracture Surgery

Christiaan N. Mamczak, DO

Assistant Professor
Department of Orthopaedic Surgery
Indiana University School of Medicine
Beacon Orthopaedic Trauma Specialists
South Bend, Indiana

Christopher S. Smith, MD

LCDR MC USN
Associate Professor, USUHS
Director of Orthopaedic Trauma
Department of Orthopaedic Surgery
Naval Medical Center Portsmouth
Portsmouth, Virginia

Michael J. Gardner, MD

Professor and Vice Chairman
Chief, Orthopaedic Trauma Service
Stanford University School of Medicine
Stanford, California

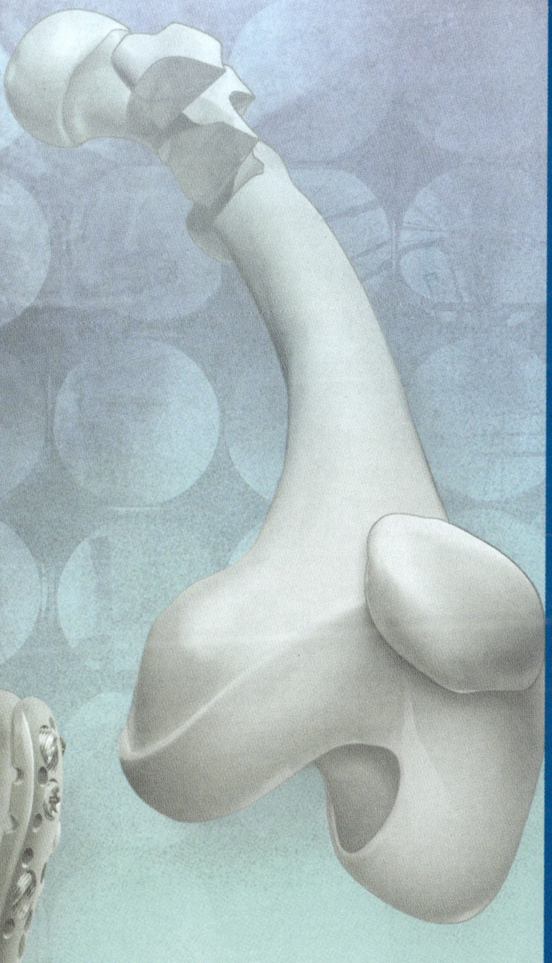

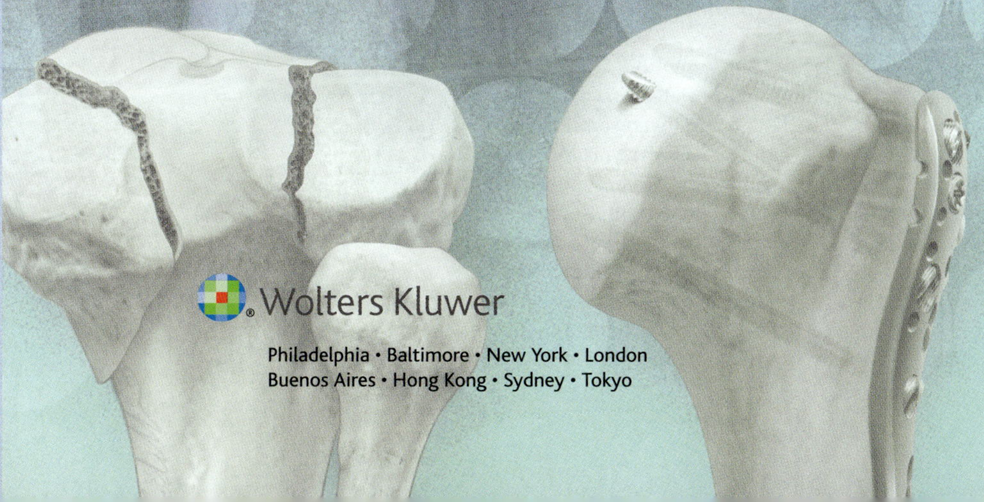

Wolters Kluwer

Philadelphia • Baltimore • New York • London
Buenos Aires • Hong Kong • Sydney • Tokyo

Acquisitions Editor: Brian Brown
Editorial Coordinator: Dave Murphy
Marketing Manager: Dan Dressler
Production Project Manager: David Saltzberg
Design Coordinator: Stephen Druding
Manufacturing Coordinator: Beth Welsh
Illustrator: Scott Bodell
Prepress Vendor: SPi Global

9 8 7 6 5 4 3 2 1

Printed in China

Library of Congress Cataloging-in-Publication Data
Names: Mamczak, Christiaan N., editor. | Smith, Christopher S., editor. | Gardner, Michael J., editor.
Title: Illustrated tips and tricks for intraoperative imaging in fracture surgery / [edited by] Christiaan N. Mamczak, Christopher S. Smith, Michael J. Gardner ; illustrations by Scott Bodell.
Description: Philadelphia : Wolters Kluwer Health, [2018] | Includes bibliographical references and index.
Identifiers: LCCN 2017040691 | ISBN 9781496328960 (hardback)
Subjects: | MESH: Fracture Fixation, Internal—methods | Fluoroscopy—methods | Intraoperative Period | Patient Positioning—methods
Classification: LCC RD101 | NLM WE 185 | DDC 617.1/5—dc23 LC record available at https://lccn.loc.gov/2017040691

LWW.com

RRS1710

I am grateful to my co-editors, Chris and Mike, and our friends (the authors) who were instrumental in composing this educational textbook. Together we have worked to create a valuable reference for orthopedic fracture surgeons. I'd also like to recognize all of the fluoro techs that I have worked with over the years.

Lastly, I would like to acknowledge and thank my family for the understanding and patience they have demonstrated in support of my career. It has been a long and tedious road with many call days and nights away from the people dearest to me. Luckily they embrace my passion for orthopedic trauma surgery and desire to publish. I have been blessed with unconditional love from my wife, Debbie, and children: Zac, Alexandra, Nadia, and Sophia. Coming home to them after each workday makes my life complete.

—Christiaan N. Mamczak

Thank you, my coeditors and chapter authors. It's been an honor and a privilege working with you to produce a great and timely practical reference. I am grateful to my mentors, who taught me the importance of getting the perfect fluoro shot and to the ortho trauma x-ray techs who performed magic in the OR. In addition, this book would not be possible if not for my residents past and present, keeping me on my toes with their thirst for knowledge. You guys continue to impress me every day.

I would like to thank my parents, Philip R. Smith and Susan E. Smith, for their encouraging support and for fostering my love for medicine and orthopaedics from an early age. Lastly, I would like to thank my family who have been by my side though numerous deployments and long hours at the hospital. To my wife Ashley, and children Andrew and Megan, thank you for your love, patience, and understanding. You guys are my rock and my life.

—Christopher S. Smith

I'd like to dedicate this book to all of my mentors at Hospital for Special Surgery, Harborview Medical Center, and Washington University who have spent countless hours and limitless energy in teaching me about all aspects of fracture care. Their passion for perfection has been awe-inspiring and has driven me to continuously search for ways to improve. And a huge thanks to my family for continuing to support me in so many ways.

—Michael J. Gardner

Contributors

Timothy S. Achor, MD
Associate Professor
Director
Orthopaedic Trauma Fellowship
Department of Orthopaedic Surgery
University of Texas Health Science Center at Houston
Memorial Hermann–Texas Medical Center
Houston, Texas

Adam Adler, MD
Fellow
Department of Orthopaedic Surgery
Stanford University School of Medicine
Stanford, California

Michael J. Beltran, MD
Chief
Orthopaedic Trauma
San Antonio Military Medical Center
San Antonio, Texas

Marschall B. Berkes, MD
Orthopaedic Surgeon
United States Air Force
Landstuhl, Germany

Julius A. Bishop, MD
Assistant Professor
Department of Orthopaedic Surgery
Associate Residency Director
Stanford University Medical Center
Stanford, California

Steven M. Cherney, MD
Resident
Department of Orthopaedic Surgery
Washington University School of Medicine
St. Louis, Missouri

Garet C. Comer, MD
Orthopaedic Hand Surgeon
Palo Alto Medical Foundation
Mountain View, California

Adam G. Cota, MD
Orthopaedic Trauma Surgeon
Rocky Mountain Orthopaedic Associates
Grand Junction, Colorado

William W. Cross III, MD
Assistant Professor
Department of Orthopedic Surgery
Mayo Clinic
Rochester, Minnesota

Jean-Claude G. D'Alleyrand, MD
LTC MC USA
Chief, Orthopaedic Traumatology
Walter Reed National Military Medical Center
Bethesda, Maryland

Gregory D. Dikos, MD
Orthopaedic Trauma Surgeon
Orthopaedics Indianapolis
Indianapolis, Indiana

Nicholas J. Erdle, MD
LT MC USN
Resident
Department of Orthopaedic Surgery
Naval Medical Center Portsmouth
Portsmouth, Virginia

Safi Faruqui, DO
Attending
Department of Orthopaedic Surgery
Mary S. Stern Hand Surgery Fellowship
TriHealth Hand Surgery Specialists
Cincinnati, Ohio

David A. Feaker Jr, DO
LT MC USN
Resident
Department of Orthopaedic Surgery
Naval Medical Center Portsmouth
Portsmouth, Virginia

Michael J. Gardner, MD
Professor and Vice Chairman
Chief, Orthopaedic Trauma Service
Stanford University School of Medicine
Stanford, California

Joshua L. Gary, MD
Associate Professor
Department of Orthopaedic Surgery
McGovern Medical School at UT Health Houston
Houston, Texas

Robert R. Gorman III, MD
Clinical Assistant Professor
Department of Orthopaedic Surgery
Director of Orthopaedic Clinical Practice Council
Western Michigan University School of Medicine
Bronson Medical Group
Kalamazoo, Michigan

Jonah Hebert-Davies, MD, FRCSC
Assistant Professor
Department of Orthopaedics and Sports Medicine
Harborview Medical Center
University of Washington
Seattle, Washington

Adam Johannsen, MD
Resident
Department of Orthopaedic Surgery
Stanford University School of Medicine
Stanford, California

Elizabeth A. King, MD
Fellow
Department of Orthopaedic Surgery
Mary S. Stern Hand Surgery Fellowship
Cincinnati, Ohio

James C. Krieg, MD
Professor and Director of Orthopaedic Trauma
Rothman Institute at Thomas Jefferson University
Philadelphia, Pennsylvania

George-Yves Laflamme, MD, FRCSC
Associate Professor
Hospital du Sacre-Coeur
University of Montreal
Montreal, Canada

Milton T.M. Little, MD
Assistant Professor
Orthopaedic Trauma Service
Cedar Sinai Medical Center
Los Angeles, California

Dean G. Lorich, MD
Associate Director
Orthopaedic Trauma Service
Hospital for Special Surgery
New York Presbyterian Hospital
New York, New York

Christiaan N. Mamczak, DO
Assistant Professor
Department of Orthopaedic Surgery
Indiana University School of Medicine
Beacon Orthopaedic Trauma Specialists
South Bend, Indiana

Theodore T. Manson, MD
Associate Professor
Department of Orthopaedic Surgery
R Adams Cowley Shock Trauma Center
University of Maryland
Baltimore, Maryland

Geoffrey S. Marecek, MD
Assistant Professor of Clinical Orthopaedic Surgery
University of Southern California Keck School of Medicine
Los Angeles, California

Ian P. McAlister, MD
Resident
Department of Orthopedic Surgery
Mayo Clinic
Rochester, Minnesota

Christopher M. McAndrew, MD, MSc
Associate Professor
Department of Orthopaedic Surgery
Washington University School of Medicine
St. Louis, Missouri

James E. Meeker, MD
Associate Professor
Department of Orthopaedic Surgery
Oregon Health and Science University
Portland, Oregon

Anna N. Miller, MD, FACS
Associate Professor
Department of Orthopaedic Surgery
Washington University School of Medicine
St. Louis, Missouri

John W. Munz, MD
Assistant Professor
Department of Orthopedic Surgery
Orthopedic Trauma Service
McGovern Medical School at UT Health Houston
Houston, Texas

Daniel A. Osei, MD, MSc
Assistant Professor of Orthopedic Surgery
Washington University School of Medicine
St. Louis, Missouri

W. Michael Pullen, MD
LT MC USN
Staff Orthopaedic Surgeon
Department of Orthopaedic Surgery
United States Naval Hospital, Yokosuka
Yokosuka, Japan

William M. Ricci, MD

Professor and Vice Chair Chief, Orthopaedic Trauma Service
Washington University School of Medicine
St. Louis, Missouri

Jason W. Roberts, MD

Clinical Assistant Professor
Department of Orthopaedic Surgery
Medical Director of Orthopaedic Trauma
Western Michigan University School of Medicine
Bronson Methodist Hospital
Kalamazoo, Michigan

Bharat Sampathi, BS

Medical Student
University of California, Irvine School of Medicine
Irvine, California

John A. Scolaro, MD, MA

Assistant Professor
Department of Orthopaedic Surgery
University of California, Irvine
Orange, California

Andrew J. Sheean, MD

Chief Resident
Department of Orthopaedic Surgery
San Antonio Military Medical Center
San Antonio, Texas

Jason L. Shewmaker, RT (R)

Senior Radiographic Technologist
Department of Radiology
University of Kentucky Chandler Medical Center
Lexington, Kentucky

Christopher S. Smith, MD

LCDR MC USN
Associate Professor, USUHS
Director of Orthopaedic Trauma
Department of Orthopaedic Surgery
Naval Medical Center Portsmouth
Portsmouth, Virginia

Tyler Snoap, MD

Resident
Department of Orthopaedic Surgery
Western Michigan University
Homer Stryker School of Medicine
Kalamazoo, Michigan

Ryan Taylor, MD

Assistant Professor
Department of Orthopaedic Surgery
University of Texas at Houston
Houston, Texas

Dominic L. Van Nielen, MD

LT MC USN
Resident
Department of Orthopaedic Surgery
Naval Medical Center Portsmouth
Portsmouth, Virginia

David S. Wellman, MD

Assistant Professor
Department of Orthopaedic Surgery
Hospital for Special Surgery, Weill Cornell Medical College
New York, New York

Matthew J. Wilson, DO

LT MC USN
Resident, Department of Orthopaedic Surgery
Naval Medical Center Portsmouth
Portsmouth, Virginia

Raymond D. Wright Jr, MD

Associate Professor
Department of Orthopaedic Surgery
University of Kentucky Chandler Medical Center
Lexington, Kentucky

Brad J. Yoo, MD

Associate Professor
Department of Orthopaedic Surgery
Oregon Health and Science University
Portland, Oregon

Foreword

Over the past 30 years, there have been countless important clinical and technical advances in orthopedic traumatology. This progress has been nothing short of amazing, and most of it has been directly correlated with improved knowledge of osteology and imaging.

In the late 1980s, Drs. Bob Winquist and S. Ted Hansen introduced closed reamed femoral medullary nailing to North America. Femoral nailing allowed early fracture stability and patient mobility and was quickly identified to be a life changing and often life-saving technique. The patient was freed from the deadly "orthopedic crucifix" position of prolonged skeletal traction. Intraoperative fluoroscopy was the key component that changed nailing procedures from extensive and morbid open operations to safe closed ones. And the game was on for intraoperative fluoroscopy as clinicians used it more and more to better assess the fracture reduction quality and implant construct safety.

The entire field of boney imaging advanced. Plain radiographs, intraoperative imaging, and computed tomography evolved as clinicians became more aware of their value to improving patient care quality. Injury imaging included traction views, oblique images, and CT scans and helped surgeons to refine their preoperative planning. As with medullary nailing, high-quality intraoperative fluoroscopy has been directly responsible for the evolution of modern percutaneous pelvic surgery. Long before any pelvic fixation screws were inserted, we had to completely understand the various osseous fixation pathways and their imaging details. The cortical surface limits had to be identified first and then the specific images necessary to reliably demonstrate them followed. Finally, the variants of pelvic osteology were defined so that the intraoperative fluoroscopic pelvic imaging would accurately assess the manipulative reductions and also guide the insertion of pubic ramus, pelvic brim, acetabular columnar, iliosacral, and other pelvic fixation screws.

Overall, intraoperative imaging serves numerous important clinical needs including (1) proper patient positioning, (2) fracture site instability and displacements, (3) reduction accuracy, (4) implant location, (5) inadvertent retained surgical devices, and (6) stability of the repair.

With this book, Drs. Mamczak, Smith, and Gardner provide practicing surgeons, residents, medical students, nurses, operating room staff, and radiology technicians with a clear, concise, detailed, and comprehensive reference for their individual intraoperative imaging needs. Each chapter has been authored by an experienced clinician and focuses on the indications, specifics, and common mistakes of modern intraoperative imaging. This book will help you to improve your overall knowledge of modern imaging, and more importantly, it will improve your awareness, abilities, and safety.

Milton L. Chip Routt, Jr, MD

It gives me great pleasure to be invited by Chris Smith to write a forward for "*Illustrated Tips and Tricks for Intraoperative Imaging in Fracture Surgery*", that is coauthored by Drs.' Mamczak, Smith, and Gardner. This, especially so, as I was honored to be one of Chris Smith's mentors, and he continues to flourish and make us all very proud!!

The more we know about orthopedic trauma the more we realize that restoration of normal anatomy, when feasible, usually assures the best outcome. Obviously, there are many variables, including the patient, timing, other injuries, soft tissues, age, comorbidities, etc., that are involved in the decision making, but when possible as determined by the preoperative plan, "perfect" must be the goal. Obviously if that can be achieved with less direct visualization/exposure, that is an advantage, that is, precisely what an intraoperative C-arm allows! In addition, the worst case scenario as a surgeon is to have a problem intraoperatively, which one cannot see, cannot even visualize adequately with the C-arm due to poor planning and being forced to expose more (unnecessarily) or accept a less than optimal outcome.

I do believe the authors have addressed those issues in "*Illustrated Tips and Tricks for Intraoperative Imaging in Fracture Surgery*" and assured with a complete preoperative plan that includes the patient, surgery, and C-arm positioning/views to allow intraoperative visualization and assessment of reduction, fixation, and hence the best chance for an optimal outcome.

Clearly this book is a must for all orthopedic surgeons but especially for those doing trauma and fracture surgery.

David L. Helfet, MD

Preface

It goes without saying that preoperative planning is a critical prerequisite for achieving optimal outcomes in fracture surgery. However, one aspect of the process that may be underappreciated and overlooked is the importance of strategically positioning the patient as a link to maximizing the efficiency of fluoroscopy. The advent of using an intraoperative C-arm has dramatically improved the quality of fracture reductions and fixation when compared to cases without imaging. Yet despite its commonplace use, a purposeful understanding of the C-arm's capabilities and limitations is paramount. This begins with proper positioning of the patient within a preferably radiolucent operative field. Various factors come into play within this decision process: fracture type, operating table, positioning adjuncts, patient body habitus, and the functional range of the fluoroscope. Surgeon preference should be a dynamic variable as one fixation technique, and method is usually not sufficient for all variations of a fracture. Although a surgeon's surgical training experience is the most influential factor in patient positioning and fluoroscopy use, continuing education is a critical component to refining one's skills, comfort level, and outcomes.

This textbook is meant to provide a valuable guide for the use of intraoperative fluoroscopy in fracture surgery. Based on the absence of such a resource, the editors envisioned an instructional manual of tips and tricks to set surgeons up for success in fracture care. We have all been taught that "one view is no view." Most of us have probably participated in a case where better preoperative planning may have optimized the ability to arrive at the desired fixation outcome. Nothing may be more frustrating during a case than the inability to achieve a symbiotic relationship between patient positioning and obtaining accurate imaging. Settling for suboptimal images because we improperly set up the case is a less than ideal outcome. Learning from our mistakes and recreating a consistent environment to allow fluoroscopy to guide fracture reduction and safe implant fixation is inherent to the development of a talented surgeon.

The chapters within this text are a culmination of recommendations for patient positioning and variations of C-arm use by experts within the field of orthopedics. The author's tips and tricks are the result of a common desire to "get it right," our mentor's teaching, and our own struggles and experience. This book is geared to any surgeon who operates on extremity and pelvic fractures, both novice and seasoned. It is a concise review of the radiographic bony anatomy and understanding of what we should be "seeing" during fracture reduction and instrumentation. We trust that you will find this reference useful for confirming your knowledge base for the most practical cases as well as the most challenging ones. It represents a teaching tool full of illustrations for educators to use at academic centers and a quick visual refresher for any surgeon to absorb right before a case. It has been a fun challenge to create this textbook as we sought to consider the different methods of fixation and their connection to fluoroscopy. We encourage the reader to never undervalue the time spent in preoperatively planning a case and to embrace fluoroscopy as complimentary adjunct to fracture surgery. Position yourself (and the patient) for success and get it right.

Christiaan N. Mamczak, Christopher S. Smith, and Michael J. Gardner

Contents

Chapter 1
Introduction

WILLIAM M. RICCI

Brief History of Fluoroscopy

Fluoroscopy is an indispensable part of the orthopedic traumatologist's armamentarium. Although it could be argued that intraoperative imaging may be overutilized, it is almost unimaginable to consider embarking on the reduction and fixation of a complex fracture, especially when using indirect reduction techniques, without fluoroscopy. This technology dates back to the very earliest days of radiography. Within 1 year of Roentgen's discovery of x-rays, in 1896, Thomas Edison developed the "fluoroscope." This real-time viewing of x-ray images utilized a simple fluorescent screen in a light-tight viewing cone. The imaging process has since been known as "fluoroscopy."[1] For the first half of the 20th century, little changes were made to this basic practice. High doses of x-ray were required, and cumulative exposure times were often minutes long rather than seconds. This combination caused excessive exposure doses to patients and staff, limiting the utilization of this technology. In 1948, John Coltman developed the image intensifier that converted x-rays to an electron beam that could be accelerated and focused on a fluorescent screen. The light emitted could be thousands of times brighter with the image intensifier than without the image intensifier, thus reducing the doses of radiation required. Fluoroscopy could then be used with reasonable safety in more routine applications, including fracture care.

Technical Considerations

Fluoroscope Components

A typical fluoroscopic system (Fig. 1-1) includes the x-ray generating tube, a collimator, an image intensifier, and a video camera. The image intensifier is a tube with a fluorescent screen (input phosphor) that glows with the image produced by the x-ray pattern that exits the patient. The light from the input phosphor causes ejection of electrons from a photoelectric material adjacent to the input phosphor. These electrons are accelerated via a high voltage (30 kV) and focused onto a small (1-inch diameter) screen (the output phosphor). The output phosphor glows much more brightly than does the input phosphor (about 3,000 times) because of the energy gain provided by the acceleration of the electrons and also because of minification of the image. The image on the output phosphor is monitored via a video camera system.

X-Ray Basic Physics

X-rays generated by fluoroscopy and plain radiography are forms of electromagnetic radiation. Other examples of electromagnetic radiation include visible light and radio waves. X-rays are produced when a heated filament (negatively charged cathode) within a tube generates electrons that are accelerated by application of high voltage (50 to 150 kVp) toward a tungsten target (positively charged anode). The electrons, repelled by the cathode and pulled toward the anode, accelerate to more than one-half the speed of light in one inch of travel. The electrons impact the anode and suddenly slow. The energy lost by the slowed electrons is converted to heat and creation of electromagnetic radiation including infrared light, visible light, ultraviolet waves, and x-rays.

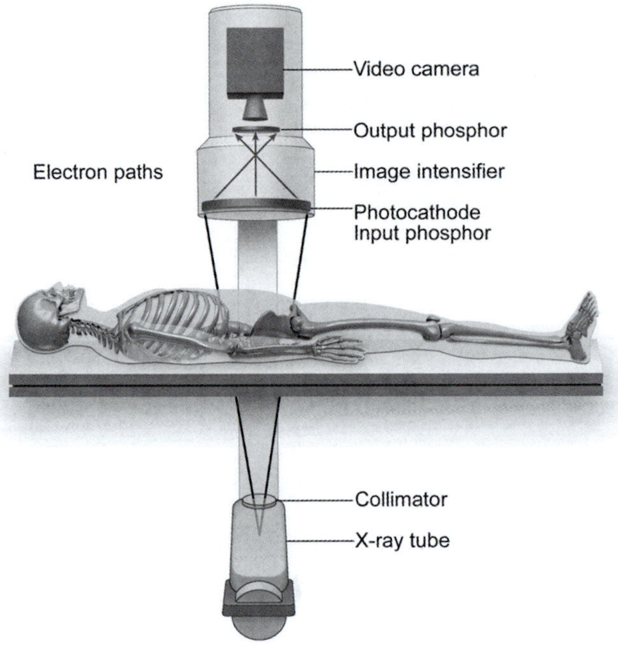

Figure 1-1 | A schematic diagram of a fluoroscopy unit.

- **X-ray generator**—Produces electrical energy and allows selection of kilovolt peak (kVp) and tube current (mA) that is delivered to an x-ray tube.
- **X-ray tube**—Converts electrical energy of x-ray generator to x-ray beam.
- **Collimator**—Contains multiple sets of shutters (round and rectangular blades) that refine the x-ray beam shape. Collimating the beam to the area of interest reduces the exposed volume of tissue and results in less scatter and better image contrast. It also reduces the overall patient and surgeon radiation dose by minimizing scatter and direct exposure.
- **Image intensifier**—Converts x-rays to photoelectric energy. Major components include an input layer (input phosphor + photocathode) to convert x-rays to electrons, an image intensifier tube to accelerate and focus the electrons, and an output layer (output phosphor) to create a visible image.
- **Video camera** system—Captures the image and displays it on a video monitor.

The flow of electrons from the filament to the target is called the tube current and is measured in milliamperes (mA). Fluoroscopy is normally performed using 2 to 6 mA and an accelerating voltage of 75 to 125 kVp. The rate of x-ray production is directly proportional to the tube current, but is more sensitive to increasing voltage than current. For example, increasing the kVp by 15% is equivalent to a 200% increase in the mA.

When x-rays traverse tissue, they can result in (1) complete penetration, (2) total absorption, or (3) partial absorption with scatter. Complete penetration means that the x-rays completely passed through the tissue, resulting in an image. Total absorption means that the x-ray energy was completely absorbed by the tissue, resulting in no image. Partial absorption with scatter involves partial transfer of energy to tissue, with the scattered x-ray possessing less energy and following a different trajectory. The scattered radiation is responsible for causing radiation exposure to the operator and staff.

Units of Radiation Exposure and Dose

Radiation exposure is defined as the quantity of x-rays required to produce an amount of ionization in air at standard temperature and pressure. The traditional unit of exposure is the *Roentgen (R)*, which is defined as R = 2.58×10^{-4} C/kg air. The SI unit is Coulombs/kilogram (C/kg). The unit Roentgen, however, is only defined for air and cannot be used to describe dose to tissue. An absorbed dose of radiation can be measured in rad *(Radiation Absorbed Dose)*. The SI unit is the Gray (Gy) where 1 Gy = 100 rad. Dose equivalent accounts for differences in biological effectiveness of different types of ionizing radiation. Dose equivalent is equal to absorbed dose (Gy or rad) multiplied by a radiation quality factor specific to the type of radiation being used. The traditional unit is the *rem (Roentgen Equivalent in Man)*; the SI unit is the *sievert (Sv)* where 1 Sv = 100 rem. In diagnostic x-ray, the radiation quality factor is 1, so 1 rad is equivalent to 1 rem. The effective dose equivalent (EDE) takes into account that the potential health effect from single organ exposure is smaller than from whole body exposure. The EDE is defined as the sum of the absorbed dose to the tissue multiplied by a weighting factor, which calculates risk of cancer from partial body irradiation versus whole body irradiation. Units are also rem or sieverts.

Radiation Exposure

Background and Direct Exposures

Exposure to intraoperative radiation is of concern to all members of the surgical team. For perspective, the average yearly exposure of the public to ionizing radiation is about 360 millirems (mrem), of which 300 mrem is from background radiation and 60 mrem from diagnostic radiographs. A chest radiograph exposes the patient to approximately 25 mrem, a hip radiograph to 500 mrem, and a hip CT 1,000 mrem. A regular C-arm exposes the patient to approximately 1,200 to 4,000 mrem/min (lower for extremity and higher for pelvis). These values represent direct exposure. Recommended yearly limits of radiation are 2 to 5 rem (depending on the governing body) to the torso, 15 rem to the eyes, 30 rem to the thyroid, and 50 rem to the extremities (e.g., hands).[2] Fetal limits, relevant to fluoroscopy in pregnant patients, are 0.5 rem over 9 months.

Surgeon Exposure

Surgeon and staff may be exposed directly, most commonly to hands in the path of the x ray beam, or exposed indirectly via scatter.[2] Those in close proximity, <36 inches, are at highest risk for exposure.[3] Sanders et al., in 1993, found that average exposure of surgeon from scatter during femoral and tibial nailing was 100 mrem per operation.[4] At this dose, yearly limits to the eyes (the most sensitive organ not typically shielded) would be reached after 150 cases. Of note, average fluoroscopy time in this study was 6.26 minutes. Similar results were found by Muller et al., in 1998, where average exposure per case to the dominant index finger was 127 mrem for nailing procedures that averaged 4.6 minutes of fluoroscopy.[5] A number of other studies[6–9] specifically evaluated exposure to the hands. Exposure varied substantially between procedure and surgeon varying from undetectable to 570 mrem per procedure. It should be noted that more recent studies have shown shorter fluoroscopy times for long bone intramedullary nailing than in the aforementioned studies that described exposure doses. Ricci et al.[10] found the average time for antegrade femoral nailing to be 153 seconds (range: 16 to 662) when using a piriformis starting point and 95 seconds (range: 20 to 375 seconds) when using a greater trochanteric starting point and in a separate study found the average fluoroscopy time for tibial nailing to be 72.4 or 82.6 seconds depending on the surgery time of day.[11] Also, more advanced newer generation C-arm devices reduce the exposure per case.

Team Exposure

Exposures to operating personnel, other than surgeon, are of concern too. Many of these individuals spend more cumulative time being exposed than do surgeons by virtue of being in the OR on a daily basis. A study utilizing simulated pelvic surgery found first assistant exposure (2 feet away) of 6 mrem/min and no detectable exposure at the scrub nurse position (3 feet away) or the anesthesia position (5 feet away).[3]

Exposure Reduction Strategies

Standard strategies to mitigate exposure to scatter include decreasing exposure time, increasing distance, shielding, and contamination control. Typical shielding techniques used by orthopedic trauma surgeons include use of lead garments that shield the body core. Thyroid shields are a common adjunct. Because eye exposure can be many times higher than central exposure, leaded glasses have been recommended.[12] There is little debate that less exposure is better than more, and a number of studies have documented strategies to reduce exposure. Use of a real-time radiation exposure feedback from the Philips DoseAware device decreased radiation exposure by 60%.[13]

Differences Between Fluoroscopy and Plain Radiography

The fluoroscopic image generally has less contrast and less resolution of fine detail than does a radiographic image. A fundamental difference between plain radiographs and fluoroscopy is that fluoroscopy machines can automatically adjust exposure based on the density of the subject. Exposure for traditional plain radiography is set by the technician and is static. Fluoroscopy units are usually operated in an automatic brightness control (ABC) mode, in which a sensor in the image intensifier monitors the image brightness. When there is inadequate brightness, the ABC increases the kVp first, which increases the x-ray penetration through the patient, and then adjusts the mA to increase the brightness. Thicker soft tissue or larger cross-sectional areas will generate greater exposure to optimize brightness. However, radiodense metallic objects may inadvertently lead to overexposed images when automatic modes are used. Conversely, a field dominated by radiolucent material, such as air in a poorly centered image, will result in an underexposed image (Fig. 1-2).

Another difference is that the area of capture for fluoroscopy is generally more limited than with plain x-rays and is round rather than rectangular. The size of most image intensifiers is approximately 12 inches in diameter, although units, often used in vascular surgery, exist with larger sized intensifiers. The relatively small size of fluoroscopy images therefore limits the ability to evaluate alignment of long bone fixation. For these purposes, plain radiography has more utility.

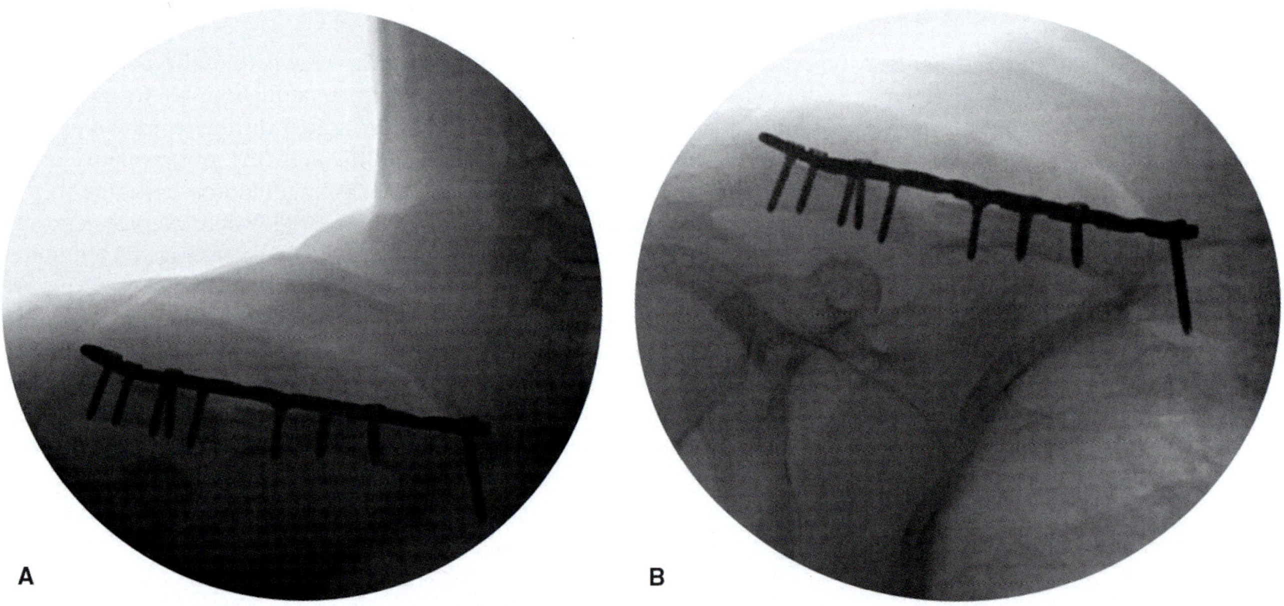

Figure 1-2 | A: This fluoroscopic image is centered such that a substantial portion of the field is air. Note that the tissue is underpenetrated due to the computer adjustments made by the fluoroscope being "fooled" to think the field is relatively radiolucent. The kVp and mA were 66 and 1.9, respectively. **B:** Centering the tissue to cover the majority of the field yields a properly exposed image with kVp and mA of 78 and 2.8, respectively.

Accuracy of Fluoroscopy

The ability to rely on fluoroscopy to definitively judge reduction has been debated. There is a general feeling in the orthopedic community that plain radiographs are more accurate than is fluoroscopy to judge fracture reduction, especially intra-articular reductions. However, critical analysis of this issue has led to varying conclusions. Several recent studies demonstrate inaccuracies of fluoroscopic evaluation of fracture reductions. Horst et al.[14] evaluated the quality of reduction and fixation based on fluoroscopy and compared results to postoperative plain radiographs. They found that in 8.2% of cases information was apparent on the postoperative plain radiographs such that a reviewer felt that the postoperative treatment plan should change. Haller et al.[15] found fluoroscopy inaccurate for evaluation of simulated tibial plateau fractures when fracture displacement was 2 mm or less. The accuracy of detecting reduction was 90% when there was a 5-mm displacement, but decreased to 37% to 83%

when displacement was 2 or 0 mm. Capo et al.[16] found that after closed reduction and percutaneous pinning of simulated Bennett's fractures in a cadaver model, the assessment of the articular gap, step-off, and displacement as detected by fluoroscopy was often in error compared to that detected by plain radiographs and direct examination.

On the other hand, there are also a number of studies that indicate fluoroscopy provides better accuracy than do plain radiographs. Norris et al.[17] found better results for fluoroscopy in evaluating positions of screws and reduction during acetabular fracture repair. Intraoperative fluoroscopy confirmed the extra-articular position of all screws evaluated. Postoperative CT scans confirmed the extra-articular placement of all screws assessed by fluoroscopy. Quality of reduction using intraoperative fluoroscopic images had a 100% correlation with reduction on final radiographs. One patient, with two screws placed without fluoroscopic evaluation, had intra-articular placement requiring revision surgery. Another study determined the accuracy of fluoroscopic imaging during closed reduction and percutaneous fixation of intra-articular thumb metacarpal fractures compared to direct vision and plain radiographs.[18] Fluoroscopy showed better correlation with direct vision than did plain radiographs for evaluation of displacement, and both fluoroscopy and plain radiographs showed excellent agreement when evaluating intra-articular step-off.

Terminology for Fluoroscopy Use in Orthopedic Trauma

There have been studies that have investigated the communication between the operative team and the fluoroscopy technician.[19,20] Poor communication can lead to unnecessary and/or poorly aligned fluoroscopy shots and therefore increased radiation exposure, frustration, and delay. Pally and Kreder[19] found that terminology used by surgeon members of the Canadian Orthopaedic Association to be tremendously diverse. They proposed that a standard lexicon be adopted and taught to orthopedic residents and technologists with the hope that efficient communication would be an unconscious part of operating the fluoroscope in every case. Although no such effort is underway in the United States at a national level, there is great utility in adopting a common terminology at the institutional level.

References

1. Quinn C. *Radiography in the Digital Age: Physics-Exposure-Radiation Biology*. 2nd ed. Springfield, IL: Charles C Thomas; 2014.
2. Singer G. Occupational radiation exposure to the surgeon. *J Am Acad Orthop Surg*. 2005;13:69–76.
3. Mehlman CT, DiPasquale TG. Radiation exposure to the orthopaedic surgical team during fluoroscopy: "how far away is far enough?". *J Orthop Trauma*. 1997;11:392–398.
4. Sanders R, Koval KJ, DiPasquale T, et al. Exposure of the orthopaedic surgeon to radiation. *J Bone Joint Surg Am*. 1993;75:326–330.
5. Muller LP, Suffner J, Wenda K, et al. Radiation exposure to the hands and the thyroid of the surgeon during intramedullary nailing. *Injury*. 1998;29:461–468.
6. Goldstone KE, Wright IH, Cohen B. Radiation exposure to the hands of orthopaedic surgeons during procedures under fluoroscopic X-ray control. *Br J Radiol*. 1993;66:899–901.
7. Noordeen MH, Shergill N, Twyman RS, et al. Hazard of ionizing radiation to trauma surgeons: reducing the risk. *Injury*. 1993;24:562–564.
8. Arnstein PM, Richards AM, Putney R. The risk from radiation exposure during operative X-ray screening in hand surgery. *J Hand Surg Br*. 1994;19:393–396.
9. Rampersaud YR, Foley KT, Shen AC, et al. Radiation exposure to the spine surgeon during fluoroscopically assisted pedicle screw insertion. *Spine (Phila Pa 1976)*. 2000;25:2637–2645.
10. Ricci WM, Schwappach J, Tucker M, et al. Trochanteric versus piriformis entry portal for the treatment of femoral shaft fractures. *J Orthop Trauma*. 2006;20:663–667.
11. Ricci WM, Gallagher B, Brandt A, et al. Is after-hours orthopaedic surgery associated with adverse outcomes? A prospective comparative study. *J Bone Joint Surg Am*. 2009;91:2067–2072.
12. Hoffler CE, Ilyas AM. Fluoroscopic radiation exposure: are we protecting ourselves adequately? *J Bone Joint Surg Am*. 2015;97:721–725.
13. Baumgartner R, Libuit K, Ren D, et al. Reduction of radiation exposure from C-arm fluoroscopy during orthopaedic trauma operations with introduction of real-time dosimetry. *J Orthop Trauma*. 2016;30:e53–58.
14. Horst TA, Mooney JF III, Hooker JA, et al. Comparison of intraoperative C-arm fluoroscopy to postoperative radiographs in operative fracture fixation. *J Surg Orthop Adv*. 2015;24:180–183.

15. Haller JM, O'Toole R, Graves M, et al. How much articular displacement can be detected using fluoroscopy for tibial plateau fractures? *Injury.* 2015;46:2243–2247.
16. Capo JT, Kinchelow T, Orillaza NS, et al. Accuracy of fluoroscopy in closed reduction and percutaneous fixation of simulated Bennett's fracture. *J Hand Surg Am.* 2009;34:637–641.
17. Norris BL, Hahn DH, Bosse MJ, et al. Intraoperative fluoroscopy to evaluate fracture reduction and hardware placement during acetabular surgery. *J Orthop Trauma.* 1999;13:414–417.
18. Greeven AP, Hammer S, Deruiter MC, et al. Accuracy of fluoroscopy in the treatment of intra-articular thumb metacarpal fractures. *J Hand Surg Eur Vol.* 2013;38:979–983.
19. Pally E, Kreder HJ. Survey of terminology used for the intraoperative direction of C-arm fluoroscopy. *Can J Surg.* 2013;56:109–112.
20. Williams TH, Syrett AG, & Brammar TJ. W.S.B.—a fluoroscopy C-arm communication strategy. *Injury.* 2009;40:840–843.

Chapter 2
Scapula Fractures

STEVEN M. CHERNEY
CHRISTOPHER M. MCANDREW

Bony Anatomy

- The scapula is a mostly flat, roughly triangular-shaped bone that is suspended off the posterolateral chest wall through the acromioclavicular articulation.
- The scapular spine arises from the upper posterior surface and gives rise superolaterally and anteriorly to the acromion.
- The coracoid process arises from the anterosuperior scapular neck. It runs in a superomedial direction before turning lateral and anterior as it thins at its "beak."
- The glenoid face is nearly perpendicular to the scapular body and forms the medial side of the glenohumeral articulation. Average glenoid version ranges from 5 degrees of anteversion to 15 degrees of retroversion.
- A majority of the scapular body bony surface area is only a few millimeters thick, limiting fixation constructs to the peripheral borders, scapular spine, glenoid neck, and coracoid.
- Imaging of the scapular body is complicated by the overlying thoracic wall and spine, while the acromion is difficult to image because of the overlying distal clavicle.
- Because of the complex anatomy and overlying structures, scapular fractures are easily missed or underestimated by plain radiographs.

Radiographic Anatomy

AP and Grashey AP View

- In the AP view, the glenohumeral articulation should be seen free from overlying structures, but the scapular body invariably overlies the thoracic wall, including the ribs and the lung fields. The medial border and inferior angle of the scapula should be included on the radiograph.
- Minimally displaced scapular body fractures, particularly over the medial half of the scapula, are difficult to appreciate secondary to overlying structures (Fig. 2-1A and B).
- To best visualize the glenohumeral joint, the beam should be rotated approximately 35 degrees aiming from the midline to lateral in order to profile the scapula, in line with the glenoid, generating a Grashey or "True AP" view (Figs. 2-2 and 2-3).
- Due to the slightly concave nature of the glenoid surface, the Grashey view allows confirmation that screws do not protrude into the glenohumeral joint (Fig. 2-4).
- The Grashey view is often best to ensure reduction of fracture fragments with spikes that exit the lateral border of the scapula. These fragments often have extension into the glenoid face, and articular reduction can be partially assessed with this view (Fig. 2-5A and B).
- The lateral and posterior displacement of the caudal fracture fragment can be due to the pull of the infraspinatus, teres major and minor, the latissimus dorsi, and the long head of the triceps, depending on the size of the fracture fragment.
- Overlying structures may obscure bony anatomy on the Grashey view, particularly toward the medial half of the scapula.

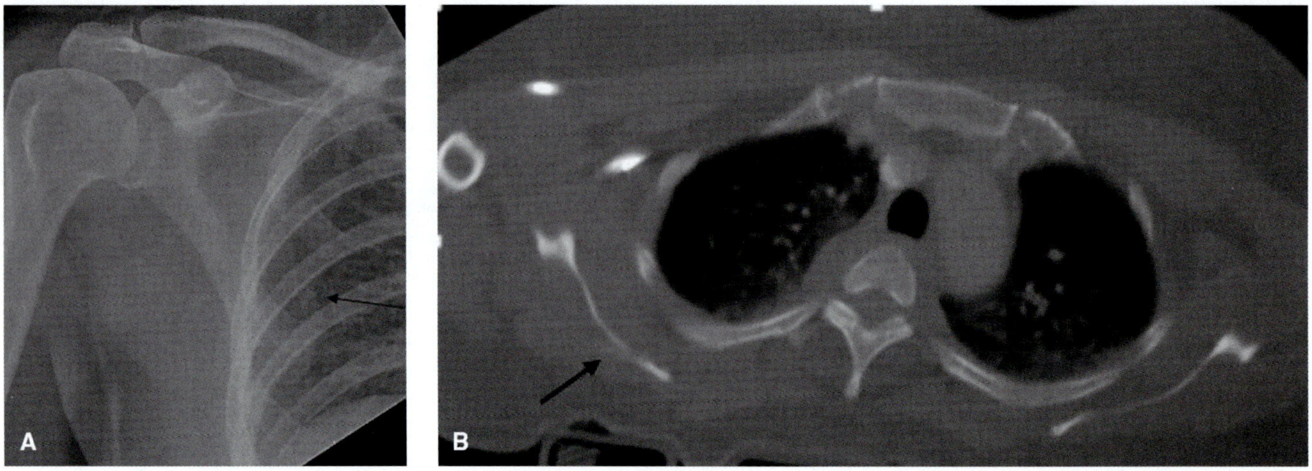

Figure 2-1 | Suboptimal technique and overlying structures resulted in a missed diagnosis of a medial scapular body fracture (*arrows*). This injury was recognized on subsequent CT scan as part of a trauma protocol.

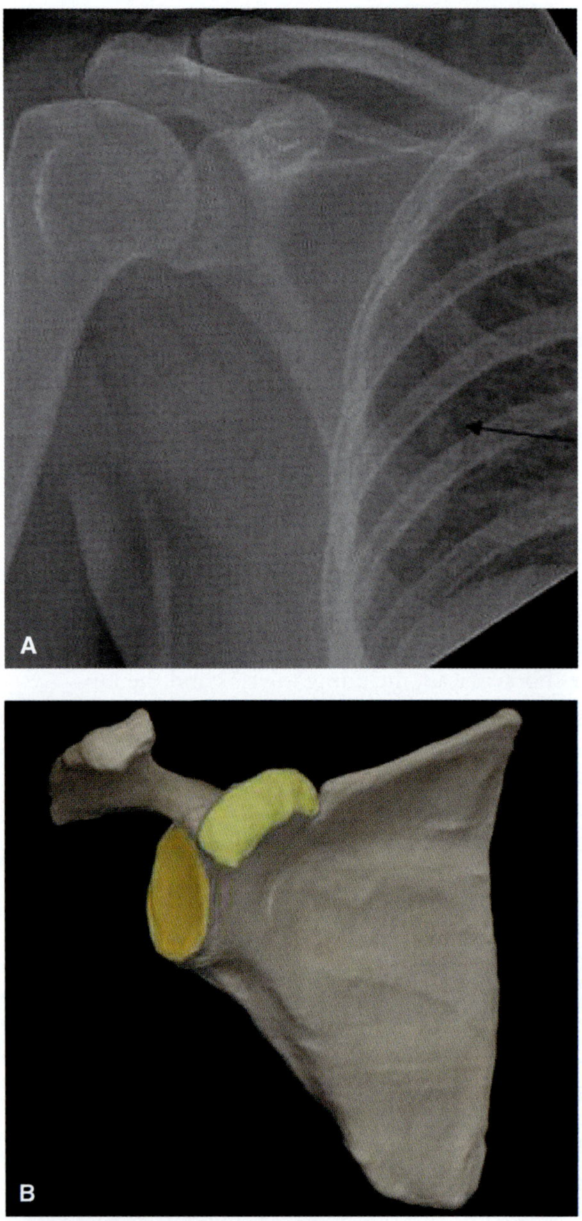

Figure 2-2 | The AP view fails to demonstrate the scapula body *en fasse* and exposes the surface of the glenoid fossa (*orange*). Note the orientation of the coracoid process (*yellow*).

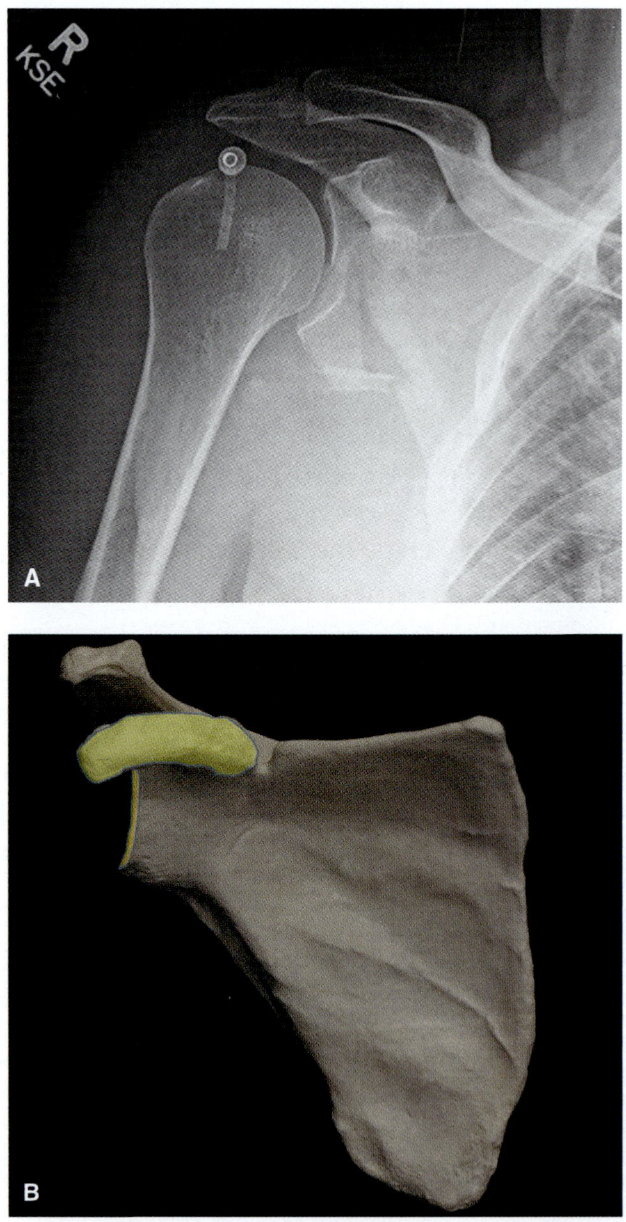

Figure 2-3 | Note the difference in orientation of the glenoid (*orange*) in profile and the coracoid process (*yellow*), as well as their radiographic representation with a Grashey AP view.

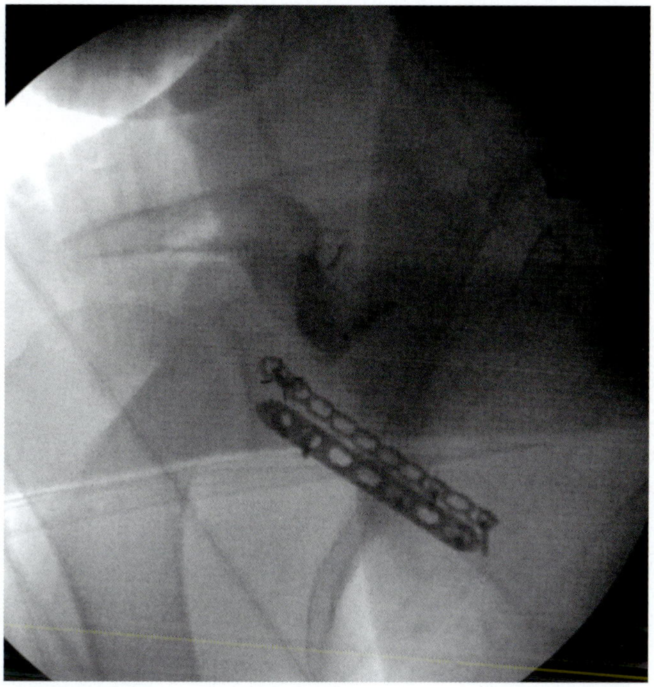

Figure 2-4 |

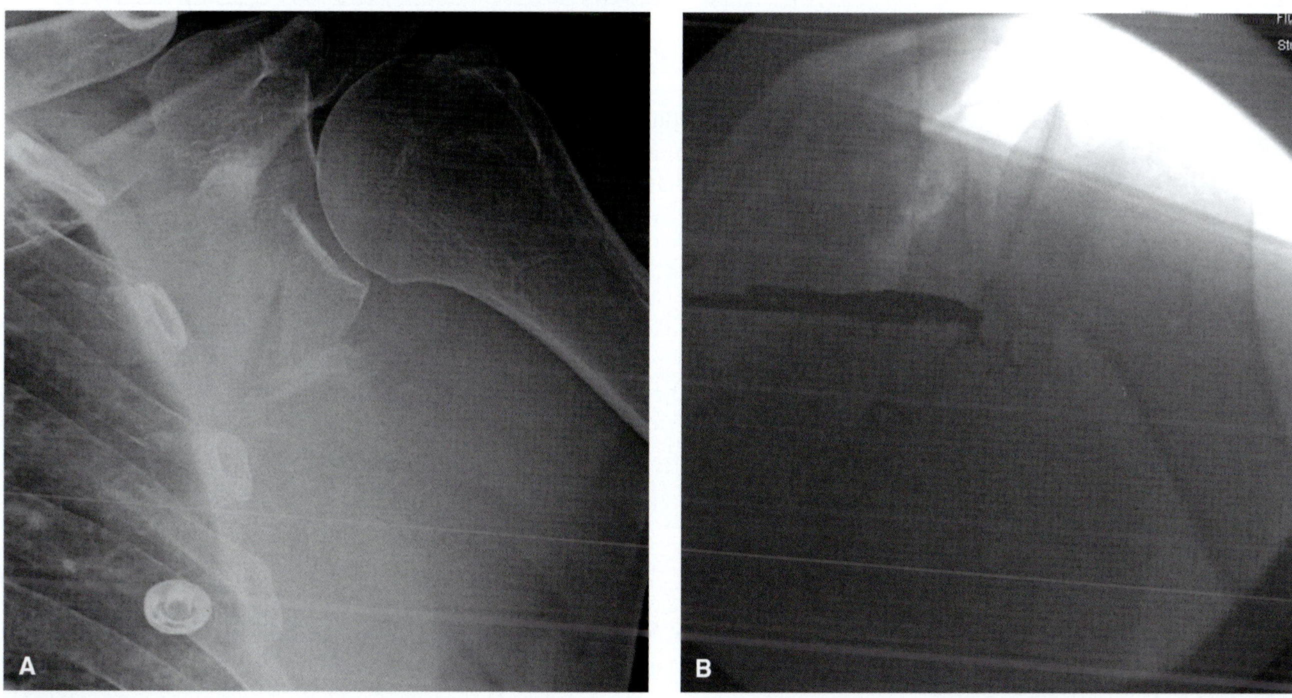

Figure 2-5 |

Lateral View (Scapular Y View)

- The humeral head should remain centralized within the bony "Y" formed from the confluence of the scapular spine (posteriorly), coracoid (anteriorly), and scapular body (inferiorly).
- From this sagittal profile, fractures of the scapular body, spine, acromion, and coracoid base can be visualized.
- The lateral view can appreciate the degree of scapular sagittal plane fracture displacement (Fig. 2-6A and B).
- Intraoperatively, the scapular Y view should be used to help ensure fracture reduction in line with the scapular body.

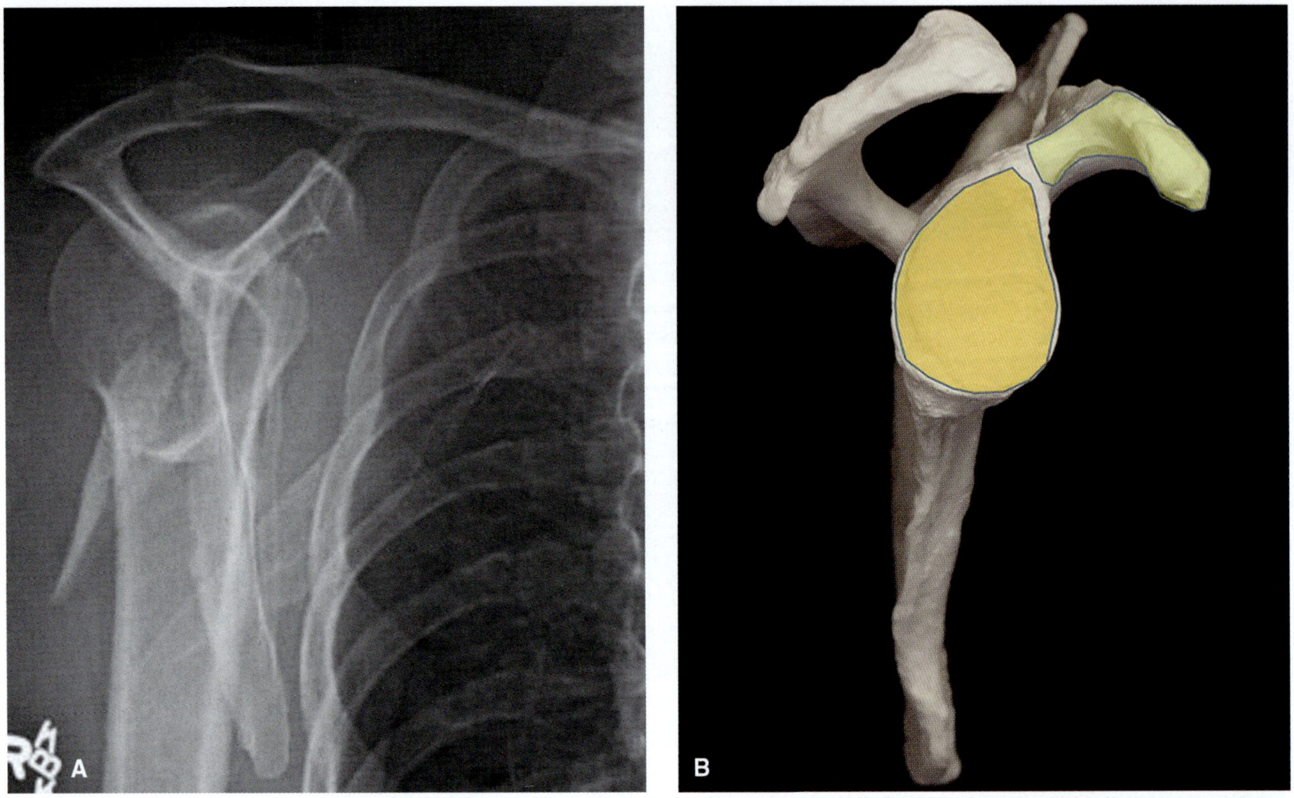

Figure 2-6 |

- The lateral view can be used as an aide to guide screw trajectory into the base of the coracoid. This screw should be placed with concomitant AP views.
- Care should be taken to make sure that screws in the scapular body are not too long, and do not impinge on the chest wall (Fig. 2-7).

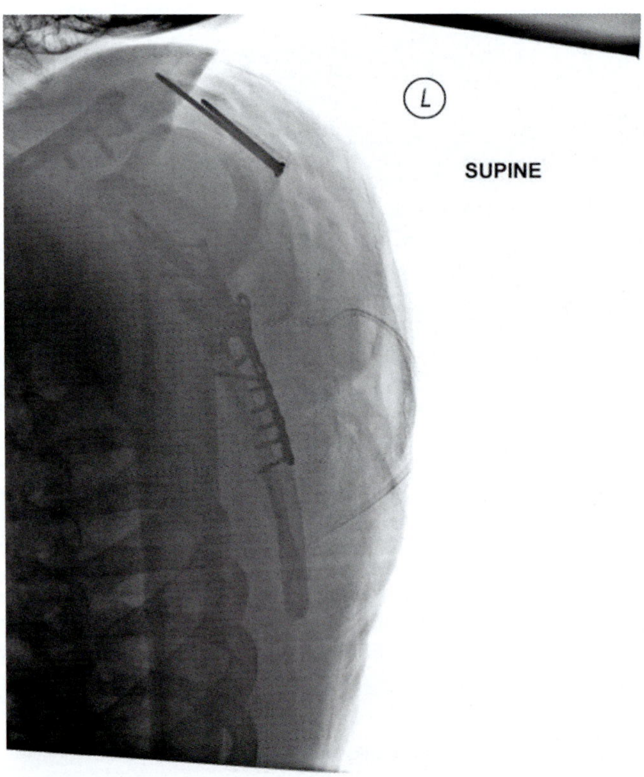

Figure 2-7 |

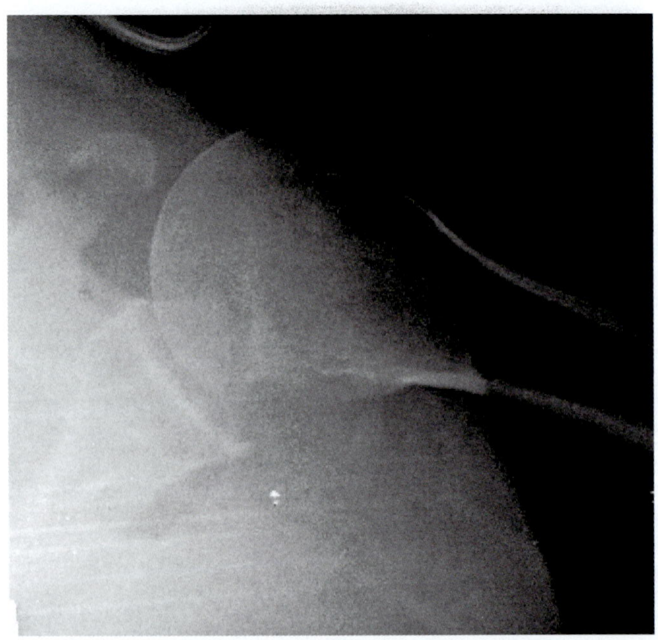

Figure 2-8 |

Axillary View

- Axillary views, including modified views, such as the Velpeau or West Point technique, can demonstrate glenohumeral dislocation, large glenoid rim fractures, and coracoid tip fractures (Fig. 2-8).

Preoperative Imaging

- The majority of scapula fractures can be managed nonoperatively; however, significant displacement and involvement of the glenohumeral joint may necessitate operative treatment.
- Standard radiographs are often inadequate to accurately delineate the fracture fragments and amount of displacement.
- The majority of these injuries occur in polytraumatized patients, and CT scans are frequently available for review. If a CT scan is not available, one should be obtained and studied prior to operative intervention.
- Three-dimensional reconstructions may be a useful adjunct for preoperative planning (Fig. 2-9A and B).

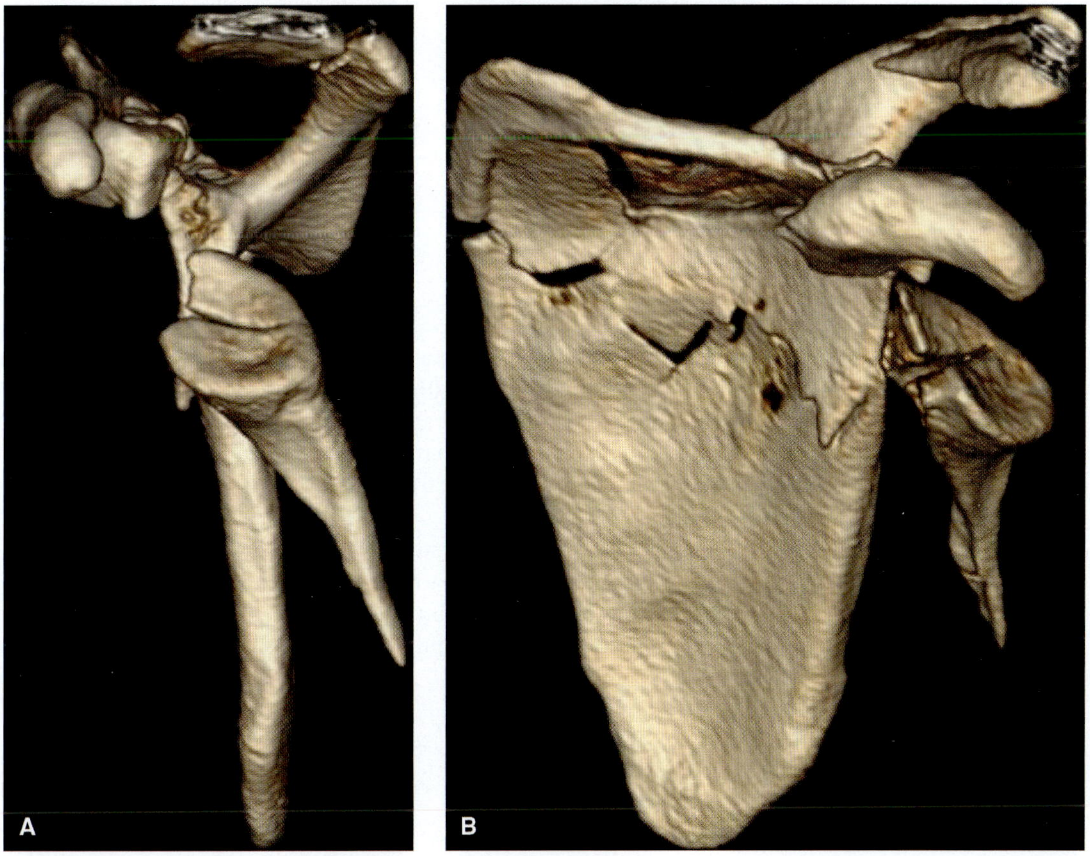

Figure 2-9 |

Intraoperative Positioning

- Lateral positioning is preferred to prone.
- Prone positioning largely prevents palpation of the coracoid tip and other anterior landmarks. Imaging is more difficult as well. The anterolateral resting position of the scapula makes the lateral view difficult to obtain.
- The patient is maintained in the lateral position with the aid of a beanbag, rolled flannel blankets, or similar positioner.

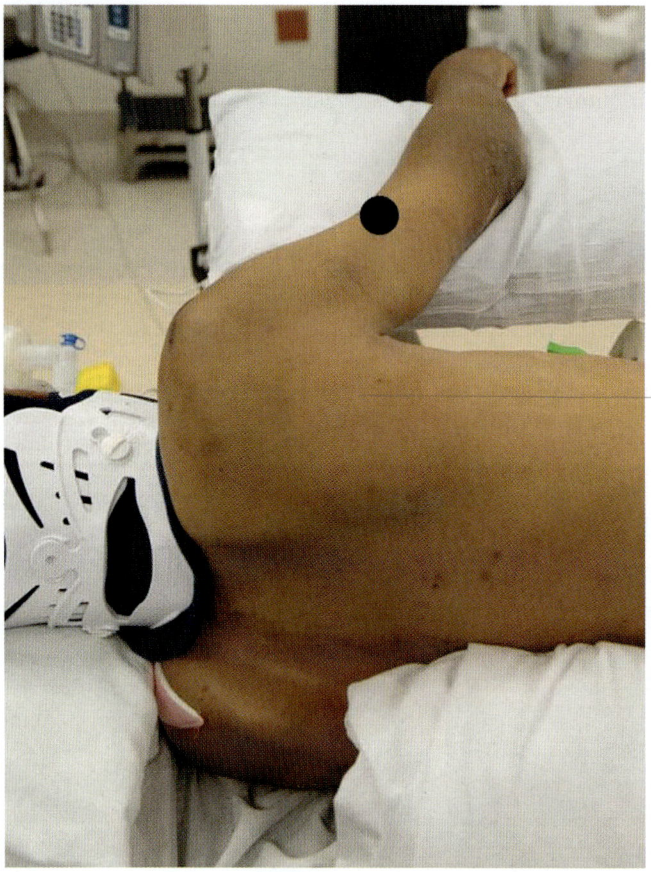

Figure 2-10 |

- The operative arm is propped up on a padded Mayo or Tenet arm board. The padded Mayo can be included in the sterile field (Fig. 2-10).
- The down arm should be supported and protected by Plexiglas, an axillary roll, blankets, and other radiolucent padding to facilitate imaging (Fig. 2-11).
- Efforts should be made to move electrodes and other radiopaque items out of the imaging field as much as possible.
- Confirm adequate imaging prior to sterile prep and drape.
- The C-arm is positioned from the patient's front.
- Posterior approaches including the Judet approach,[1] modified Judet approach,[2] and lateral border approach[3] are used to access the scapula's posterior surface (Figs. 2-12–2-14).

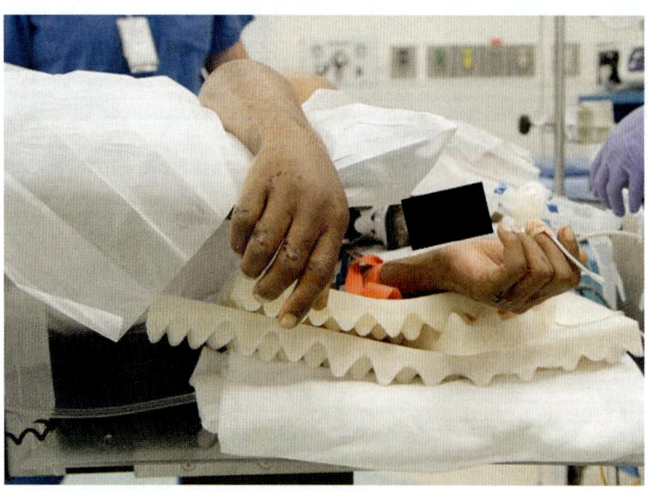

Figure 2-11 |

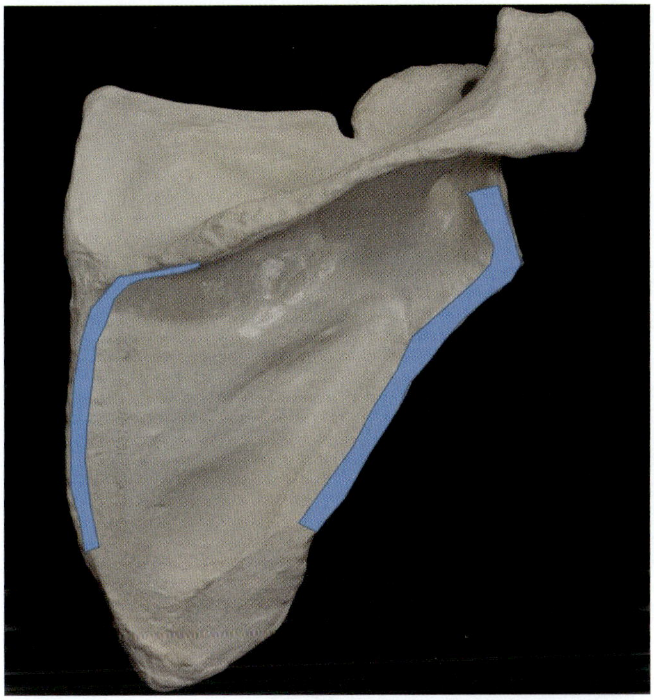

Figure 2-12 | A posterior view of the scapula model demonstrates the surfaces available for plate application (*light blue*) on the lateral border, inferior and posterior glenoid, medial border, and undersurface of the spine.

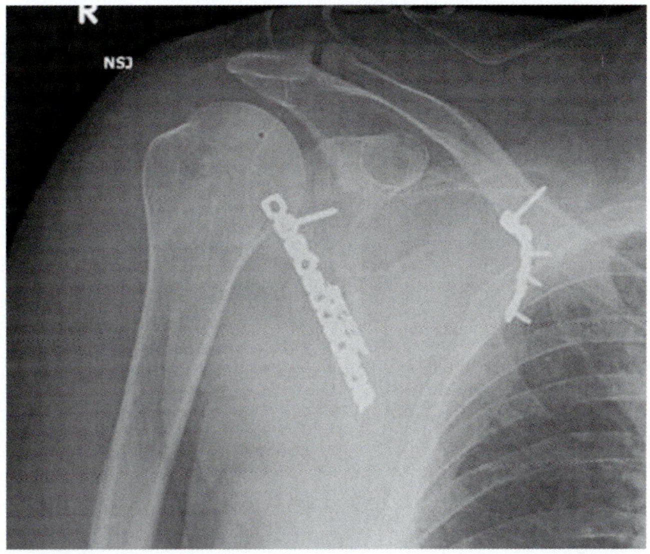

Figure 2-13 | Radiographic representation of plates applied to the lateral border, medial border, and undersurface of the scapular spine.

- The Grashey AP view is obtained by rotating the C-arm over the patient. Protraction and retraction of the scapular can be performed manually or with adjustment of the Mayo stand to improve the position of the scapula in relation to the beam (Fig. 2-15A and B).
- An excellent Grashey AP view assists the surgeon by profiling the glenoid so that the course of instruments and implants can be confirmed in an extra-articular position.

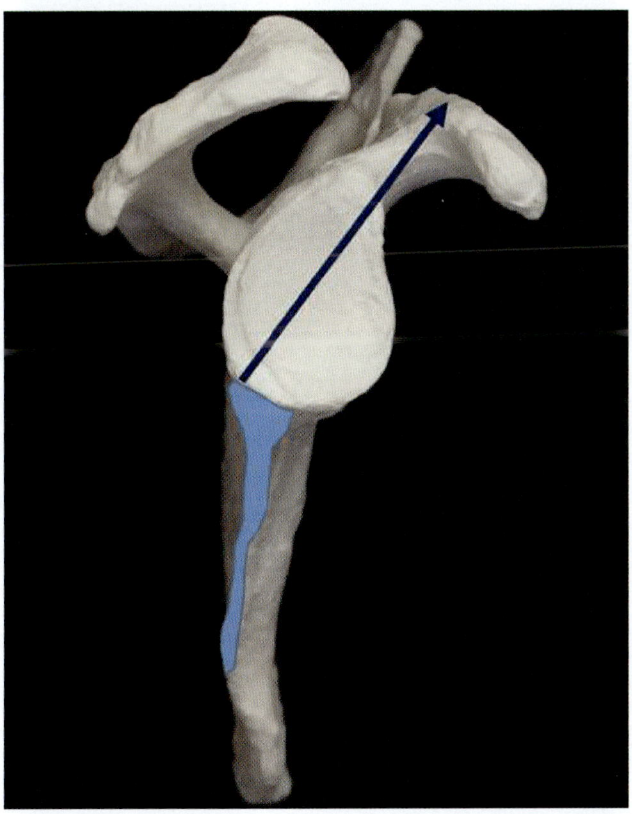

Figure 2-14 | A scapular Y view of the model demonstrates the surface available for plate application on the lateral border (*light blue*) and the orientation of the screw (*dark blue*) for fixation from the lateral border to the base of the coracoid.

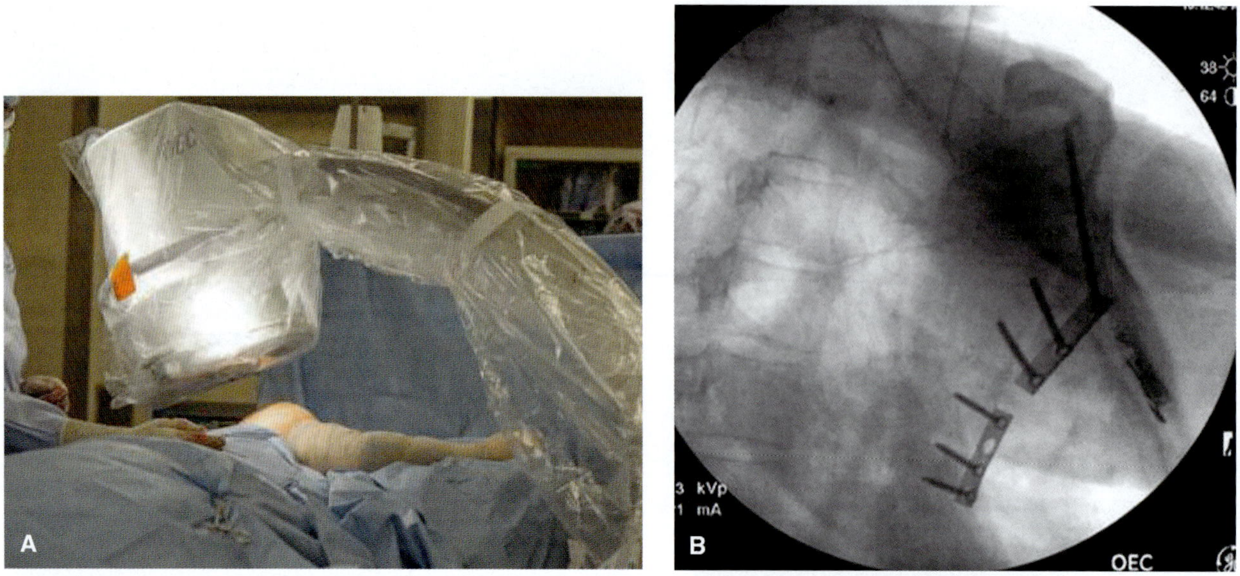

Figure 2-15 |

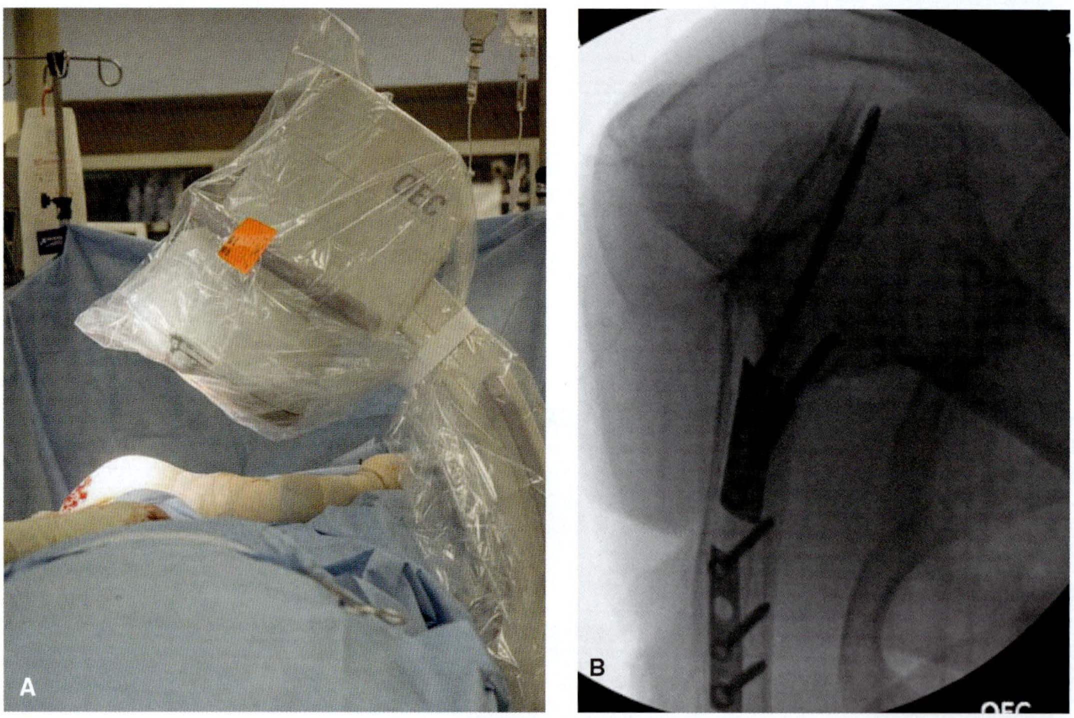

Figure 2-16 |

- The lateral (Y view) is obtained by canting the C-arm back approximately 30 degrees. Again, protraction and retraction can be fine-tuned manually or with adjustment of the Mayo stand (Fig. 2-16A and B).
- A well-positioned lateral Y view demonstrates the relative alignment of the spine, coracoid, and glenoid to confirm anatomic reduction, as well as confirming the safe course of instruments and implants into the base of the coracoid.[4]

References

1. Judet R. Surgical treatment of scapular fractures. *Acta Orthop Belg.* 1964;30:673–678.
2. Obremskey WT, Lyman JR. A modified Judet approach to the scapula. *J Orthop Trauma.* 2004;18(10):696–699.
3. Cole PA, Dubin JR, Freeman G. Operative techniques in the management of scapular fractures. *Orthop Clin North Am.* 2013;44(3):331–343.
4. Nork SE, Barei DP, Gardner MJ, et al. Surgical exposure and fixation of displaced type IV, V, and VI glenoid fractures. *J Orthop Trauma.* 2008;22(7):487–493.

Chapter 3
Clavicle Fractures

CHRISTIAAN N. MAMCZAK
MICHAEL J. GARDNER
CHRISTOPHER S. SMITH*

Bony Anatomy

- The clavicle is an S-shaped curvilinear bone with varying degrees of curvature within adult and pediatric patients.
- With articulations at the sternoclavicular (SC) and acromioclavicular (AC) joints, imaging can be challenging due to bony overlap with the ribs, vertebrae, and scapula.
- Single AP views of the clavicle do not accurately depict its anatomy or intraoperative reduction. Like any other bone, multiple views are necessary to delineate the restoration of length and alignment.

Radiographic Anatomy

AP View

- In traditional AP views, the intact clavicle will have a gentle S-shaped orientation sweeping cranially and laterally from the SC joint.
- With displaced middle and lateral third fractures, the medial segment is typically translated cranially due to the deforming forces of the sternocleidomastoid muscle (Fig. 3-1).
- Postreduction AP images should restore the gentle AP S-shaped anatomy, particularly with an apex superior bow. Flattening of the contour or apex deformity may be concerning for malreduction (Fig. 3-2).

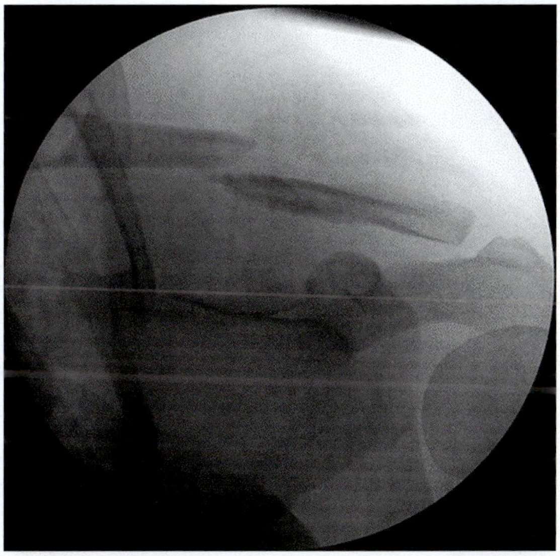

Figure 3-1 AP fluoro view of midshaft clavicle fracture with >100% displacement.

*The views expressed in this chapter are those of the author(s) and do not necessarily reflect the official policy or position of the Department of the Navy, Department of Defense or the United States Government. Christopher S. Smith is a military service member and this work was prepared as part of his official duties. Title 17 U.S.C. 105 provides that 'Copyright protection under this title is not available for any work of the United States Government.' Title 17 U.S.C. 101 defines a United States Government work as a work prepared by a military service member or employee of the United States Government as part of that person's official duties.

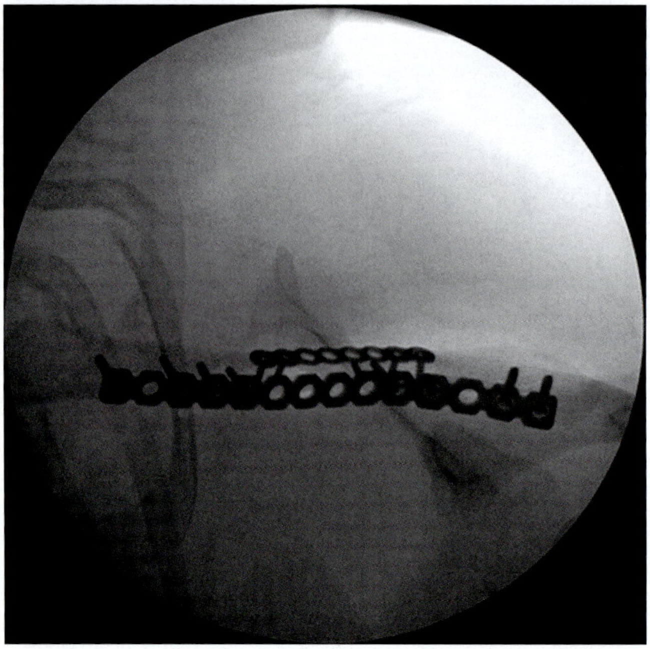

Figure 3-2 I AP fluoro view demonstrating anatomic restoration of the clavicular length and contour.

Inlet/40 to 45-Degree Caudal View

- This view accentuates the true S-shaped degree of curvature thus demonstrating that the clavicle is not a simple, straight bone.
- The x-ray/fluoro beam is directed 40 to 45 degrees caudal from the true AP with the patient supine (see figures below).
- The typical anterior butterfly fragment seen in comminuted midshaft fractures can be better delineated with this view, but posterior and inferior comminution should be expected and is not uncommon (Fig. 3-3).
- Proper screw lengths for anterior-inferior plating can be confirmed with the clavicular inlet view.
- Postreduction inlet images should restore the S-shaped anatomy. Flattening of the contour or apex deformity may be concerning for malreduction (Fig. 3-4).

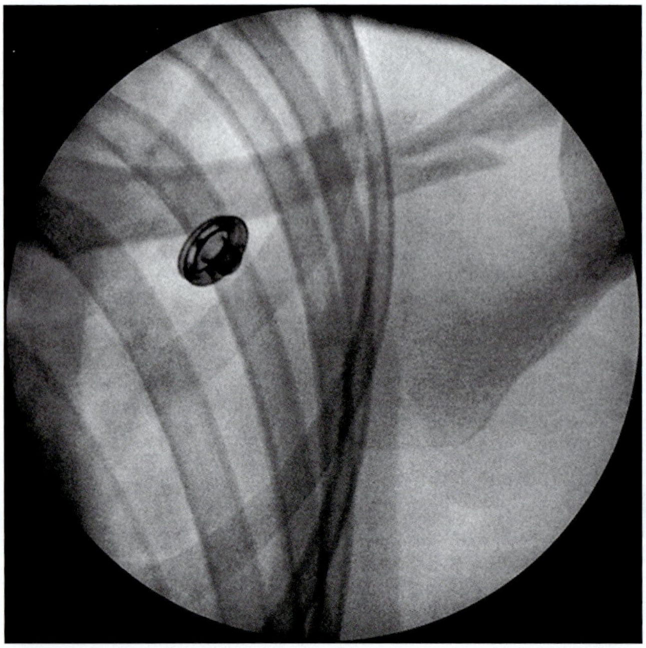

Figure 3-3 I Clavicle inlet fluoro view depicts fracture displacement and anterior comminution.

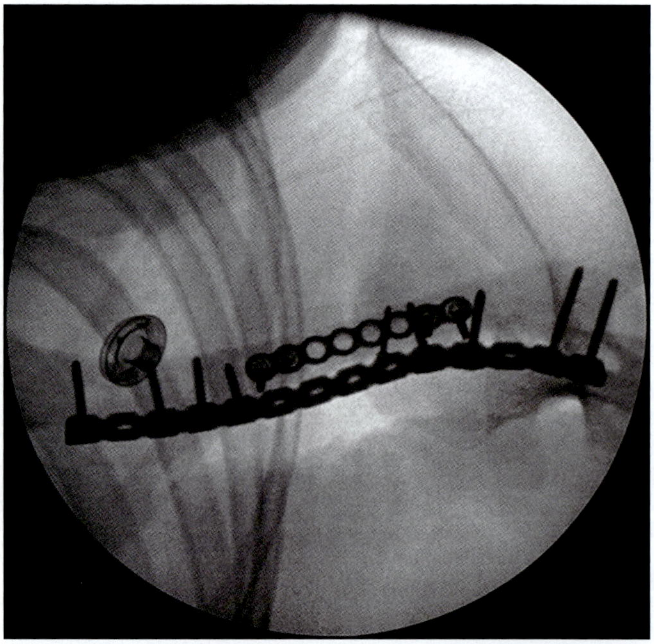

Figure 3-4 I Clavicle inlet fluoro view demonstrating anatomic restoration of the clavicular length and S-shaped contour.

Outlet/15 to 30-Degree Cranial View

- The intact clavicle is typically most linear in this view.
- The degree of cranial tilt is variable and predicated on patient anatomy and positioning.
- The x-ray/fluoro beam is directed approximately 15–30 degrees cranial or cephalad from the true AP with the patient supine.
- Medial fragment cranial displacement and inferior comminution are best imaged with the clavicular outlet view.
- Reduction and displacement of far lateral clavicle fractures with and without AC joint ligamentous injury are also well visualized with the outlet view (Fig. 3-5).
- Proper screw lengths for superior plating are appreciated with this view.
- Postreduction outlet images should restore the linear anatomy. Apex deformity may be concerning for malreduction, although some clavicles have physiologic apex superior morphology (Fig. 3-6).

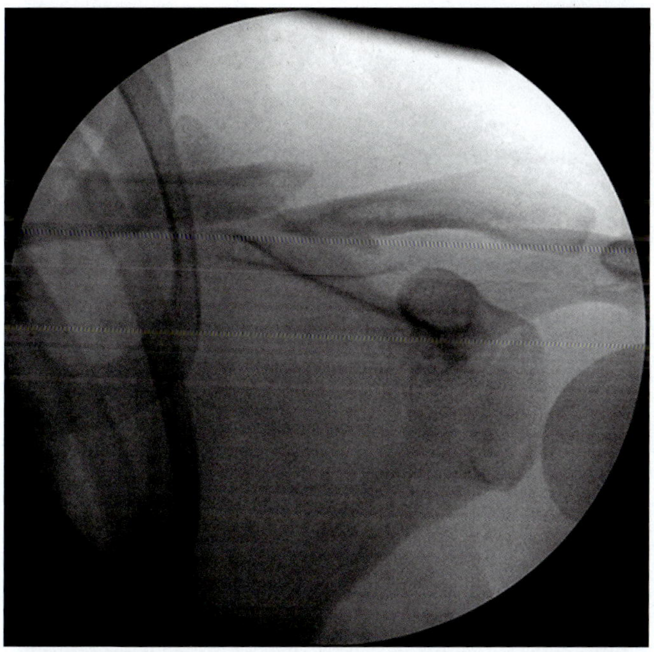

Figure 3-5 | Clavicle outlet fluoro view depicts fracture displacement and inferior comminution.

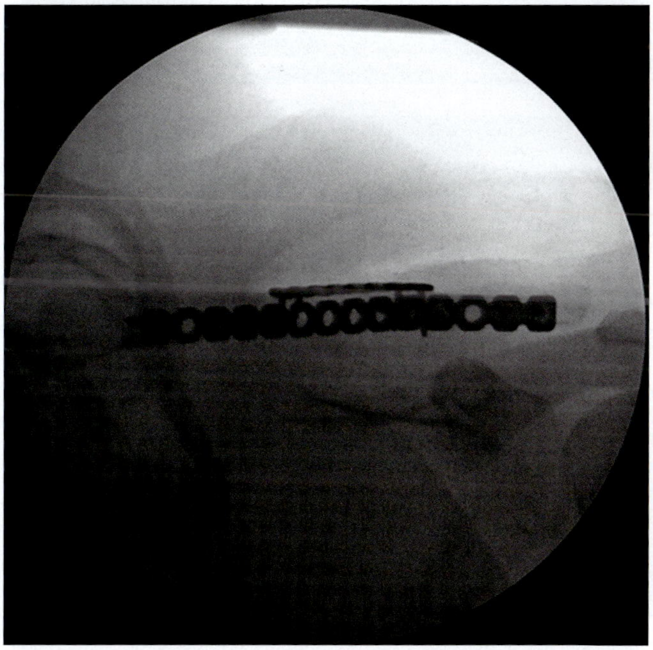

Figure 3-6 | Clavicle outlet fluoro view demonstrating anatomic restoration of the clavicular length and straight axial contour.

Serendipity 40-Degree Cranial SC View

- Medial clavicular fractures and dislocations of the SC joint are best depicted on this midline view of the clavicles. Imaging technique is similar to the outlet view (Fig. 3-7).
- Note that advanced imaging (i.e., CT scan) offers better anatomic orientation of SC dislocations because orthogonal views of the SC joint anatomy are obscured by overlap of surrounding medial bony and soft tissue structures. 3D CT can also better demonstrate the multiplanar deformity associated with an acute clavicle fracture (Fig. 3-8).

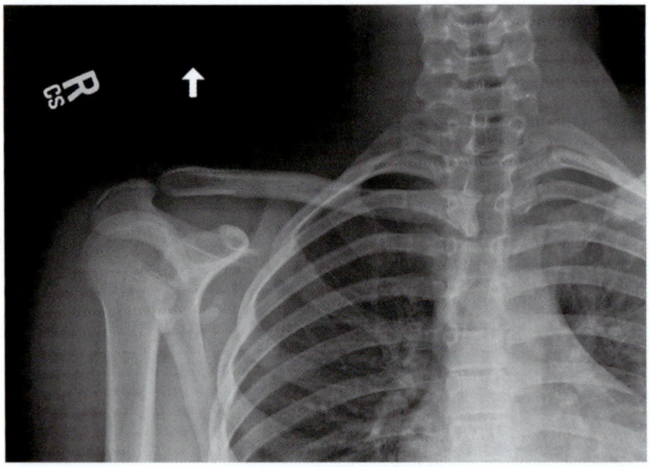

Figure 3-7 I SC Serendipity radiograph demonstrates posterior and superior dislocation of the the right SC joint.

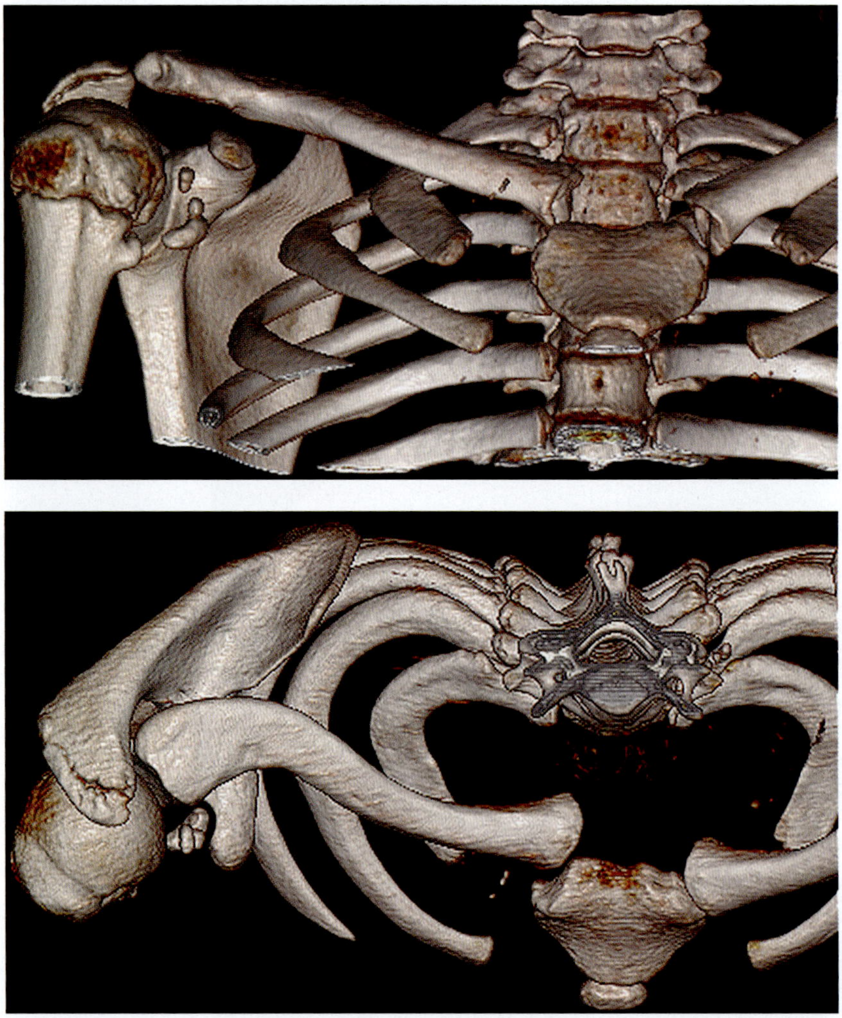

Figure 3-8 I 3D CT reconstructions better delineate the posterior and superior dislocation of the the right SC joint.

Preoperative Imaging

- The radiographic indications for operative treatment of middle third clavicle fractures are predicated on shortening, displacement, and comminution.[1]
- Standard AP views of the clavicle are good screening radiographs for middle and lateral third fractures. However, they offer limited information about the degree of displacement or shortening.
- Recently described, a comparison of supine and standing upright AP radiographs can offer additional information about gravity-dependent fracture displacement.[2] Standing PA views of both clavicles are valuable for measuring the degree of shortening as the clavicles are well defined because they are closer to the imaging cassette and the intact clavicle can be used as a reference length when measured from medial to lateral.
- The addition of clavicular inlet and outlet views (as described above) can offer more information on fracture deformity, but due to the previously mentioned variability, standardized imaging angles have not been described.

Intraoperative Positioning

- Surgical fixation of clavicle fractures is dependent on the fracture pattern, surgical approach, fixation preference (i.e., superior versus anteroinferior plating or intramedullary nail/screw) and surgeon preference.
- There are inherent pros and cons of supine versus mild reverse Trendelenburg versus beach chair positioning. This includes advantages or limitations with intraoperative fluoroscopy.
- The beach chair position proves to be the most obtrusive to obtaining clavicular inlet and outlet views due largely to limitations of the interface with the C-arm and the operative table.
- Ideally, a fully radiolucent table permits the most degrees of freedom for flouro imaging.

1. Supine Position

- The supine position is largely used for the anteroinferior plating approach but also offers access to the superior clavicle.
- Note that a superior surgical approach can be difficult from this position due to patient position.
- Adding 30+ degree of reverse Trendelenburg (head up/feet down) tilt with the table will utilize gravity to your advantage and allow greater superior approach access.
- Patients may be placed onto a radiolucent table such as a Maquet diving board or an OSI/Jackson. The patient should be at the end of the Maquet table diving board with the table rotated 90 degrees relative to anesthesia to allow C-arm imaging coming in over the patient's head. This allows unobstructed AP, inlet, and outlet views throughout the case (Figs. 3-9 and 3-10).

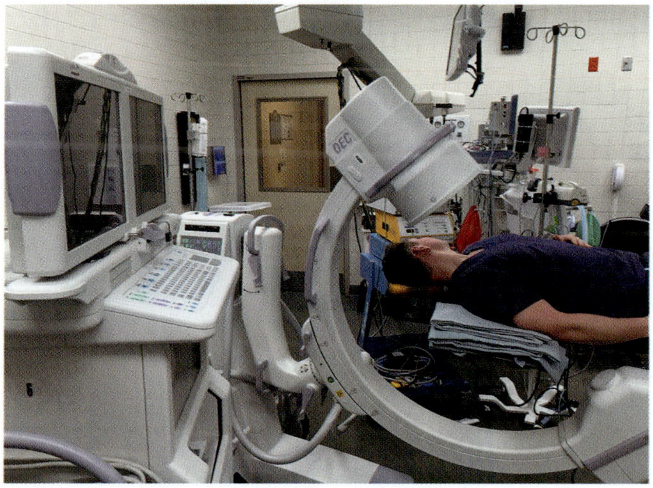

Figure 3-9 | Inlet view 40-degree caudal tilt.

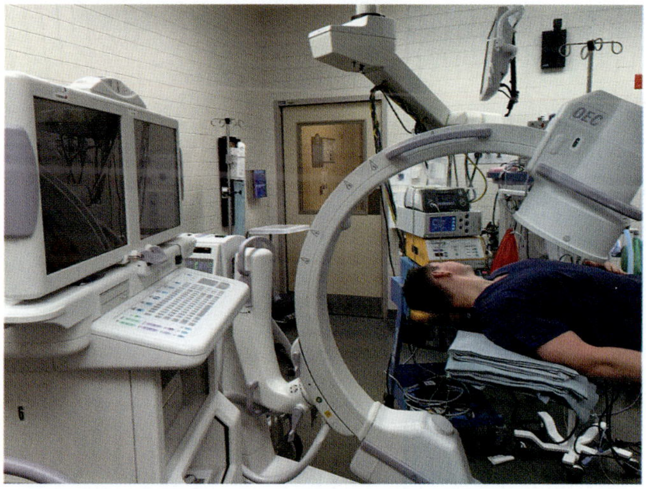

Figure 3-10 | Outlet view 15–30-degree cephalad tilt.

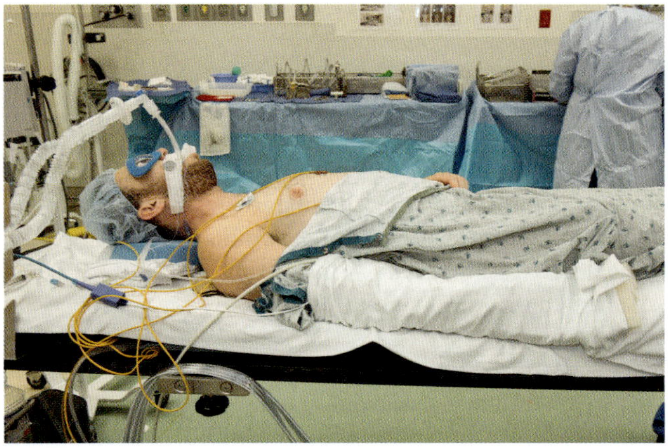

Figure 3-11 I The elbow of the operative arm should be resting on a radiolucent (e.g., Plexiglas) board padded with blankets.

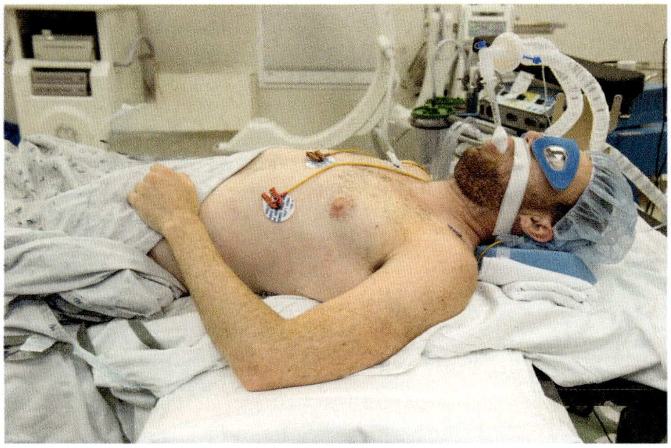

Figure 3-12 I The C-arm then comes in from across the table and allows for unencumbered "inlet" and "outlet" views of the clavicle.

- Use of an OSI/Jackson table requires the patient to be positioned with the feet at the end of the table and the head away from the proximal table post. With the C-arm located at the contralateral side, AP and inlet/outlet views can typically be captured with little interference between the C-arm and the table.
- Pull the patient toward the injured side so that the uninjured can be tucked without an arm board, allowing the C-arm to image the injured extremity (Figs. 3-11–3-14).

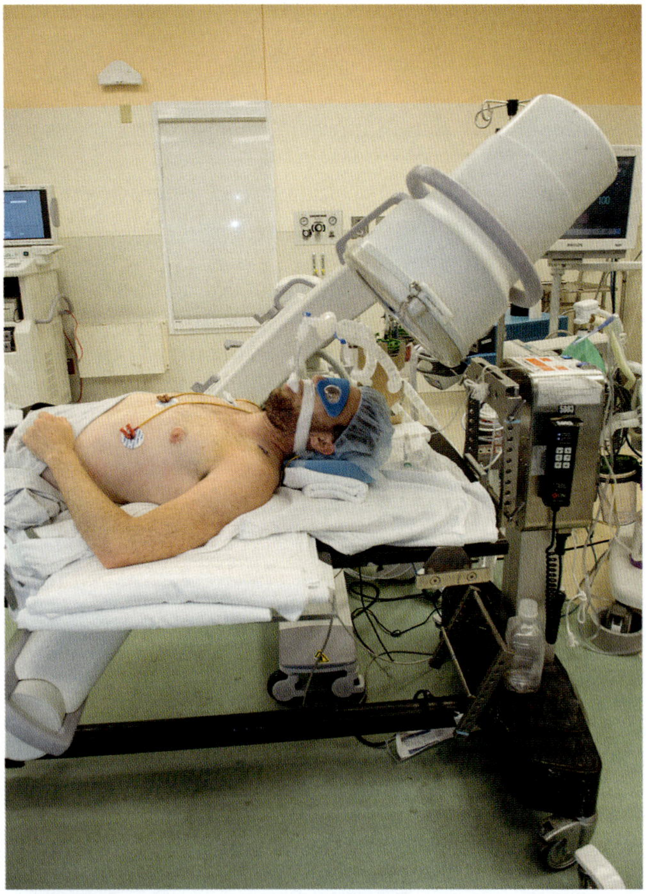

Figure 3-13 I Inlet view 40-degree caudal tilt.

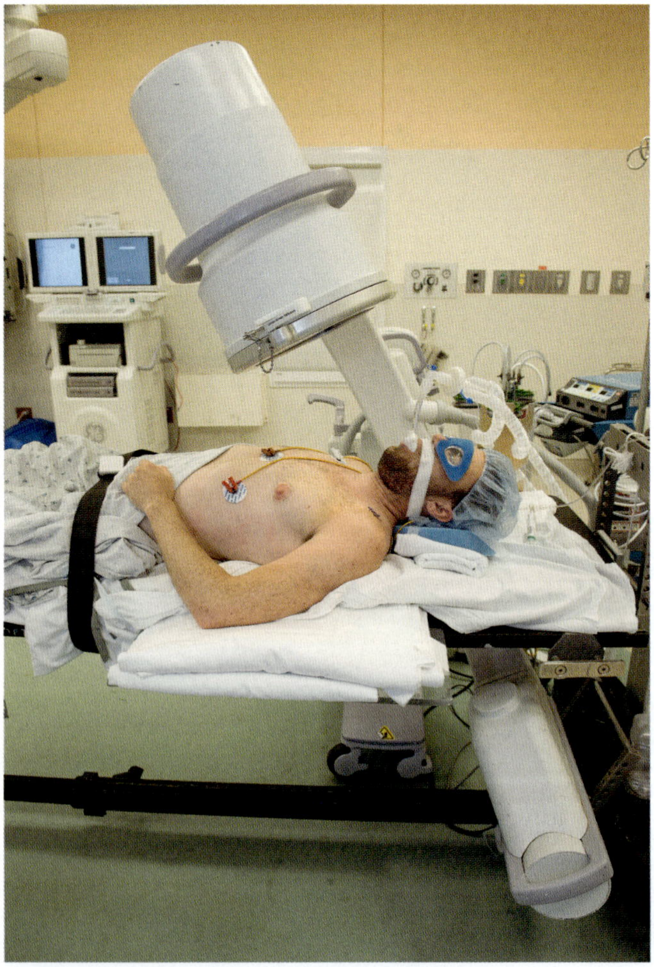

Figure 3-14 I Outlet view 15–30-degree cranial tilt.

2. Beach Chair Position

- This position is most commonly used for a superior approach and plating of the clavicle. Various beach chair tables are available for use; some are equipped with a radiolucent backboard.
- The patient is typically positioned with varying degrees of reverse Trendelenburg tilt (60 to 80 degrees).
- The C-arm can be positioned from either over the patient's head or coming in from the ipsilateral side (contralateral side obstructs the anesthesiologist's access to the patient) (Figs. 3-15 and 3-16).

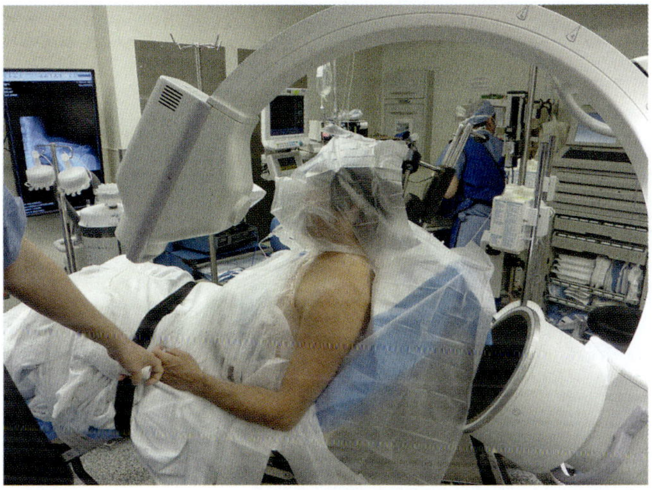

Figure 3-15 | Beach chair position.

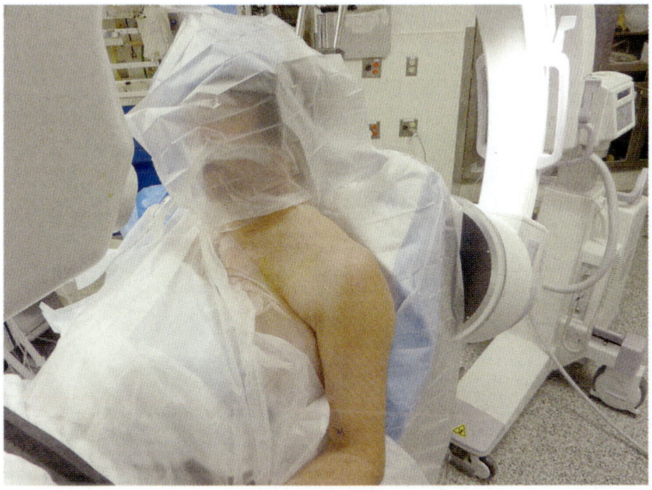

Figure 3-16 | Inlet and outlet clavicular imaging is least reliable with this position due to interference of the table and C-arm, limitations of C-arm excursion, and the ability to maintain a sterile field with awkward C-arm positions.

Additional Positioning Tips

- Politely educate anesthesia on your positioning requirements and request that the endotracheal tube be taped to the contralateral side and that the anterior and posterior upper chest is free of radiopaque-obscuring EKG leads/lines.
- Avoid the use of standard armboards that may obstruct the C-arm. When in doubt, securely pad and tuck the uninjured, contralateral upper extremity against the body.
- Widely prep and drape the entire upper extremity and upper chest across the SC notch to allow complete access to the clavicle.

- A small rolled sheet bump placed underneath the upper thoracic spine can allow the scapula to retract, thereby "elongating" the clavicle and assisting with the reduction of shortening.
- Before prepping and draping, obtain AP clavicle, inlet view (40 degrees caudal tilt), and outlet view (40 degrees cephalad tilt). Have the x-ray tech place tape on the floor to mark the position of the base of the C-arm (Figs. 3-17–3-19).

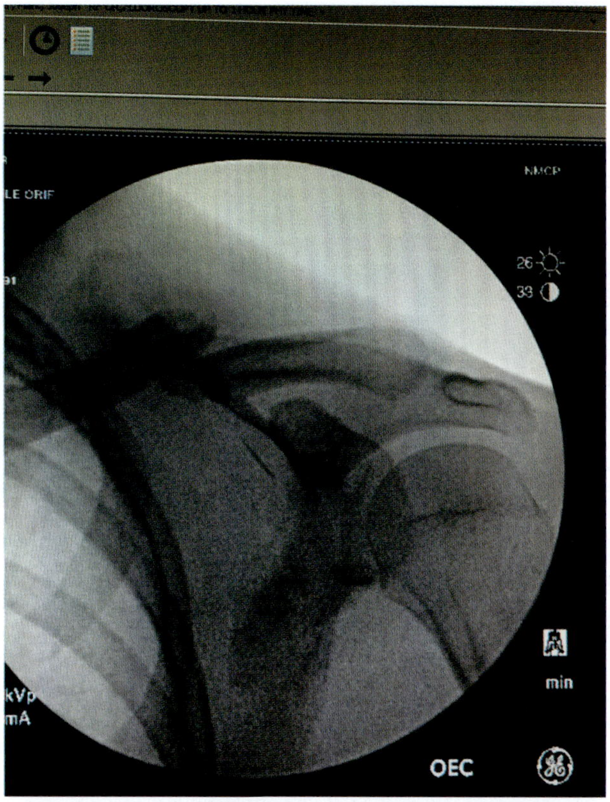

Figure 3-17 | AP left clavicle prior to prepping and draping.

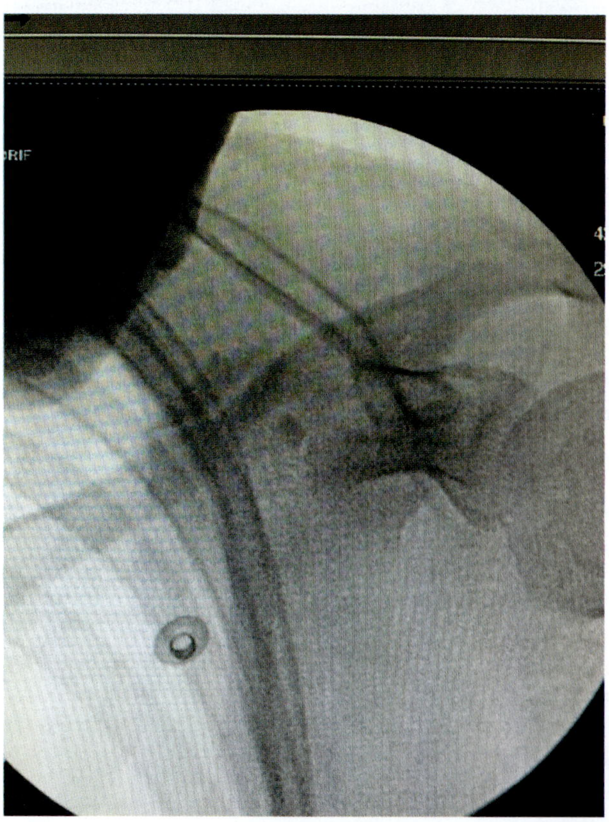

Figure 3-18 | Inlet view (40-degree caudal tilt) left clavicle prior to prepping and draping.

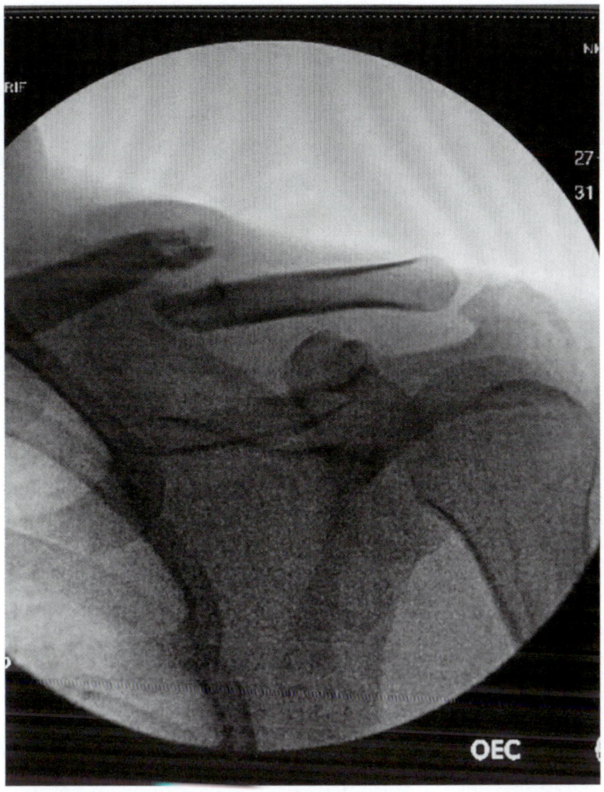

Figure 3-19 | Outlet view (40-degree cephalic tilt) left clavicle prior to prepping and draping.

- One can place the desired plate over the skin prior to incision, to assist in proper incision placement.
- In order to accurately view screw lengths of a superiorly based clavicle plate, one needs a perfect "edge view" of the plate, which can be obtained by the outlet clavicle view (40 degrees cephalic tilt), which also reveals an AP of an anterior inferiorly based plate (Fig. 3-20).

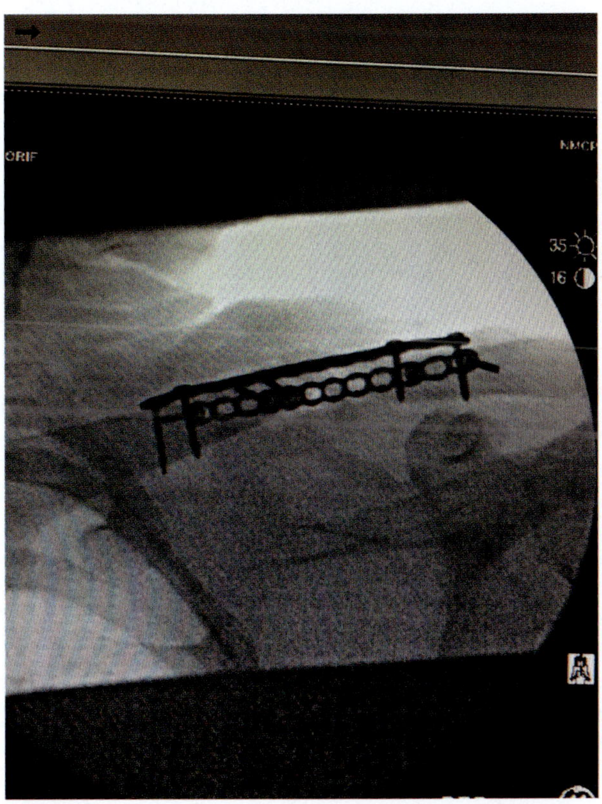

Figure 3-20 | Outlet view (40-degree cephalic tilt) left clavicle post fixation. Note this view provides a true lateral of the superiorly based plate, which reveals accurate screw lengths.

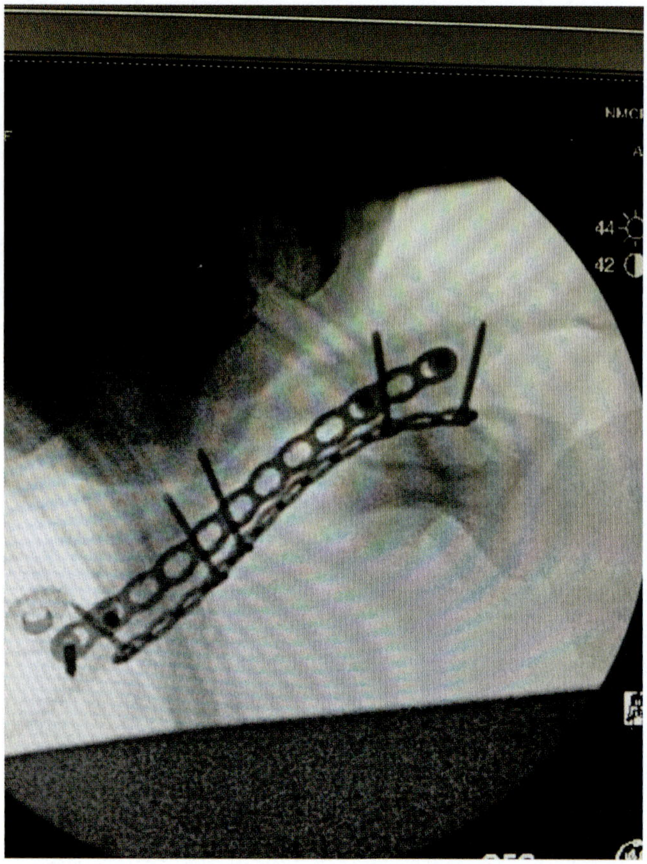

Figure 3-21 | Inlet view (40-degree caudal tilt) left clavicle post fixation. Note this view provides a true lateral of the anterior inferiorly based plate, which reveals accurate screw lengths.

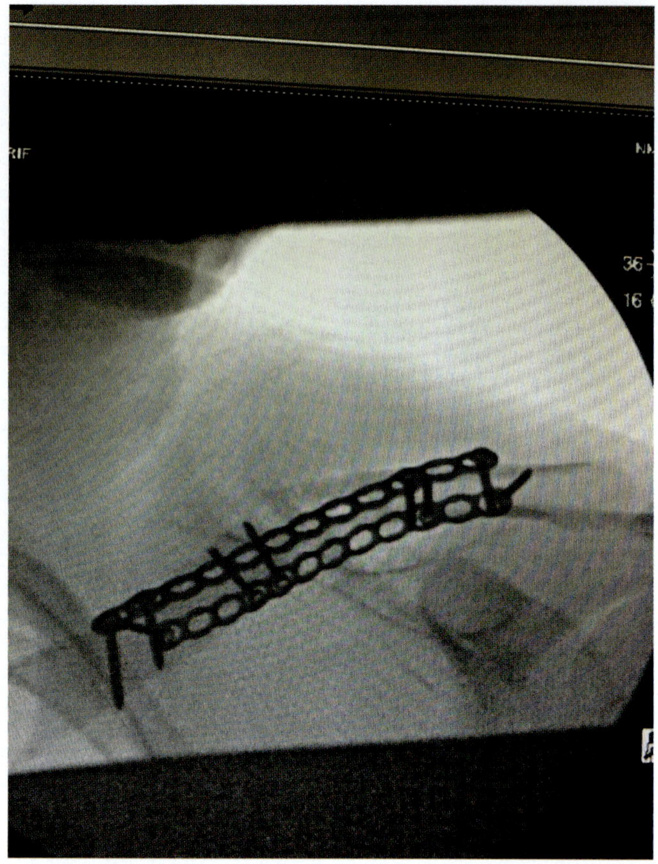

Figure 3-22 | AP view left clavicle post fixation. Note the inability difficulty in gauging accurate screw lengths of either plate.

- In order to accurately view screw lengths of an anterior based clavicle plate, one needs a perfect "edge view" of the plate, which can be obtained by the inlet clavicle view (40 degrees caudal tilt), which also reveals an AP of superiorly based plate (Figs. 3-21 and 3-22).

References

1. Robinson CM, Court-Brown CM, McQueen MM, et al. Estimating the risk of nonunion following nonoperative treatment of a clavicle fracture. *J Bone Joint Surg Am.* 2004;86:1350–1365.
2. Backus JD, Merriman DJ, McAndrew CM, et al. Upright versus supine radiographs of clavicle fractures: does positioning matter? *J Orthop Trauma.* 2014;28:636–641.

Chapter 4
Proximal Humerus Fractures

JONAH HEBERT-DAVIES
GEORGE-YVES LAFLAMME

Bony Anatomy

- The proximal humerus is composed of the head (articular surface), the lesser and greater tuberosities, and the surgical neck.
- The lesser tuberosity is the attachment for the subscapularis, which can lead to medial fragment displacement in multipart proximal humeral fractures. The greater tuberosity is where the supra- and infraspinatus muscles insert; superior and posterior displacement of this fragment is not uncommon.
- The height of the greater tuberosity is important to recreate accurately. It is approximately 5.6 mm above the pectoralis major tendon insertion.
- The glenohumeral joint is extremely mobile and can lead to confusing imaging.
- The scapula is typically internally rotated 20 to 30 degrees. The humeral head is also retroverted approximately 30 degrees relative to the elbow joint axis.

Radiographic Anatomy

AP Shoulder View

- The standard AP view of the shoulder is in fact an AP view of the ipsilateral chest wall.
- This view allows good visualization of the proximal humeral neck and shaft.
- Because the proximal humerus is internally rotated relative to the arm, the greater tuberosity is visualized *en face*, and this can highlight the typically posterior and superior displacement.
- The standard AP view also allows for a linear view of the acromioclavicular joint (Fig. 4-1).

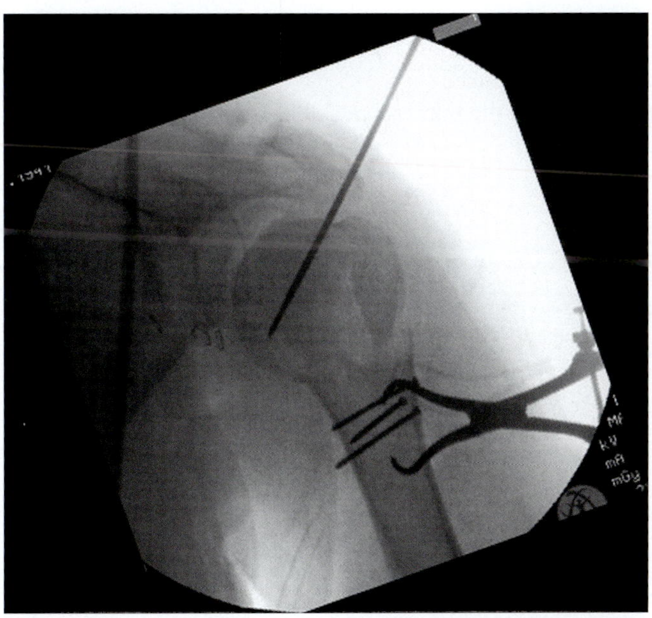

Figure 4-1 | AP view of the shoulder. The AC joint is seen parallel to the fluoroscopy beam. Note that the head is still in varus with GT fragment superior to the articular surface.

Grashey or True AP View

- This view best demonstrates the profile of the glenohumeral joint. It is performed with the fluoroscopic beam in 30 degrees of internal rotation in order to match the position of the scapula/glenoid.
- The congruity of the humeral head can also be better appreciated on this view along with the restoration of the medial calcar.
- Performing this view in 30 to 40 degrees of abduction will help recreate normal anatomy.
- On final fluoroscopic films, the lengths of screws, and especially the proximal screws, should be checked to ensure iatrogenic perforation has not occurred (Fig. 4-2).

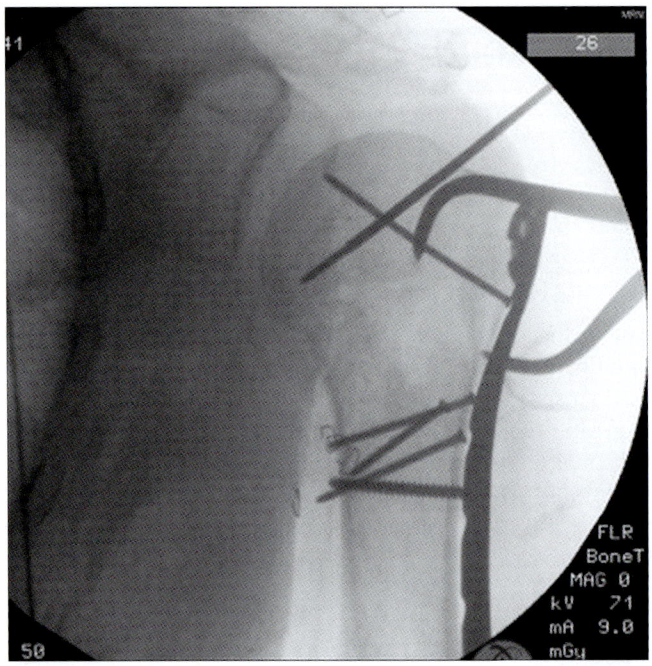

Figure 4-2 | Grashey view of the shoulder with an excellent profile of the glenohumeral joint. Note that the reduction k-wire and clamp have restored the neck-shaft angle and calcar.

Axillary View

- The image is obtained by shooting through the axilla with the shoulder in neutral flexion and 30 to 90 degrees of abduction.
- This view is rarely useful until most of the reduction has been completed. It allows the surgeon to ensure that (Fig. 4-3):
  - The glenohumeral joint is concentric.
  - The lesser tuberosity is reduced.
  - The greater tuberosity is reduced.
  - Sagittal plane reduction of the humeral neck has been achieved.

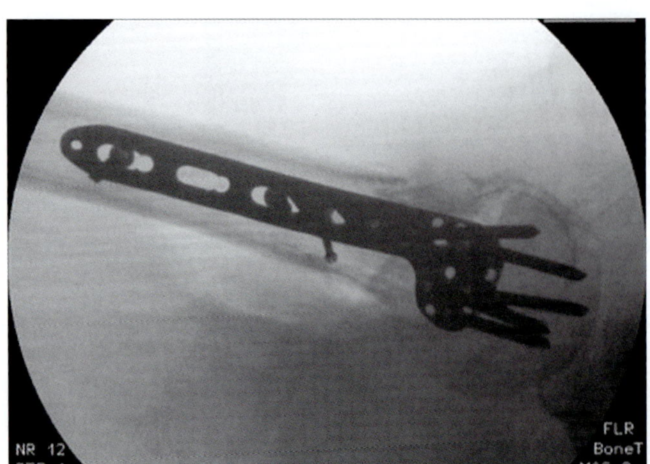

Figure 4-3 | Axillary view of the shoulder. The lesser tuberosity reduction can be seen. This view also helps confirm proper plate position on the humeral head and shaft.

- Humeral head retroversion has been restored.
- The plate is appropriately located on the proximal humerus.
- The screw lengths and trajectories are appropriate.

Preoperative Imaging

- Preoperative imaging for all proximal humerus fractures should include AP, Grashey, and an axillary view.
- Indications for surgery include displaced three and four part fractures, severely displaced two-part fractures in active patients, head split–type fractures, and any irreducible fracture dislocation.
- Often, a CT scan is useful in assessing the fracture pattern. A head split may be difficult to discern on the plain films, but becomes obvious on CT scan. Also, the extent and displacement of tuberosity comminution can be quantified prior to surgery. Finally, the concentricity of the glenohumeral joint can be appreciated if a preoperative axillary view was not done or unclear.

Intraoperative Positioning

- Operative treatment of proximal humerus fractures can be achieved in several ways. Most commonly open reduction and internal fixation is performed; however, in some cases the humerus is unrepairable and arthroplasty is necessary. Some authors have also started advocating newer humeral nailing systems with numerous interlocking options.
- If internal fixation is chosen, this can be achieved through two different operative approaches (deltopectoral and deltoid splitting).
- Open reduction and internal fixation can be performed in either the supine or beach chair positions. Arthroplasty is typically done in the beach chair position.
- Therefore, fractures that may not be amenable to fixation should be placed in the beach chair position if an intraoperative decision to perform arthroplasty is taken.
- Advantages to the supine position include easier fluoroscopic imaging and avoidance of cerebral hypotension issues associated with beach chair position.
- Another advantage of the supine position is it can be used in the polytrauma patient for multiple site fracture fixation (i.e., simultaneous upper and lower extremity fractures).
- The beach chair position is more versatile, and surgeons should be familiar with optimal positioning if required.

1. Supine Position

- This position should be used for ORIF as mentioned. Optimal position can allow for easier imaging and subsequently more efficient surgery.
- A radiolucent table should be used with the head elevated slightly (20 to 30 degrees).
- The patient should be moved over completely to the operative side so that the head is flush with the proximal corner of the table.
- It is important to fix the patients head in this position, because it may shift during surgery, especially with longitudinal traction of the arm, which is often necessary for reduction.
- A padded radiolucent board (i.e., Plexiglas with blankets) approximately 8 to 12 inches in width can be placed underneath to support the arm. This ensures clear imaging by eliminating the table side, which can sometimes interfere with fluoroscopy.
- The uninjured side can be padded and placed on the operative table safely.
- The table is rotated 90 degrees into the room, and the C-arm is brought in from the head and preoperative fluoroscopy is done to ensure proper positioning (Fig. 4-4).
- Alternatively, the C-arm can be brought in from the opposite side in the polytrauma context where multiple fracture sites will be operated on (Fig. 4-5).
- The AP view is achieved by shooting with a perpendicular beam, which require some rollover (cranial tilt) to match the tilt of the table.
- The Grashey view is then obtained in the same fashion but by adding 30 degrees of lateral tilt to match scapular rotation.
- Finally, the axillary view is produced with the C-arm rolled back parallel with the patient in both planes. Sometimes a small amount of internal rotation and abduction of the beam is necessary to clear the head adequately.

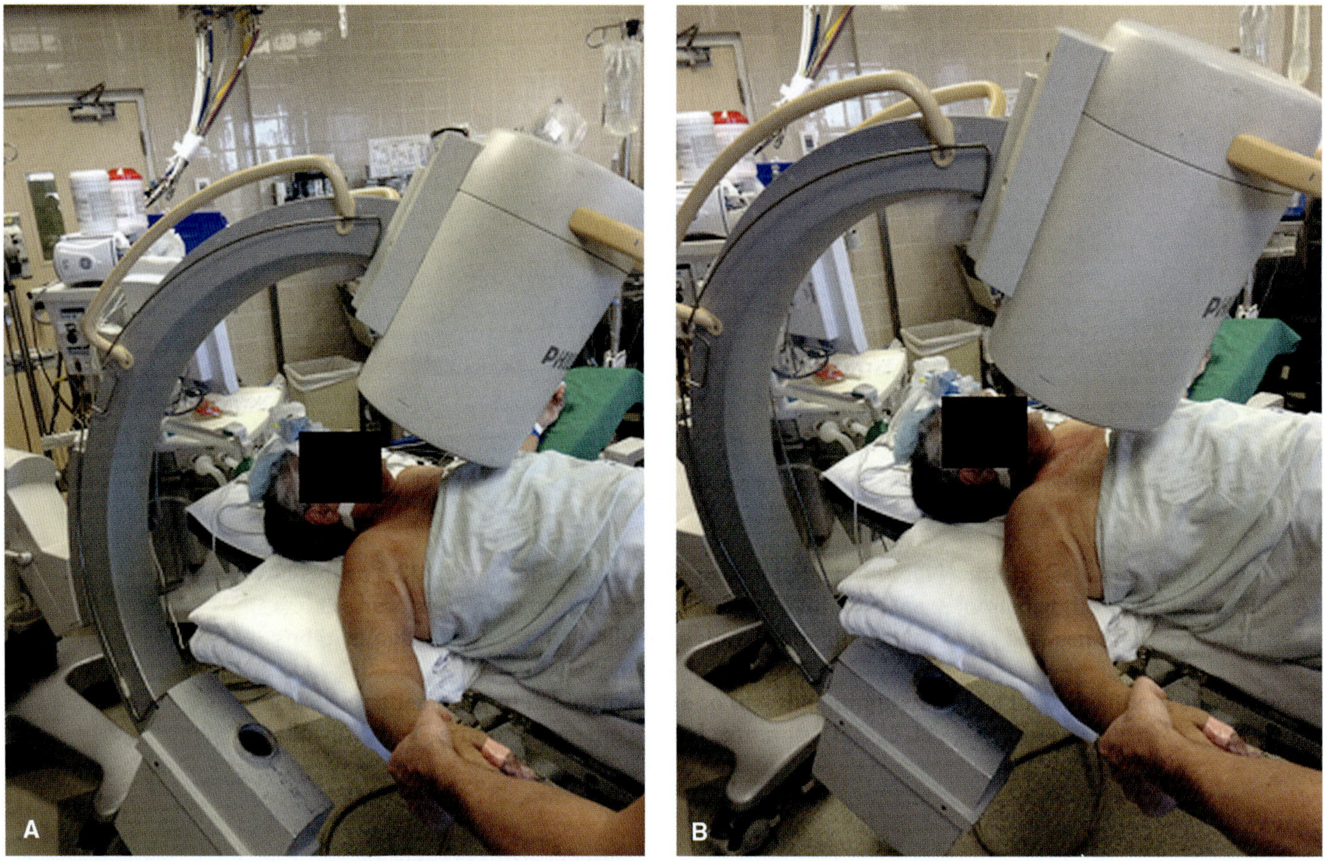

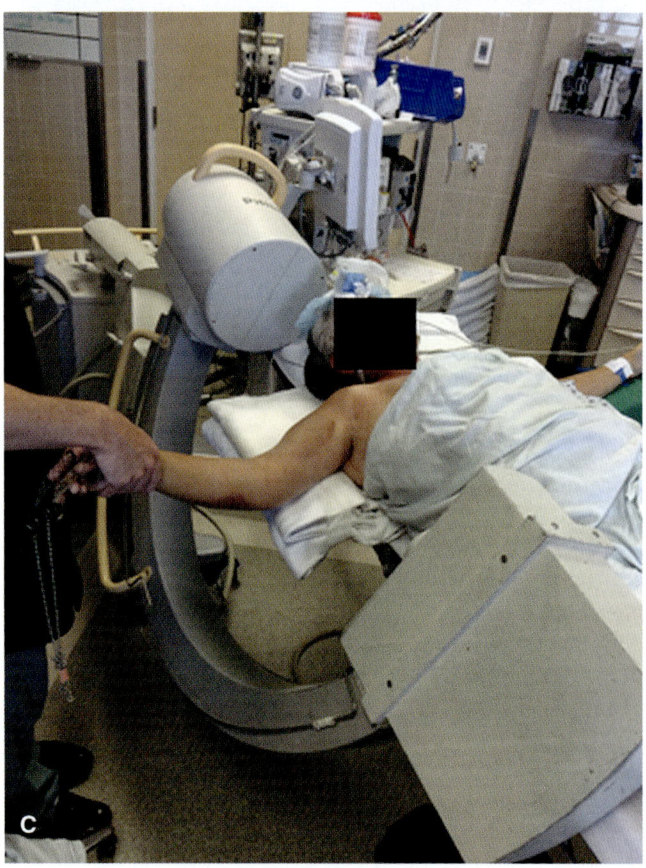

Figure 4-4 | A–C: A Grashey, AP, and axillary view in the supine position. Note the rotation of the C-arm to produce the axillary view.

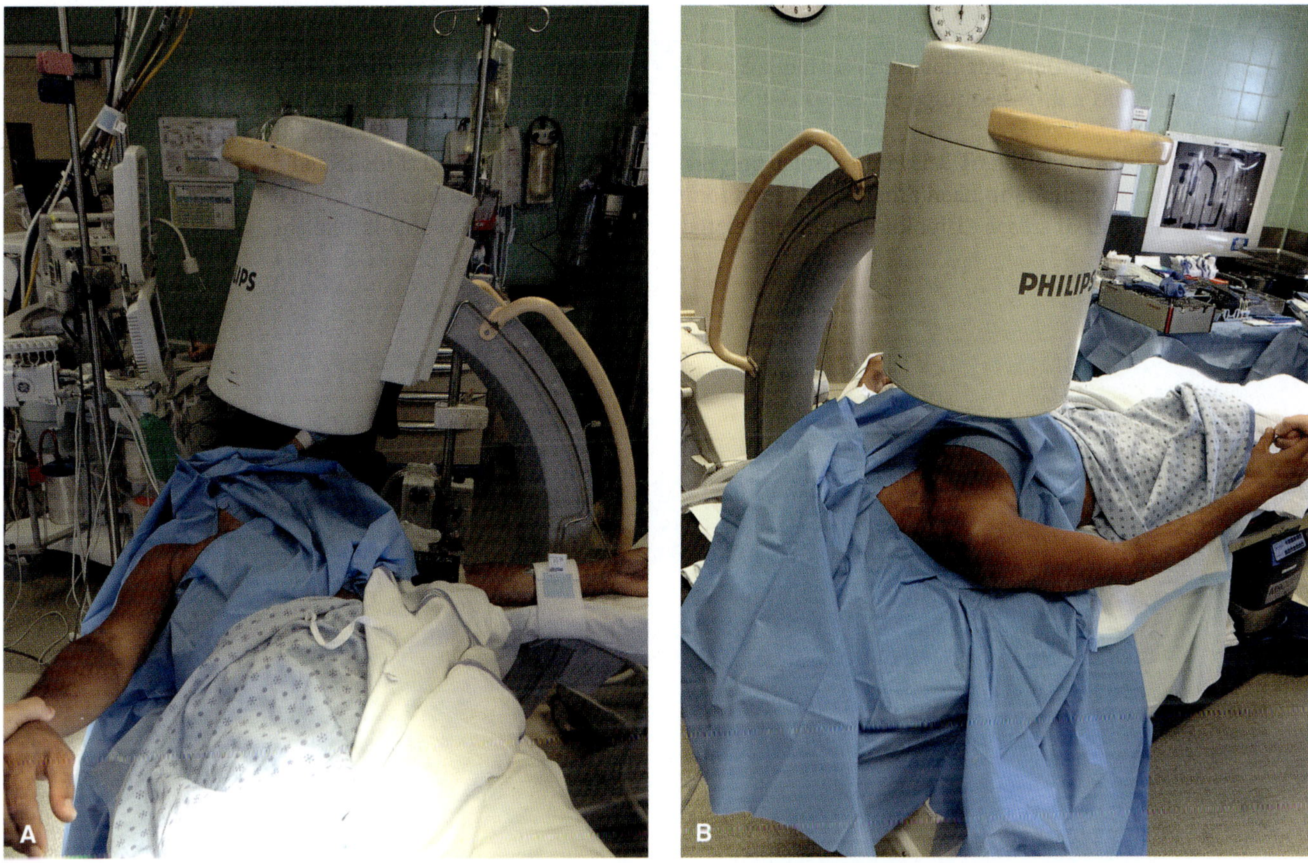

Figure 4-5 | A and B: AP and Grashey views obtained with the C-arm coming in from the contralateral side. The opposite arm can be placed along the body or out as seen in the picture.

2. Beach Chair Position

- This position can be used for ORIF, nailing, or arthroplasty.
- Various models of positioners exist, and it is essential to be familiar with the available system. Some models have a back that pushes over and other a removable back under the operative side. Either way, it is important to ensure the shoulder is completely free both for manipulation during surgery and for proper imaging.
- The patient is sat up according to surgeon preference, although it is generally easier to be more supine for ORIF (45 degrees) and more upright for arthroplasty (80 degrees).
- A pillow is placed underneath the knees to prevent the patient from sliding.
- The endotracheal tube is positioned away from the operative side to avoid contact with the fluoroscopy.
- The head is placed in a neutral flexed position with a slight lateral flexion and rotation away from the operative side. This makes obtaining the Grashey view less cumbersome.
- An arm positioner (e.g., Spider, McConnell) can be used or the arm can be placed free on the patients lap during surgery.
- The nonoperative arm is placed on a well-padded armboard.
- The C-arm is positioned coming from proximal to distal on the ipsilateral side.
- AP, Grashey, and axillary views are obtained similarly to what has been described for the supine position, however with the addition of the rollover (caudal tilt) of the beam to match the elevation of the table. This can be problematic if the patient is seated upright at too great an angle due to the rotation limit of different fluoroscopic machines.

Additional Positioning Tips

- Ensuring proper visualization during this surgery is key. Optimal positioning and thorough removal of all potentially radiopaque accessories (including bed positioners, EKG leads, armboards) is important.
- Obtain all fluoroscopic views prior to prepping and draping. Often, there will be something unforeseen obstructing the view, especially in the beach chair position.

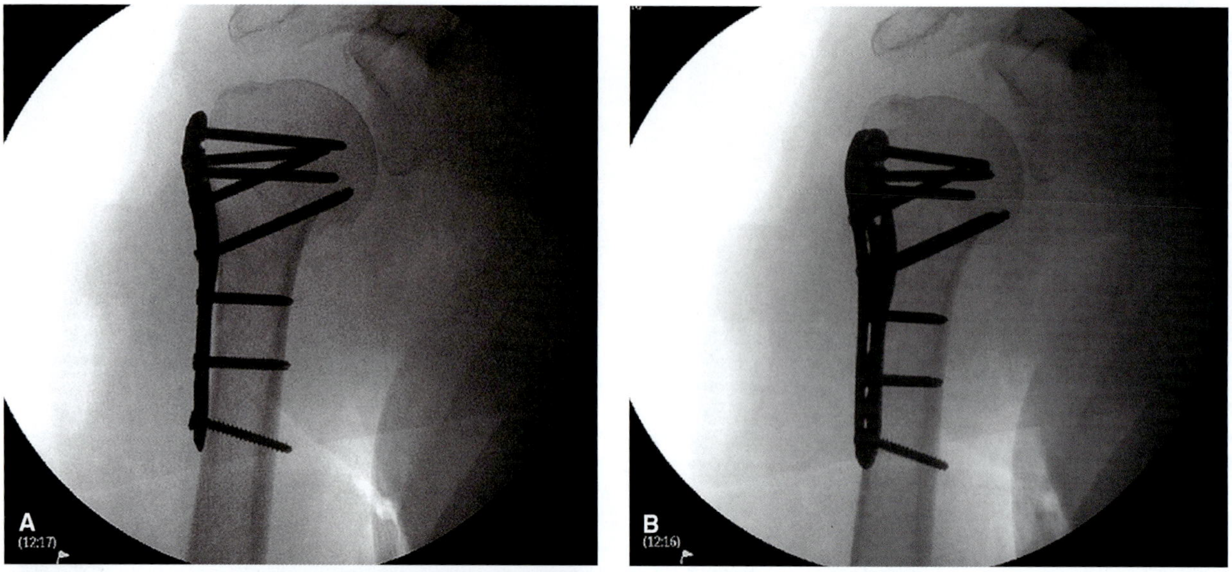

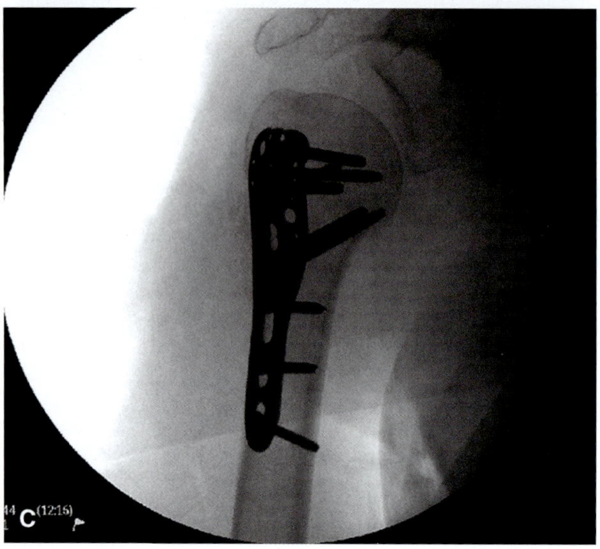

Figure 4-6 | A–C: Screws can be seen getting closer and further away from the articular margin with continuous motion from maximum external rotation to maximal internal rotation.

- A preoperative view of the contralateral side may be useful in particularly difficult cases where normal anatomic landmarks may be lost.
- After initial reduction, gentle internal rotation of the humerus in the AP/Grashey views will allow better visualization of the greater tuberosity. This can sometimes reveal more significant posterior displacement than was initially thought.
- The position of the lesser tuberosity is easiest to appreciate on the axillary view, although one should rely on intraoperative anatomic landmarks.
- Screw penetration is a serious complication associated with ORIF; therefore, screw lengths should be checked in multiple views. Once fixation is finished, fluoroscopic images should be obtained in various degrees of rotation. The final test should be done using live imaging and bringing the humerus from maximal external rotation to maximal internal rotation. The surgeon should look at the screw tips and see them getting closer to the articular margin and then getting further away. Screws are considered safe if the closest point between the tip of the screw and the articular margin is >2 to 3 mm (Fig. 4-6A–C). Because the humeral head is convex, if the screw appears out on any view, it has penetrated the joint.
- The same result can be obtained using multiple angles of inclination and rollback in combination to view the entire head from posterior to anterior in both planes.[1]

Reference

1. Lowe JB, Monazzam S, Walton B, et al. How to use fluoroscopic imaging to prevent intra-articular screw perforation during locked plating of proximal humerus fractures: a cadaveric study. *J Orthop Trauma.* 2015;29(10):e401–e407.

Chapter 5
Humeral Shaft ORIF

NICHOLAS J. ERDLE*
DOMINIC L. VAN NIELEN*
CHRISTOPHER S. SMITH*
MICHAEL J. GARDNER
CHRISTIAAN N. MAMCZAK

Bony Anatomy

- The humerus is a tubular-shaped long bone whose shaft is defined from the proximal border of the pectoralis major insertion to the supracondylar ridge distally.[1]
- Proximally, the diaphysis is uniformly cylindrical changing to a conical shape in the midshaft and then more flattened distally in the coronal plane.
- Typically, the anterior and posterior cortices represent the flatter sides of the bone for plating, but any surface is amenable to plate fixation assuming adequate protection of the neurovascular structures.
- The deltoid tuberosity is located laterally at the junction of the proximal and middle thirds of the diaphysis and represents a potential director of deforming varus forces.
- The spiral groove is a posterior bony landmark on the humerus corresponding to the path of the radial nerve and deep brachial artery. Proximally, the medial aspect of the spiral groove is approximately 10 to 14 cm distal to the acromion with the lateral edge at 14 to 21 cm. From the distal landmark of the lateral epicondyle, it can be found medially at 16 to 20 cm and laterally around 10 to 15 cm.[2]
- Proximally, the axillary nerve is encountered 5 to 7 cm distal to the lateral edge of the acromion.[2]
- Manipulation of the fractured humerus preoperatively and intraoperatively may have clinically important neurovascular implications.

Radiographic Anatomy/Preoperative Imaging

Typically, two orthogonal views are sufficient for imaging fractures of the humeral diaphysis. Fracture patterns that extend into the proximal or distal thirds may also benefit from dedicated views of the shoulder and elbow. Advanced CT imaging is rarely necessary unless pathological fracture or intra-articular extension is suspected.

Anteroposterior (AP) View

- The AP view is performed with the greater tuberosity and medial epicondyle oriented 180 degrees to each other in the coronal view such that an AP of the distal humerus serves as a reference for rotation of the unstable distal fragment.

Lateral View

- In cases of humeral shaft fracture, the proximal lateral view is performed with an "on face" view of the glenoid and a lateral of the distal humerus demonstrating overlap of the capitellar and trochlear cortices forming a "teardrop" (cortical overlap of the coronoid and olecranon fossae).

*The views expressed in this chapter are those of the author(s) and do not necessarily reflect the official policy or position of the Department of the Navy, Department of Defense or the United States Government. Nicholas J. Erdle, Dominic L. Van Nielen, and Christopher S. Smith are military service members and this work was prepared as part of their official duties. Title 17 U.S.C. 105 provides that 'Copyright protection under this title is not available for any work of the United States Government.' Title 17 U.S.C. 101 defines a United States Government work as a work prepared by a military service member or employee of the United States Government as part of that person's official duties.

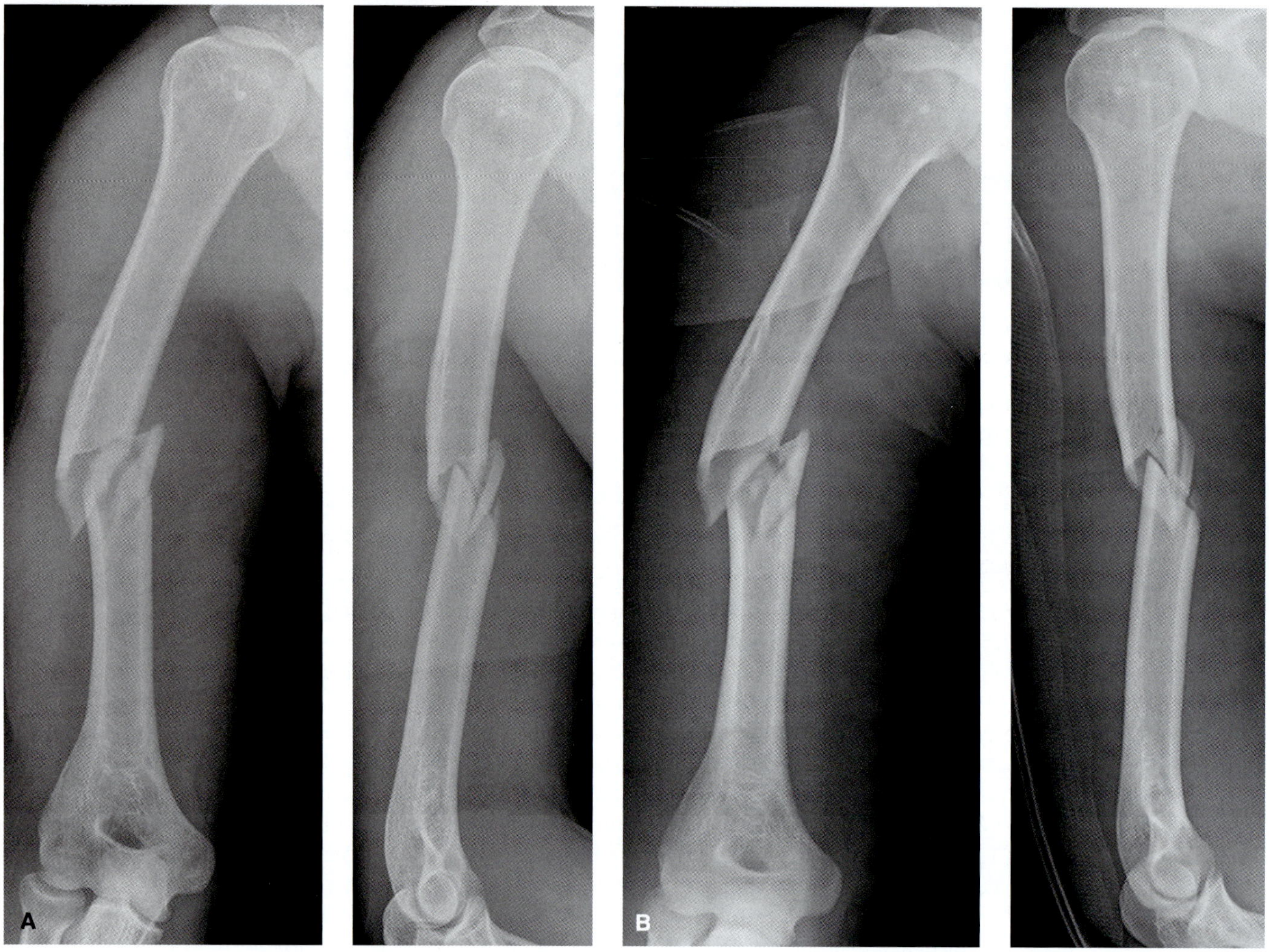

Figure 5-1 | A: Rotation of the distal fragment in the fractured extremity leads to rotation through the fracture site, placing neurovascular structures at risk. **B:** The splinted arm shows better concomitant rotation of the proximal and distal fragments. A transthoracic view, changing the orientation of the x-ray beam instead of the fractured extremity, would be the safest manner to show orthogonal views of both the proximal and distal fragments.

- In order to prevent rotation through the fracture site, a transthoracic view should be obtained with the arm held at against the chest wall. Alternatively, with adequate anesthesia, the arm can be abducted over a cassette for lateral imaging (Fig. 5-1A and B).

In patients with a fracture of the humeral shaft, additional considerations must be taken while obtaining orthogonal views to avoid rotation through the fracture site. (A) Note that rotation of the brachium to obtain a lateral of the distal humerus results in rotation through the fracture site in close proximity to the radial nerve and deep brachial artery, with the humeral head maintaining the same orientation at the glenohumeral joint. (B) With supported abduction of the extremity, both AP and lateral views of the humerus can be obtained with less theoretical risk of insult to the structures in the spiral groove.

Although important in the decision-making process, the radiographic appearance of a displaced humerus fracture is not an indication for operative treatment. With coronal angulation <30 degrees, sagittal angulation <20 degrees, and shortening <3 cm, a majority of humeral shaft fractures are amenable to conservative treatment and bony union. Relative indications for operative treatment include open fractures, associated articular fractures, neurovascular injury, "floating elbow" injuries, polytrauma, pathologic fractures, and failure of closed management to achieve alignment within the tolerances (Fig. 5-2A–C).[1]

Intraoperative fluoroscopic images demonstrate the utility of obtaining orthogonal views to ensure angular alignment of humeral shaft fracture. A lag screw placed in the butterfly fragment and a smaller compression plate assist in obtaining reduction and provisional stabilization prior to placement of the larger plate (Fig. 5-3A and B).

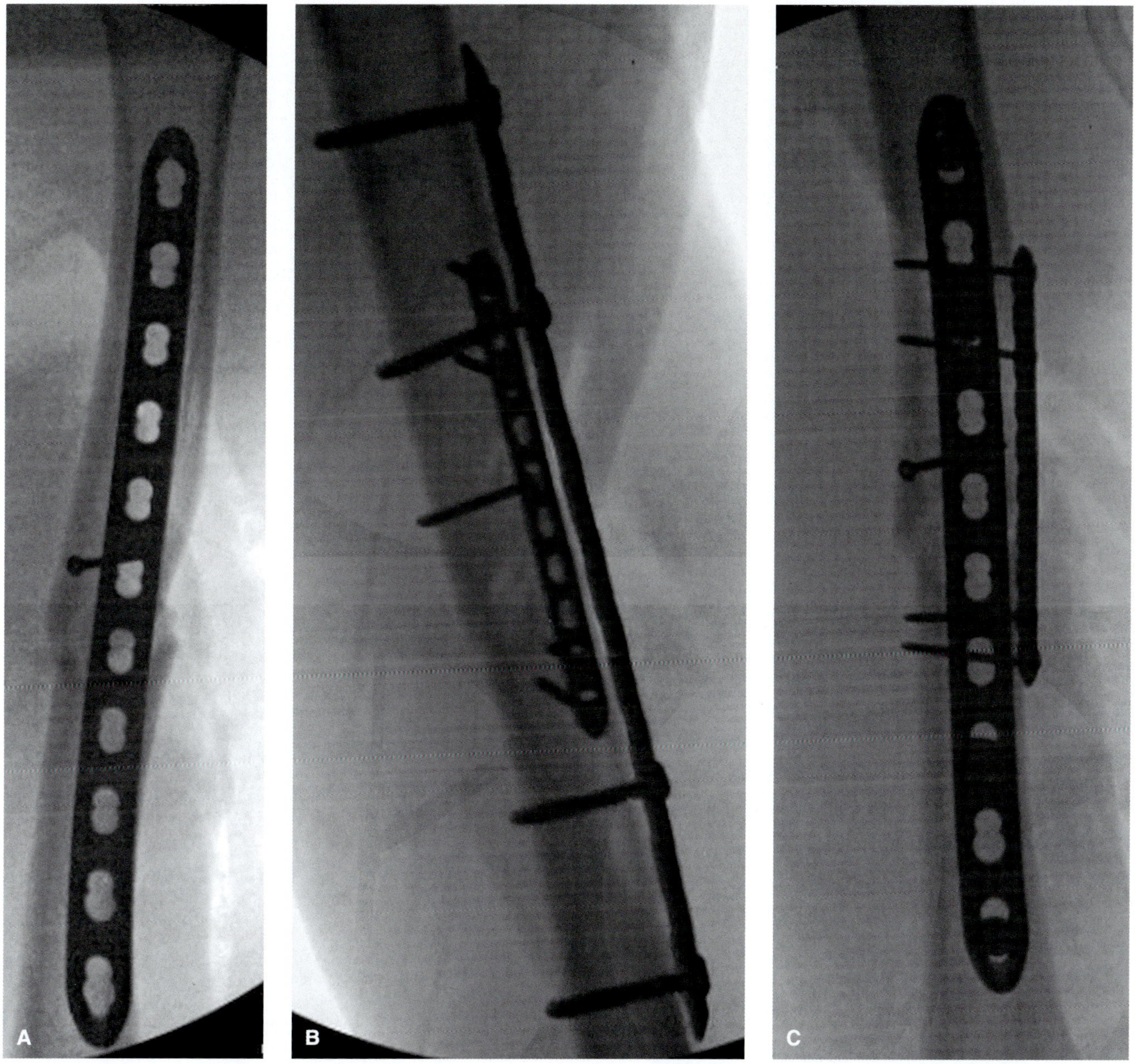

Figure 5-2 | Orthogonal views obtained intraoperatively.

Intraoperative Positioning

Fracture pattern, surgical approach, associated injuries, and surgeon experience help dictate the operative decision for patient positioning, exposure, reduction, and fixation. The humeral shaft is typically approached via anterolateral, direct lateral, or posterior methods.

Supine Positioning—Option 1

- The patient is secured supine on radiolucent table (Jackson, OSI) with the C-arm entering perpendicularly from the opposite side permitting adequate imaging without encroachment into the space occupied by surgeons or anesthesia providers.
- A radiolucent armboard and rolled blanket are placed under the affected extremity to elevate and facilitate manipulation on the field.
- Using rotation of the C-arm in an axis perpendicular to the table, AP and lateral views can be obtained with minimal telescoping in and out of the field with the base of the fluoroscopy machine locked. The AP view is achieved with C-arm rollback and lateral with rollover as depicted below (Fig. 5-4).
- Intraoperatively, the shoulder can be flexed and internally rotated with the forearm flexed over the chest of the patient to facilitate a posterior approach to the humerus (if necessary).

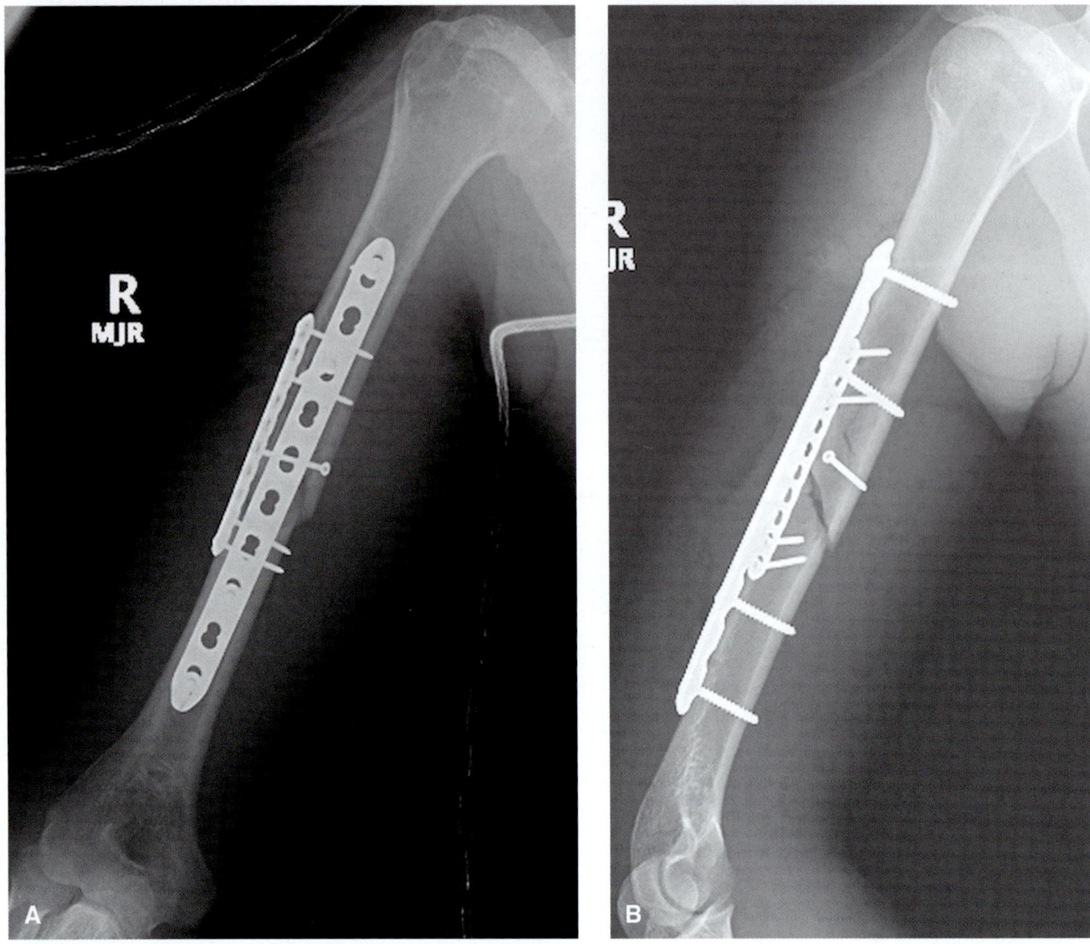

Figure 5-3 | A and B: Postoperative radiographs.

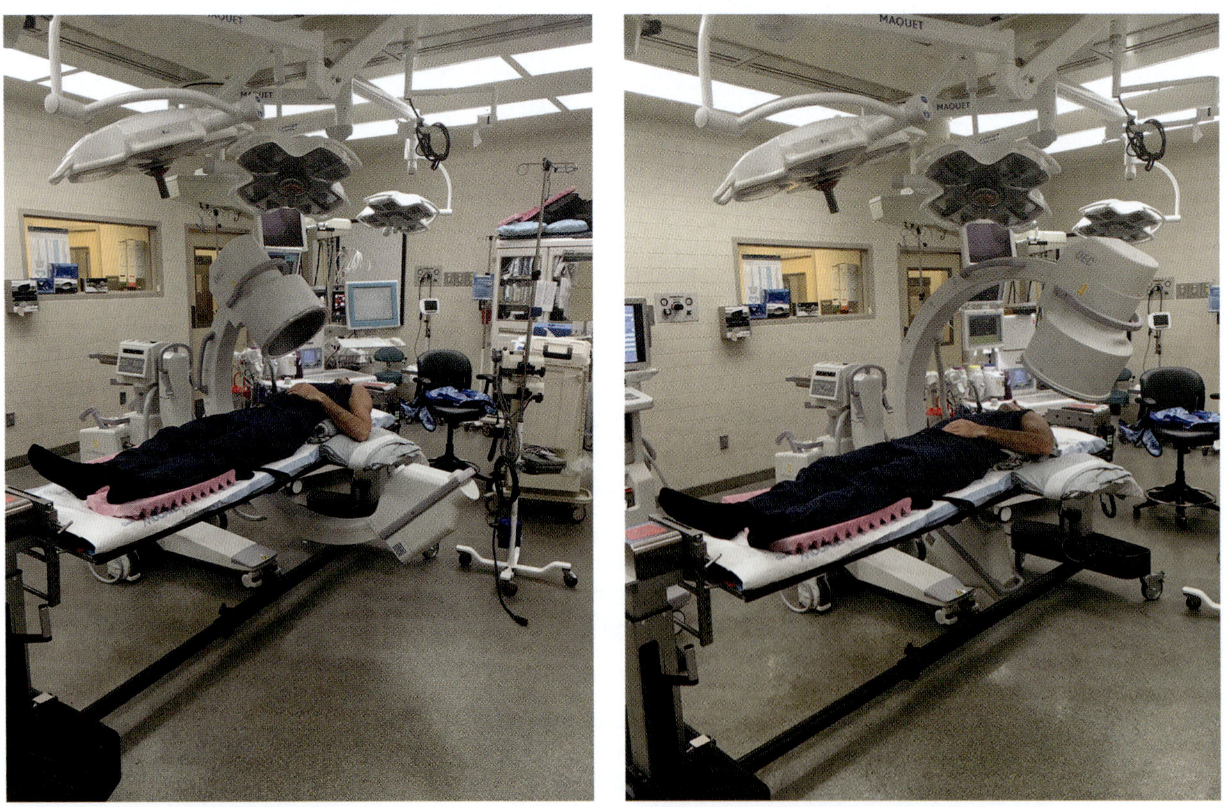

Figure 5-4 | Orthogonal views can be obtained intraoperatively with minimal manipulation of the fractured extremity.

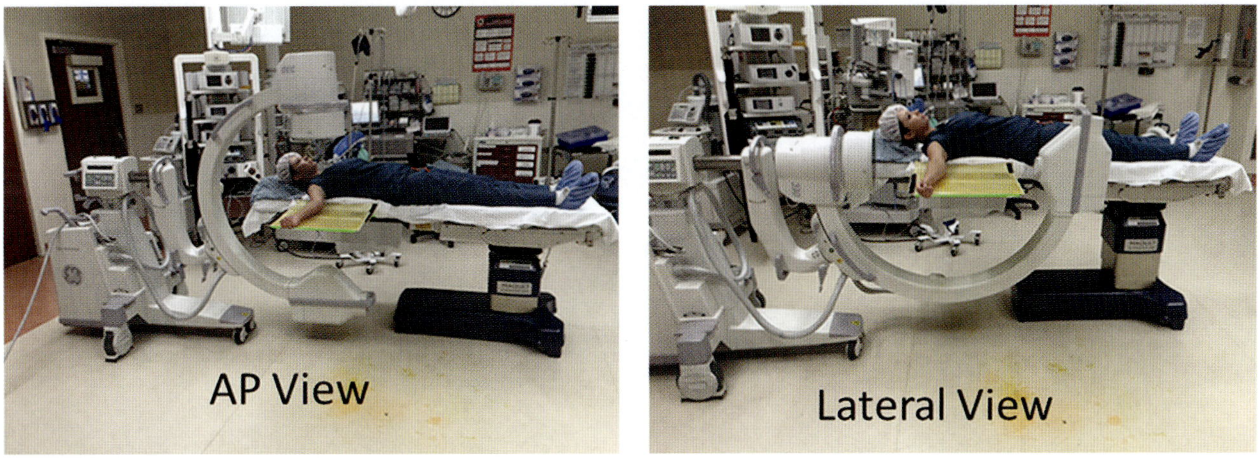

Figure 5-5 | Alternative positioning and fluoroscopic approach for imaging in the supine position.

Supine Positioning—Option 2

- The patient is secured on a radiolucent table (i.e., Maquet diving board) with a large radiolucent working arm table.
- The table is rotated 90 degrees within the room and the C-arm approached from the patient's head for standard AP views of the abducted arm and 90 degrees rollover for lateral images as depicted below (Fig. 5-5):

Lateral Positioning

- The patient is placed in the lateral decubitus position or the semilateral position and stabilized using either a beanbag or chest rolls. An axillary roll or thoracic wedge should be used under the down upper extremity, which is well padded and secured to a radiolucent arm table.
- The affected extremity is draped over a padded radiolucent arm positioner (i.e., Bone Foam) to facilitate a posterior exposure.
- The table is rotated 90 degrees within the room, and the C-arm enters from the front of the patient's head and orientated perpendicular to the hand table to facilitate AP and rollover lateral imaging as depicted below (Fig. 5-6).

Prone Positioning

- The prone position can be used to facilitate the posterior approach to the humerus while decreasing the need to reposition the arm for intraoperative fluoroscopy.
- Following a stabilized intubation, the patient is placed prone onto a radiolucent table (i.e., Maquet diving board) with the use of chest rolls or onto a Wilson frame with an additional cross roll to pad the iliac crests.

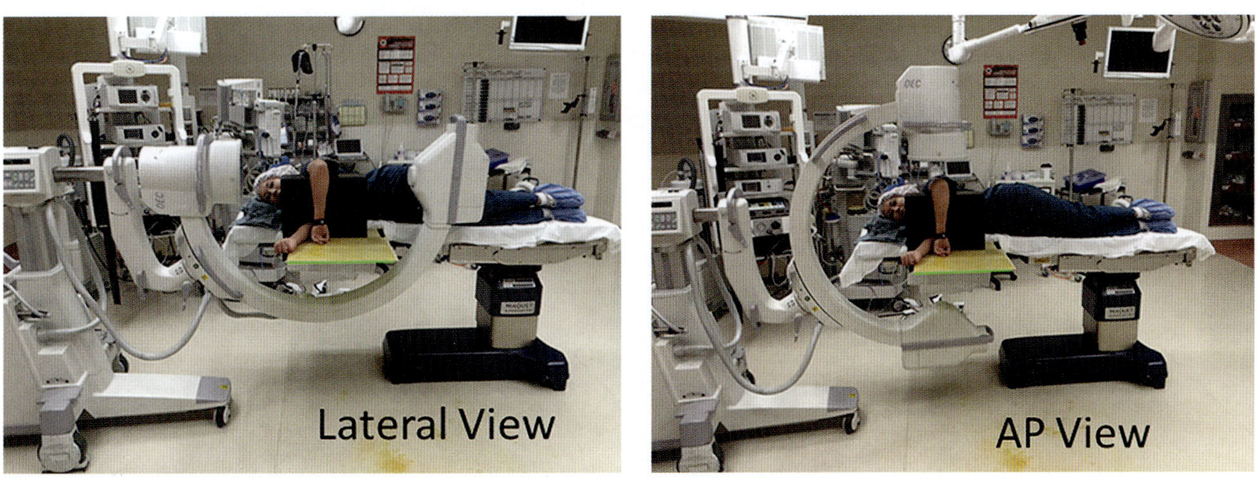

Figure 5-6 | Fluoroscopic approach in the lateral position.

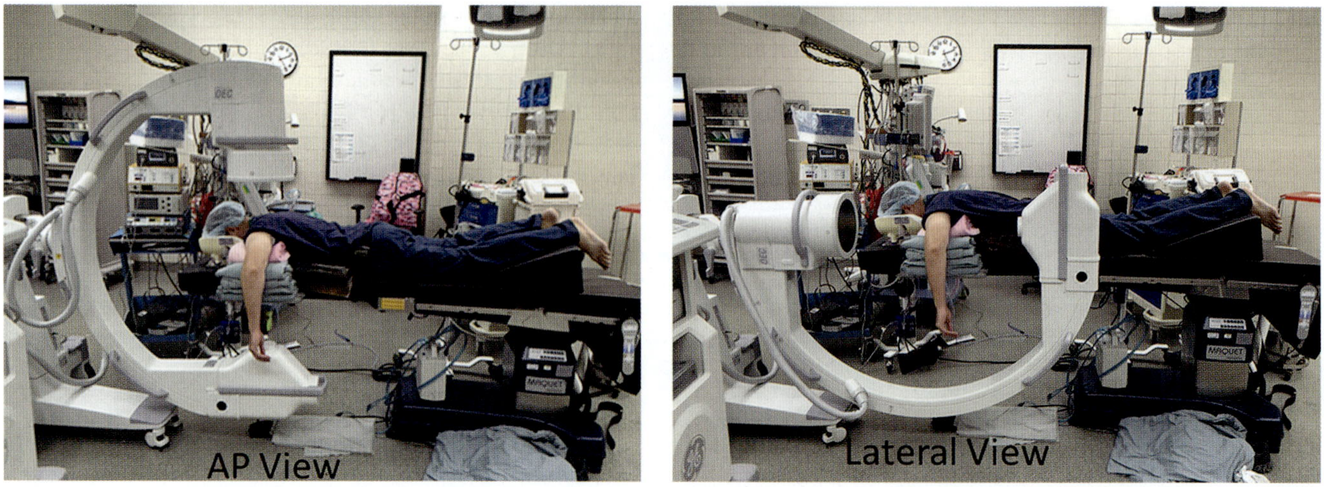

Figure 5-7 | AP and lateral imaging in the prone position. Chest rolls, foam pillows, and Plexiglas arm table are used with blankets to support and pad the arm in a safe position. Adequate fluoroscopic access is confirmed prior to completion of draping.

- The operative extremity is shoulder abducted 90 degrees away from the body and positioned over a short Plexiglas table extending 5 to 8 inches beyond the edge of the table with radiolucent rolls and/or blankets.
- The table is rotated 90 degrees within the room, and the C-arm enters from the front of the patient's head and orientated perpendicular to the hand table to facilitate AP and rollover lateral imaging as depicted below (Fig. 5-7).

Additional Positioning and Imaging Tips

- Discussing positioning needs with anesthesia and operating room staff preoperatively is integral for ensuring patient safety and efficiency following the administration of anesthesia.
- Placement of a tourniquet will obscure the field proximally and is typically not used in fractures of the humeral shaft.
  - However, a sterile tourniquet will allow for exposure of the distal shaft, proximally to where the radial nerve crosses the humeral shaft. This can be useful for expediting ORIF of distal humeral shaft fractures prior to identification of the nerve.
- Use of a radiolucent arm table or radiolucent Plexiglas allows freedom of fluoroscopic imaging.
- Obtaining adequate AP and lateral views of the humerus prior to draping ensures fluoroscopic access.
- Preoperative radiograph with the planned implant superimposed over the humerus can guide incision length.
- Minimizing manipulation of the humerus and its fractured segments until it is stabilized may decrease insults to the important neurovascular structures that are inherently at risk with midshaft fractures.

Intraoperative Imaging Tips

- Preoperative traction fluoro shots can help delineate the complexity of comminuted fracture patterns and assist with the determination to proceed with primary reduction and bone healing versus bridge plating (Figs. 5-8 and 5-9).
- Transverse humerus diaphyseal fractures not amenable to conservative treatment can also pose a challenge to achieve adequate intraoperative compression. Standard AO technique advocates for overbending the plate at the transverse fracture line to achieve far-cortical compression as depicted in the fluoroscopic sequence below (Fig. 5-10).
- Spiral fracture factures typically require numerous reduction clamps at different vectors to achieve anatomic reduction. The resulting lag screw compression and reduction should be checked

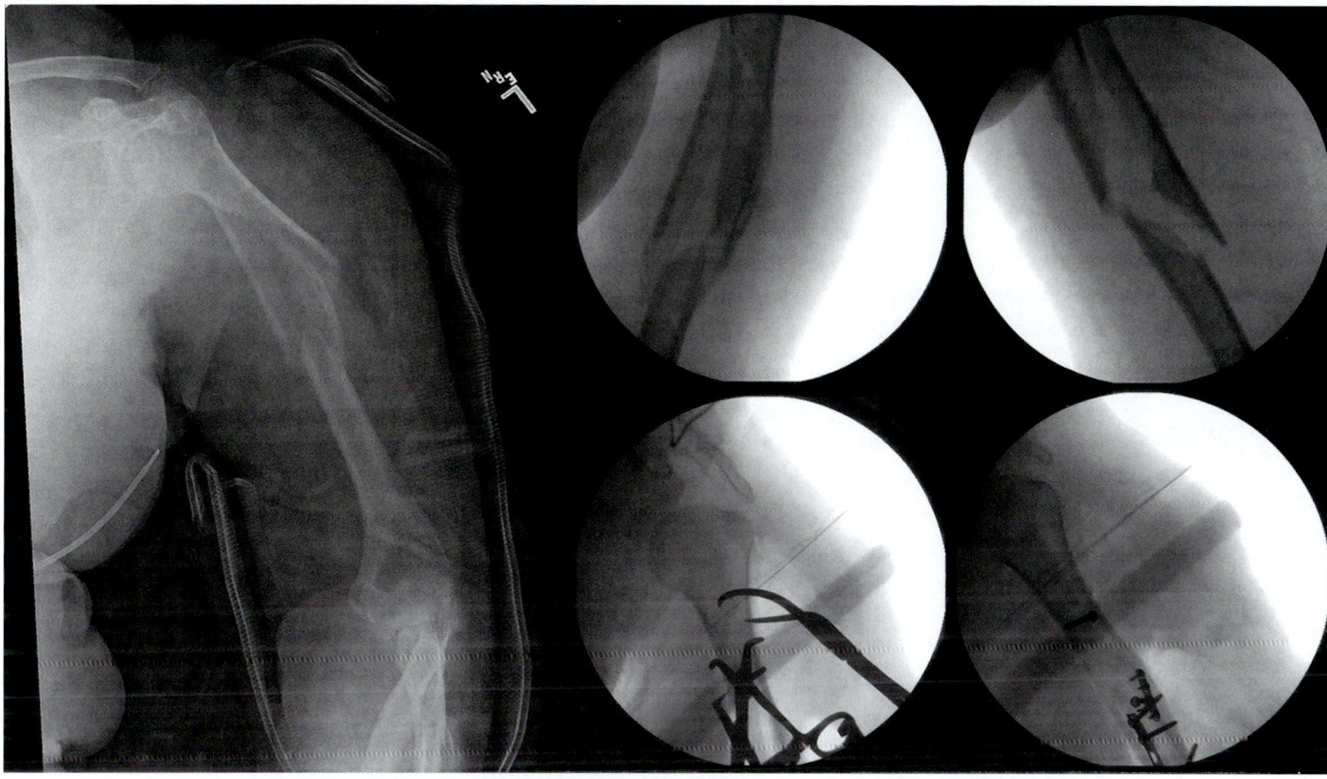

Figure 5-8 | Intraoperative traction shots assist add information that can be helpful to the surgeon.

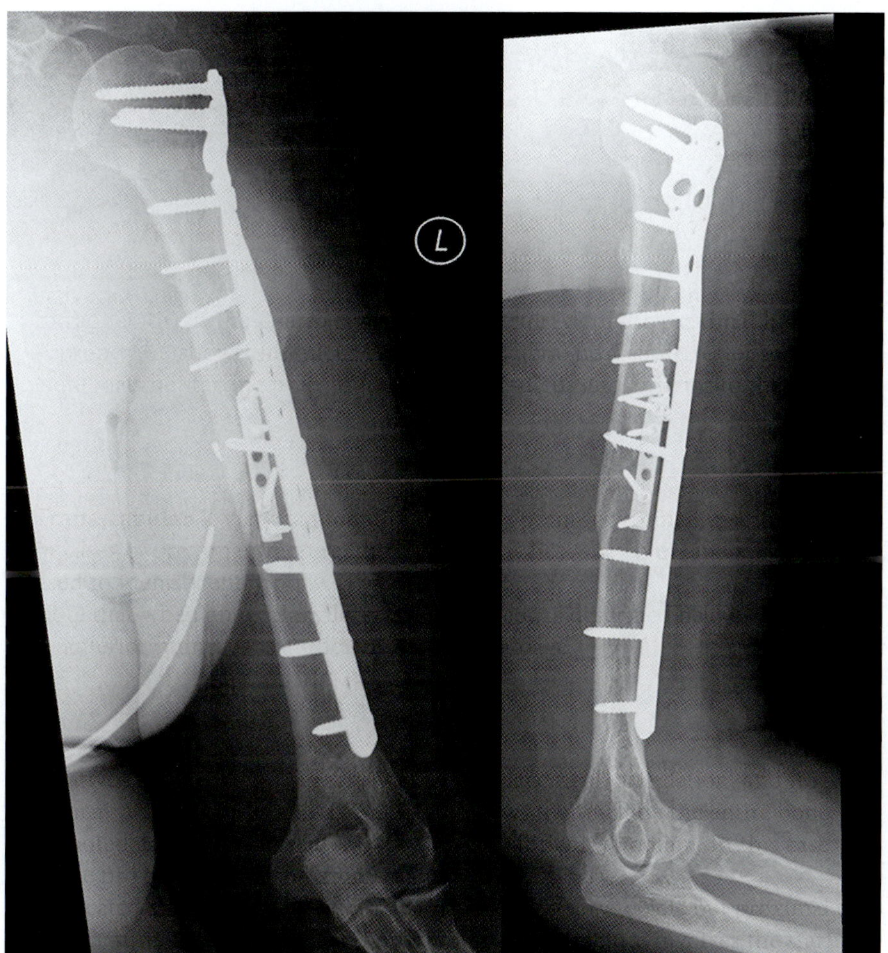

Figure 5-9 | Postoperative radiographs.

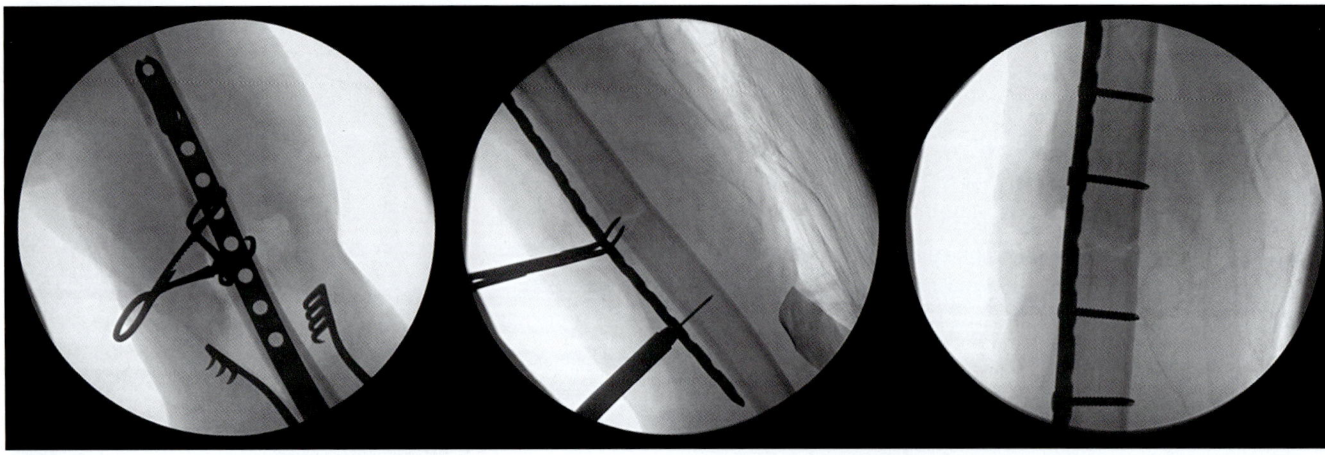

Figure 5-10 | Plate contouring techniques can assist with reduction and compression.

standard orthogonal AP and lateral fluoro views along with oblique images to assure anatomic alignment before neutralization plating (Fig. 5-11).

- Proper plate alignment should be confirmed when spanning a long segment of the humerus. Provisional pinning of the plate position, especially in distal fracture patterns, verifies the absence of plate impingement at the posterior ulnohumeral joint. Final fluoro shots should confirm unrestricted elbow motion and fracture alignment (Fig. 5-12).
- It is helpful to dictate the operative location of the radial nerves path crossing posterior to the plate. In this case, the nerve courses from medial to lateral over the plate near the 4th and 5th proximal holes (Fig. 5-13).

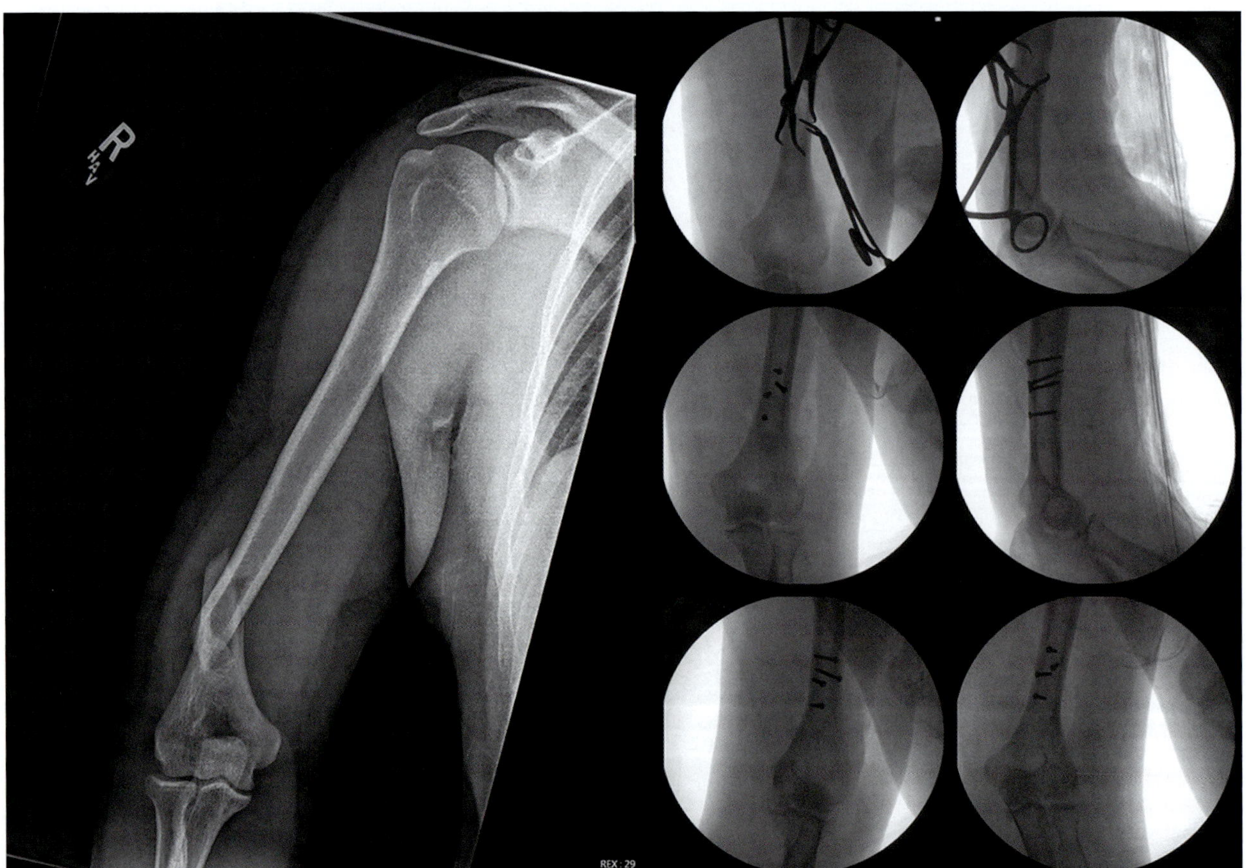

Figure 5-11 | Anatomic reduction with clamps and lag screws can be confirmed prior to plating.

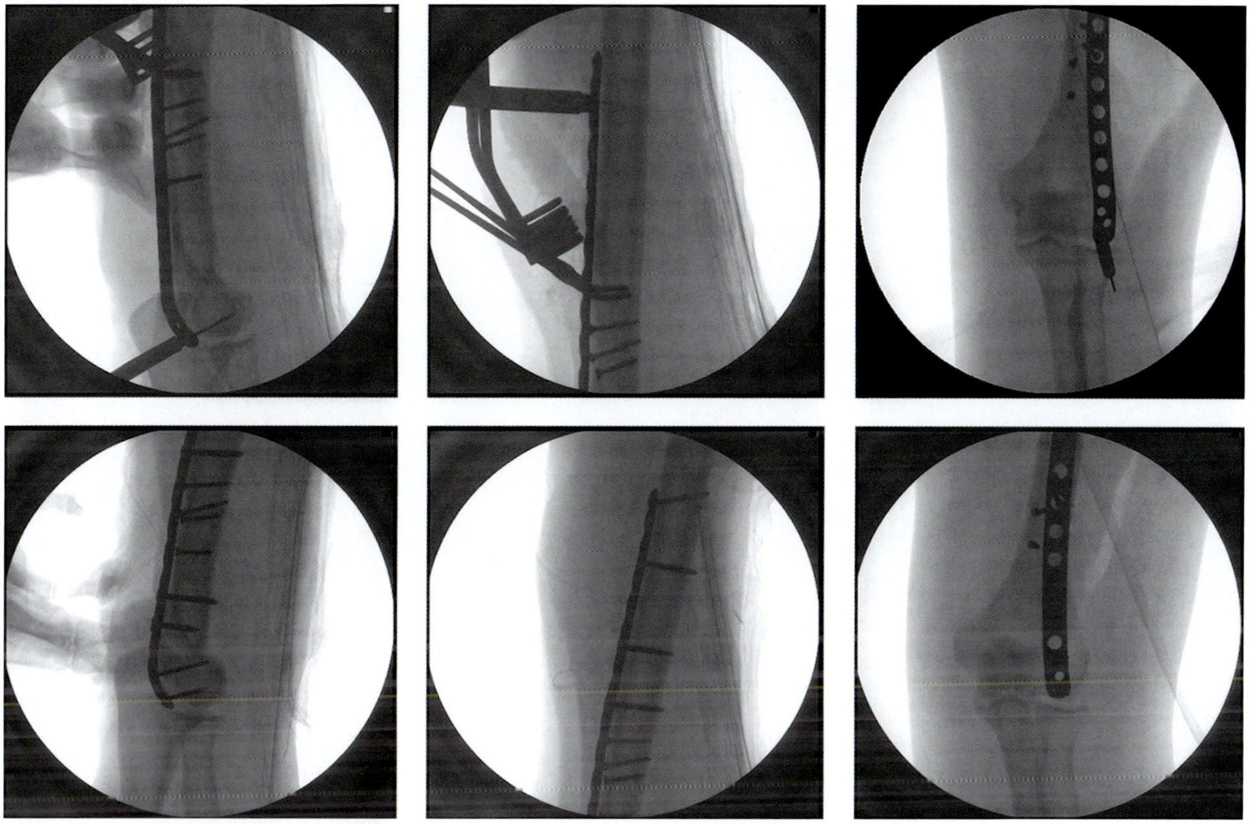

Figure 5-12 | Final intraoperative images.

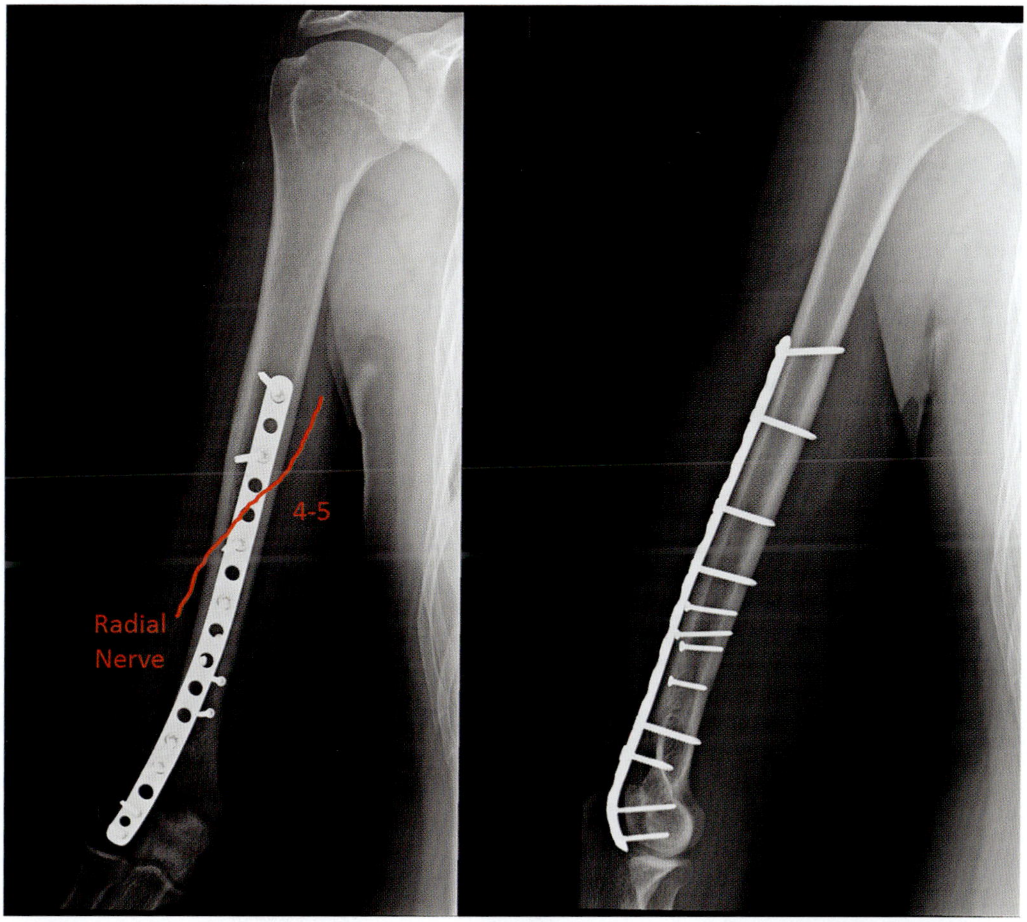

Figure 5-13 | A dictation that includes the location of important neurovascular structures relative to implanted hardware may be helpful to the surgeon revising the fixation or removing the hardware.

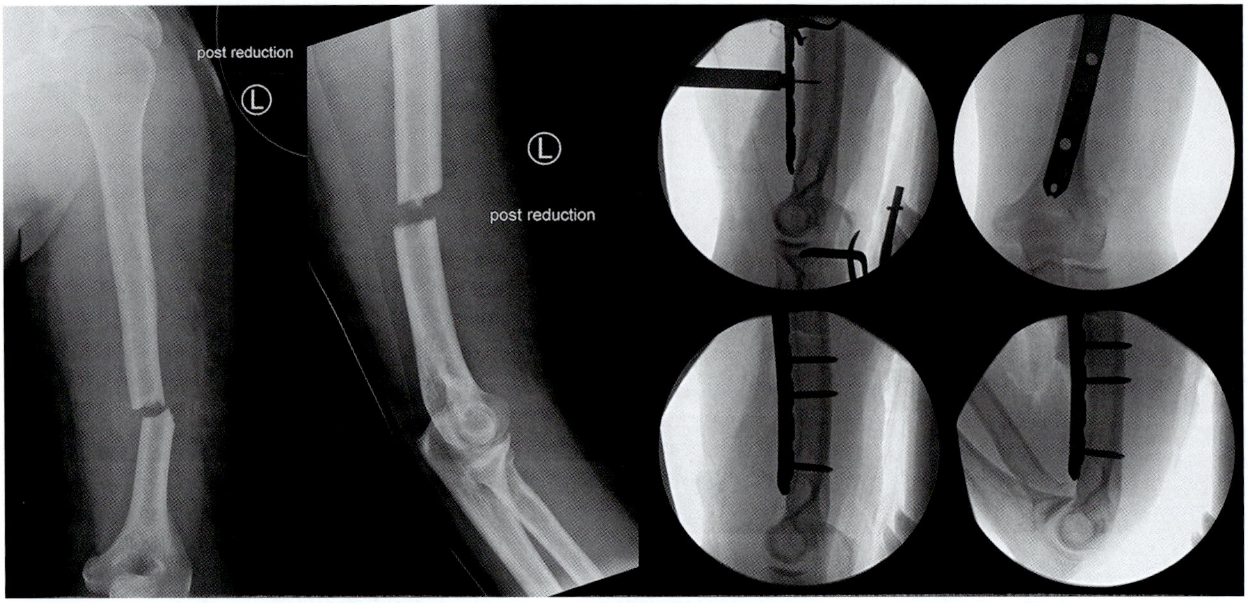

Figure 5-14 | Range of motion can be assessed intraoperatively on fluoroscopy.

- Intraoperative assessment of joint range of motion adjacent to plate constructs can be beneficial to document the absence of plate impingement and the presence of full joint motion (useful to encourage patients' post-op therapy). In this case, anterior plating was performed on a distal fracture due to demand for a supine position to address an open contralateral wrist fracture during the same anesthetic (Fig. 5-14).
- When spanning the entire humerus with a plate, proper coronal and sagittal position can be assessed using sequential, overlapping fluoro shots to assure that the plate is on bone with the desired alignment (Fig. 5-15).

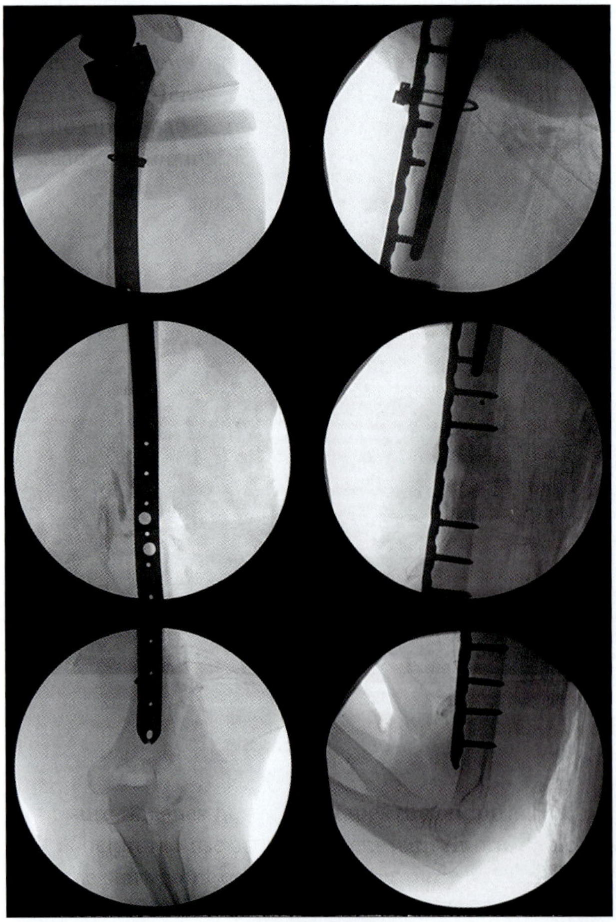

Figure 5-15 | The extremity is immobilized while the fluoroscopy machine is rolled in a single direction to allow imaging of the whole bone in one plane.

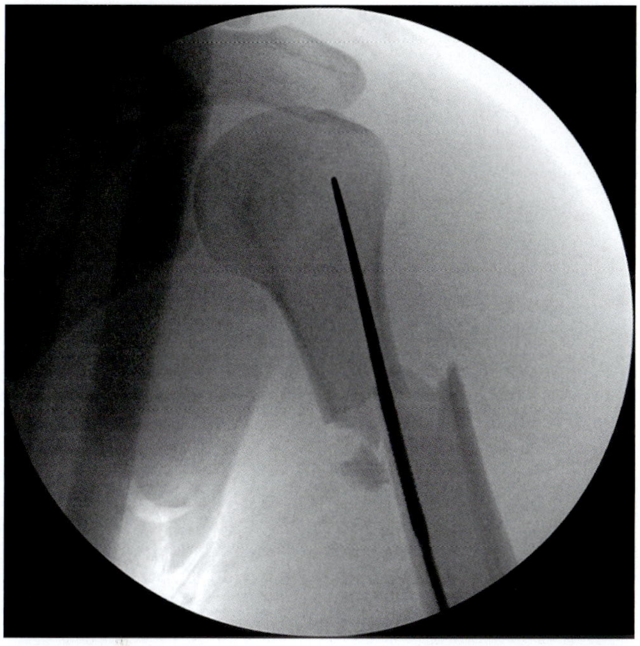

Figure 5-16 | A preoperative fluoroscopic image with a freer laid on the patients skin assists with determining incision location and length. Alternatively, the implant/plate could be used to better predict incision length.

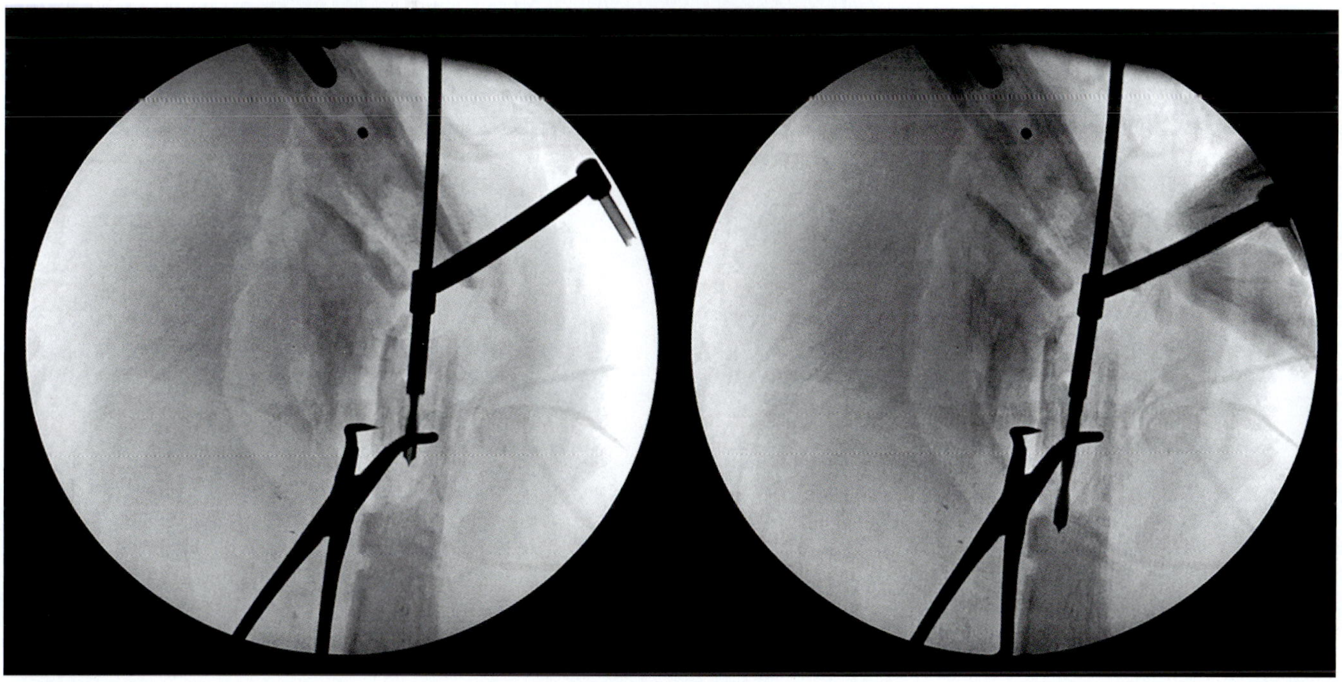

Figure 5-17 | Fluoroscopy in nonunion.

- Preincision spot fluoro shots can assist in localizing the correct location for incision, especially in patients with a generous soft tissue envelope (Fig. 5-16).
- During nonunion cases, fluoroscopic images can depict adequate recanalization of the humeral diaphysis in atrophic patterns. This sequence demonstrates the intramedullary stenosis of the nonunion with advancement of the drill to establish a new medullary canal, which assists in atrophic bone debridement, vascularization of the nonunion repair, and options for intramedullary grafts (Fig. 5-17).

References

1. Carroll EA, Schweppe M, Langfitt M, et al. Management of humeral shaft fractures. *J Am Acad Orthop Surg.* 2012;20:423–433.
2. Zlotolow DA, Catalano LW, Barron OA, et al. Surgical exposures of the humerus. *J Am Acad Orthop Surg.* 2006;14:754–765.

Chapter 6
IM Nailing of Humerus Shaft Fractures

JAMES C. KRIEG

Bony Anatomy

- The bony anatomy of the proximal humerus consists of the shaft, the head, and the greater and lesser tuberosities, which are separated by the bicipital groove (Fig. 6-1).
- The articular surface of the head and the greater tuberosity are separated by a sulcus, where the insertions of the infraspinatus and supraspinatus tendons begin (Fig. 6-2).

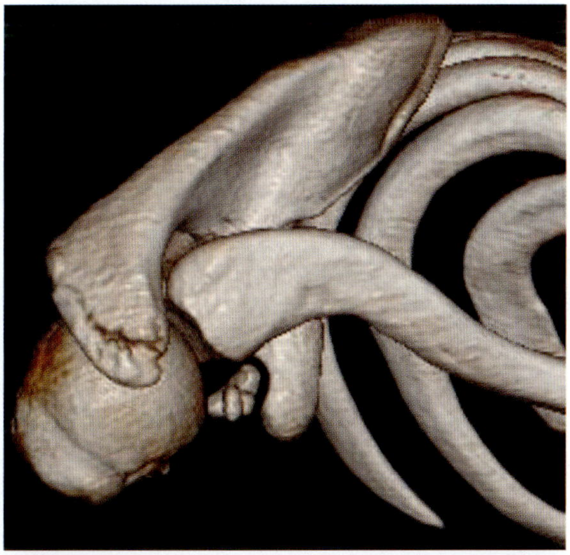

Figure 6-1 | The bony anatomy of the shoulder shows the head is anterior to the acromion, and the bicipital groove separates the greater and lesser tuberosities.

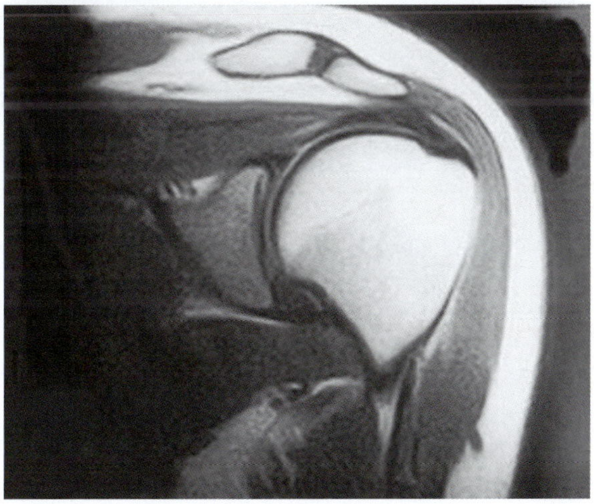

Figure 6-2 | MRI of the shoulder shows the relevant soft tissue anatomy. Note how the supraspinatus tendon inserts in the sulcus at edge of articular surface.

- The proximal humerus articulates with the glenoid and is partially covered by the acromion. The acromion overlies the posterior portion of the humeral head, and a significant portion of the humeral head is anterior to the acromion.
- The head is retroverted from the shaft, generally around 30 degrees.
- The humeral shaft has a posterior bow.
- The medullary canal of the humerus tapers and ends several centimeters proximal to the olecranon fossa.

Radiographic Anatomy

AP View Humerus

- The AP view is obtained with the arm in neutral rotation. There is a tendency to get internally rotated views, with the forearm on the abdomen, and often the arm needs to be held for proper positioning (Fig. 6-3).
- AP of the entire arm is helpful in determining deformity as well as fracture pattern (Fig. 6-4).
- Postoperative x-rays are easier to obtain, with an intact limb.

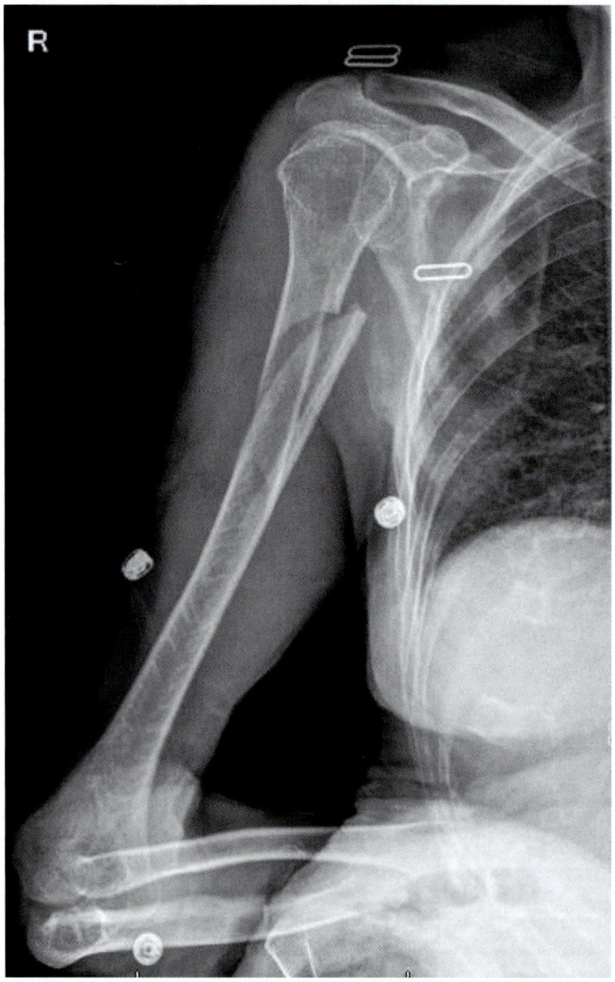

Figure 6-3 | Injury AP film. Note how internally rotated it is.

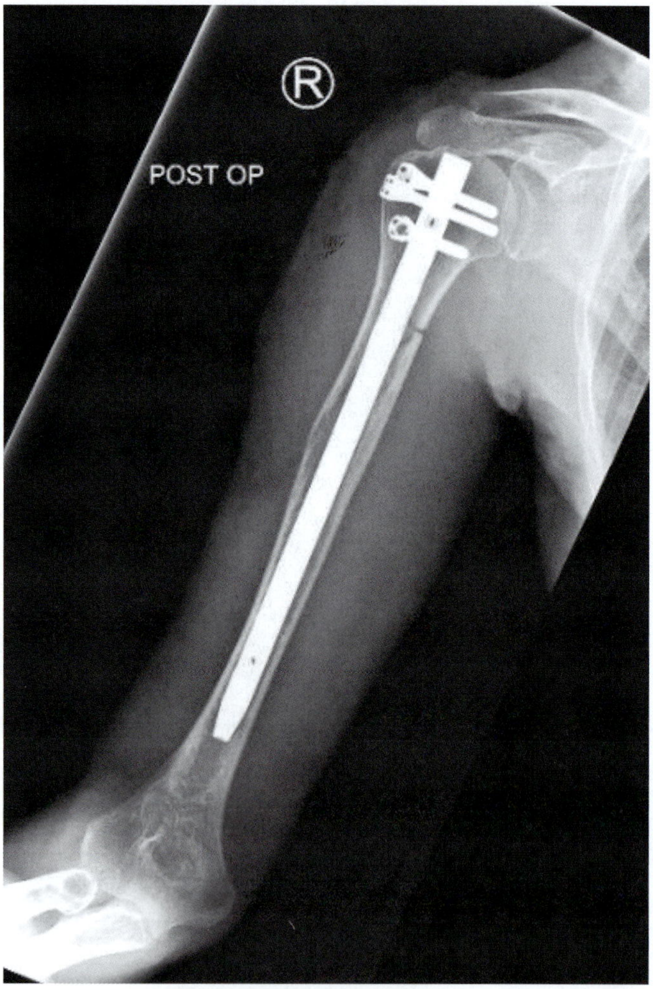

Figure 6-4 | Postoperative AP view is in neutral rotation, and makes it easier to see the bony landmarks.

Lateral View Humerus

- Lateral view of the entire humerus can be difficult to obtain in case of fracture.
- Lateral of the proximal humerus can be obtained with axillary lateral of the shoulder or as a transscapular Y view.
- Caudal portion best obtained as cross-table lateral with arm held in neutral (Fig. 6-5).
- Postoperatively, a single view can be obtained.

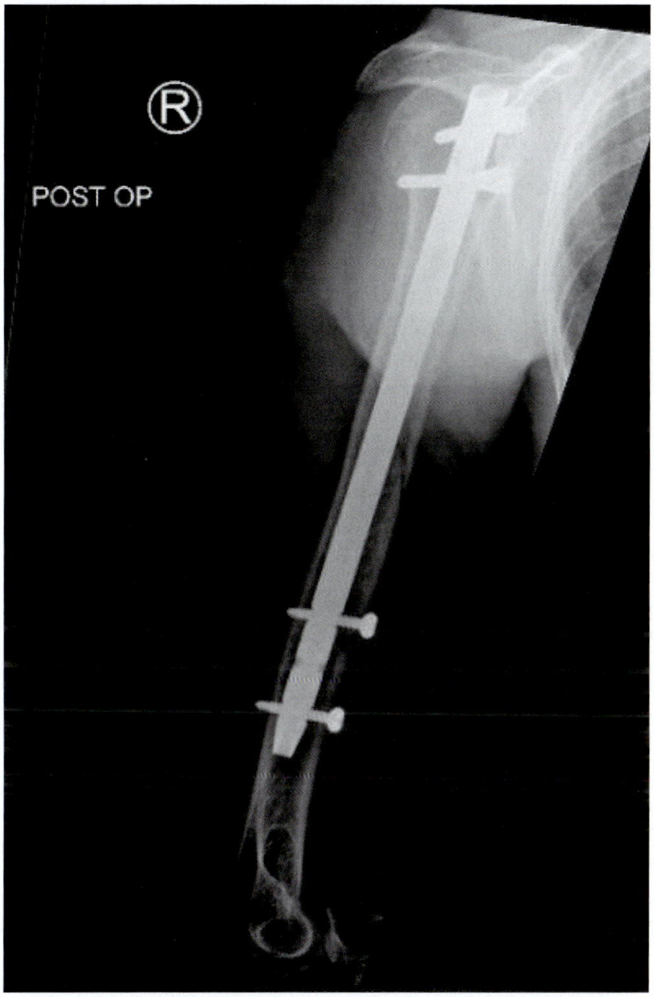

Figure 6-5 I The lateral view can be obtained by fully internally rotating the arm, or cross table.

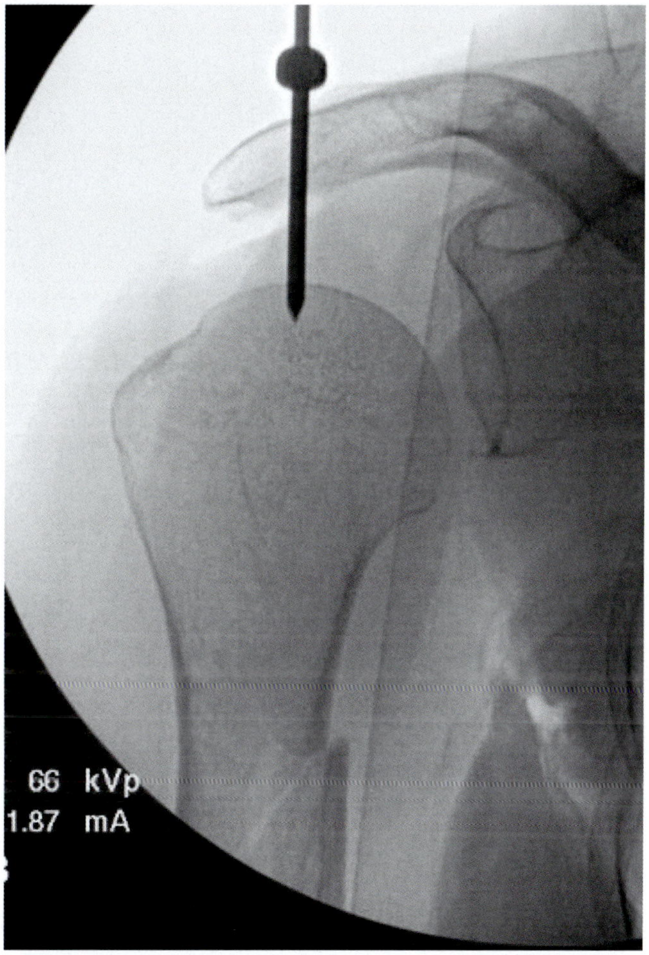

Figure 6-6 I A neutral AP view, with the sulcus seen at the edge of the joint, will guide placement of the guidewire for nail entry hole placement.

AP View Shoulder

- Intraoperatively, the C-arm is used to get a true AP of the proximal humerus (Fig. 6-6).
- A proper AP shows the sulcus between the lateral head and greater tuberosity at its deepest profile.
- Note that the starting point is medial to the sulcus and anterior to the acromion.

Lateral View Proximal Humerus

- **Transscapular Y view** can identify the entry point for IM nail insertion (Fig. 6-7).
- In cases of proximal fracture, the reduction is best shown on an axillary view, which can also be used to identify entry point (Fig. 6-8).
- Note that when an **axillary lateral** is obtained, as described below, the image is upside down, that is, anterior humerus is at the bottom of the image.

Preoperative Imaging

- Relative indications for surgery include displacement, angulation, and fracture pattern. The deformity is seen best on AP and lateral views that include the entire bone, when possible.
- As noted earlier, a single lateral view can be difficult to obtain. In this case, separate lateral images of the proximal and distal segments may be necessary.
- Dedicated shoulder or elbow x-rays may be necessary to rule out proximal or distal extension of the fracture. It is important to know whether the fracture involves the start point or whether it extends too distal to accommodate a nail.

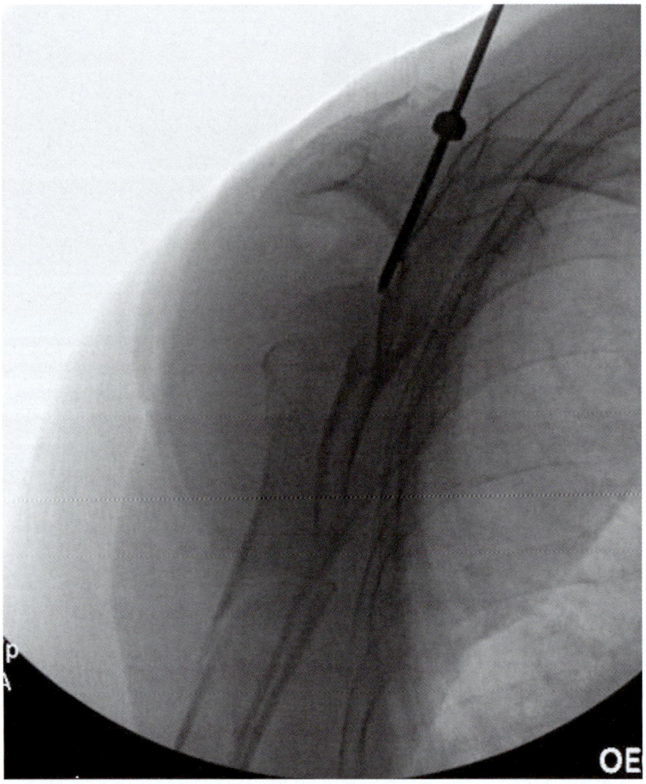

Figure 6-7 I The transcapular Y view is the easiest way to show the entry point in the lateral view.

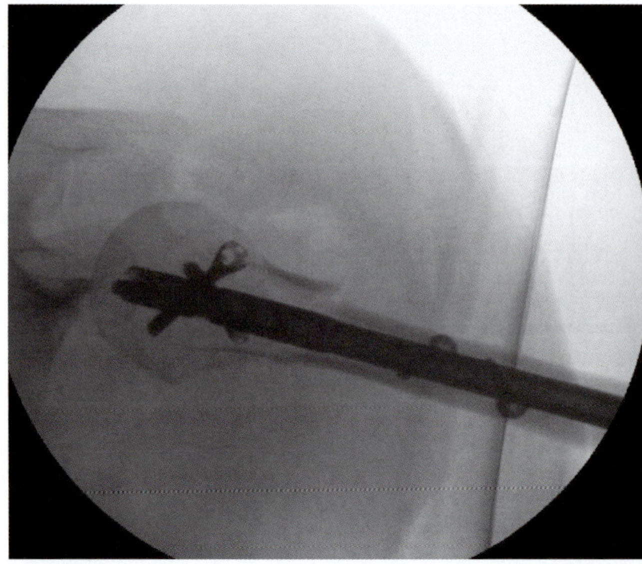

Figure 6-8 I The axillary view shows reduction as well as entry point, both of which are essential in the proximal fracture. Note that the image is inverted, and the lesser tuberosity (anterior) is at bottom of the image.

Intraoperative Positioning

- IM nailing of humerus fracture requires full access to the limb and free mobility of the shoulder and elbow in all planes. This will facilitate the reduction, surgical approach, and nail insertion. Thus, the arm should be prepped free.
- Supine positioning can be modified to allow for the surgical approach to the entry site and also allow for reduction.
- The position allows for full imaging of the entire humerus in at least two planes. This is best done without having to move the limb when placing an IM nail.

1. Supine Position

- The advantages of the modified supine position include easier imaging in orthogonal views, without moving the limb.
- Patients may be placed onto a radiolucent table such as a Maquet diving board or an OSI/Jackson. The patient should be at the end of the Maquet table diving board.
- The C-arm is placed on the contralateral uninjured side and comes across the body to image the operative limb.
- The patient is brought to the edge of the table. If brought over the edge, then the C-arm may have a hard time reaching the limb.
- The unaffected limb is padded and tucked at the side. There cannot be an arm board on the uninjured side, as this will prevent the C-arm from coming in far enough to image the injured limb.
- By placing folded blankets under the hip and shoulder on the operative side, the body is actually rotated 10 to 15 degrees from the fully supine position (Figs. 6-9 and 6-10).
- By supporting the operative side with folded blankets, the shoulder can be extended as needed to better access the starting point.

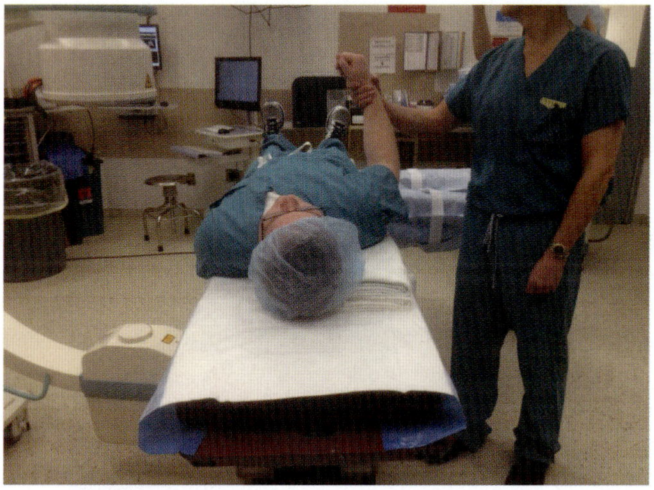

Figure 6-9 | Semisupine position with blanket bump, and patient at edge of bed. Well arm is tucked.

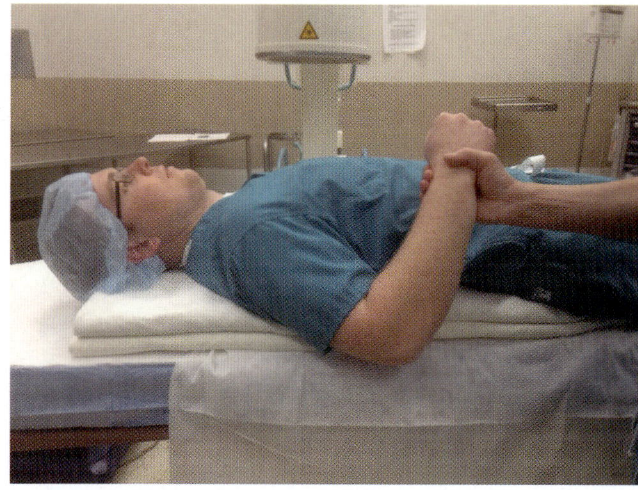

Figure 6-10 | Bump allows for shoulder extension, which can help with entry point access anterior to the acromion.

2. The AP View

- The AP view is obtained by rolling the C-arm back until the sulcus between the head and greater tuberosity is seen maximally. Because of the position of the C-arm, this is often called the "rollback" view for the C-arm technologist (Fig. 6-11).
- Note that the forearm is in line with the beam. This ensures that the same position will allow for an AP of the entire humerus and elbow.

3. Transscapular Y View

- The simplest lateral view is the transscapular Y view. This is obtained simply by rolling over the C-arm, without moving the limb (Fig. 6-12).
- Some C-arms do not roll over sufficiently, and this is another reason that placing a small bump under the operative side can help.
- Fluoroscopy is used to identify the entry point for IM nail insertion.
- By identifying the radiographic entry point on C-arm before incision, the approach can be directed to the optimal entry point with a minimum of soft tissue dissection.

4. Axillary View

- Axillary lateral view is obtained by positioning the C-arm as you would for an inlet view of the pelvis, with maximal side tilt of the C-arm. The shoulder can be slightly abducted and extended to facilitate it (Fig. 6-13).

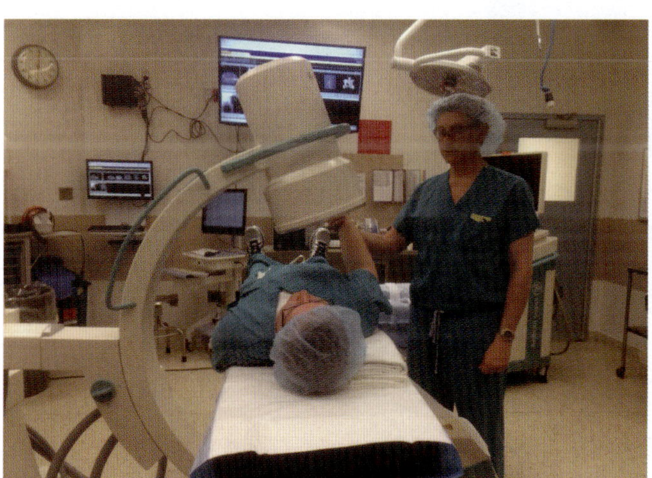

Figure 6-11 | The C-arm is rolled back to get the AP view.

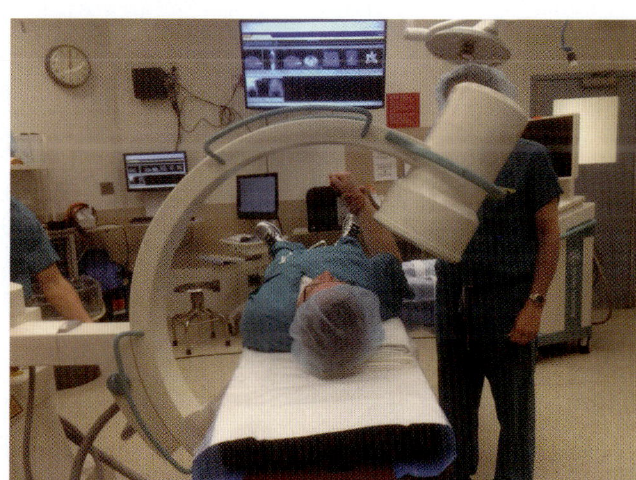

Figure 6-12 | Rolling the C-arm over the top obtains the transcapular Y-view. The arm has not moved.

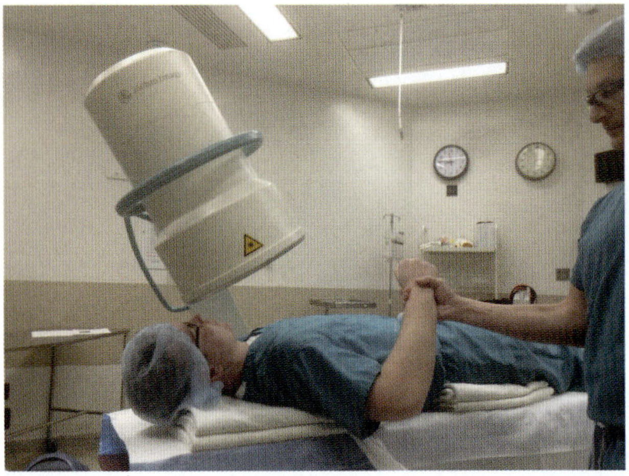

Figure 6-13 I The C-arm is tilted to get the axillary view. Shoulder extension can help with this.

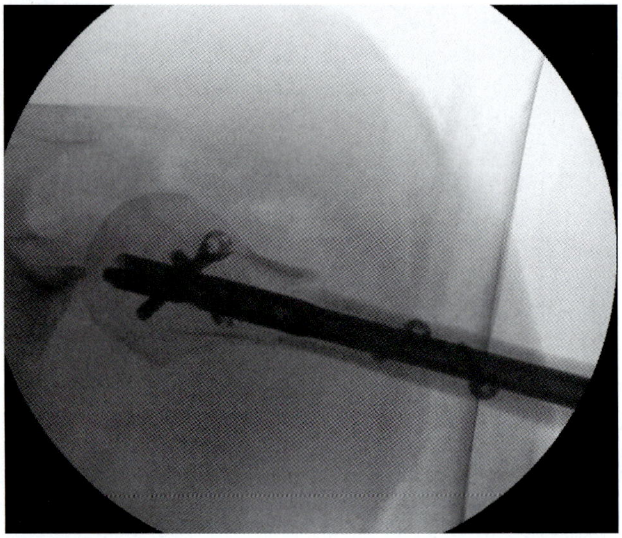

Figure 6-14 I Axillary view. The image is inverted and the anterior humerus is at the bottom of the image.

- The forearm is rotated to neutral position (Fig. 6-14).
- Because of the position of the C-arm, the image is inverted. Note that the lesser tuberosity is seen at the bottom of the image.
- The axillary view can be helpful to determine reduction of proximal humerus fractures, in addition to the IM nail entry point. It can also be used to assess version of the head.

5. Views of the Distal Humerus

- The entire humerus can be imaged by using the rollover and rollback views. This can be done to assess reduction.
- When imaging the distal humerus for freehand interlocking, the arm is gently rotated to neutral. Because screws are generally inserted anterior to posterior, having the arm in neutral rotation makes it easier, as the surgeon is working straight up and down (Fig. 6-15).
- The elbow can be rested on the padded edge of a Mayo stand, to position the arm and keep it steady during interlock insertion.

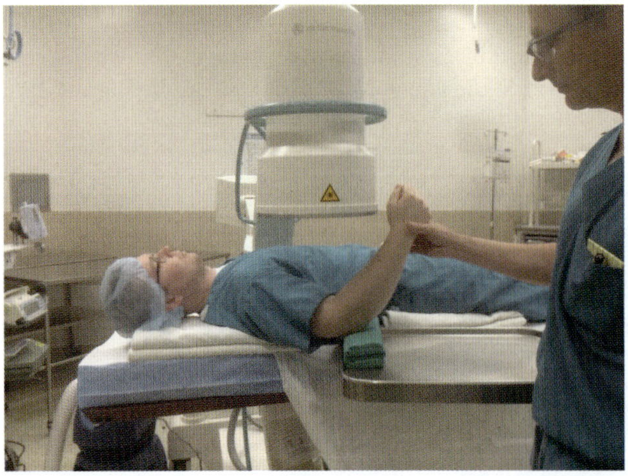

Figure 6-15 I AP view of entire humerus is easily obtained.

Additional Tips

- Be sure the anesthesiologist tapes the endotracheal tube to the unoperated side.
- It is helpful to use an instrument with fluoroscopic imaging to identify the ideal place for exposure of the start point before each layer of dissection. This ensures that the minimum amount of dissection is done to expose the ideal starting point.

Chapter 7
Distal Humerus Fractures

DOMINIC L. VAN NIELEN*
NICHOLAS J. ERDLE*
CHRISTOPHER S. SMITH*
MICHAEL J. GARDNER
CHRISTIAAN N. MAMCZAK

Bony Anatomy[1-3]

- The distal humerus articulates with the sigmoid notch of the ulna (ulnohumeral joint) for flexion/extension at the elbow and the radius (radiocapitellar joint) to allow for pronation/supination.
- The highly congruent joint allows for excellent bony stability but also requires anatomic alignment of intra-articular fracture fragments to minimize early-onset traumatic arthritis.
- The ulnohumeral joint is positioned in 3 to 9 degrees of external rotation, 4 to 8 degrees of valgus in relation to the humeral shaft.
- The medial column is oriented 45 degrees from longitudinal axis of the humeral shaft, while the lateral column diverges at a more acute 20-degree angle.
- The medial epicondyle serves as attachment for both anterior and posterior bundles of medial collateral ligament as well as the origin of the flexor/pronator mass. Therefore, its anatomic reduction and fixation is paramount to joint stability. Inferiorly, the ulnar nerve courses from posterior to anterior under the bony sulcus of the medial epicondyle and is at risk for injury with fractures and surgical fixation.
- The posterior surface of the distal humerus is relatively wide and flat, making it easier to apply plate fixation.
- The anterior surface is more irregular and largely covered by articular cartilage with the convex capitellum laterally and the undulating trochlear joint surface medially. Both surfaces project approximately 45 degrees distal and anterior from the long axis of the humerus sharing a common center arc of rotation in the sagittal plane (thus directly influencing joint congruity and motion with malreduction of either column).

Radiographic Anatomy

1. AP View

- The AP view is obtained with the elbow fully extended and forearm supinated; this allows a clear view of the joint surface while minimizing overlap of the radius and ulna.
- The joint surface is best visualized on AP view. Ulnohumeral and radiocapitellar joints should be symmetric without any intra-articular step-off.
- The radial head should line up with the center of the capitellum in AP, lateral, and oblique views (Figs. 7-1 and 7-2).

2. Lateral View

- The lateral view is obtained with the elbow in 90 degrees of flexion.
- A "true" lateral radiograph demonstrates concentric overlap of three bony circles: the capitellum and the narrowest and widest portions of the trochlea (dashed yellow circle below).

*The views expressed in this chapter are those of the author(s) and do not necessarily reflect the official policy or position of the Department of the Navy, Department of Defense or the United States Government. Dominic L. Van Nielen, Nicholas J. Erdle, and Christopher S. Smith are military service members and this work was prepared as part of their official duties. Title 17 U.S.C. 105 provides that 'Copyright protection under this title is not available for any work of the United States Government.' Title 17 U.S.C. 101 defines a United States Government work as a work prepared by a military service member or employee of the United States Government as part of that person's official duties.

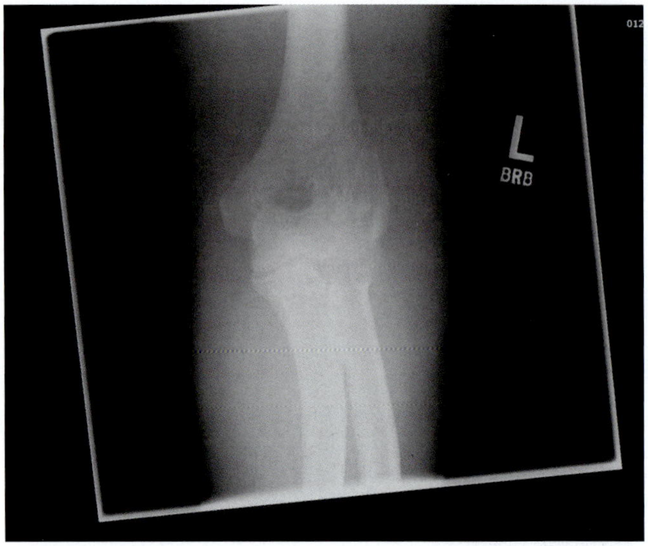

Figure 7-1 | AP view of elbow/distal humerus demonstrates a lateral condyle fracture with intra-articular extension but without step-off.

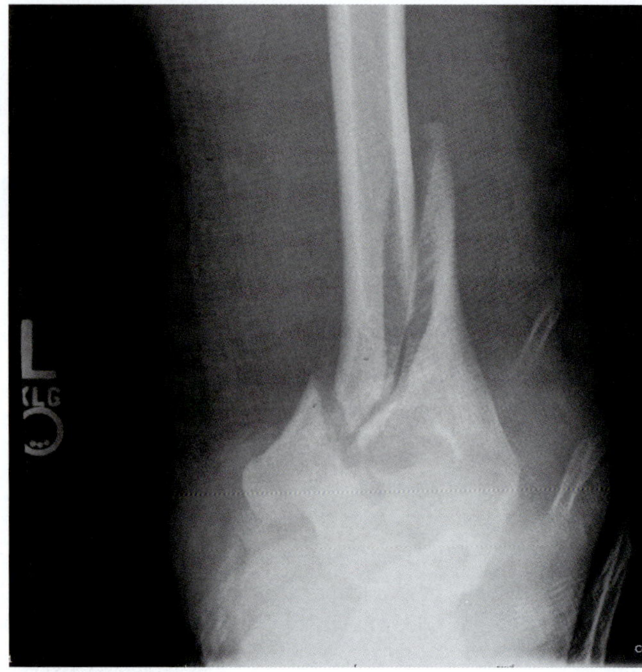

Figure 7-2 | AP of distal humerus: bony detail is obscured by splinting material, but intra-articular involvement as well as the degree of articular displacement and fracture comminution are easily visualized.

- The "figure of 8" or "hourglass" (blue inset) is made from superimposition of bone forming the sagittal trochlear cortical surface and the distal termination of the humeral medullary canal. The narrow neck of the hourglass corresponds to the olecranon fossa.
- The radius should directly line up with the center of the capitellum (light blue arrow). Any subluxation should be critically evaluated for fracture or ligamentous injuries.
- A joint effusion, or "sail sign," can be demonstrated radiographically. An anterior capsular lucency may be normal, but a posterior sail sign is always pathologic for an intra-articular process.
- The double-arc sign is pathognomonic for a coronal shear fracture (Figs. 7-3 and 7-4).

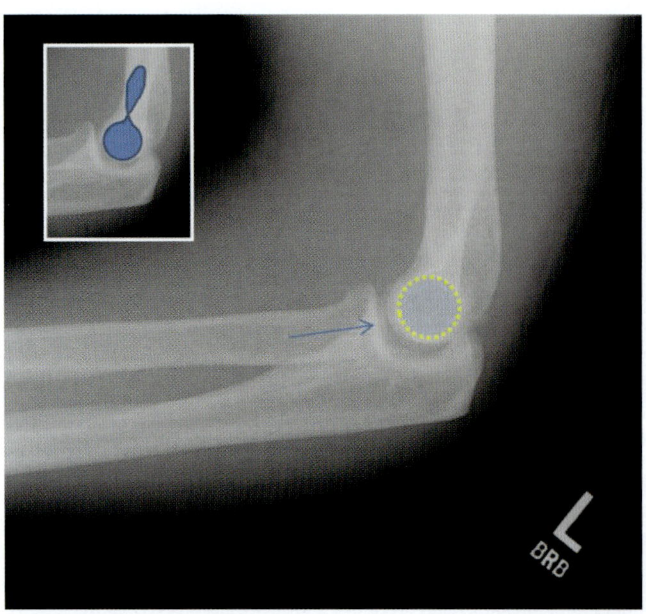

Figure 7-3 | Lateral view of an intact elbow/distal humerus.

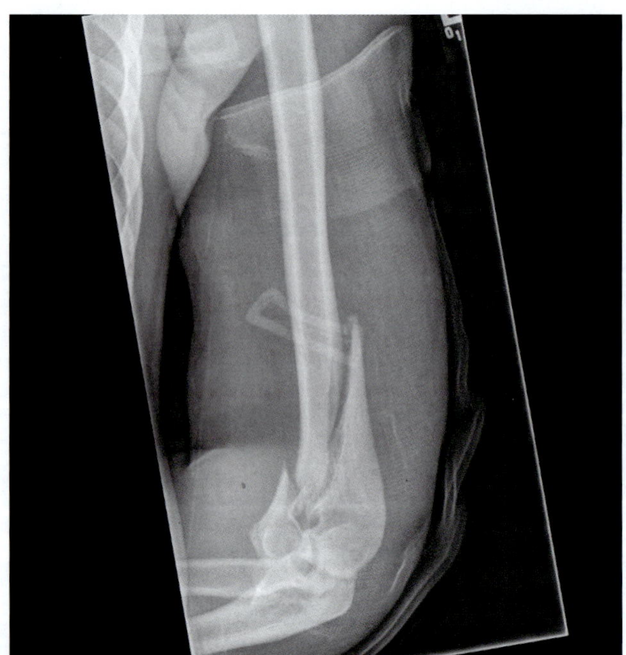

Figure 7-4 | Rotation through fracture site can make obtaining "true lateral" difficult, but proximal extension is clearly visualized.

3. Oblique Views

- The patient is positioned with elbow extended and forearm supinated.
- Oblique views can be helpful to better visualize condylar fractures.
  - Internal rotation (medial rotation) view is obtained with entire arm rotated medially 45 degrees to beam. This view better demonstrates medical epicondyle fractures (Fig. 7-5).
  - External rotation (lateral rotation) view is obtained with entire arm rotated laterally approximately 45 degrees to beam; this view better visualizes lateral epicondyle fractures (Fig. 7-6).

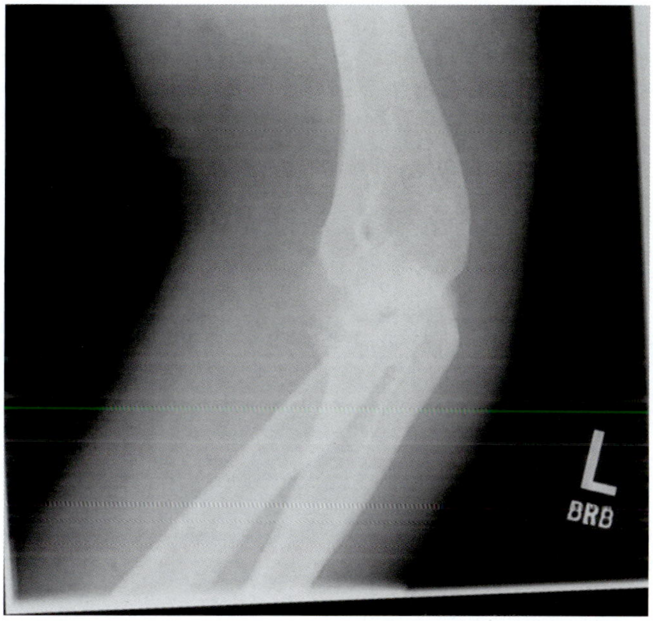

Figure 7-5 | Internal oblique.

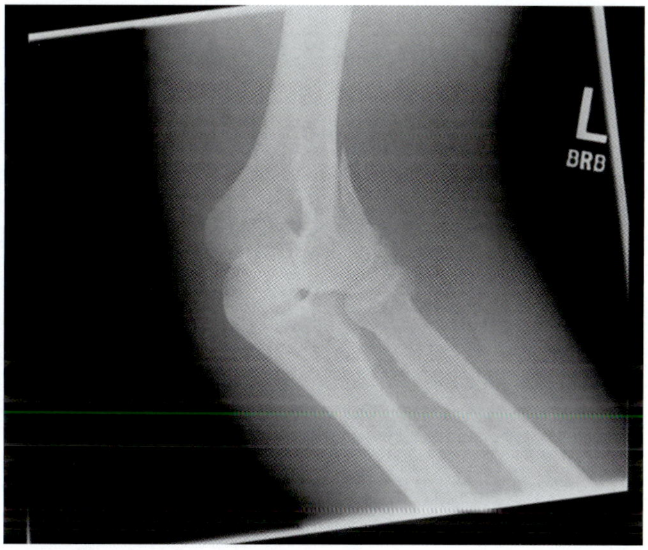

Figure 7-6 | External oblique.

4. Traction Views

- In severely comminuted or shortened fractures, traction views can be helpful in preoperative planning: plating orientation, surgical approach (i.e., olecranon osteotomy), or total elbow replacement (Fig. 7-7A and B).
- Distal humerus fracture with and without a traction view.

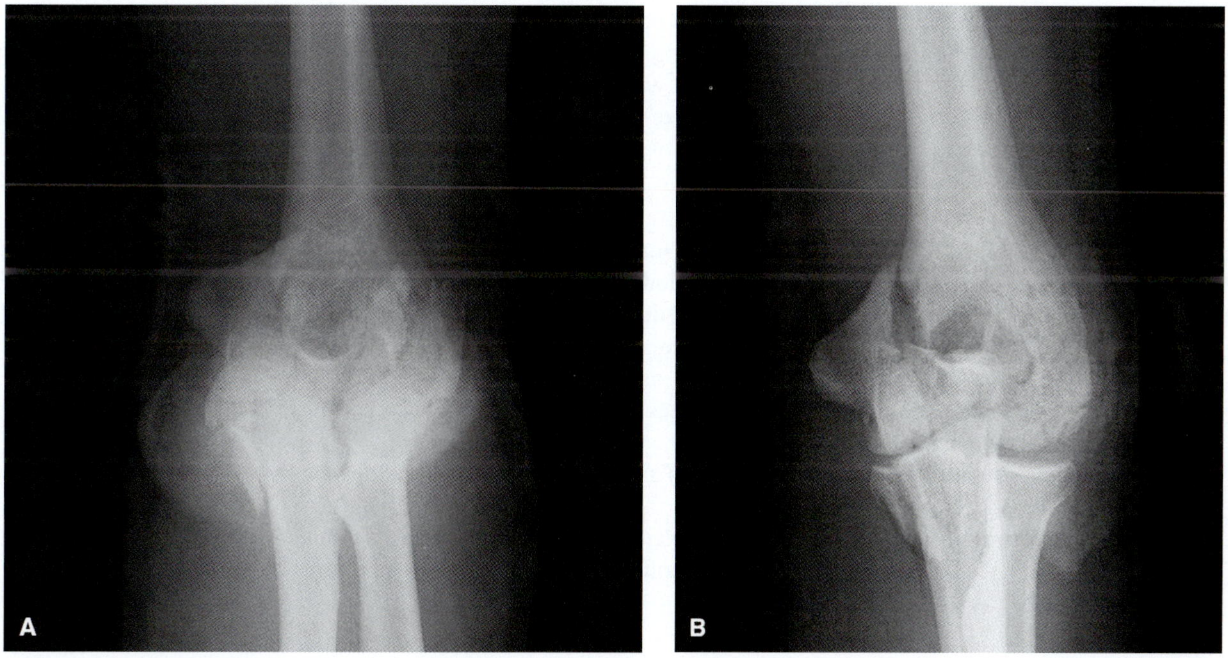

Figure 7-7 | **A:** AP without traction. **B:** AP with traction.

Preoperative Imaging

- The operative indication for distal humerus fractures includes articular involvement with displacement >2 mm of the articular surface, shortening, displacement, and comminution. Most skeletally mature fracture patterns are treated operatively to restore joint congruity and allow early range of motion.
- Surgical fixation of distal humerus fractures is dependent on fracture pattern, choice of surgical approach, and fixation preference (Fig. 7-8).

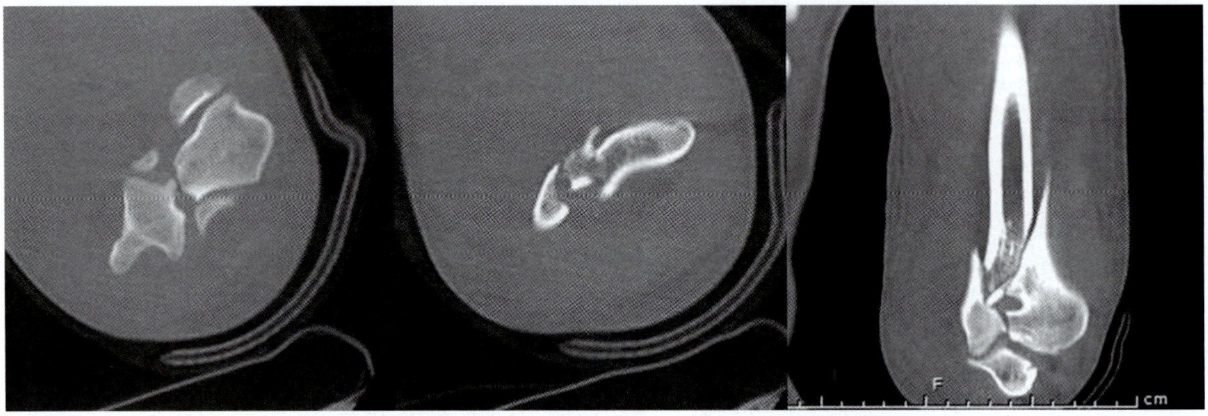

Figure 7-8 I Axial and coronal images from CT scan further demonstrating the degree of intra-articular comminution and step-off.

Intraoperative Positioning

1. Prone Position

- Used for posterior approach to humeral shaft as well as proximal ulna fractures.
- Chest rolls are used in order to reduce pressure on the patient's abdomen; alternatively, a Wilson frame can be used. Care should be taken to pad any bony prominences.
- The operative arm should be abducted 90 degrees over a well-padded Plexiglas board with towels or blankets taped to match the height of OR table. Plexiglas should be positioned perpendicular to table with only 5 to 8 inches exposed to allow for proper 90 degrees of elbow flexion and radiolucency.
- The contralateral arm can be adducted to lay on the armboard parallel to the table or abducted <90 degrees on a "prone" positioning armboard to prevent excessive external rotation (<70 degrees).
- Preferably, the operating table should be turned 90 degrees within the room. Position the C-arm at the head of table, parallel to the long axis of the table. This allows swinging from PA to lateral images without moving the extremity and potentially losing fracture reduction.
- Utilize a sterile tourniquet to minimize bleeding and provide for better visualization (Fig. 7-9).

2. Lateral Position

- Useful for a standard posterior distal humeral approach and for patients unable to be positioned prone or in fractures with extensive bone loss, which may require iliac crest bone graft.
- Safely position the patient in a lateral decubitus position and stabilized using a padded bean bag, chest rolls, or peg-board positioner with posts. An axillary roll should be used to prevent neurapraxia. Preferably, a radiolucent arm holder is utilized to position the affected extremity in 90 degrees of abduction and 90 degrees of elbow flexion. The well arm is positioned on a padded radiolucent arm board.
- The operative arm should be prepped and draped proximally to deltoid insertion, utilizing a sterile tourniquet.
- C-arm should be positioned perpendicular to table (again rotated 90 degrees within the room) to facilitate AP and lateral imaging without moving the operative extremity (Fig. 7-10).

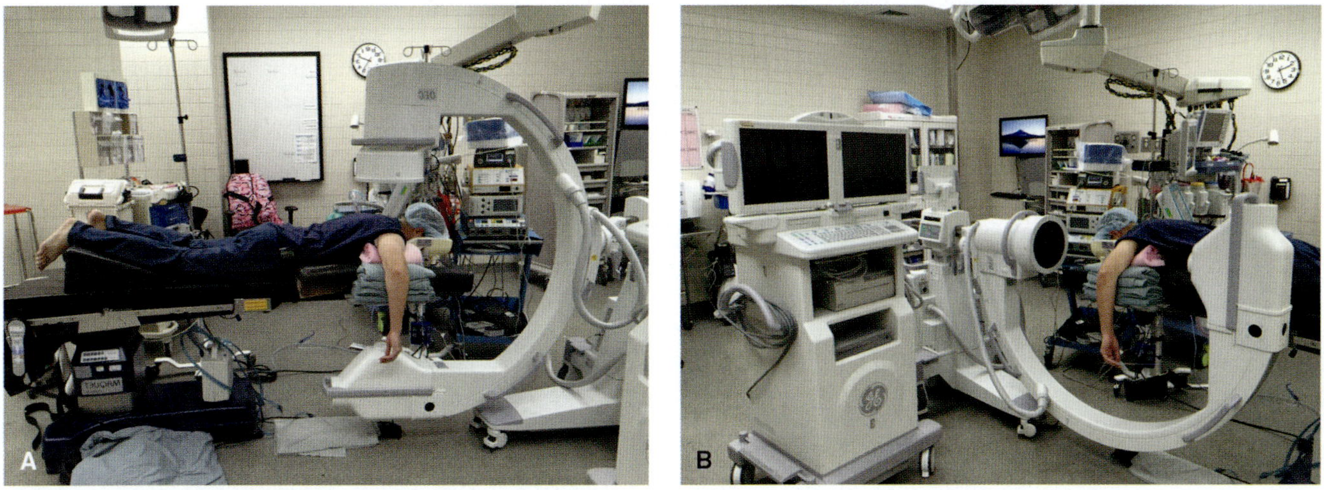

Figure 7-9 | **A:** Operating table with chest rolls and blanket with foam pillow and Plexiglas in place to facilitate transfer to prone position following intubation. **B:** Patient prone with appropriate padding. Adequate fluoroscopic access is confirmed prior to completion of draping.

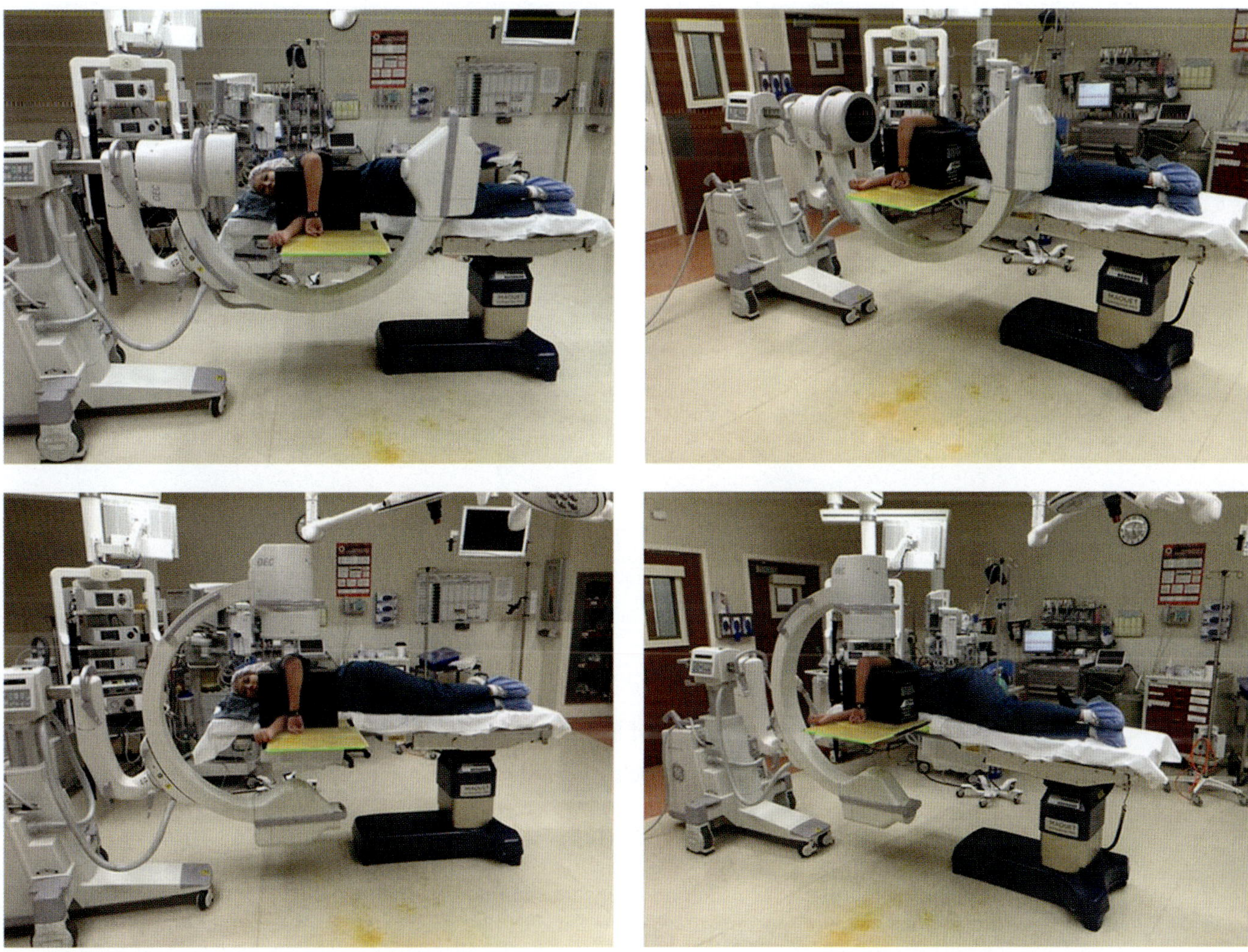

Figure 7-10 | Lateral positioning for a distal humerus fracture ORIF.

3. Supine Position

- While not generally recommended for open reduction and internal fixation of distal humerus fractures, the supine position can also be used in cases where prone or lateral positioning is not possible.
- Intraoperatively, the shoulder can be flexed and internally rotated with forearm flexed over the chest to facilitate a posterior approach.
- The sterile draped C-arm should enter from approximately a 45-degree angle to maximize space efficiency within the room. The operative extremity must be rotated in order to obtain AP and lateral radiographs (Fig. 7-11).

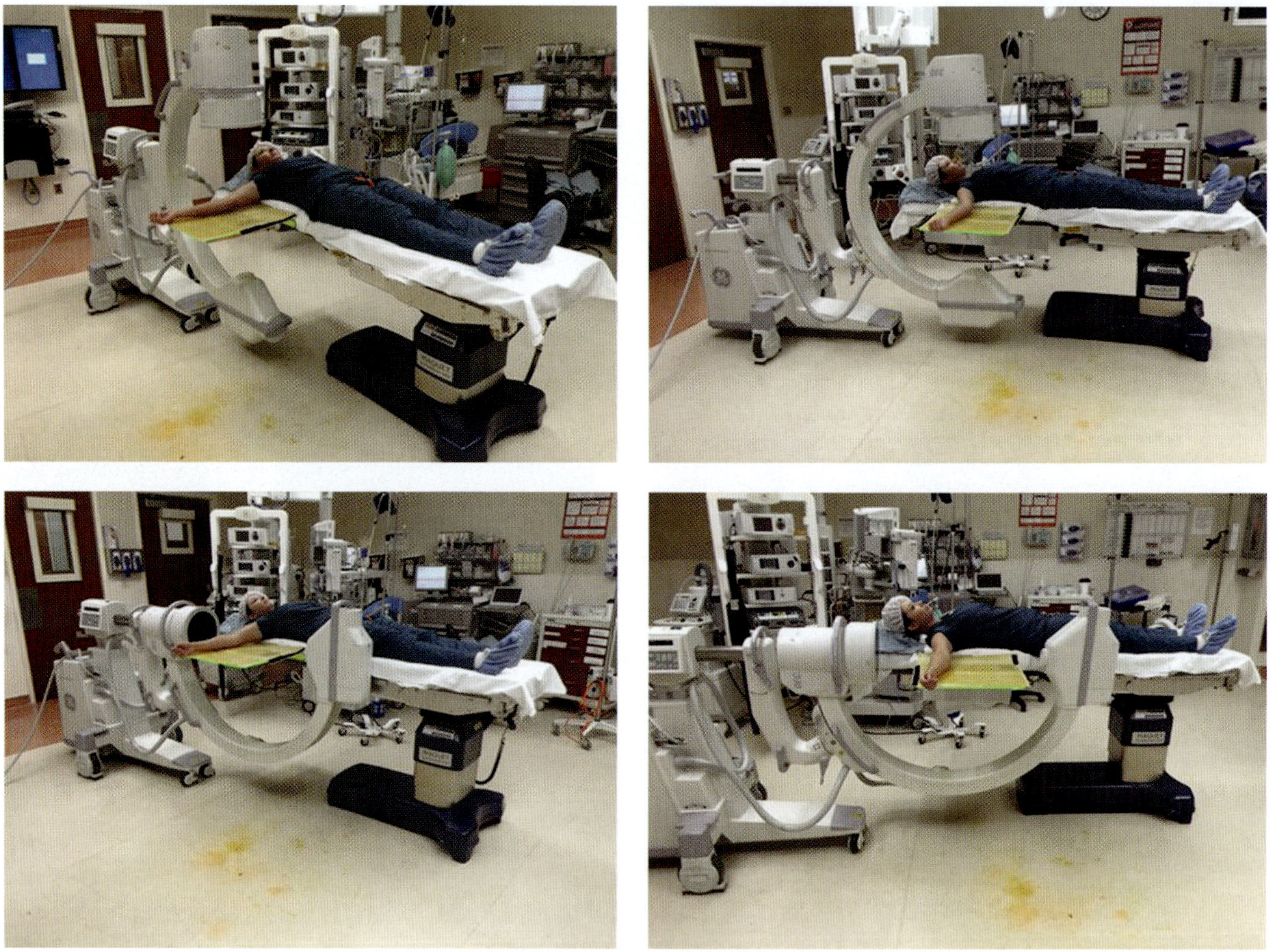

Figure 7-11 | Supine positioning and fluoroscopy.

Intraoperative Imaging

- Provisional fluoro (traction) views help define the fracture while the patient is under anesthesia (Figs. 7-12–7-14).
- Elbow stiffness is typically expected postoperatively, but it is important to document a stable full range of motion in the OR. Flexion and extension fluoroscopic views of the elbow should be obtained following final fixation to ensure stability and maintenance of a concentric joint throughout range of motion and to show patients that they can safely range the joint (Fig. 7-15).
- Highly comminuted fracture patterns can be challenging, but a systematic sequence of reducing the articular fragments first and then restoring length, alignment, and rotation is attainable along with proper fluoroscopic imaging (Fig. 7-16).

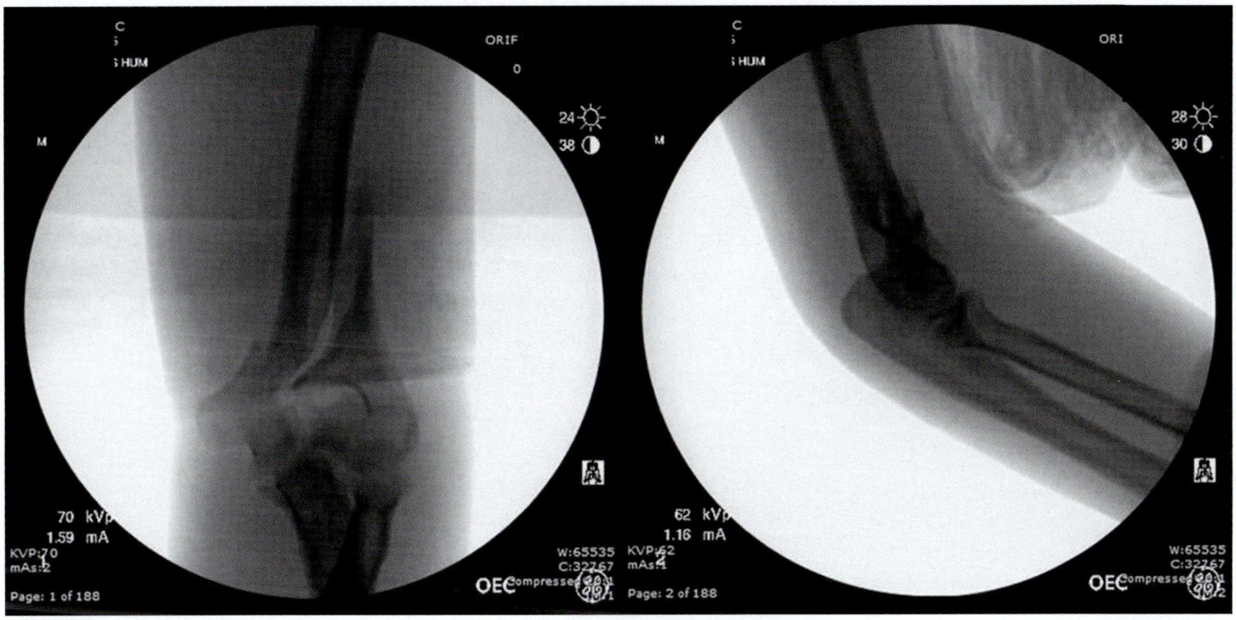

Figure 7-12 | Intraoperative AP fluoroscopic image demonstrates the intra-articular comminution and displacement necessitating an open approach for direct visualization of the joint surface and anatomic reduction. The lateral image shows loss of concentric circles of trochlea and capitellum as well as distortion of the "hourglass" due to a displaced fracture through olecranon fossa.

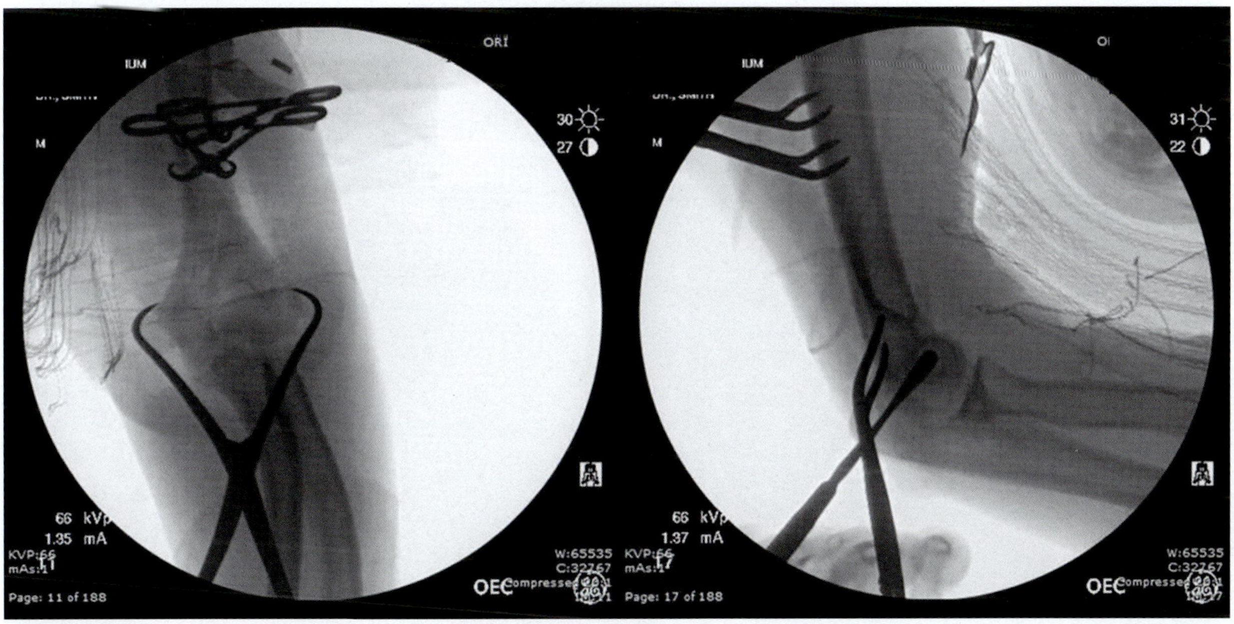

Figure 7-13 | After posterior triceps sparing approach to distal humerus, anatomic reduction of the articular surface was first obtained and then clamped using point-to-point reduction forceps: the AP image confirms varus-valgus reduction and the lateral demonstrates restoration of the teardrop and reduced sagittal plane alignment.

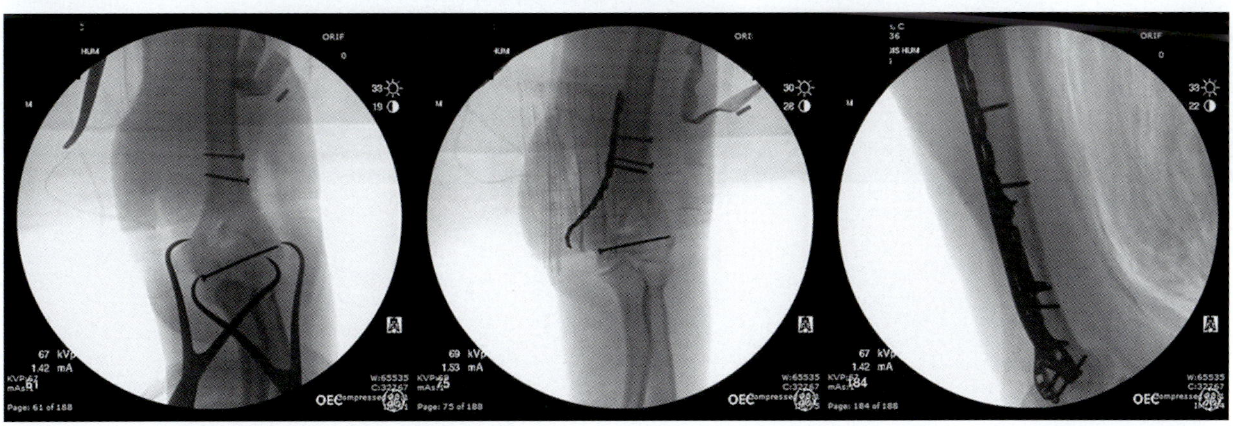

Figure 7-14 | Once reduction is achieved, lag screw fixation is utilized for absolute stability of both the articular surface as well as maintaining reduction of the articular block to the humeral shaft before application of definitive neutralization plates (which can be placed in 90–90 or 180-degree constructs depending upon the fracture pattern).

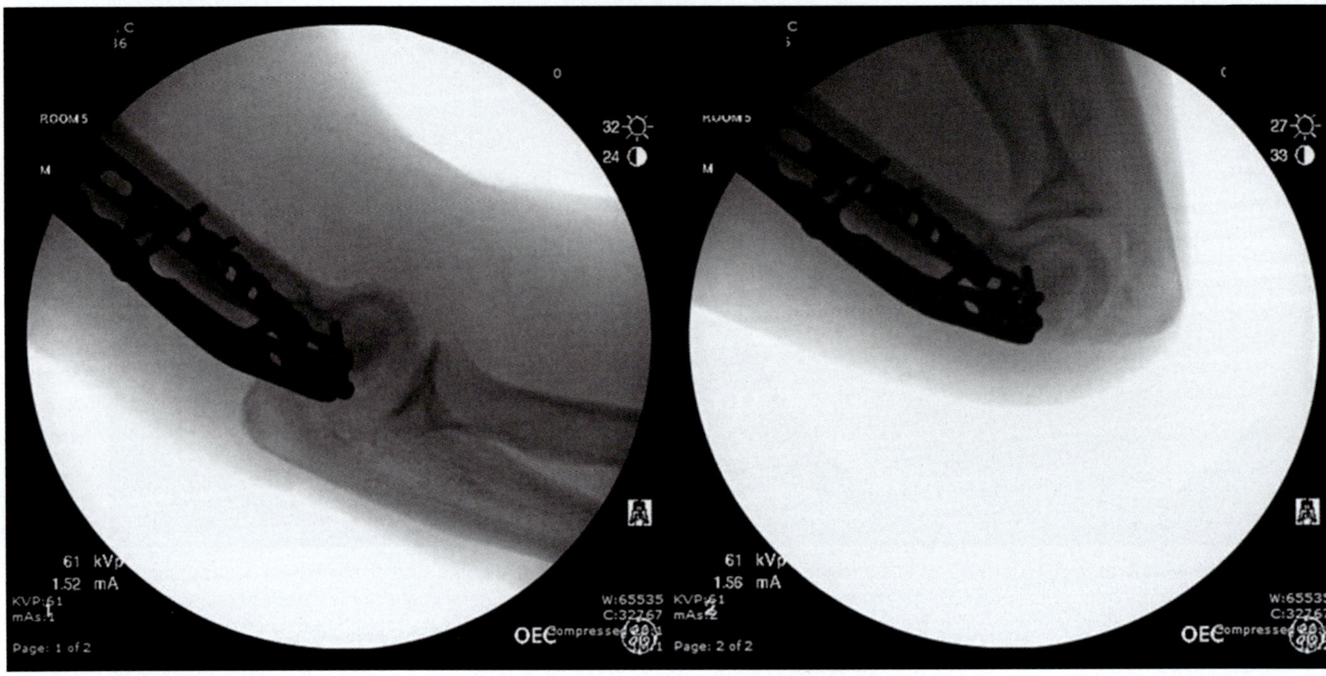

Figure 7-15 | Range of motion evaluation.

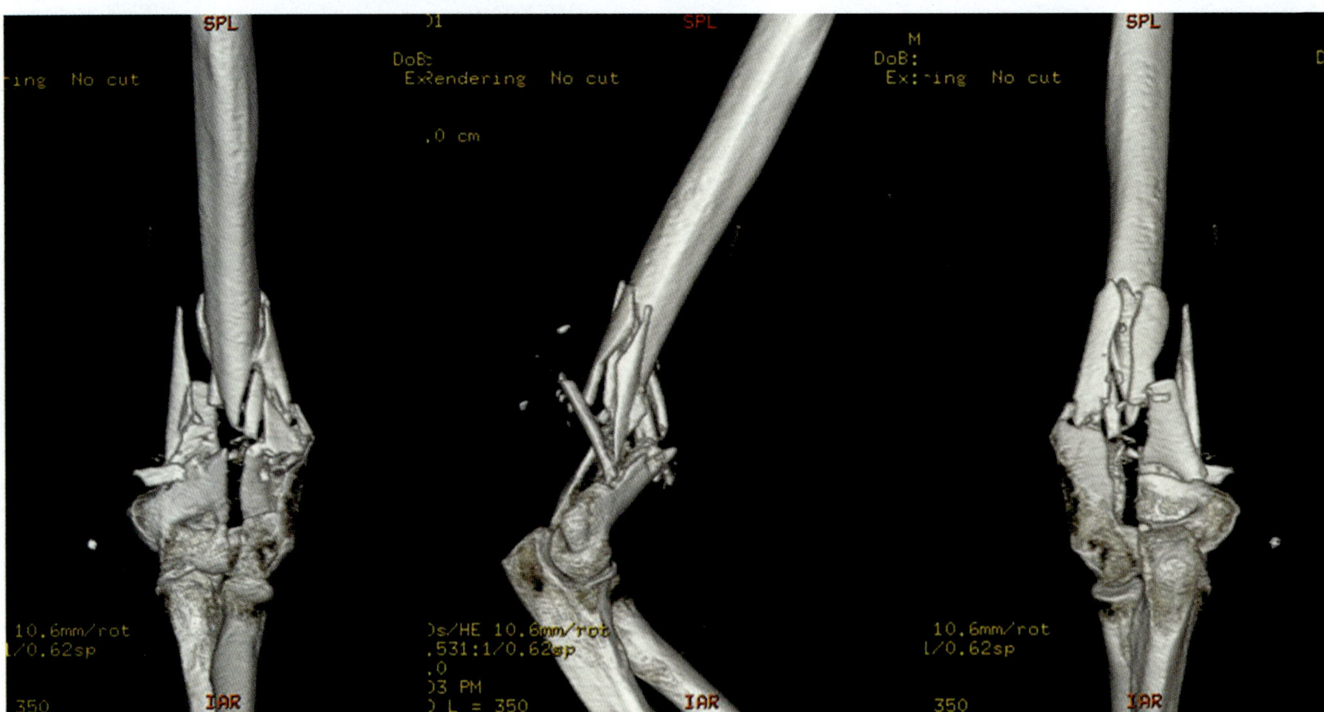

Figure 7-16 | CT with 3D reformatting.

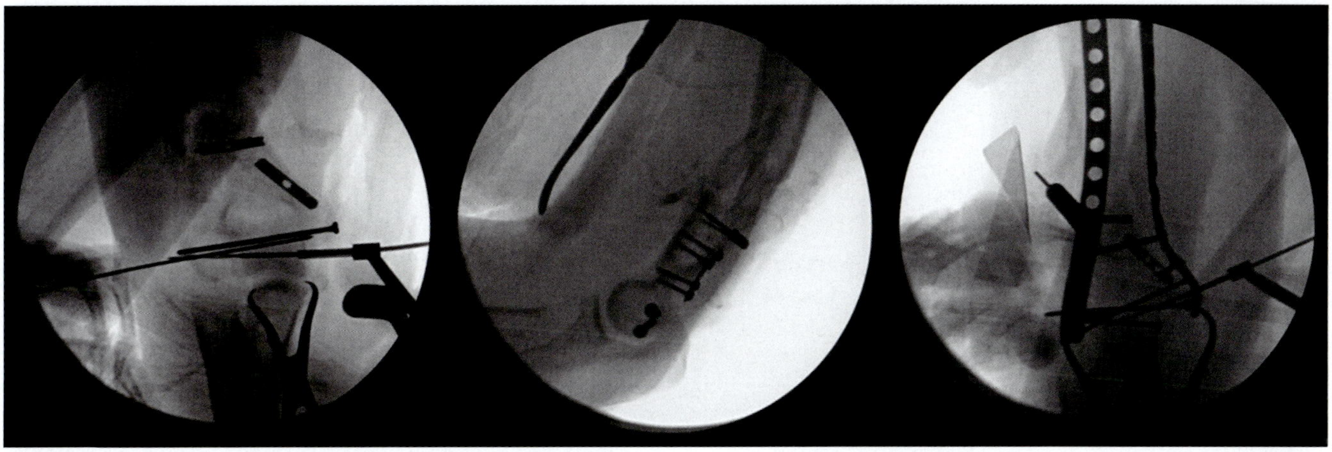

Figure 7-17 | Articular reduction.

- Perfect AP and lateral fluoro sequences depict anatomic reduction of the articular segment and metaphysis prior to bridge plating the zone of comminution (Fig. 7-17).
- Fluoro scanning shots up and down the fracture fixation can confirm proper restoration of length, alignment, and rotation (as seen on the post-op radiographs) (Fig. 7-18).

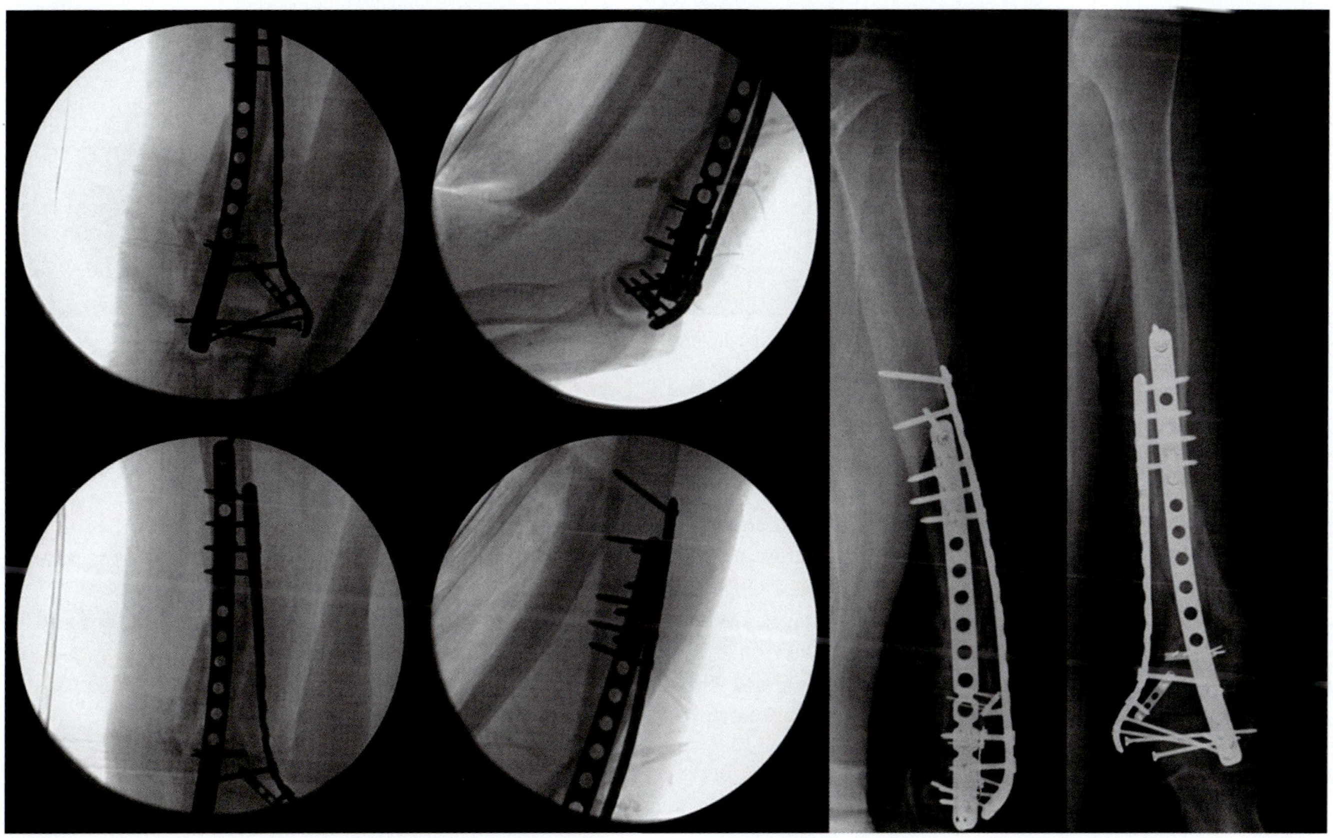

Figure 7-18 | Fluoroscopic intraoperative and postoperative evaluation of length, alignment, and rotation.

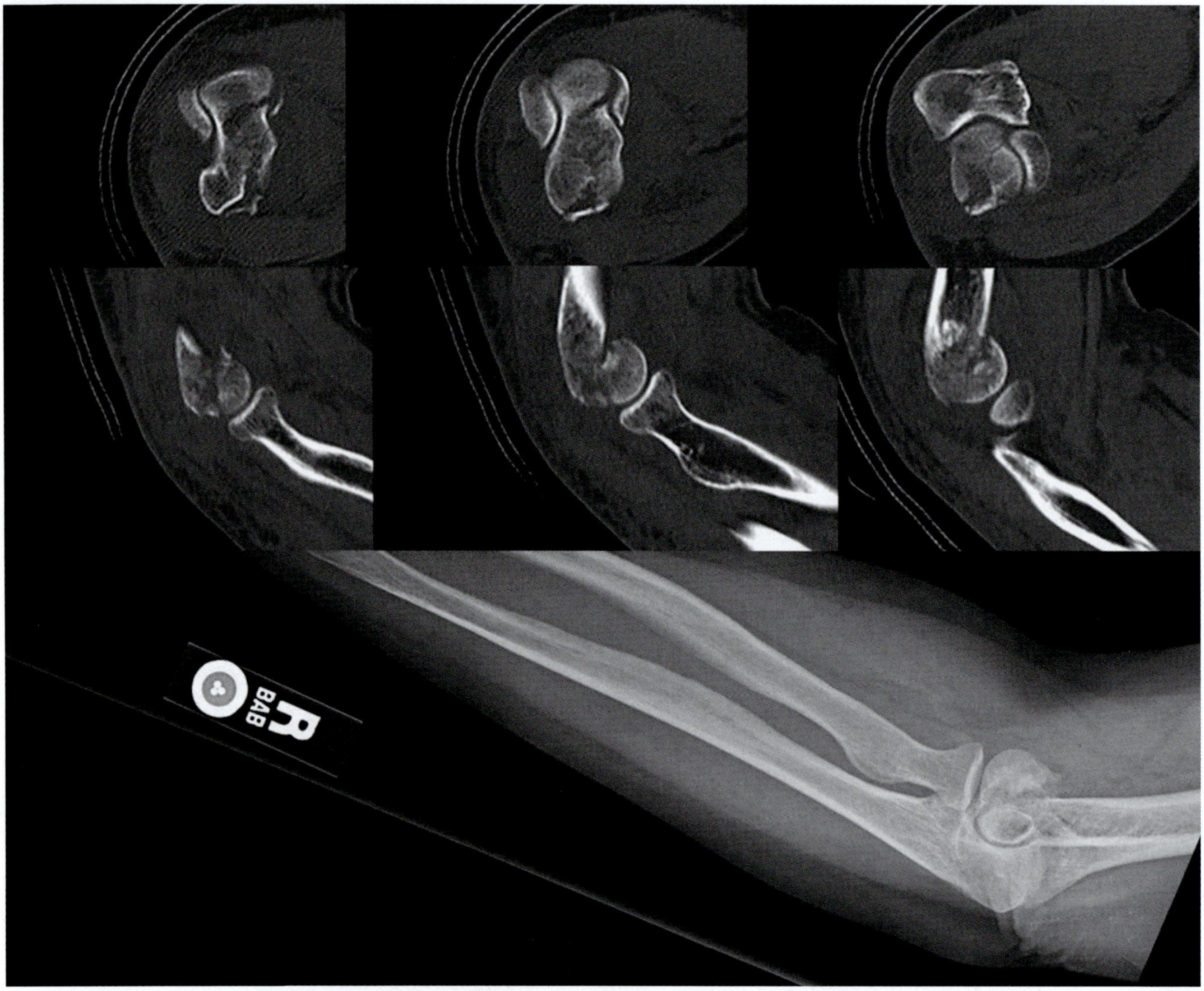

Figure 7-19 | CT can add additional information to guide surgical plan.

- Capitellar shear fracture patterns often require adjunctive CT imaging for preoperative planning (Fig. 7-19).
- Intraoperative fluoroscopic imaging before incision demonstrates atypical extension of the capitellar fragment but does not fully demonstrate a sagittal split of the capitellum that is seen on the preoperative CT (Fig. 7-20).
- Perfect lateral fluoro images are necessary to assure proper reduction of the fracture pattern and safe placement of hardware that does not overpenetrate the articular surface (Fig. 7-21).
- Range of motion images along with dynamic stress images document stability and the need for lateral collateral ligament repair prior to closure (Fig. 7-22).

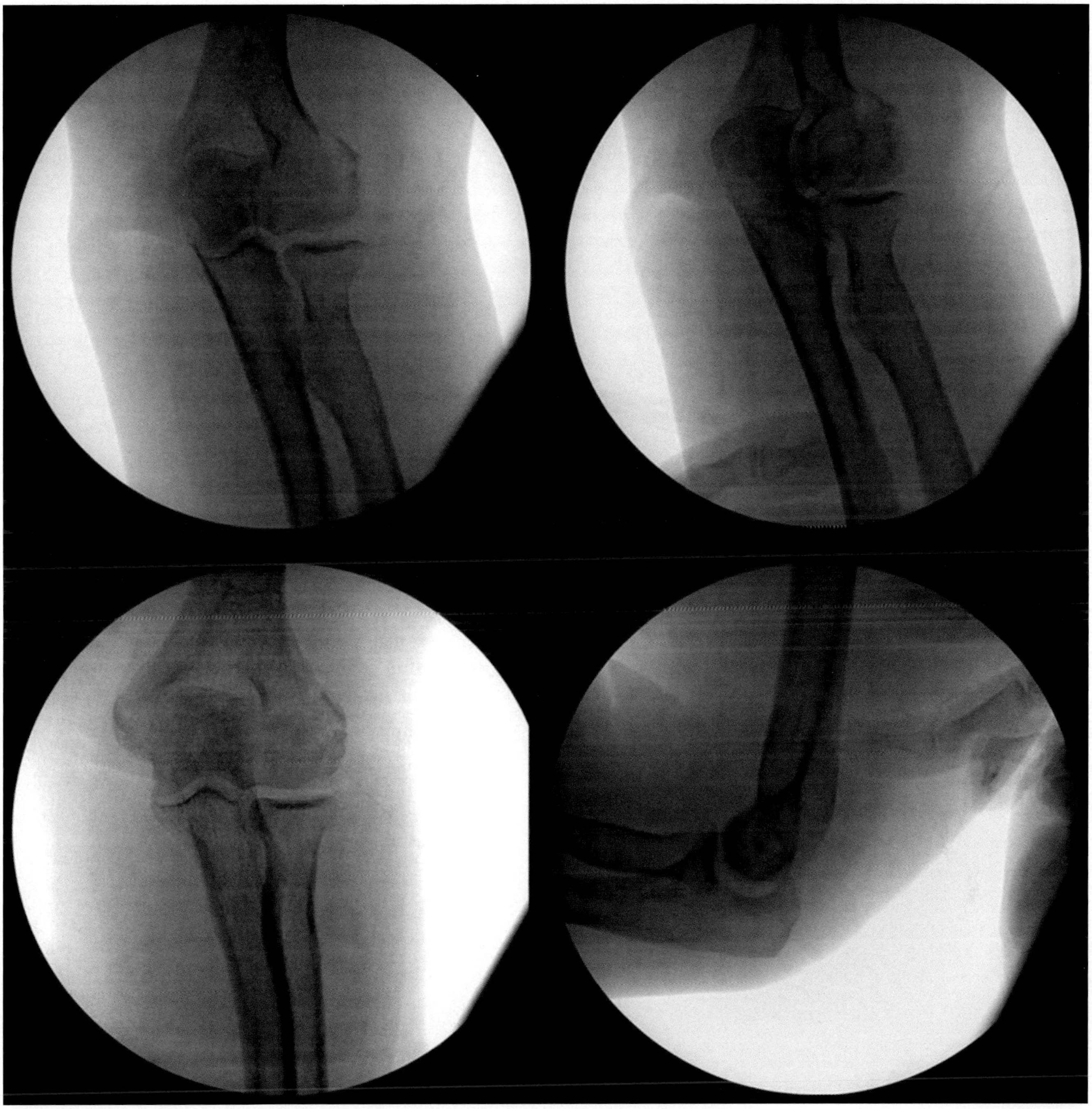

Figure 7-20 ‖ Fluoroscopic exam under anesthesia.

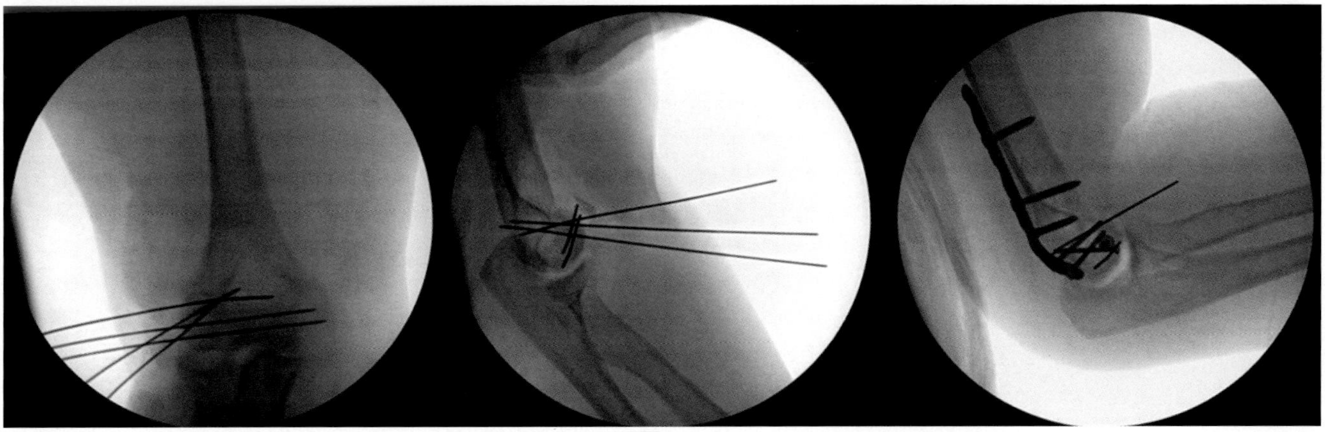

Figure 7-21 ‖ Intraoperative fluoroscopy.

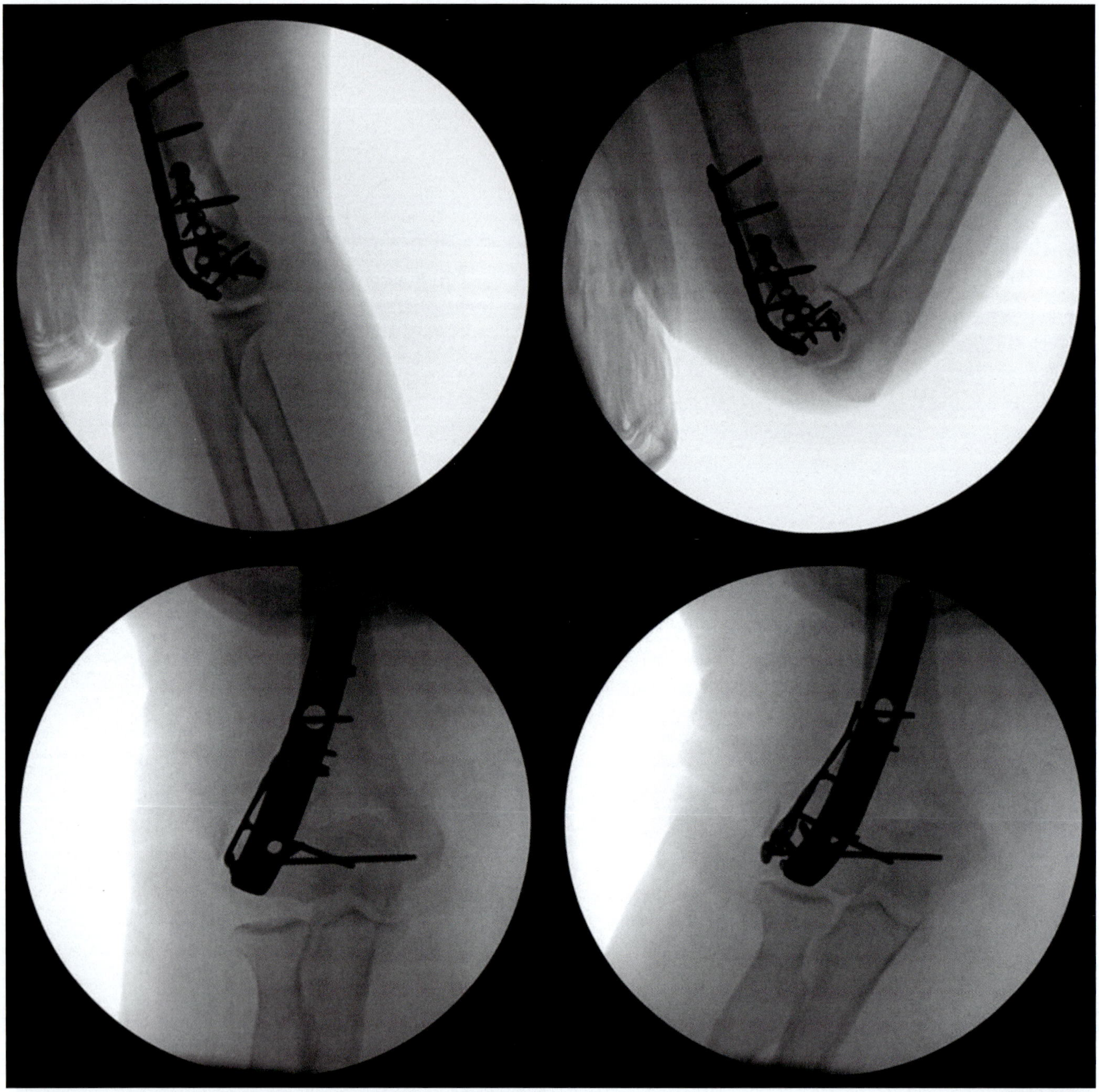

Figure 7-22 | Range of motion, varus, and valgus stress exams performed prior to closure.

References

1. Anglen J. Distal humerus fractures. *J Am Acad Orthop Surg.* 2005;13:291–297.
2. Galano GJ, Ahmad CS, Levine WN. Current treatment strategies for bicolumnar distal humerus fractures. *J Am Acad Orthop Surg.* 2010;18:20–30.
3. Nauth A, McKee MD, Ristevski B, et al. Distal humeral fractures in adults: current concepts review. *J Bone Joint Surg Am.* 2011;93:686–700.

Chapter 8
Terrible Triad Elbow Injuries

GARET C. COMER
JULIUS A. BISHOP

Bony Anatomy

- The elbow is a complex structure arising from the articulations of the ulna, radius, and humerus.
  - Ulna
    - The proximal ulna has two articular facets:
      - The greater sigmoid notch of the ulna articulates with the humeral trochlea along its 190-degree arc.
      - The radial notch is a groove along the proximal ulna that allows for articulation with the radial head.
    - The coronoid process projects anteriorly from the greater sigmoid notch and provides an anterior and varus buttress to the ulnohumeral joint. It consists of four parts:
      - The coronoid tip serves as an insertion point of the anterior capsule.
      - The coronoid base provides an anterior buttress.
      - The anteromedial facet, which contains the sublime tubercle on which the anterior bundle of the medial collateral ligament inserts.
      - The anterolateral facet along which sits the radial notch of the ulna and supinator crest on which the lateral ulnar collateral ligament inserts.
  - Radius
    - The radial head is slightly elliptically shaped in the axial plane with a central convexity to allow for articulation with the concave capitellum.
    - The radial neck forms a 15-degree angle with respect to the radial shaft and is encircled by the annular ligament.
  - The humerus
    - The distal articular surface of the humerus sits in 5 degrees of valgus and projects anteriorly 30 degrees relative to the humeral shaft.
    - The distal articular surface is composed of three convexities including the trochlea, the capitellum, and a central ridge between the two.
    - The center of rotation in the sagittal plane passes from the anteroinferior portion of the medial epicondyle to the center of the lateral surface of the capitellum where the lateral ulnar collateral ligament originates.

Radiographic Anatomy

AP View

- The traditional AP view is performed in forearm supination to minimize overlap of the radius and ulna (Fig. 8-1).
- Joint congruency
  - The lines drawn along the distal humeral articular surface and along the anterior surfaces of the ulnohumeral and radiocapitellar articular surfaces should be perfectly parallel.

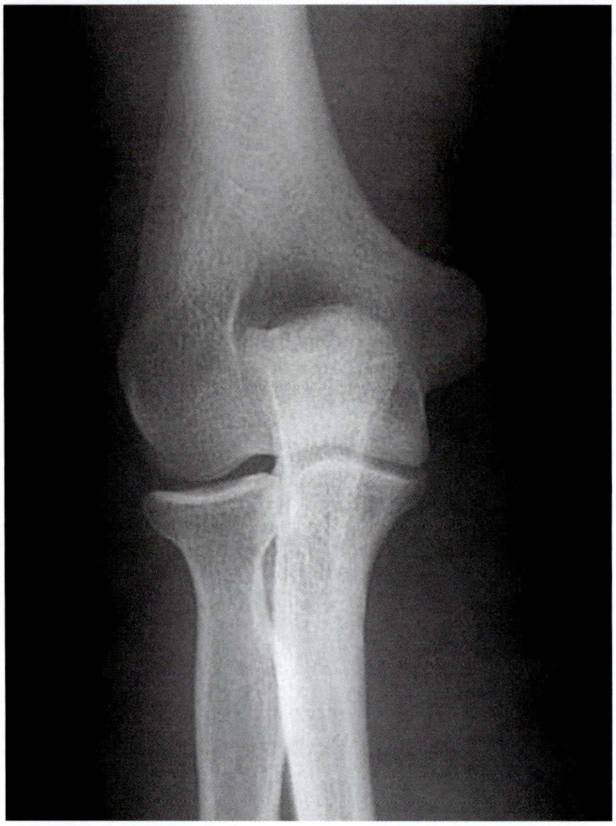

Figure 8-1 | A normal AP elbow x-ray.

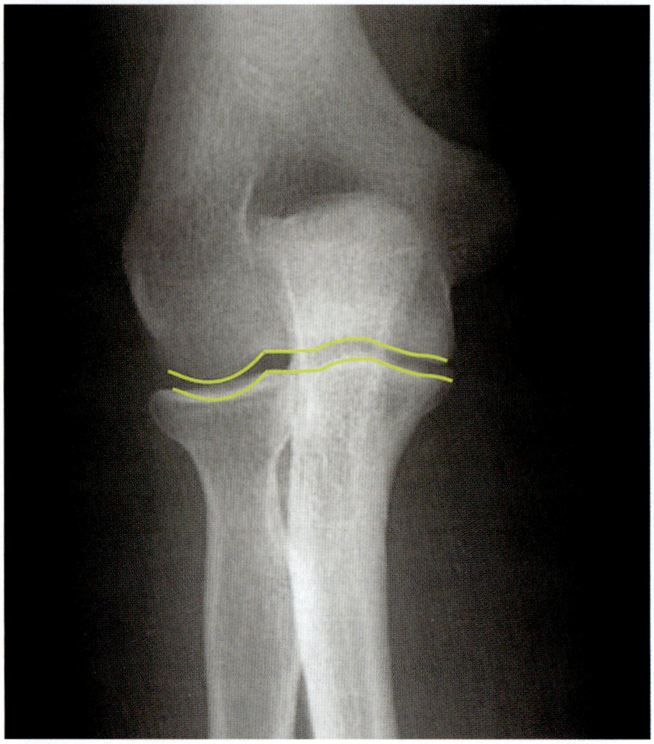

Figure 8-2 | A normal AP elbow x-ray with concentric lines drawn along the articular surfaces.

- Any divergence of these lines (indicating asymmetry of the ulnohumeral joint) is an indication that the elbow is not concentrically reduced or—in the case of radial head arthroplasty—may be "overstuffed" with too prominent an implant (Figs. 8-2 and 8-3).

- The AP view should be examined for the extent of coronoid fracture with special attention toward evaluating for anteromedial facet involvement. Ultimately, though, CT is the most reliable modality for evaluating the coronoid.
- Small avulsion fractures from the lateral ulnar collateral ligament footprint are frequently visible with proximal LUCL disruption much more common than midsubstance or ulnar avulsions.

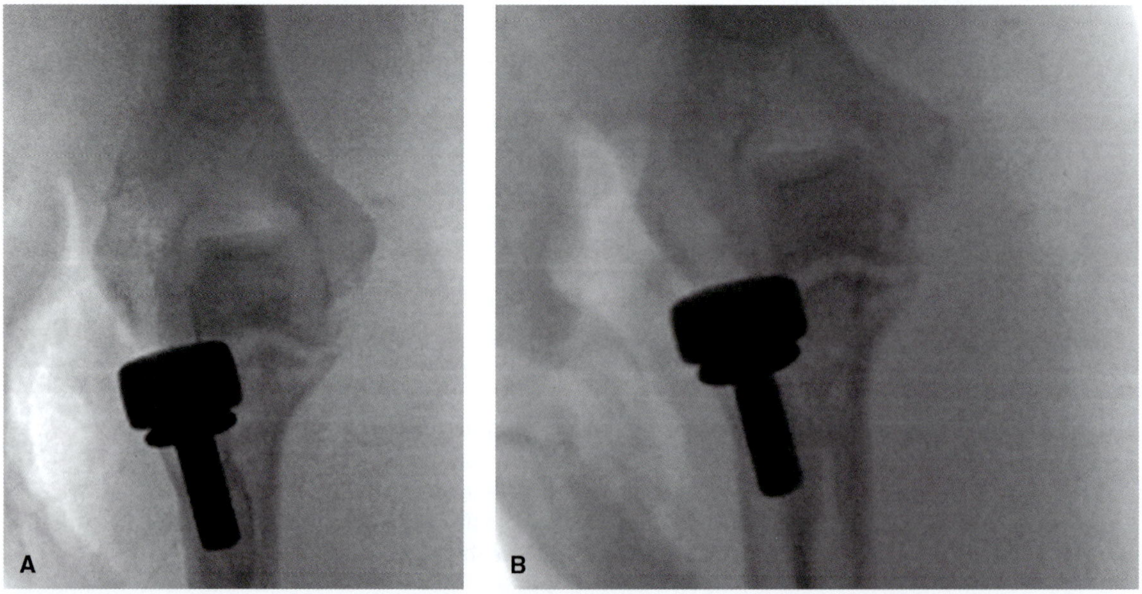

Figure 8-3 | Intraoperative fluoroscopic views demonstrating divergence of the ulnohumeral lines due to an overstuffed radial component in the image on the left **(A)** and an appropriately sized implant in the right image **(B)**.

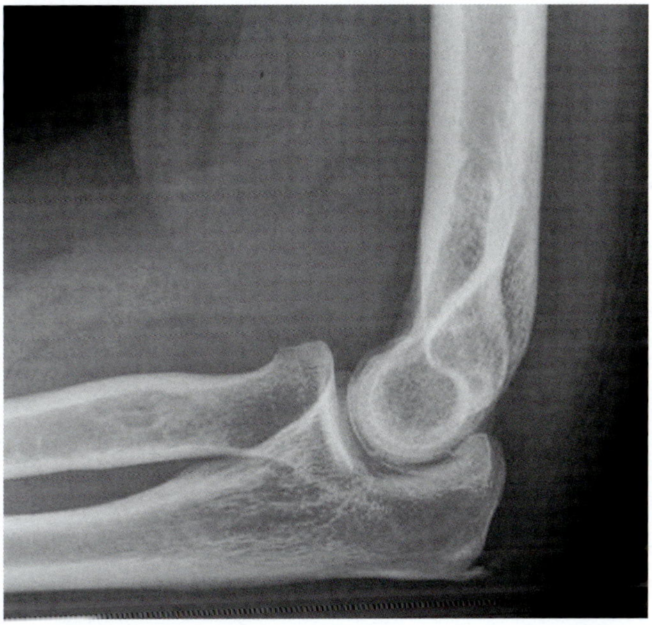

Figure 8-4 | A normal lateral elbow x-ray.

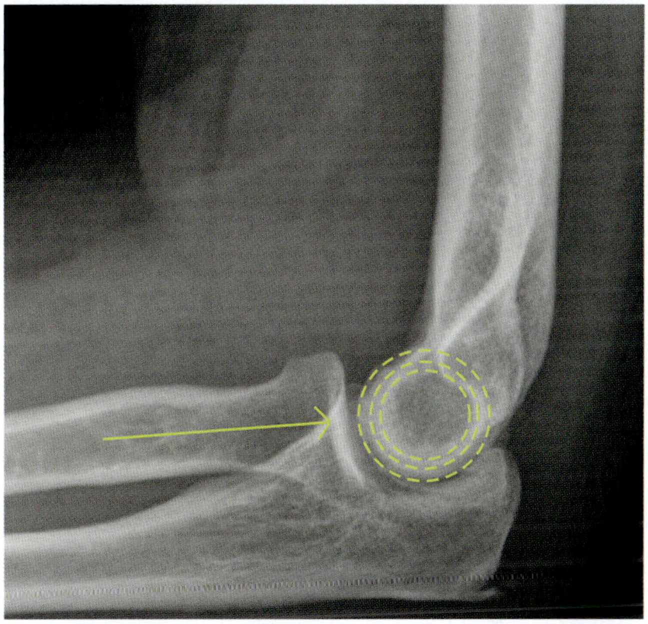

Figure 8-5 | A normal lateral elbow x-ray with the three concentric *circles* represented with *dashes* and a *line* drawn along the radial neck pointing to the center of the capitellum indicating a concentric radiocapitellar reduction.

- The AP view is also useful to evaluate the radial head fracture morphology to determine if ORIF or radial head replacement is appropriate.

Lateral View

- The traditional lateral view is performed with the elbow flexed to 90 degrees and the forearm in neutral rotation (Fig. 8-4).
- A true lateral view will produce three perfectly concentric circles over the distal humerus corresponding to the medial lip of the trochlea, the trochlear sulcus, and capitellum (Fig. 8-5).
- Joint congruency
    - The greater sigmoid notch and humeral surface should be concentrically aligned.
    - On all projections, a line drawn through the radial head should bisect the capitellum, which is especially important on the lateral view given the posterolateral mechanism of terrible triad injuries.
    - The radiographic landmark for the origin of the lateral ulnar collateral ligament is identified at the center of the three concentric circles of the distal humeral articular surface.
    - The tip of the coronoid should lie just proximal to the radial head, which may assist in determining appropriate radial height.
- The lateral projection is useful to estimate the depth of the coronoid fracture.
- The lateral projection is also useful to evaluate the radial head fracture morphology to determine if ORIF or radial head replacement is appropriate.
- Intraoperatively, the lateral view is utilized to confirm the correct location for suture button repair of the lateral ulnar collateral ligament to its origin. The origin is represented as the center point of the three concentric circles of the lateral image (Fig. 8-6).

Radial Head View

- The radial head view is performed in neutral forearm rotation with the beam oriented 45 degrees internally rotated in the axial plane.
- This view allows an unencumbered view of the proximal radius (Fig. 8-7).

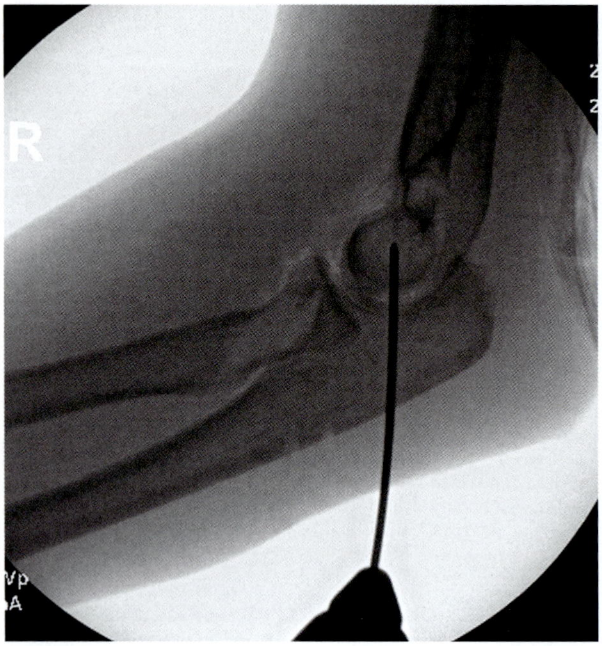

Figure 8-6 | Intraoperative fluoroscopic image with a K-wire marking the LUCL origin at the center of the three concentric circles of the lateral elbow view.

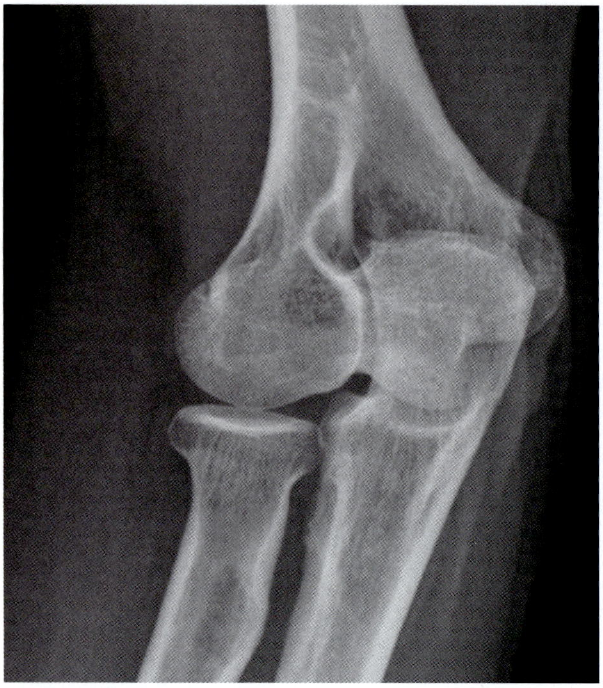

Figure 8-7 | Normal radial head view.

Lateral Hanging Arm View

- The lateral hanging arm or drop view is a stress view used to examine joint stability.
- The view is obtained in full extension and supination with a bump under the humerus and the beam oriented for a lateral projection. The weight of the hand and forearm stresses the joint, and a positive drop sign indicative of persistent instability indicated by ≥4 mm of ulnohumeral distance.[1]
- This view must be obtained at the end of terrible triad reconstruction to evaluate stability (Figs. 8-8 and 8-9).

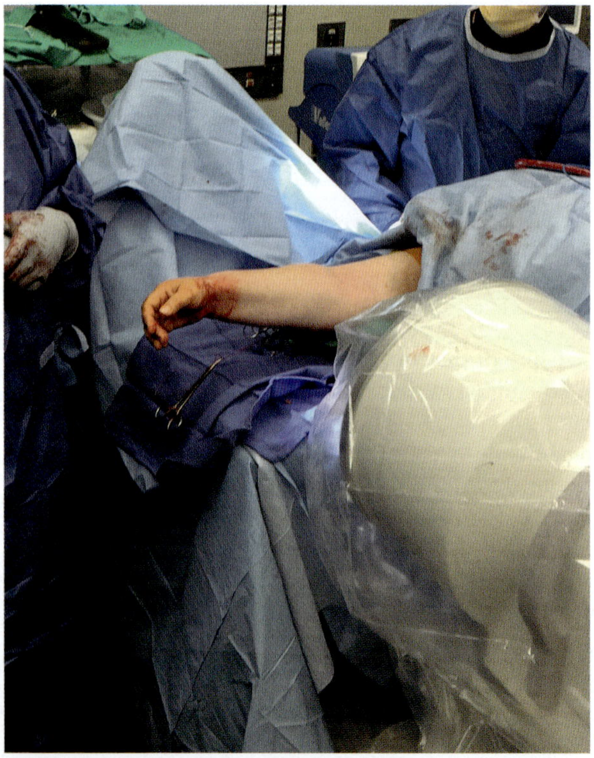

Figure 8-8 | Supine patient with a towel bump under the arm positioned for the lateral hanging arm view.

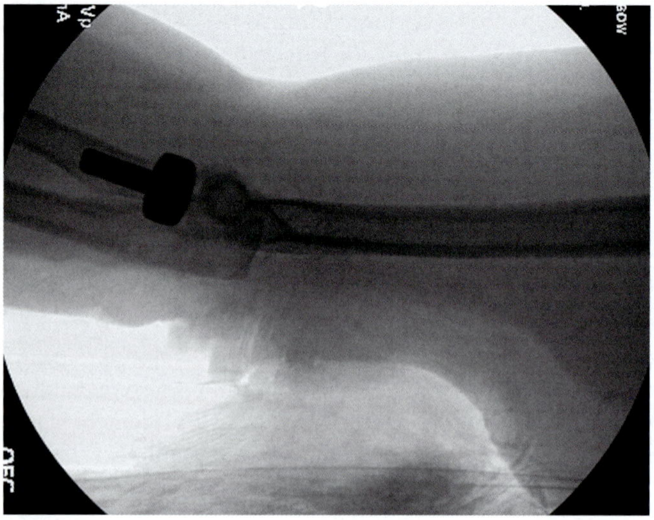

Figure 8-9 | Intraoperative fluoroscopic lateral hanging arm view with concentric ulnohumeral reduction.

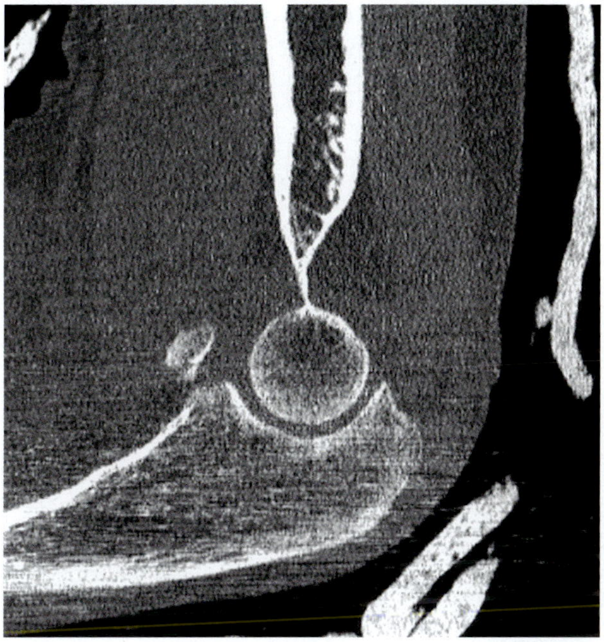

Figure 8-10 | Sagittal CT reconstruction demonstrating a coronoid tip fracture.

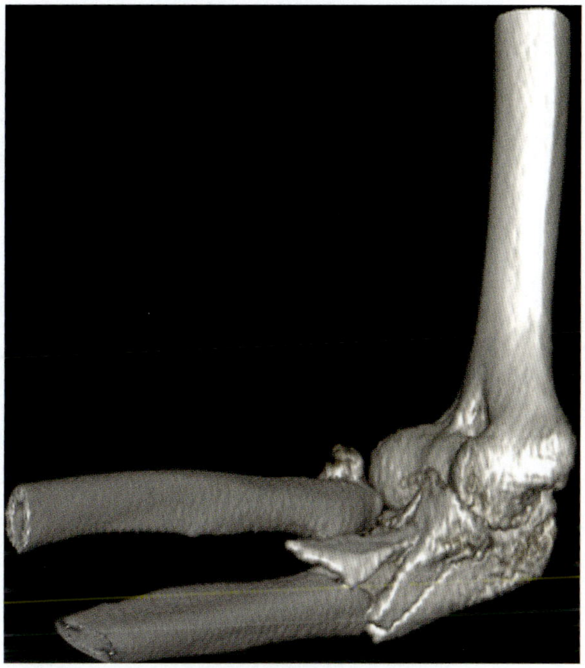

Figure 8-11 | Three dimensional CT reconstruction of a complex elbow fracture dislocation allows an improved assessment of the coronoid fracture.

Preoperative Imaging

- Standard AP and lateral views are obtained before and after closed reduction.
- A CT scan is also obtained primarily to evaluate the coronoid fracture morphology.
- Three-dimensional reconstructions are particularly useful in cases with complex coronoid involvement (Figs. 8-10 and 8-11).

Intraoperative Positioning

- Proper patient positioning and draping is essential to allow for adequate surgical exposure, C-arm access, and anesthesia access.
- The patient may be positioned in supine, lateral decubitus, or prone position depending upon pathology and surgical plan.
- A radiolucent flat-top table or conventional table turned backward can be utilized according to surgeon preference, but unencumbered C-arm access must be ensured.
- Supine
  - We utilize a regular table with a radiolucent armboard (Carter Hand Surgery Table, Instrument Specialist, Inc., Boerne, TX).
  - The C-arm is positioned to enter the surgical field from the foot of the bed in line with the patient's body. In this manner, AP and lateral views may be obtained without manipulating the extremity.
  - Furthermore, the lateral hanging arm view is easily obtainable by resting the humerus on a stack of towels. The importance of obtaining this view at the end of terrible triad reconstruction to ensure appropriate stability cannot be overemphasized.
- Lateral
  - We utilize an inverted regular table with a radiolucent attachment. Rolled blankets or a beanbag can be used for patient positioning.
  - A narrow radiolucent armboard is attached over which the patient's elbow is flexed (Fig. 8-12).
  - The C-arm is positioned to enter the surgical field from the head of the bed. AP and lateral views can be taken with the elbow in the flexed or extended position (Fig. 8-13).
- Prone
  - We infrequently utilize the prone position for terrible triad injuries but position the patient with a similar narrow armboard or padded radiolucent Plexiglas over which the elbow is flexed.
  - C-arm positioning is the same as for lateral position.

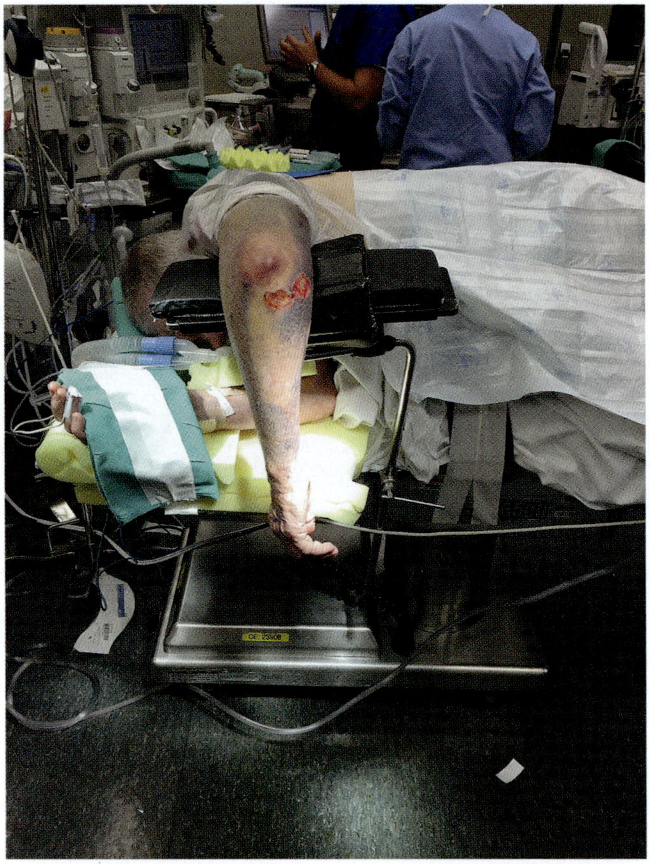

Figure 8-12 | Lateral positioning with the use of a radiolucent armboard.

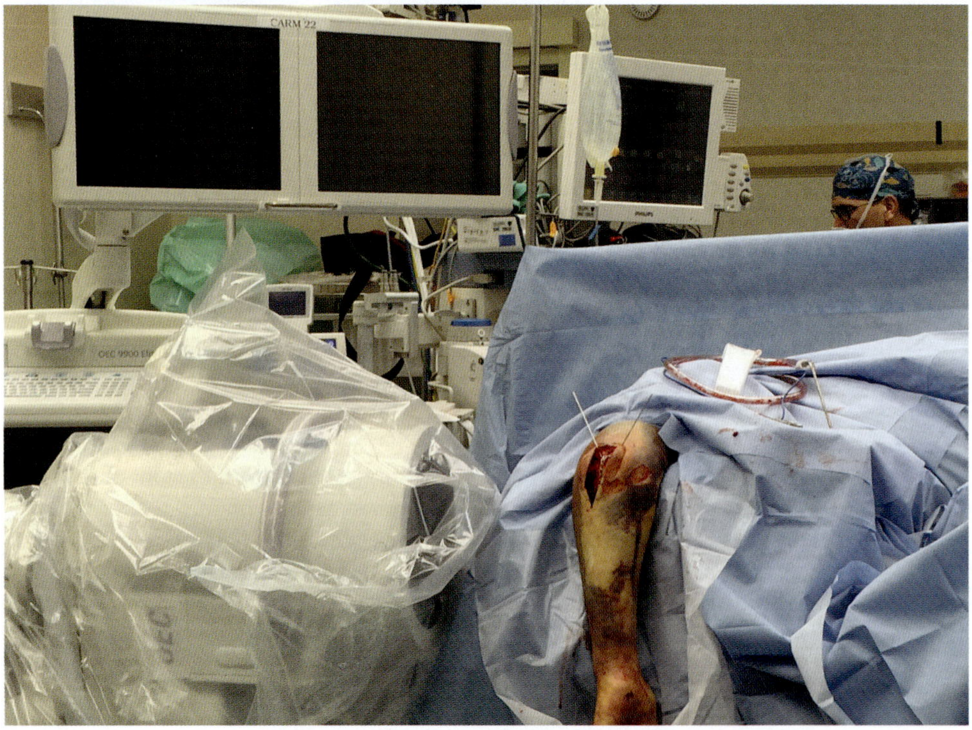

Figure 8-13 | Lateral positioning demonstrating appropriate C-arm and monitor positioning.

Reference

1. Coonrad RW, Roush TF, Major NM, et al. The drop sign, a radiographic warning sign of elbow instability. *J Shoulder Elbow Surg.* 2005;14:312–317.

Chapter 9
Olecranon Fractures

NICHOLAS J. ERDLE*
DOMINIC L. VAN NIELEN*
CHRISTOPHER S. SMITH*
DAVID S. WELLMAN

Anatomy

- The elbow is a complex ginglymus, or hinge joint, that permits flexion and extension of the forearm, while the proximal radioulnar articulation is a pivot joint that permits pronation and supination of the forearm.[1]
- The anterior band of the ulnar collateral ligament and the radial head resist valgus stresses on the elbow.[2]
- The lateral collateral ligament complex, which includes the ulnohumeral ligament, resists varus stresses.
- The coronoid process and olecranon process of the ulna resist anterior and posterior translation of the ulna at the ulnohumeral joint.[1]
- The olecranon is subcutaneous on its posterior surface, and its most proximal aspect is the insertion point of the triceps tendon.
- Direct trauma, such as a fall onto the elbow, can result in comminuted fracture of the olecranon.
- Indirect trauma, such as a fall onto an outstretched hand, can result in transverse or short oblique fractures of the olecranon due to forceful triceps contraction.[2]
- Olecranon fractures are intra-articular, requiring anatomic reduction of the articular surface with more than 2 mm of displacement.[1]
- A reported 2% to 30% of olecranon fractures are open, due to the very superficial nature of the bone.
- Posterior Monteggia lesions are typically the result of low-energy trauma but can still be associated with coronoid process fractures (25%), ipsilateral humeral shaft fractures (23%), radial shaft fractures (68%), and also ligamentous injury about the elbow.[3]

Radiographic Anatomy

Anteroposterior (AP) View

- The AP view is performed with the elbow extended and the arm in supination.
- The AP view demonstrates radiocapitellar alignment as well as congruent articular surfaces of the ulnohumeral joint and the radiocapitellar joint (Fig. 9-1).

Lateral View

- The lateral view is performed with the elbow in 90 degrees of flexion.
- The lateral view demonstrates radiocapitellar alignment, and in intra-articular trauma, it can demonstrate the presence of effusion through displacement of intra-articular fat pads (Fig. 9-2).

---

*The views expressed in this chapter are those of the author(s) and do not necessarily reflect the official policy or position of the Department of the Navy, Department of Defense or the United States Government. Nicholas J. Erdle, Dominic L. Van Nielen, and Christopher S. Smith are military service members and this work was prepared as part of their official duties. Title 17 U.S.C. 105 provides that 'Copyright protection under this title is not available for any work of the United States Government.' Title 17 U.S.C. 101 defines a United States Government work as a work prepared by a military service member or employee of the United States Government as part of that person's official duties.

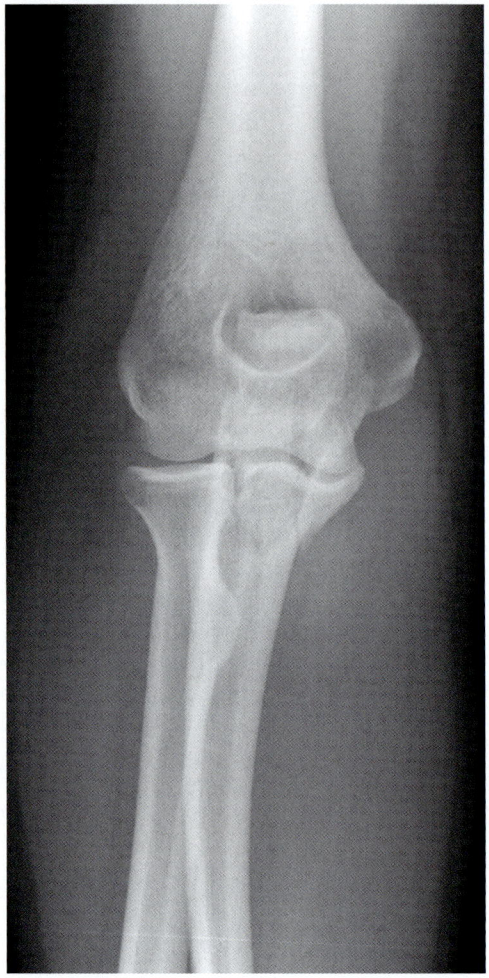

Figure 9-1 | AP radiograph of the elbow demonstrating comminuted olecranon fracture with joint space narrowing on the medial aspect of the ulnohumeral joint.

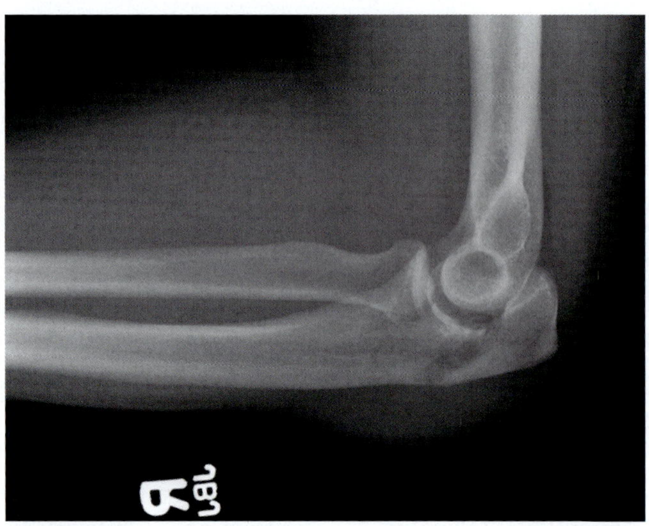

Figure 9-2 | Lateral radiograph of the same elbow shown above demonstrates comminuted olecranon fracture with joint effusion and intra-articular impaction.

Radiocapitellar View

- The radiocapitellar view is performed in the same positioning as the lateral view, with 45-degree inclination of the beam.
- The radiocapitellar view is useful in characterizing coronoid process fractures, radial head fractures, and capitellar sheer fractures (Fig. 9-3).

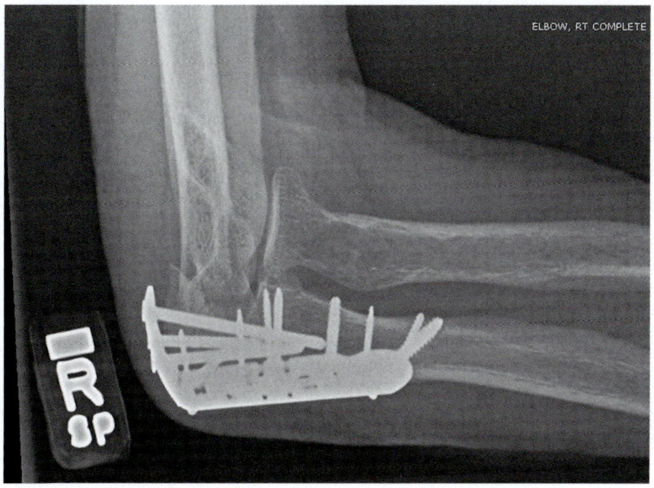

Figure 9-3 |

Oblique Views

- Obtained by rotating extremity 45 degrees internally or externally in relation to the beam.
- The internal oblique view of the humerus is useful in visualizing medial epicondylar fractures.
- The external oblique view of the humerus is useful in visualizing lateral epicondylar fractures.

Preoperative Imaging

- The radiographic indication for operative treatment of an olecranon fracture is >2 mm displacement of the fracture, which causes intra-articular incongruity.
- Due to the strong pull of the triceps attachment, even minimally displaced fractures are likely to need operative fixation to prevent delayed displacement with active or passive range of motion.[4]
- Standard radiographic views include AP, lateral, and radiocapitellar views to ensure the treating surgeon sees all aspects of the injury pattern.
- In comminuted olecranon fractures, computed tomography (CT) is useful in demonstrating impaction and displacement of fracture fragments and characterizing intra-articular fragments that may contribute to posttraumatic arthritis (Figs. 9-4–9-6).

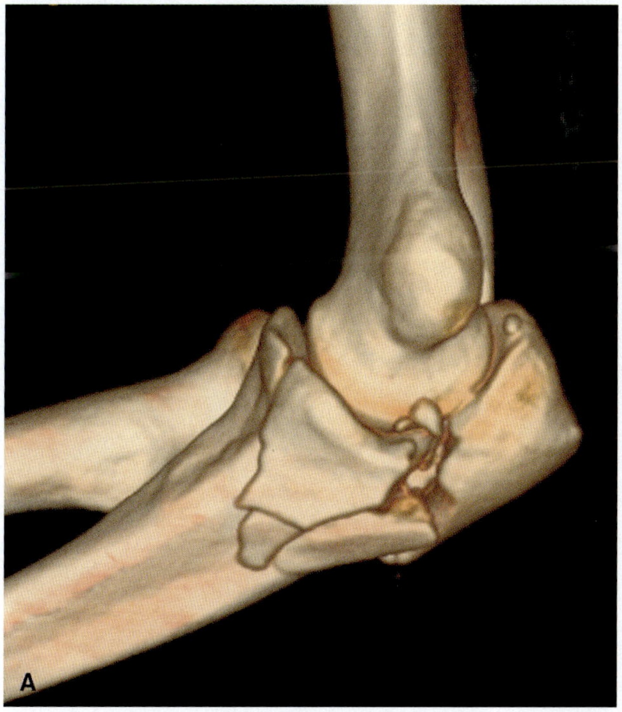

Figure 9-4 | **A:** CT 3D reconstruction. **B1:** Axial cuts in the plane of the distal humerus. **B2:** Coronal in the plane of the proximal ulna. **C1 and C2:** Sagittal cuts of the elbow. **D1:** Axial cuts in the plane of the proximal ulna. **D2:** Coronal in the plane of the distal humerus CT demonstrates degree of comminution, impaction, and intra-articular fracture fragments.

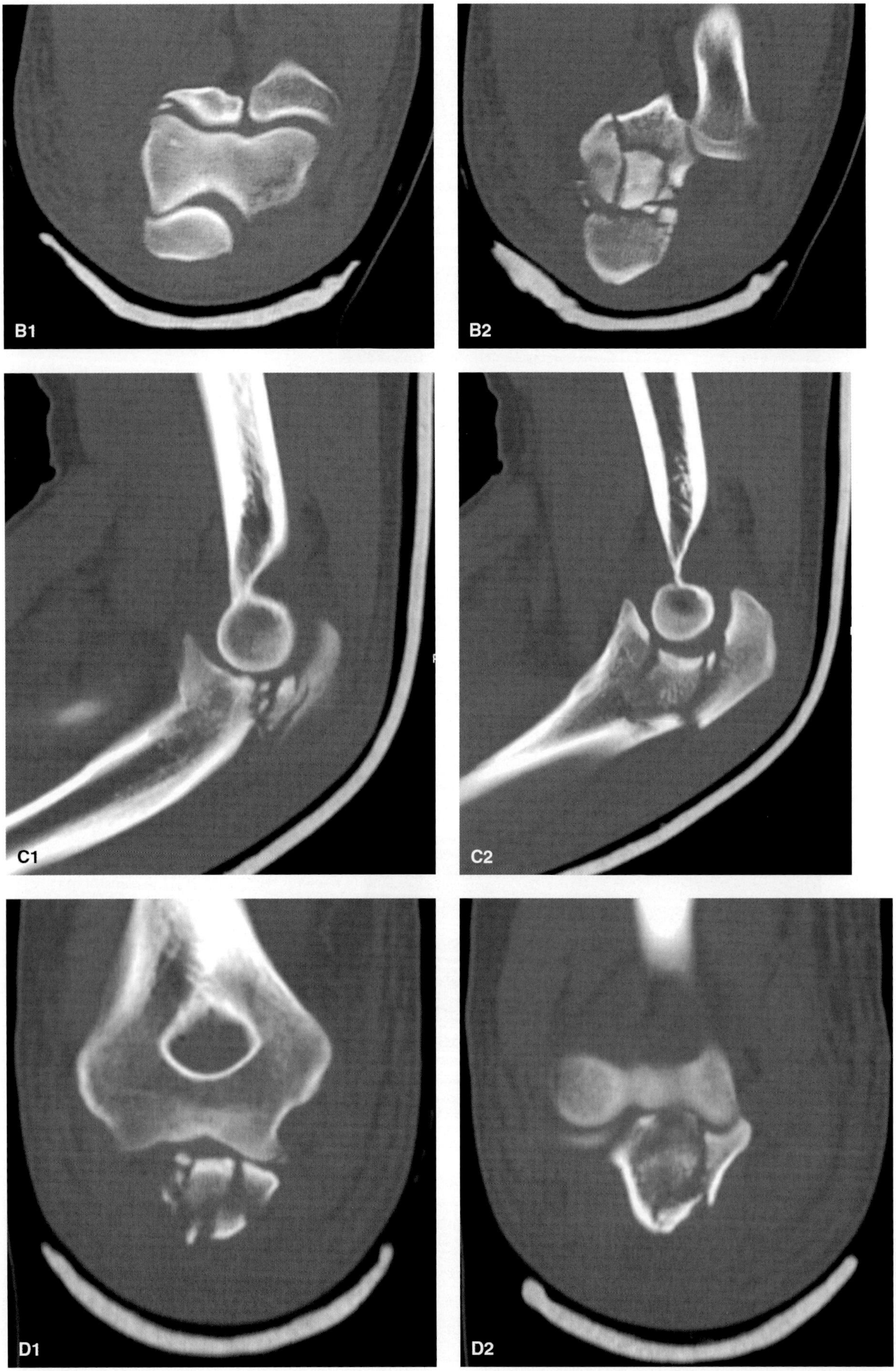

Figure 9-4 | (*Continued*)

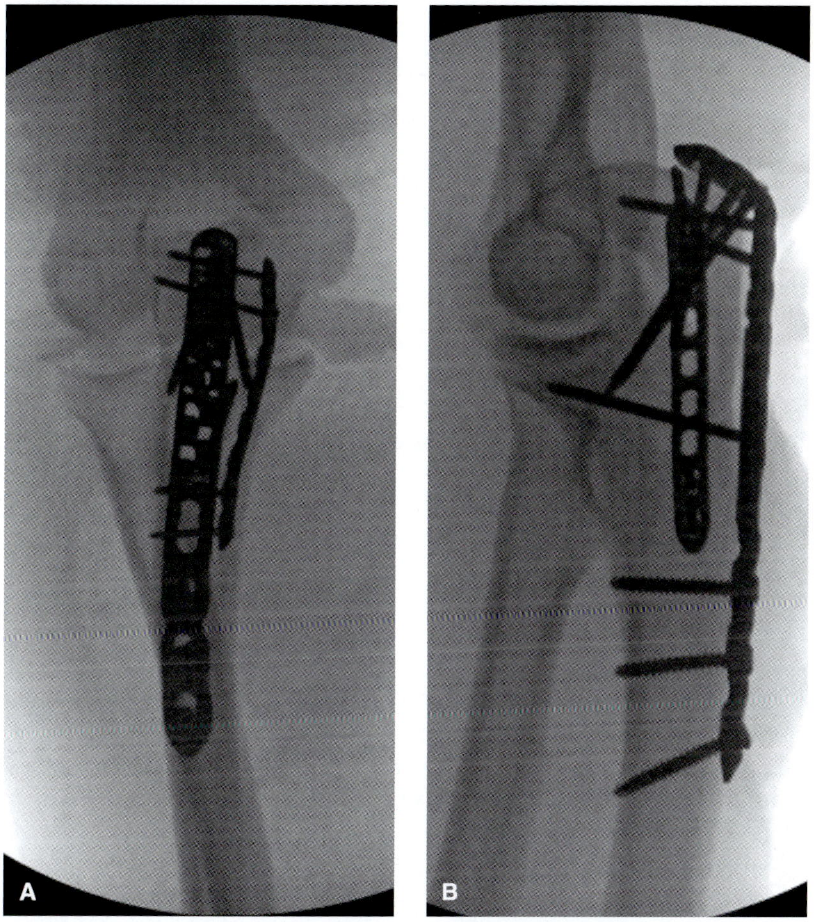

Figure 9-5 | A and B: AP and lateral fluoroscopic images obtained with the patient in prone position following open reduction and internal fixation of olecranon fracture.

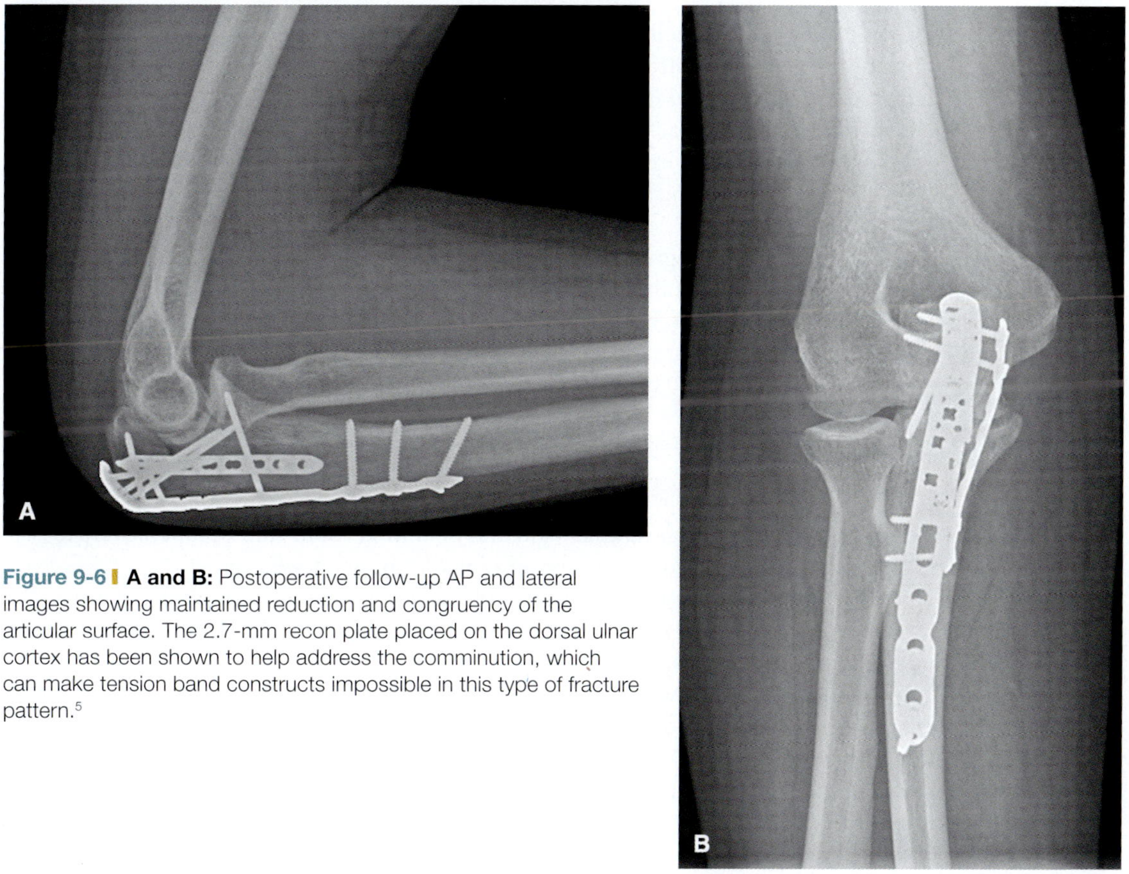

Figure 9-6 | A and B: Postoperative follow-up AP and lateral images showing maintained reduction and congruency of the articular surface. The 2.7-mm recon plate placed on the dorsal ulnar cortex has been shown to help address the comminution, which can make tension band constructs impossible in this type of fracture pattern.[5]

Intraoperative Positioning

Supine and 45-Degree Lateral Positioning

- The supine position or semilateral position can be used to easily perform preparatory sterilization and draping of the operative extremity, as well as perform intraoperative imaging. This allows the anesthesiologist direct access to the patient's airway, allowing for regional anesthesia without the need for intubation. This position is also useful for polytrauma patients with positioning restrictions.
- Intraoperatively, the shoulder can be flexed and internally rotated with the forearm flexed over the chest of the patient to facilitate a posterior approach to the distal humerus and proximal ulna. To support the operative arm, a bump or a well-padded Mayo stand placed from the contralateral side of the patient can be used.
- The operating table can be rotated 90 degrees in the room to facilitate use of fluoroscopy and maximize space for multiple surgeons while still enabling anesthesia staff to have appropriate access to airway and intraoperative monitoring devices.
- The draped C-arm should enter from a 45-degree angle with one of the surgeons positioning the arm appropriately to obtain either true AP or lateral views of the arm on the arm table (Fig. 9-7).

Lateral Positioning

- The patient is placed in the lateral decubitus position and stabilized using either a beanbag or chest rolls. An axillary roll or thoracic wedge should be used for the down upper extremity.
- The down extremity is well padded and secured to an armboard.
- The C-arm should enter from the front of the patient orientated perpendicular to the table to facilitate AP and lateral imaging with positioning of the operative extremity on an elevated armboard or well-padded Mayo stand (Fig. 9-8).

Prone Positioning

- The prone position can be used to facilitate the posterior approach to the elbow while decreasing the need to reposition the arm for intraoperative fluoroscopy.
- The patient is placed prone following intubation with the use of chest rolls or a Wilson frame with an additional cross roll to pad the iliac crests if using rolled blankets and an additional roll under the operative shoulder to elevate the extremity.
- The contralateral arm is adducted and laid parallel to the table or abducted less than 90 degrees to prevent excessive external rotation.
- The operative arm is abducted 90 degrees over Plexiglas armboard that is positioned with 5 to 8 inches exposed beyond the edge of the table to enable greater than 90 degrees of elbow flexion.
- AP and lateral views of the elbow can be obtained by extending the elbow for the AP view and by rotating the C-arm 90 degrees so that it parallels the long axis of the table.
- The operating table can be rotated 90 degrees to facilitate fluoroscopic access (Fig. 9-9).

Additional Positioning and Imaging Tips

- Discuss positioning needs with the anesthesia team and operating room staff preoperatively to ensure patient safety and efficiency following the administration of anesthesia.
- Placement of a sterile tourniquet as proximal on the brachium as possible to minimize the risk of draping the patient in a manner that obstructs the operative field. This will facilitate intraoperative manipulation of the extremity for imaging.
- Use a radiolucent arm table that allows freedom of fluoroscopic imaging.
- Obtain contralateral stress views following administration of anesthesia and prior to draping if ligamentous injury is suspected.
- Obtain preoperative radiograph with the planned implant superimposed over the olecranon to guide incision length.

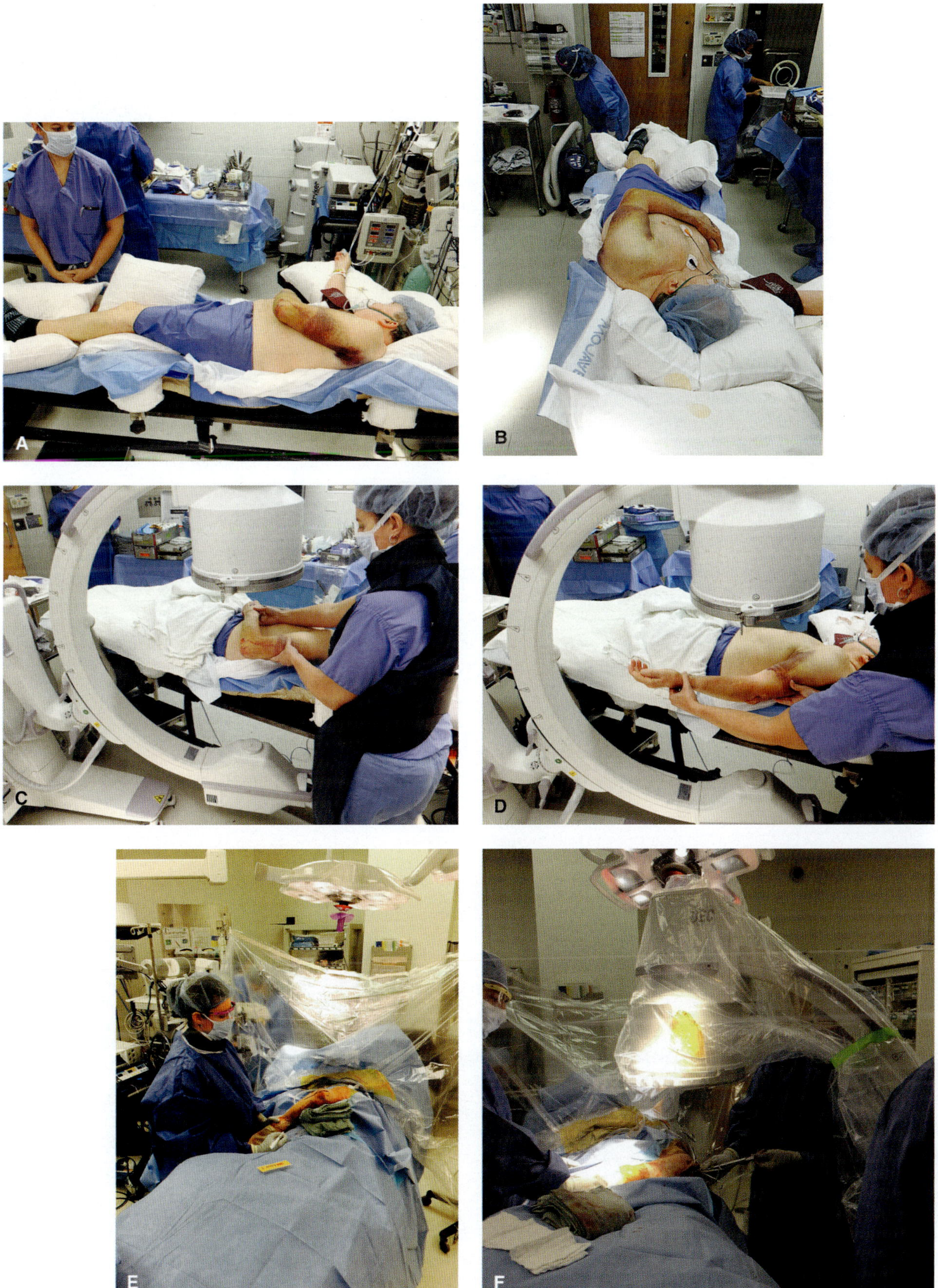

Figure 9-7 | A: Before preparation and draping, a beanbag with padded soft tissue protection is used to obtain a 45-degree lateral positioning with the arm resting over the body. **B:** View from the head of the bed. **C:** Method of obtaining a lateral intraoperative film with fluoroscopy on the ipsilateral side of the body. **D:** AP intraoperative film positioning. **E:** View of the patient from the foot of the bed after preparation and draping; the surgeon stands on the ipsilateral side of the table with the first assistant on the contralateral side. Both team members have excellent access during the case. **F:** Hardware insertion with the fluoroscopic machine ipsilateral.

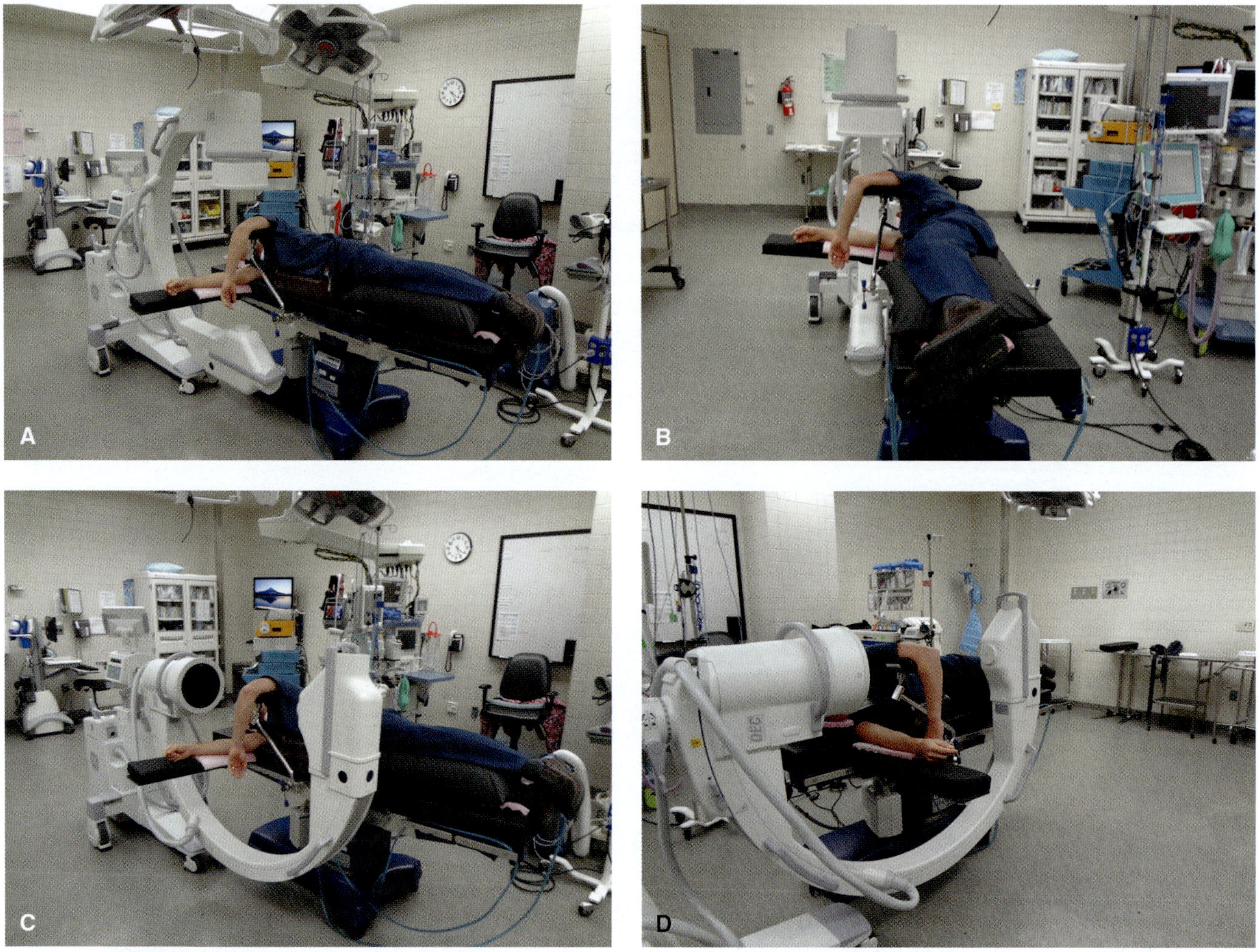

Figure 9-8 | A and B: Demonstration of padding and positioning for an AP view in the lateral position. **C and D:** Demonstration of positioning for a lateral view in the lateral position.

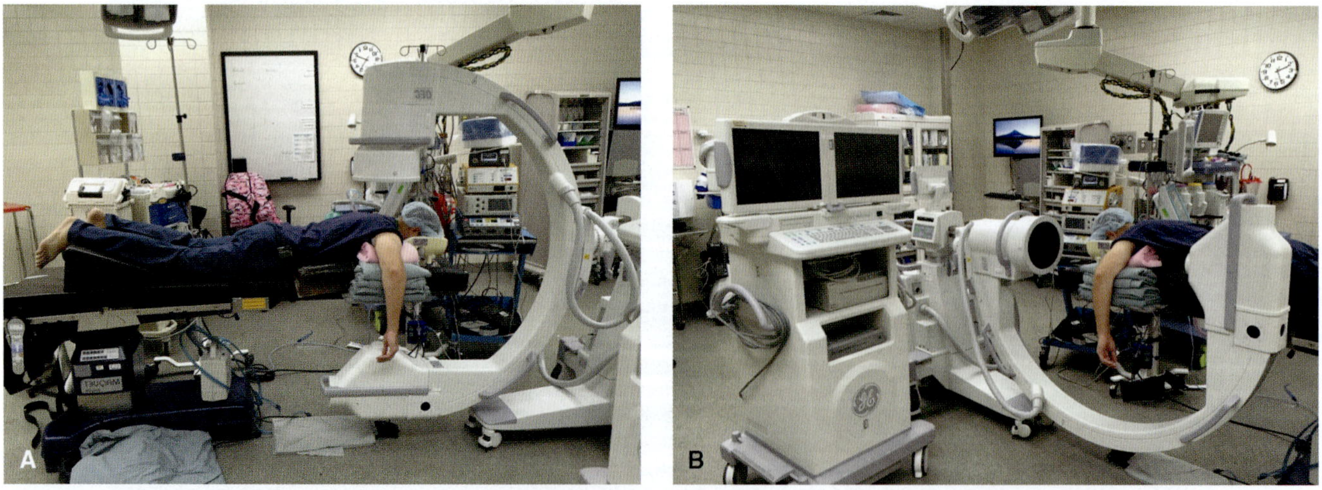

Figure 9-9 | A: Operating table with chest rolls and blanket with foam pillow and Plexiglas in place to facilitate transfer to prone position following intubation. **B:** Patient prone with appropriate padding. Adequate fluoroscopic access is confirmed prior to completion of draping.

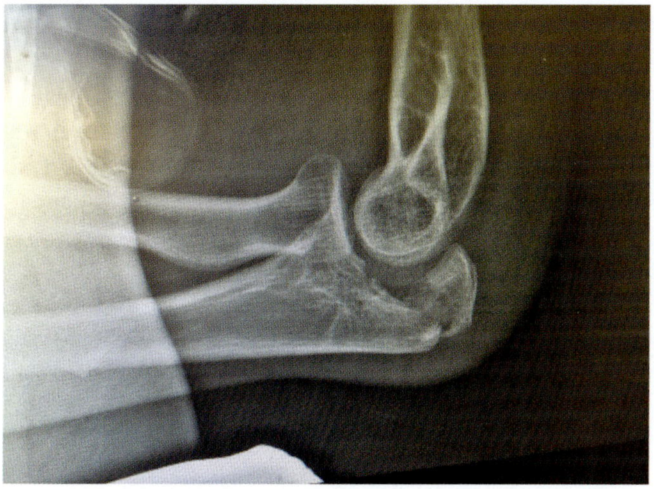

Figure 9-10 | Lateral elbow.

Intraoperative Imaging

- Intraoperative stress radiographs, performed with varus and valgus loading, can elucidate ligamentous instability that may need to be addressed at the time of fracture fixation in more complex fracture-dislocations of the elbow.

Case Examples

Case 1

- A 27-year-old female fell onto her left elbow sustaining a closed left intra-articular olecranon fracture.
- Preoperative lateral x-ray and sagittal CT images (Figs. 9-10 and 9-11)
- The patient was positioned in the 45-degree lateral position, as described above.
- During surgery, a fully threaded rafting K-wire was used to secure the reduction of the central articular surface depression, which can be reduced using the humerus as a template for fragment position. As this bone fragment is quite small, attempting to pass a large screw through the piece can be destructive. The threaded wire can be kept as part of the final construct. Fully threaded wires are used in this scenario to prevent late migration (Fig. 9-12).
- The pointed reduction clamps used to reduce the principal proximal fragment have been removed to highlight the trajectory of the threaded K-wire, which is placed outside the footprint of the planned plate.
- With the wire retained, plating can progress around the wire (Figs. 9-13 and 9-14).
- With the plate in acceptable position, a cortical screw is placed in a distal hole to control plate height and rotation.
- Next, a bicortical screw into the coronoid is placed, crossing the fracture fragments (Fig. 9-15).
- A second interfragmentary screw with bicortical purchase is then passed through the proximal segment followed by placement of the distal cortical screws (Fig. 9-16).
- Final result with the K-wire cut flush with the proximal bone (Figs. 9-17 and 9-18)

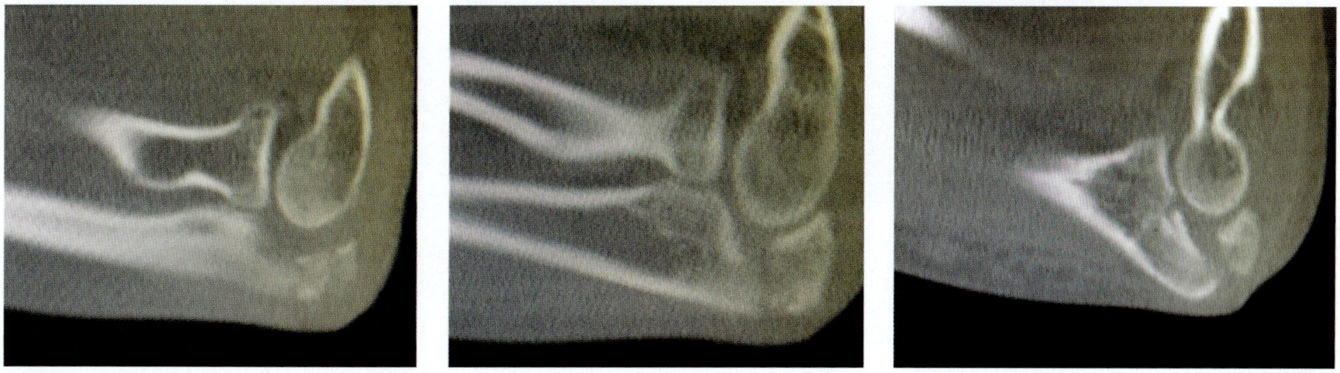

Figure 9-11 | Sagittal CT.

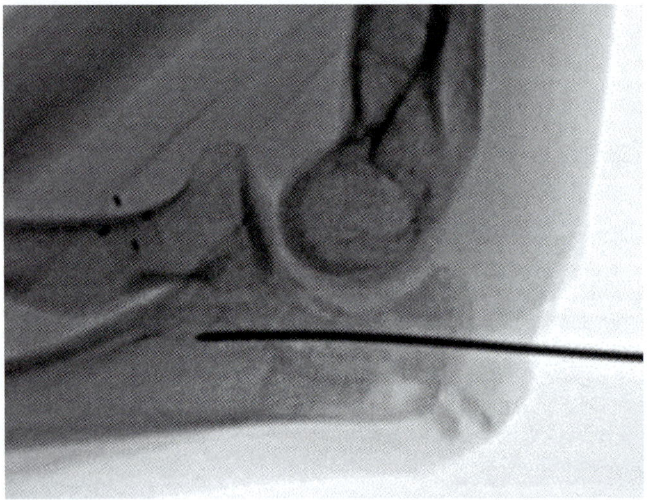

Figure 9-12 | Threaded K-wire to prevent migration.

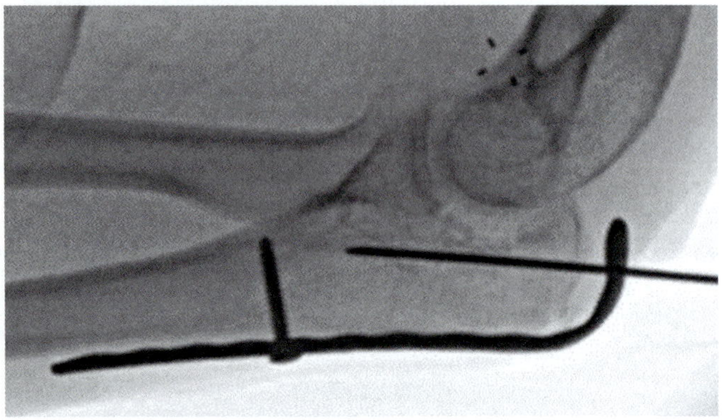

Figure 9-13 | Plating can be performed around the wire.

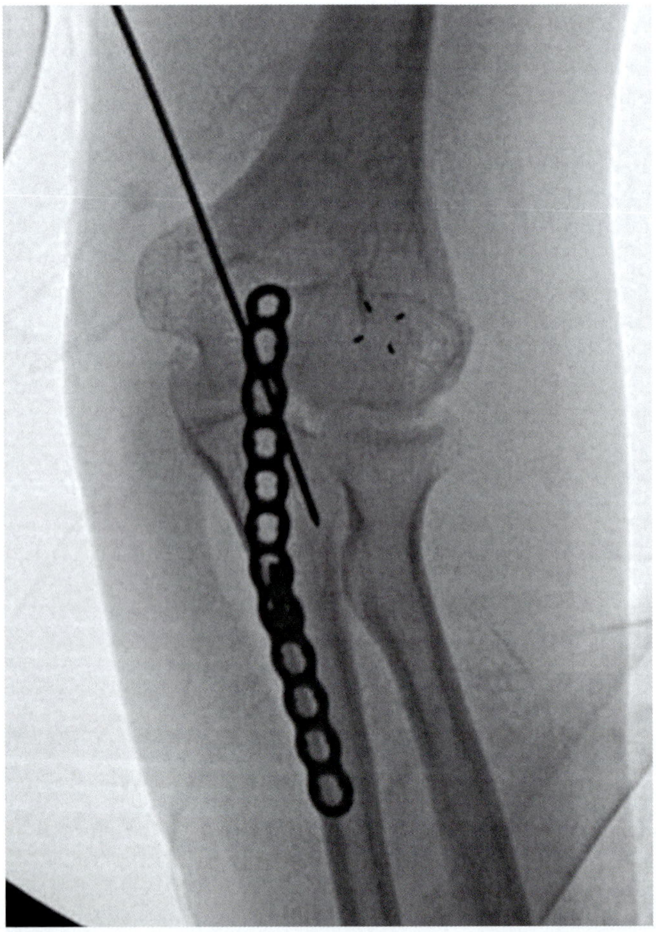

Figure 9-14 |

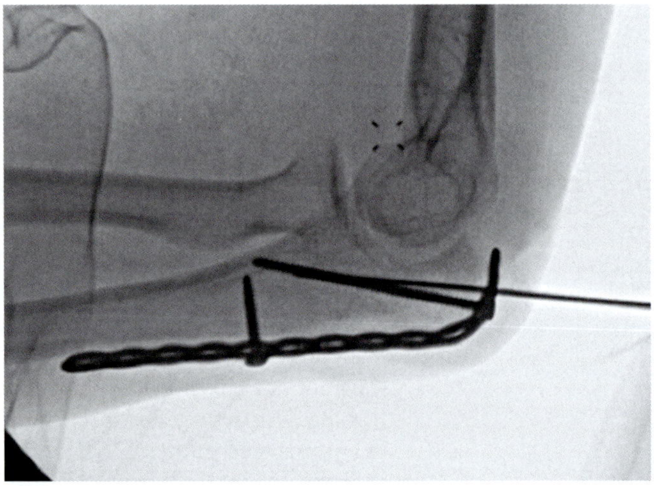

Figure 9-15 |

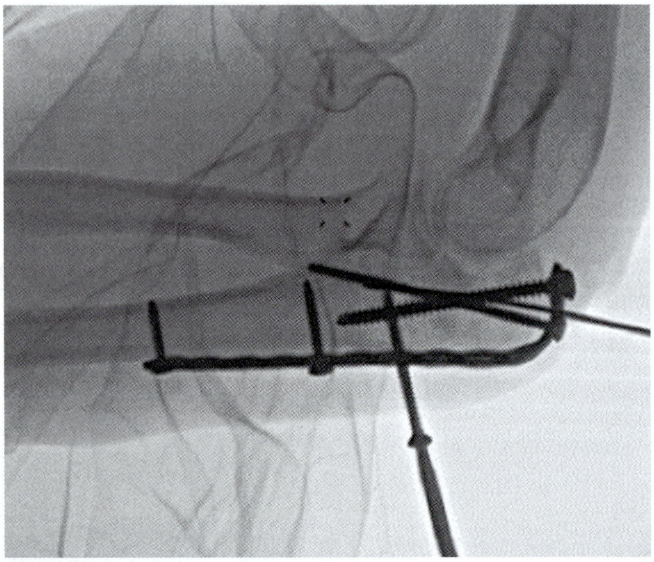

Figure 9-16 |

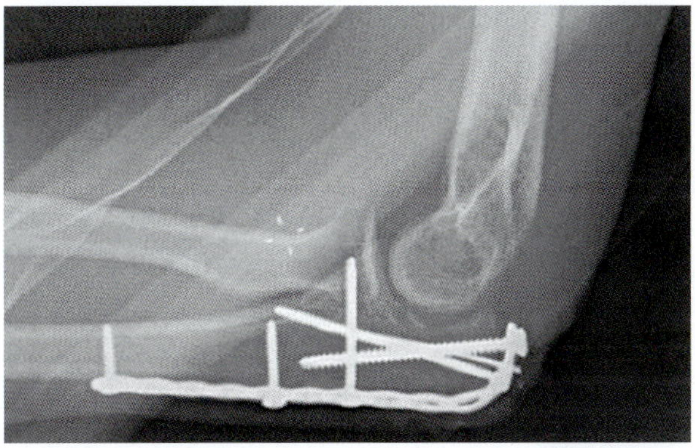

Figure 9-17 | K-wire can be cut flush and retrained. Lateral postoperative radiograph.

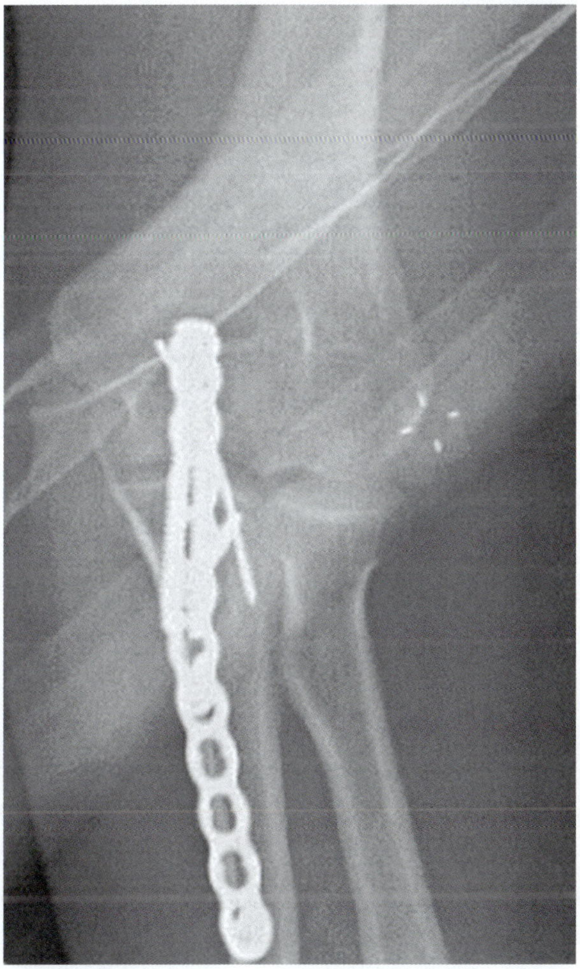

Figure 9-18 | AP postoperative radiograph.

Case 2

Lateral and oblique radiographs of a 47 y/o male with a comminuted, displaced olecranon fracture sustained from a fall from 5 foot height directly onto R elbow. Note how oblique image demonstrates medial-sided comminution not appreciated on the initial lateral image (Figs. 9-19 and 9-20).

Note provisional K-wire fixation to provisionally hold comminuted fragments. Fragment-specific fixation is used for absolute stability at the articular surface. Once the reduction is verified, plates can be threaded over or around the K-wires and contoured to the specific anatomy. Comminuted fracture patterns such as this are difficult or impossible to treat with a large partially threaded screw or tension band wire construct[3] (Fig. 9-21).

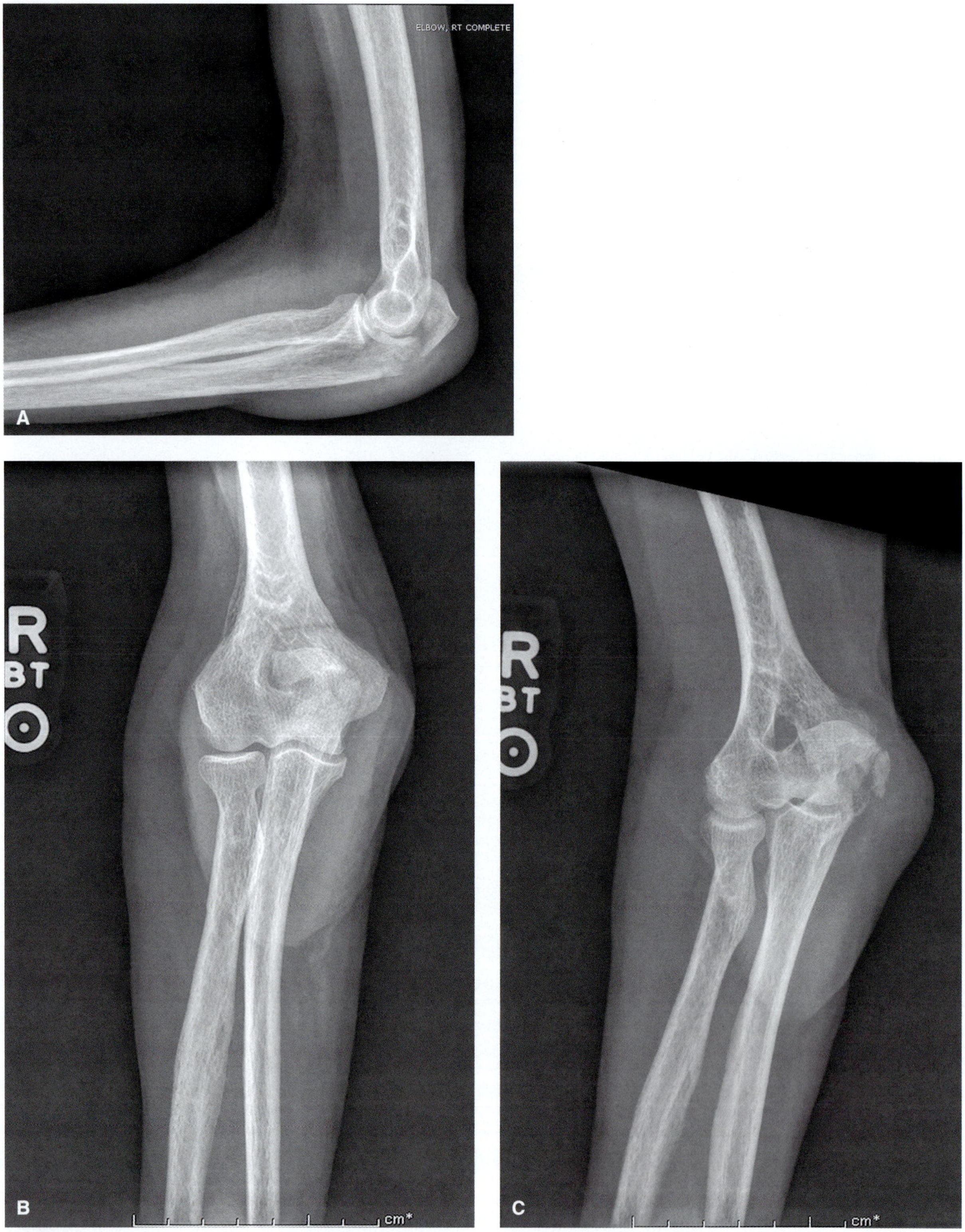

Figure 9-19 | Lateral **(A)**, AP **(B)**, oblique **(C)** view demonstrating medial comminution and displacement less appreciable on AP and lateral views.

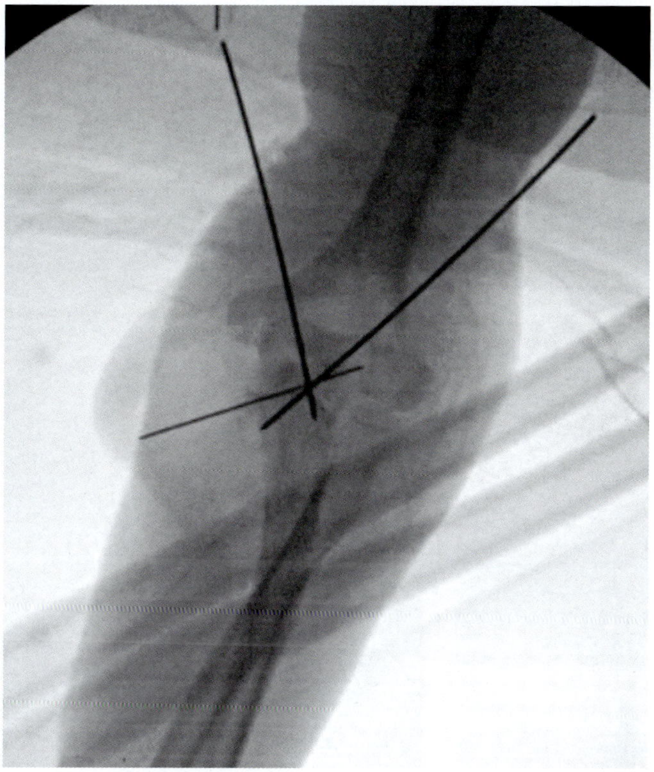

Figure 9-20 | Intraoperative fluoroscopy of olecranon pinning to obtain reduction.

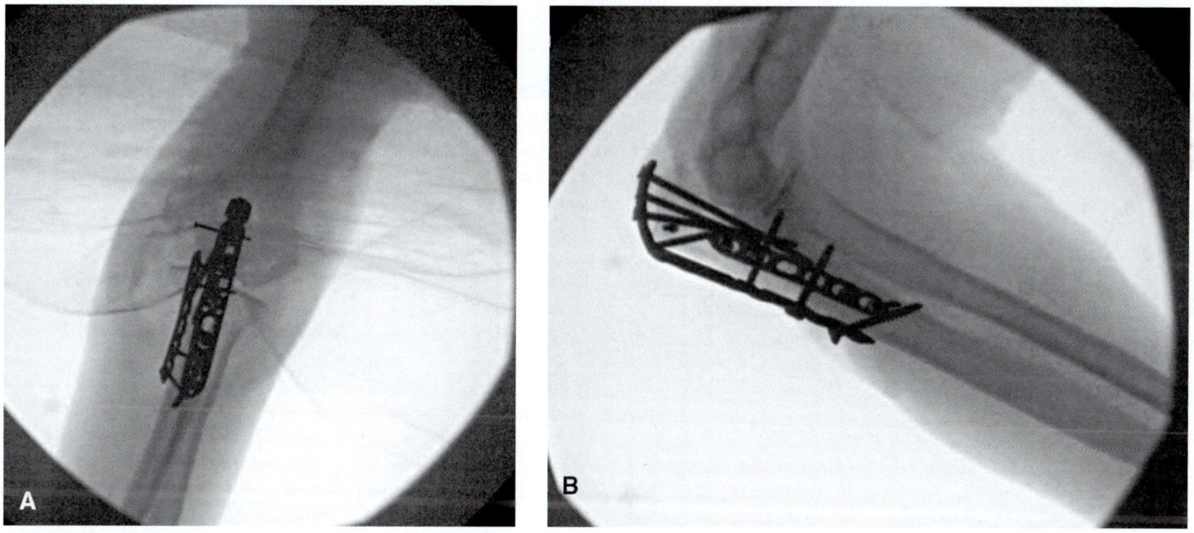

Figure 9-21 | Plates placed around pins. Pins can later be removed or cut flush and retained.

Intraoperative AP and lateral images showing the placement of a 3.5 proximal contoured olecranon plate as well as a 2.7-mm recon plate to provide fixation and compression to the ulnar comminution. Wellman et al. demonstrated that this technique prevented late malunion and provided stability for early range of motion. Of note, 18 of 35 patients requested hardware removal after fracture union.[5] This is on par with rates reported elsewhere in the literature (Fig. 9-22).

AP, lateral, and oblique images obtained in the postoperative recovery unit demonstrate dual-plate fixation of comminuted olecranon fracture. Patients are placed in posterior plaster splint postoperatively for 2 weeks to allow incisions to heal. At the 2-week postoperative appointment, sutures are removed and gentle passive elbow range of motion is encouraged. Stable fixation allows for early active and passive range of motion, preventing elbow stiffness and leading to better overall outcomes.[6]

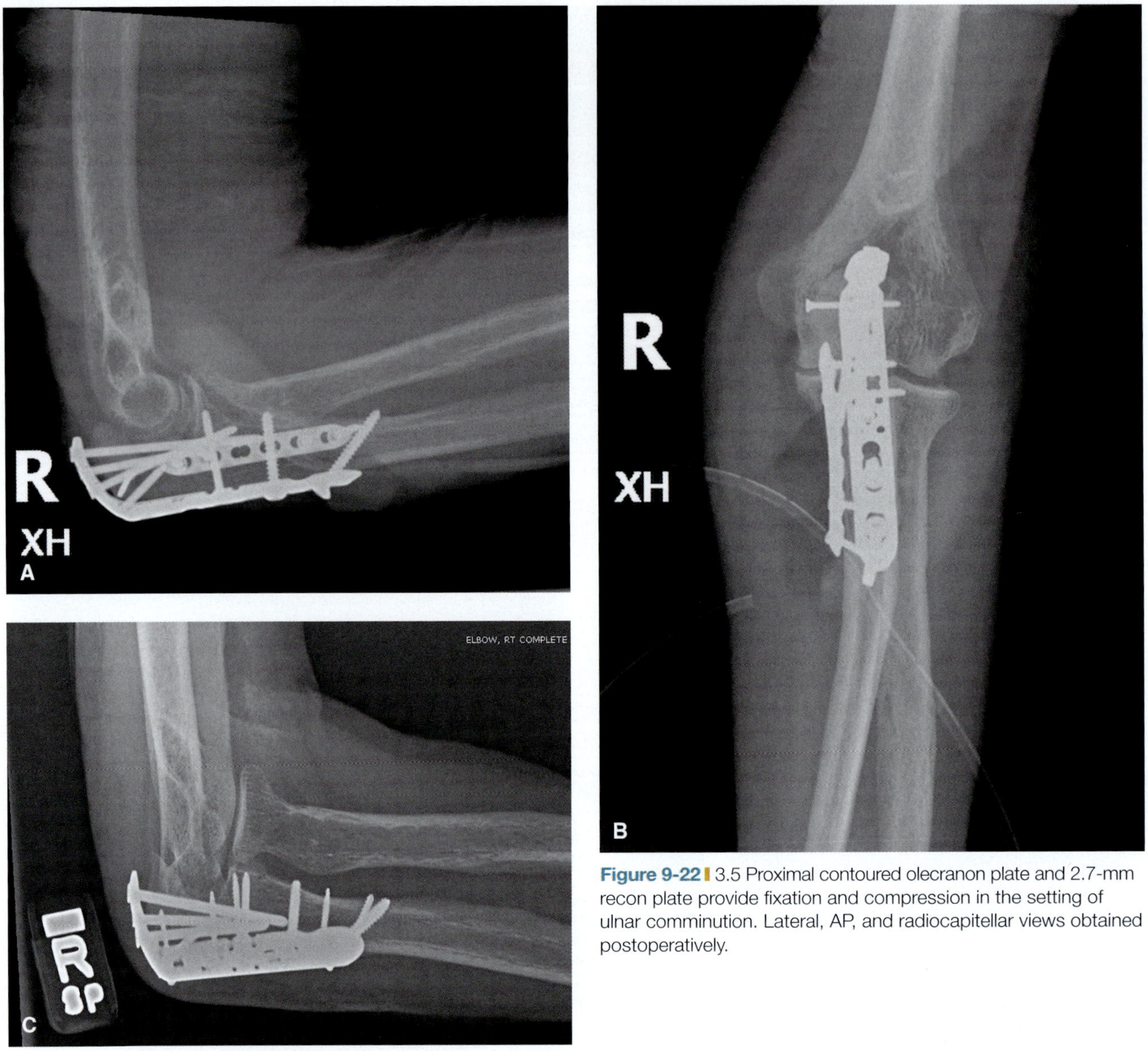

Figure 9-22 | 3.5 Proximal contoured olecranon plate and 2.7-mm recon plate provide fixation and compression in the setting of ulnar comminution. Lateral, AP, and radiocapitellar views obtained postoperatively.

References

1. Hak DJ, Golladay GJ. Olecranon fractures: treatment options. *J Am Acad Orthop Surg.* 2000;8:266–275.
2. Rouleau DM, Sandman E, Van Reit R, et al. Management of fractures of the proximal ulna. *J Am Acad Orthop Surg.* 2013;21(3):149–160.
3. Beingessner DM, Pollock JW, King GJW. *Elbow Fractures and Dislocations. Rockwood and Green's Fractures in Adults.* Philadelphia, PA: Lippincott Williams & Wilkins; 2015.
4. Baecher N, Edwards S. Olecranon fractures. *J Hand Surg.* 2013;38(3):593–604.
5. Wellman D, Lazaro LE, Cymerman RM, et al. Treatment of olecranon fractures with 2.4 and 2.7 mm plating techniques. *J Orthop Trauma.* 2015;29(1):36–43.
6. Nieto H, Billaud A, Rochet S, et al. Proximal ulnar fractures in adults: a review of 163 cases. *Injury.* 2015;46:18–23.

Chapter 10
ORIF Forearm Fractures

DAVID A. FEAKER JR*
MATTHEW J. WILSON*
CHRISTOPHER S. SMITH*
MICHAEL J. GARDNER

Bony Anatomy[1-6]

- The forearm is composed of the radius and ulna. Proximally, the radius articulates with the capitellum as well as the ulna at the lesser sigmoid notch while the ulna articulates with the trochlea via the trochlear notch, which is formed by the olecranon and coronoid.
- Distally, the radius articulates with the scaphoid and lunate at the scaphoid fossa and lunate fossa. The radius and ulna articulate distally at the sigmoid notch.
- The radius rotates about the axis of the ulna. The bow of the radius allows for supination and pronation about the ulna and must be restored with ORIF of the radius. The radius also has a minor anterior bow.
- The ulna is rather straight in comparison to the radius with a minimal anterior bow. The ulna is subcutaneous in its position along the medial forearm.
- Important bony landmarks of the radius proximally are the radial head, which is palpable on the lateral aspect of the elbow as well as the radial tuberosity, which is oriented on the lateral aspect of the radius in supination and the dorsal aspect in pronation. The radial shaft is distal to the radial tuberosity.

Radiographic Anatomy

- On an AP of the forearm (Fig. 10-1), the wrist should be positioned in supination and the elbow should be extended against the table. Distally, the radial styloid should appear in profile, and there should be minimal overlap of the radius and ulna. Proximally, the radial tuberosity should slightly overlap the ulna and should be 180 degrees from the radial styloid. The radiocapitellar joint should be well visualized with minimal overlap of the proximal ulna. If the elbow is unable to be fully extended, then two AP views should be taken. One AP is taken with the humerus parallel with the tabletop and the second radiograph is taken with the forearm parallel with the tabletop.[7-9]
- A good lateral of the forearm (Fig. 10-2) is evident when there is a good lateral of the elbow as well as a good lateral of the wrist. Elbow is placed in 90-degree flexion, and humeral epicondyles are superimposed and perpendicular to the image receptor. The humerus and the forearm are positioned in the same plane, which may require the distal forearm to be slightly elevated using a radiolucent sponge or towel. The wrist is placed in a true lateral position with elbow in 90-degree flexion, ulnar side down, and radius and ulna superimposed. The wrist is positioned neutral (without flexion or extension) and the radius and ulna superimposed by aligning the second and third metacarpals with the radius.[7-9]
- Intraoperatively, it is difficult to view both the forearm and wrist within the same radiograph due to a limited viewing field provided by fluoroscopy (Figs. 10-3 and 10-4). We recommend obtaining a perfect lateral of the wrist and then repositioning the fluoroscopy without changing the position of the upper extremity to assess the placement of the hardware. When working proximally, obtain a perfect lateral of the elbow and then move the beam distally.

*The views expressed in this chapter are those of the author(s) and do not necessarily reflect the official policy or position of the Department of the Navy, Department of Defense or the United States Government. David A. Feaker, Matthew J. Wilson, and Christopher S. Smith are military service members and this work was prepared as part of their official duties. Title 17 U.S.C. 105 provides that 'Copyright protection under this title is not available for any work of the United States Government.' Title 17 U.S.C. 101 defines a United States Government work as a work prepared by a military service member or employee of the United States Government as part of that person's official duties.

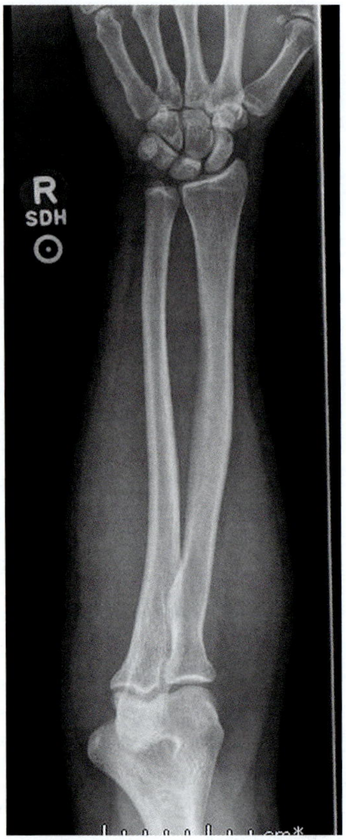

Figure 10-1 I The AP view of the forearm shows the radial styloid in profile with minimal overlap of the radius and ulna. Note that the radial tuberosity slightly overlaps the ulna and the radial styloid and radial tuberosity are separated by 180 degrees.

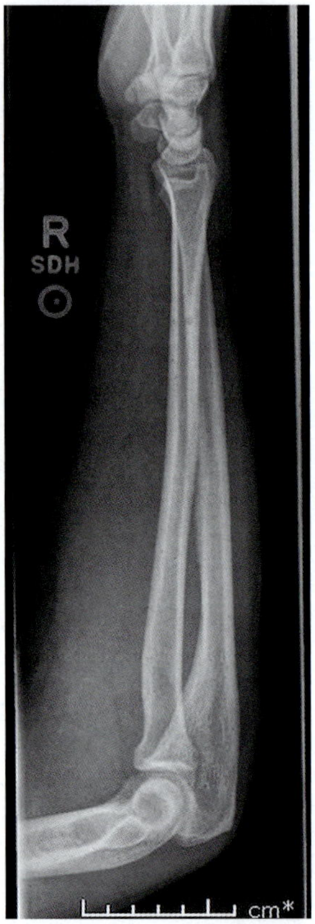

Figure 10-2 I A perfect lateral of the forearm is defined by obtaining a good lateral of the wrist combined with a good lateral of the elbow.

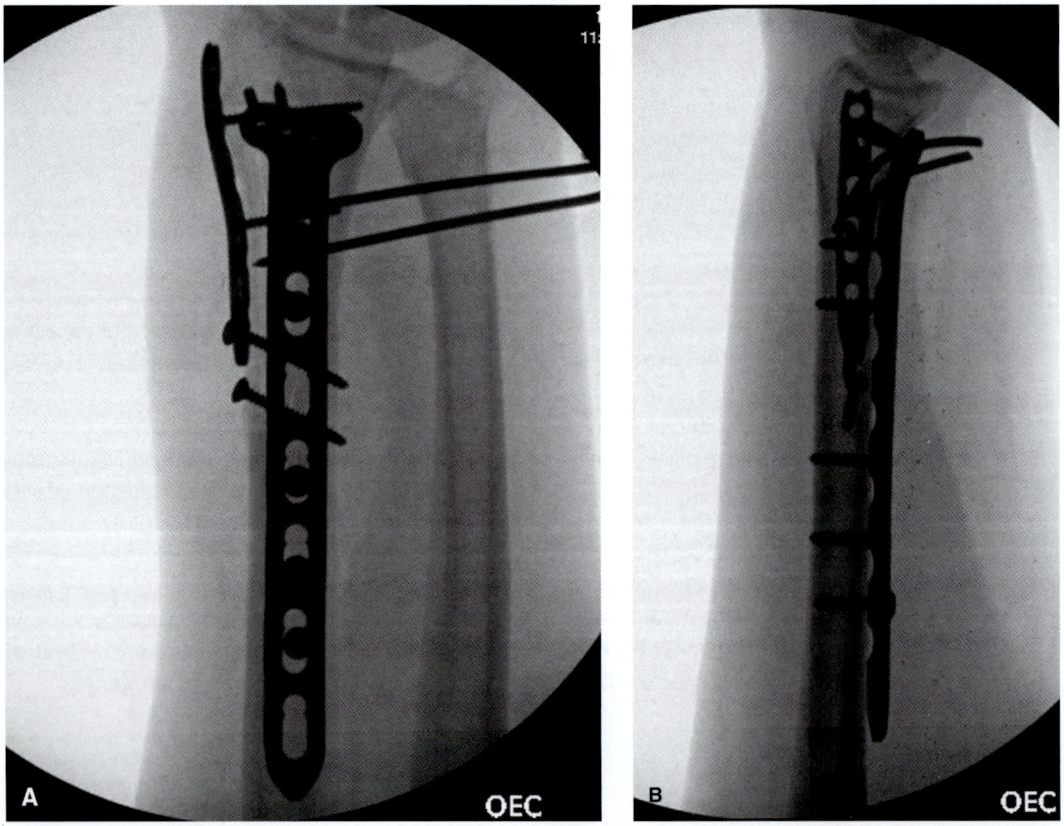

Figure 10-3 I A and B: Intraoperative imaging does not allow for simultaneous visualization of wrist and forearm on a lateral view. Obtain a perfect lateral of the wrist prior to imaging the forearm.

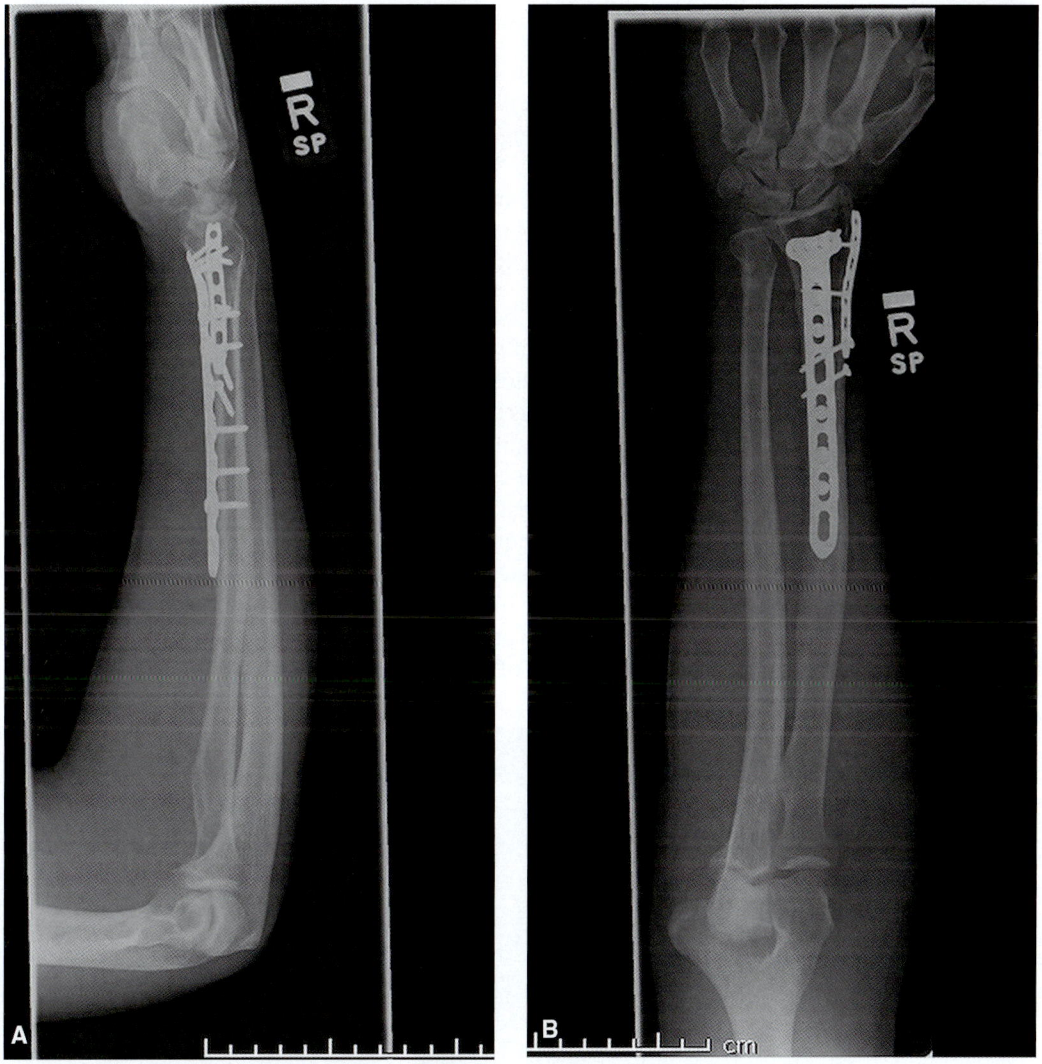

Figure 10-4 | **A and B:** Post ORIF films obtained with portable x-ray intraoperatively or postoperatively in the PACU.

Preoperative Imaging

- Preoperative imaging should include wrist and elbow films in addition to forearm radiographs with suspected radial and ulnar shaft fractures.[3]
- In all cases of forearm fracture, we recommend obtaining contralateral forearm radiographs for preoperative planning as well as comparison of the radial bow following ORIF.
- Associated injuries with diaphyseal fractures of the forearm include elbow dislocations, PRUJ/DRUJ disruptions, and injury to the interosseous membrane. Obtaining proper distal and proximal imaging is crucial to avoid missing other associated injuries.[3,10–13]
- Visualizing the radial bow is important to evaluating proper reduction for functional biomechanics postinjury. The major radial bow extends distally from the bicipital tuberosity to the distal radioulnar joint. The apex of the bow is found just distal to the midpoint of the distance of the radius. Restoration of this bow with surgical intervention is of the utmost importance to allow pronation and supination.[2]
- Deforming forces on the radial and ulnar diaphyses play a major role in fracture patterns and displacement. Depending on where the fracture occurs, the net forces of supination and pronation will exert the displacement seen on injury films. The primary pronators of the forearm are the pronator quadratus and the pronator teres. The primary supinators of the forearm are the supinator and biceps muscles. If a fracture of the radius occurs distal to the supinator forces, but proximal to the insertion of the pronators, the resulting force will lead to a rotational deformity of unopposed supination of the proximal segment and pronation of the distal segment. Fractures distal to the pronator teres will have more balanced net forces and be less deformed rotationally.[7]

Indications for Surgery[1,3,7,10,14–17]

- Fractures of the proximal two-thirds of the ulna with >50% displacement.
- Monteggia/Galeazzi fracture dislocations.
- Greater than 10 degrees of angulation.
- Loss of the radial bow.
- Both bone forearm fractures are considered fractures of necessity for ORIF.

Imaging in Galeazzi Fractures

- The uninjured DRUJ should be assessed with a shuck test prior to prepping and draping to ascertain the patient's normal motion.[3,18]
- Following fixation of the radius, the DRUJ of the injured side may then be assessed and compared to the uninjured. If stability is achieved with the wrist in a supinated position, the forearm may be casted in supination. If stability is not achieved, an appropriate reduction should be confirmed using radiography[3,18] (Fig. 10-5A and B).
- Imaging is focused at the wrist rather than the forearm.
  - A lateral of the wrist is adequate when the 2nd and 3rd metacarpal overlap or the pisiform is contained between the volar lip of the scaphoid tubercle and volar aspect of the capitate head.[19]
  - It is important to critically inspect the image (Fig. 10-6) as overlap of the radius and ulna can be achieved by adjusting the rotation of the forearm, but if this is not done utilizing a true lateral radiograph, malreduction of the DRUJ may occur.[18]

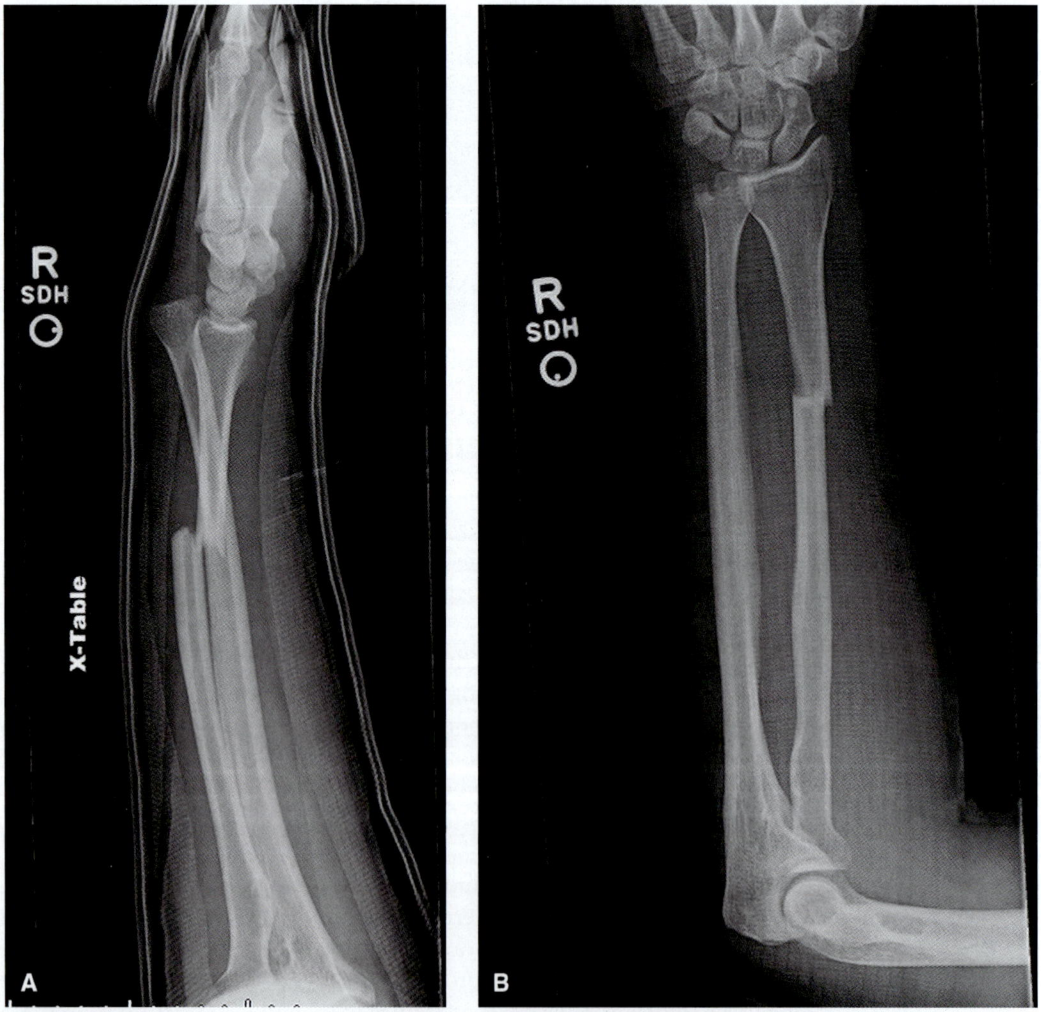

Figure 10-5 | A: A lateral image of a Galeazzi fracture. In this image, note the obvious dislocation of the DRUJ. The 2nd and 3rd metacarpals are not perfectly overlapped, and the pisiform is not fully contained within the volar aspect of the scaphoid tubercle and capitate head. **B:** AP image of the same patient.

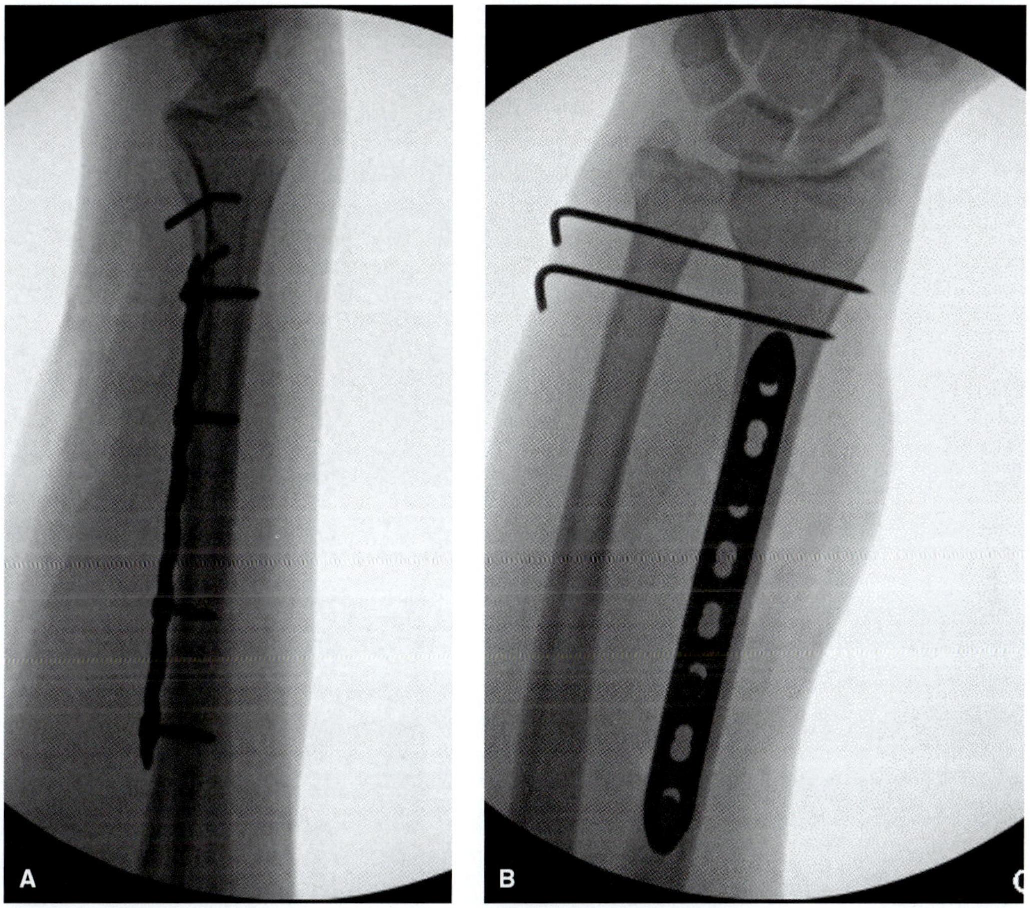

Figure 10-6 | **A and B:** Care must be taken when obtaining a lateral prior to fixation of the DRUJ with a Galeazzi fracture-dislocation. A perfect lateral of the wrist should first be obtained as the radius and ulna can easily be made to overlap with rotation of the forearm, which would lead to malreduction of the DRUJ.

- Once an adequate lateral has been obtained and manual reduction is confirmed, two 1.6-mm or 2-mm K-wires are inserted percutaneously proximal to the fovea through the ulna and both cortices of the radius.[4,7]
  - When placing these K-wires and utilizing a large C-arm, the patient's elbow can be flexed to 90 degrees while the large C-arm is placed in a lateral position. This will allow real-time assessment of the positioning of the K-wire (Fig. 10-7).
  - A similar setup may be done with the mini C-arm though you must ensure that the underportion of the mini C-arm has remained sterile to this point of the case. Mini C-arms are occasionally utilized for pediatric forearm fractures, with the benefit of reducing radiation exposure.[20]

Intraoperative Positioning

- The patient is placed supine on a Maquet table.
- A radiolucent arm table is used for the operative extremity; an armboard is used for the nonoperative extremity with the elbow padded with egg crate and secured.
- The extremity should be positioned such that the wrist is centered on the arm table with the patient's shoulder near the edge of the bed.
- In both-bone forearm fractures and isolated radius fractures, the forearm is positioned on a radiolucent arm side table to permit the appropriate radial approach. The ulnar fixation is performed with the forearm held vertically and the elbow resting on the side table.
- An unsterile 18 inches (or appropriate size based upon patient anatomy) tourniquet is placed on the operative upper arm followed by an unsterile 1015 clear U-drape around the circumference of the operative extremity just distal to the tourniquet.
- Shave the operative wrist and forearm with clippers followed by an appropriate and thorough scrub with alcohol and chlorhexidine. SCD and TED hose are placed on the lower extremities, which are then covered with a sheet and taped to the bed.

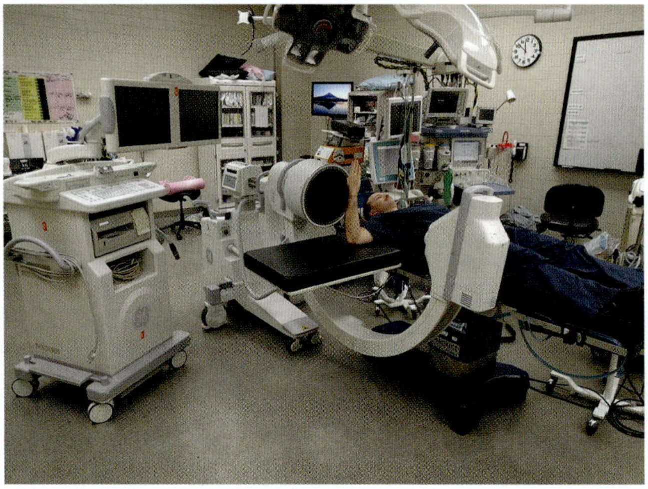

Figure 10-7 | The large C-arm may be placed in standard lateral positioning for live assessment.

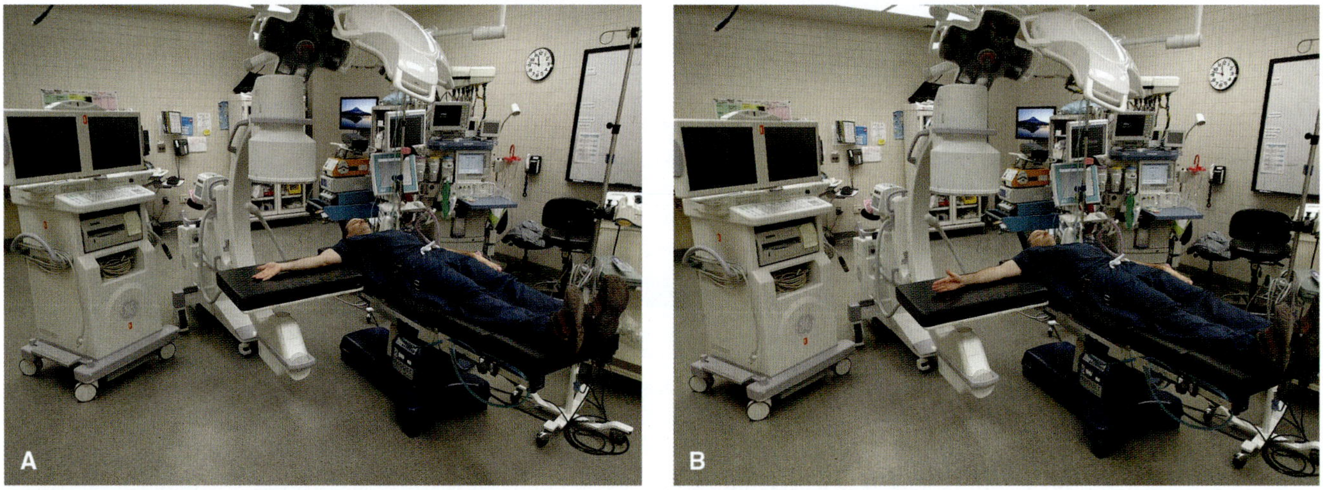

Figure 10-8 | A and B: An example of intraoperative setup with a radiolucent armboard. The surgeon is positioned in the axilla. The fluoroscope enters from the head where the assistant is seated. The viewfinder should be placed in a location easily viewed by the surgeon. Positioning for an AP is shown in figure **(A)**, and a lateral positioning is shown in figure **(B)**. A perfect lateral of the wrist should be obtained when imaging the forearm.

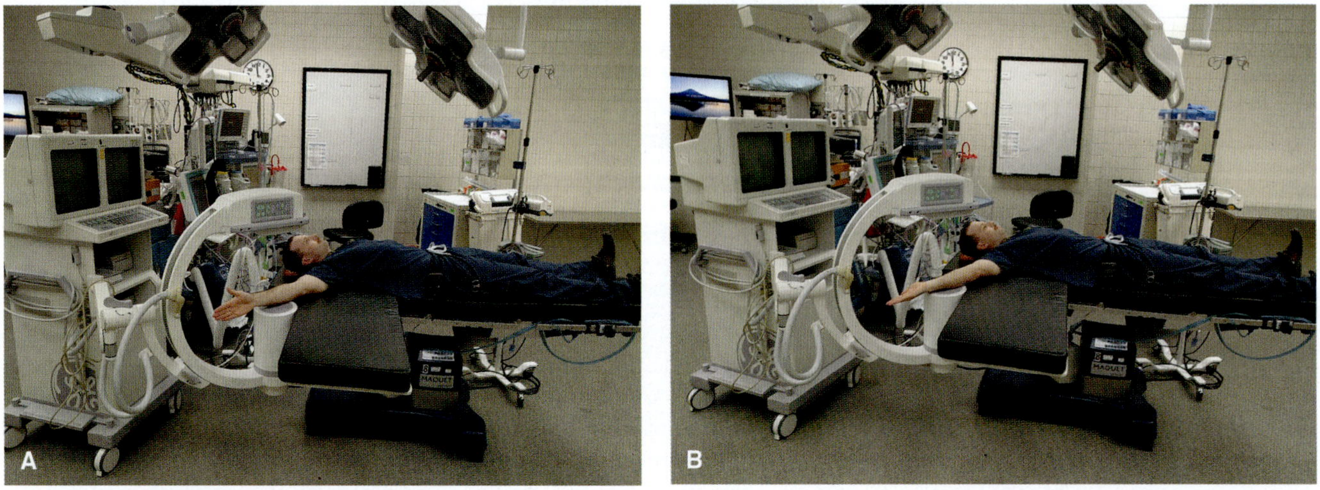

Figure 10-9 | A and B: Alternative setup utilizing a mini C-arm.

- The large C-arm is sterilely draped to enter from the head side of the arm table. The surgeon is either seated or standing in the axilla (Fig. 10-8A and B).
  - Alternatively, a mini C-arm may be used and is brought in from either the head or foot side of the armboard depending on mobility of the patient's shoulder and fracture location (Fig. 10-9A and B).
- Many surgeons recommend initial fixation of simplest fracture in a both-bone forearm fracture, which may help obtain length and aid in reduction of the more difficult fracture. When possible, it is recommended that ORIF of the radius be completed first as this will provide a strut for fixation of the ulna with the elbow placed at 90 degrees (Figs. 10-10 and 10-11).[7,17]

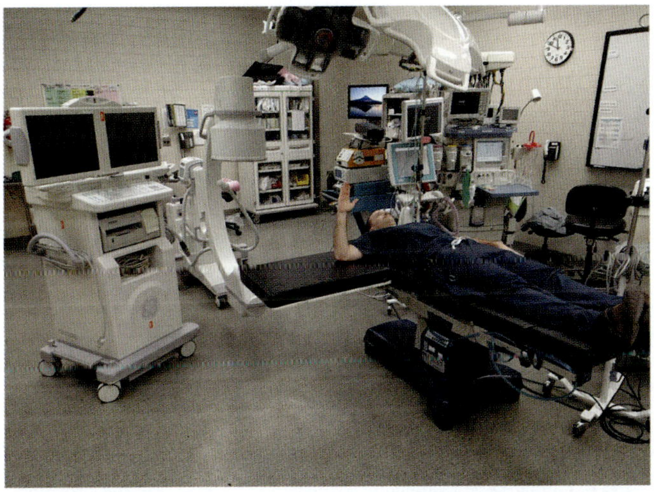

Figure 10-10 | After ORIF of the radius, it is much easier to perform ORIF of the ulna with the patient's elbow bent 90 degrees.

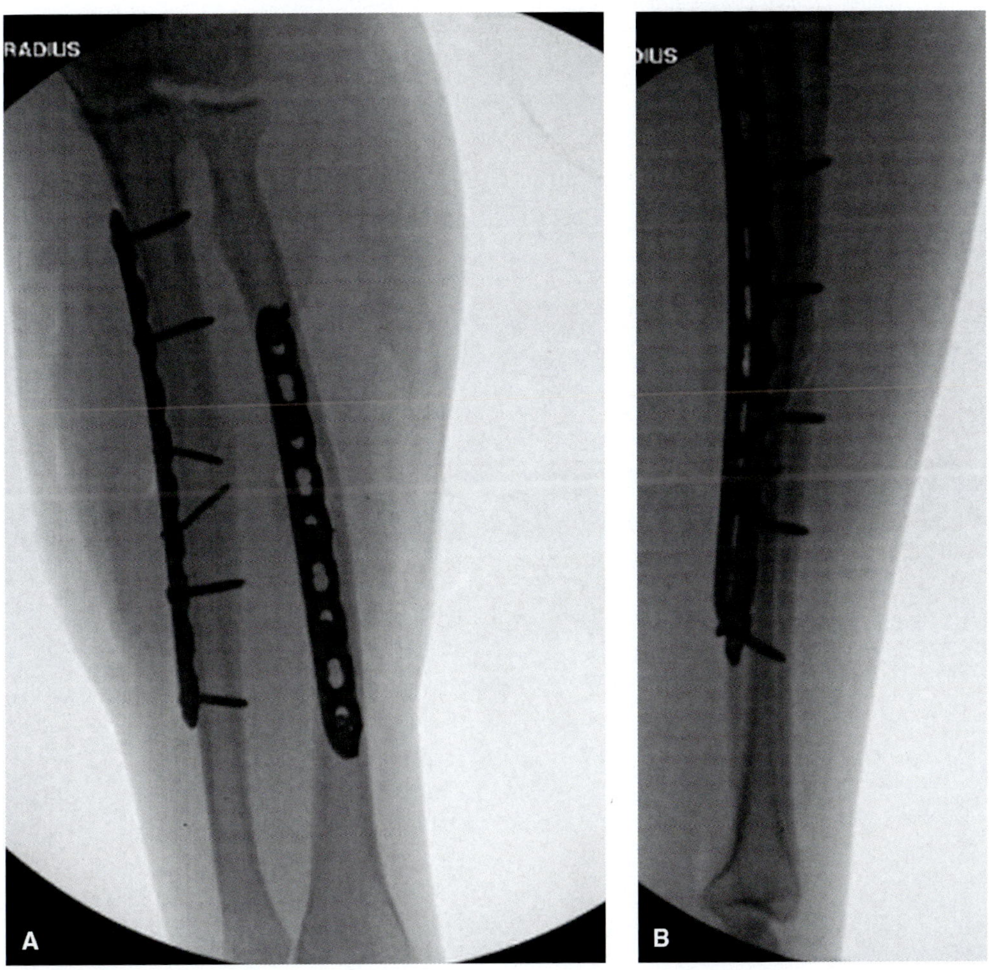

Figure 10-11 | A and B: An example of a both-bone forearm fracture. The radius was fixed first, which allowed the elbow to be flexed (as pictured above) for fixation of the ulna.

References

1. Schulte LM, Meals CG, Neviaser RJ. Management of adult diaphyseal both-bone forearm fractures. *J Am Acad Orthop Surg.* 2014;22(7):437–446.
2. Schemitsch EH, Richards RR. The effect of malunion on functional outcome after plate fixation of fractures of both bones of the forearm in adults. *J Bone Joint Surg Am.* 1992;74(7):1068–1078.
3. Means K, Graham T. Disorders of the forearm axis. In: Wolfe S, Hotchkiss R, Pederson W, et al. eds. *Green's Operative Hand Surgery*. 6th ed. Philadelphia, PA: Elsevier; 2010:837–868.
4. Kleinman WB, Graham TJ. The distal radio-ulnar joint capsule: clinical anatomy and role in posttraumatic limitation of forearm rotation. *J Hand Surg Am.* 1998;23:588–599.
5. Doyle JR, Botte MJ. *Surgical Anatomy of the Hand and Upper Extremity*. Philadelphia, PA: Lippincott Williams & Wilkins; 2003.
6. Hotchkiss RN, An KN, Sowa DT, et al. An anatomic and mechanical study of the interosseous membrane of the forearm: pathomechanics of proximal migration of the radius. *J Hand Surg Am.* 1989;14(2 Pt 1):256–261.
7. Streubel PN, Pesantez RF. Diaphyseal fracture of the radius and ulna. In: Rockwood CA, Bucholz RW, et al. eds. *Rockwood and Green's Fractures in Adults*. 8th ed. Philadelphia, PA: Wolters Kluwer Health; 2015:1121–1177.
8. Greenspan A, Steinbach LS. Chapter 6: Upper limb II. 5th ed. *Orthopedic Imaging: A Practical Approach*. Philadelphia, PA: Lippincott Williams & Wilkins; 2010:93–167.
9. Helms CA. *Fundamentals of Skeletal Radiology*. 4th ed. Philadelphia, PA: Elsevier/Saunders; 2014:76–110.
10. Bado JL. The Monteggia lesion. *Clin Orthop.* 1967;50:71–86.
11. Givon U, Pritsch M, Levy O, et al. Monteggia and equivalent lesion. *Clin Orthop.* 1997;337:208–215.
12. Ring D, Jupiter JB, Simpson NS. Monteggia fractures in adults. *J Bone Joint Surg Am.* 1998;80:1733–1744.
13. Giannoulis FS, Sotereanos DG. Galeazzi fractures and dislocations. *Hand Clin.* 2007;23(2):153–163.
14. Mikik ZDJ. Galeazzi fracture-dislocations. *J Bone Joint Surg Am.* 1975;57:1071–1080.
15. Sauder DJ, Athwal GS. Management of isolated ulnar shaft fractures. *Hand Clin.* 2007;23(2):179–184.
16. Barquet A. Fracture of the shaft of ulna and radius with associated dislocation of the radial head. *Injury.* 1981;12(6):471–476. PMID:7275290
17. Gaulke R. Diaphyseal fracture of the forearm. In: Browner BD, Jupiter JB, Krettek C, et al. eds. *Skeletal Trauma: Basic Science, Management, and Reconstruction*. 5th ed. Philadelphia, PA: Saunders; 2015:1313–1346.
18. Atesok KI, Jupiter JB, Weiss AP. Galeazzi fracture. *J Am Acad Orthop Surg.* 2011;19(10):622–633.
19. Schreibman KL, Freeland A, Gilula LA, et al. Imaging of the hand and wrist. *Orthop Clin North Am.* 1997;28(4):537–582.
20. Sumko MJ, Hennrikus W, Slough J, et al. Measurement of radiation exposure when using the mini C-arm to reduce pediatric upper extremity fractures. *J Pediatr Orthop.* 2016;36(2):122–125. PMID: 25730377.

Chapter 11
Distal Radius Fractures

ELIZABETH A. KING
DANIEL A. OSEI
SAFI FARUQUI

Bony Anatomy

- The distal end of the radius is a plateau that articulates with the scaphoid and lunate as well as the ulnar head.
- The concave articular surface of the distal radius is divided distally into two articular facets: one for the scaphoid and one for the lunate. These are separated by a longitudinal sagittal ridge.
- Medially, a concave articular surface articulates with the ulnar head. This is where forearm rotation occurs as the radius rotates around the ulna during pronation and supination. Restoration of each of these articular surfaces is paramount for success in treating distal radius fractures.
- Multiple views of the wrist are needed to accurately assess displacement, angulation, rotation, and shortening of the fracture.
- The dorsal cortex of the distal radius has a bony prominence at Lister's tubercle with many undulations that support the extensor compartments (Fig. 11-1).
  - Knowledge of this anatomy is vital to avoid dorsal cortex screw penetration and irritation of the extensor tendons with volar plate fixation.

Radiographic Anatomy

- **PA**
  - Standard PA views show the distal radius and its carpal and ulnar articulations, which normally are smooth and congruent.
  - Radial height (12 mm), radial inclination (average 23 degrees), coronal shift, and ulnar variance (average 1 mm negative) are measured on this view (Fig. 11-2).

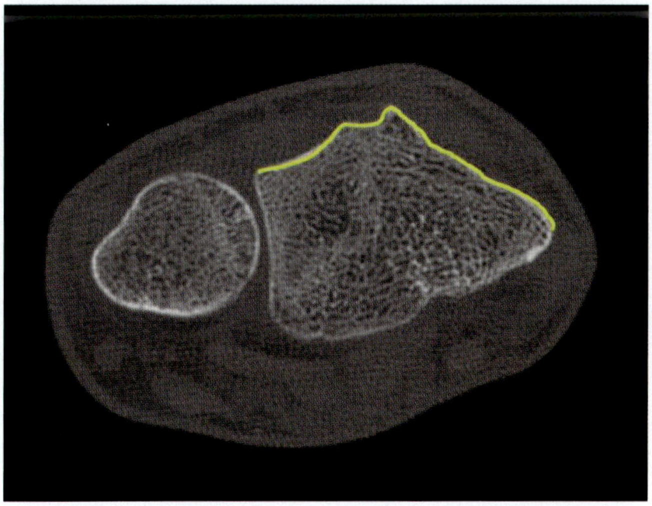

Figure 11-1 Axial CT image demonstrates the bony undulations of dorsal cortex of the distal radius.

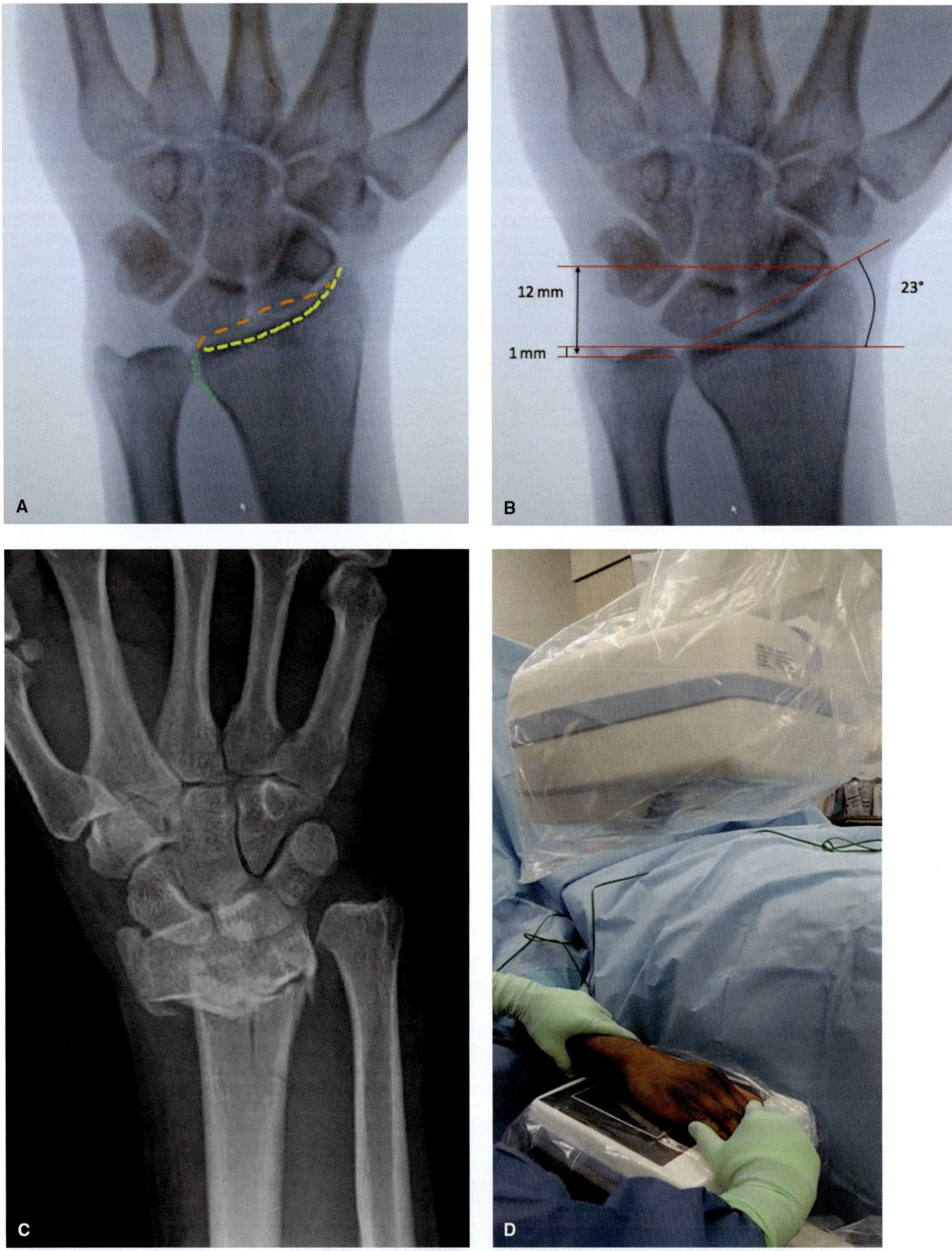

Figure 11-2 | A: AP view of the wrist demonstrates dorsal cortex (*orange*), volar cortex (*yellow*), and DRUJ articulation/sigmoid notch (*green*). **B:** Radial length, radial inclination, and ulnar variance. **C:** Distal radius fracture with loss of radial height and inclination, with a clear radial coronal shift and disruption of articular surface. **D:** Wrist positioned on fluoroscopy unit to obtain AP view.

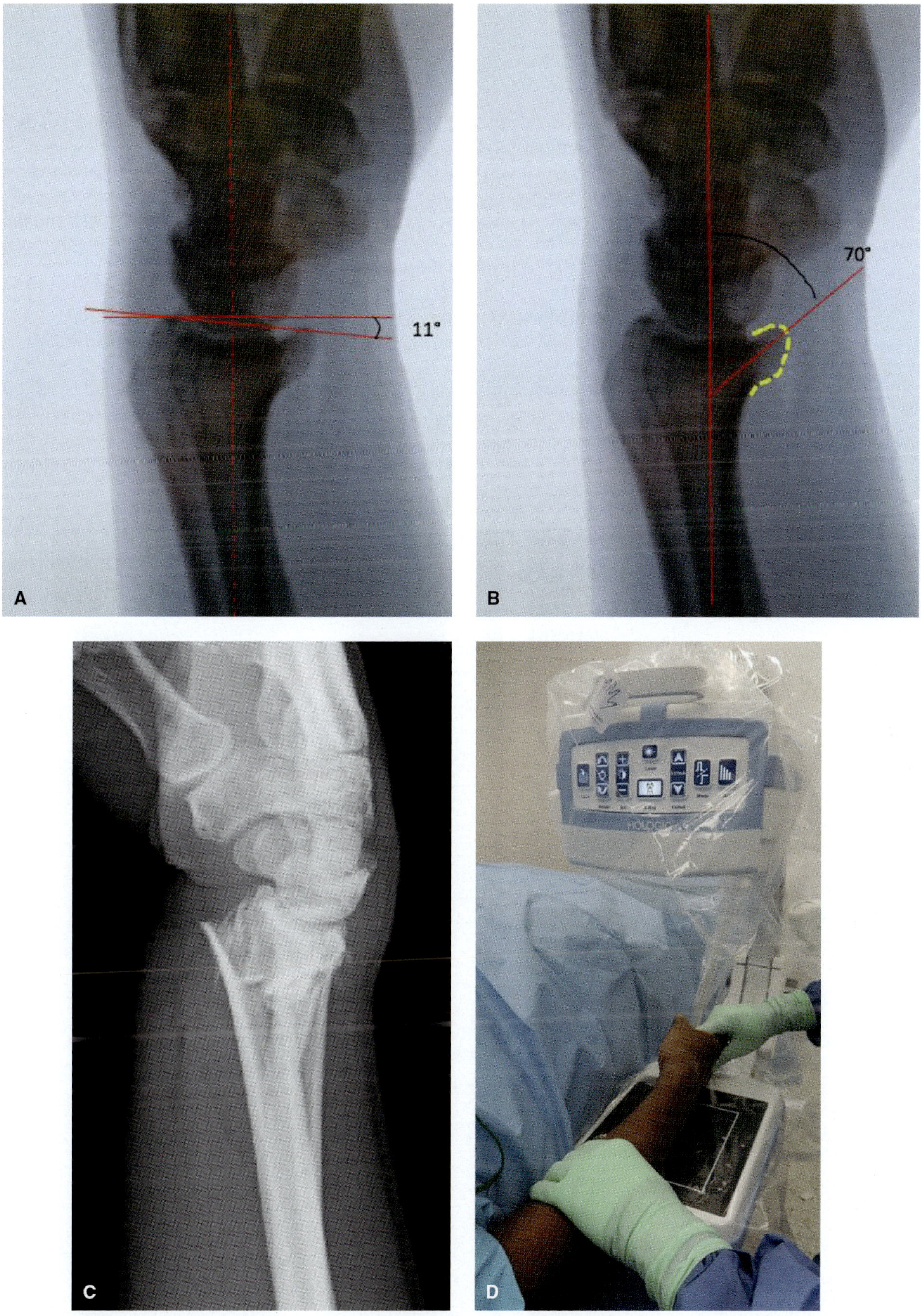

Figure 11-3 | A: Lateral view of the wrist, volar tilt 11 degrees. **B:** Teardrop, represents volar rim of lunate facet, and teardrop angle, approximately 70 degrees. **C:** Dorsally angulated, shortened, distal radius fracture. **D:** Wrist position to obtain lateral view.

- Coronal fracture displacement can be assessed in this view, though various images in different planes are necessary to quantify intra-articular involvement, displacement, and angulation.
- Neutral PA view is useful in identifying radioulnar joint disruption.

- **Lateral**
  - This view is important in assessing the radiocarpal articulation, dorsal/volar displacement of the fracture fragment(s), and any corresponding carpal abnormalities.
  - On a true lateral view, the palmar cortex of the pisiform should overlie the central third of the interval between the distal scaphoid pole and the capitate head.[1]
  - Volar tilt (average 11 degrees), AP distance (average 20 mm in males, 18 mm in females), and the teardrop angle are measured on this view (Fig. 11-3).
    - The teardrop represents the volar rim of the lunate facet, the mechanical buttress for subluxation of the lunate.[2]
    - Teardrop angle is measured between a line drawn along the central axis of the teardrop and a line along the central axis of the radial shaft. Normal teardrop angle is approximately 70 degrees.[2]
  - VISI (volar intercalated segmental instability) and DISI (dorsal intercalated segmental instability) deformities of the lunate can signify lunotriquetral or scapholunate ligament injury, respectively (Fig. 11-4).
  - Smith, Colles, and Barton fractures are best confirmed on this view (Fig. 11-5).

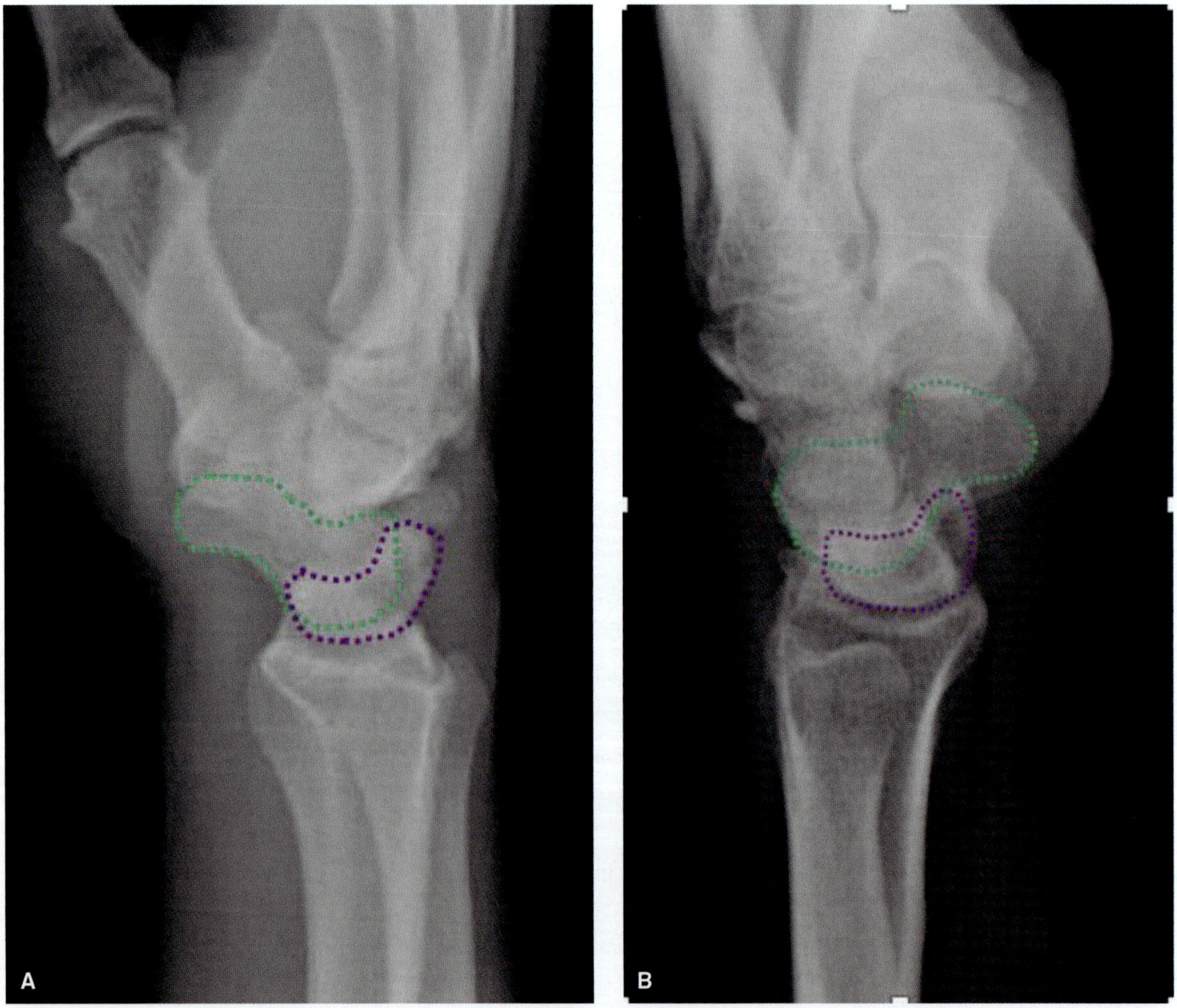

Figure 11-4 | A: VISI deformity, with volar flexion of the lunate, scapholunate angle <30 degrees. **B:** DISI deformity, with dorsal tilt of the lunate and scaphoid flexion, scapholunate angle >70 degrees.

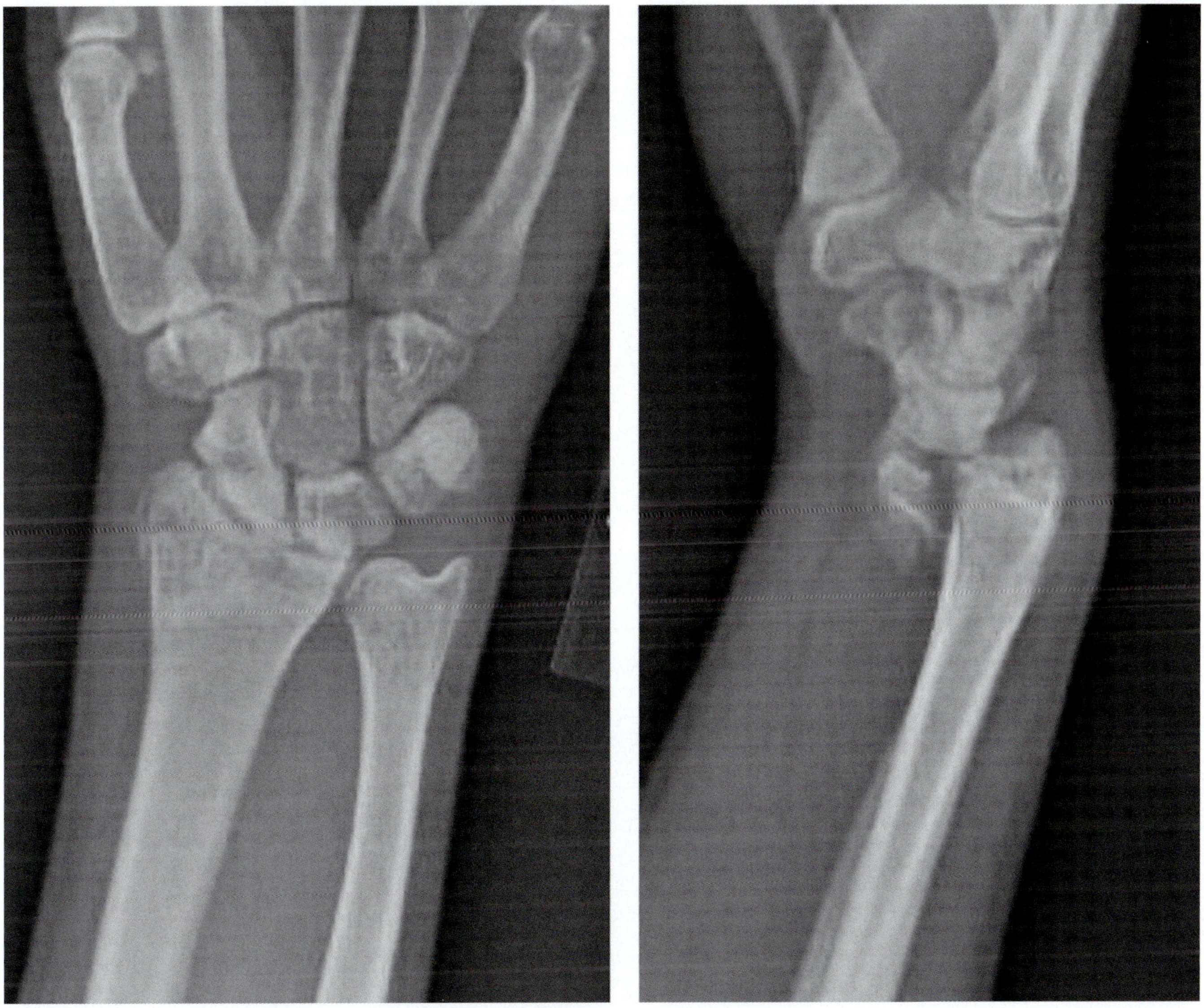

Figure 11-5 | Volar Barton's fracture, AP and lateral views.

- **Pronation/supination PA oblique**
  - Oblique views are taken with the forearm and wrist in 45 degrees of pronation or supination (Fig. 11-6).
  - These are important views that can show intra-articular involvement not seen on standard AP and lateral views.
  - Pronation oblique view best visualizes the radial styloid and is useful in assessing subchondral screw placement after plate placement.[3]
  - Supination oblique view allows evaluation of the dorsal ulnar facet of the lunate fossa.
- **PA tilt view**
  - Taken by directing the PA view 10 degrees from distal to proximal (Fig. 11-7).
  - View is parallel to the radiocarpal joint and accounts for the dorsal lip of the radius.
  - Proven to be an effective view to verify subchondral screw placement, especially for radial styloid screws.[4]

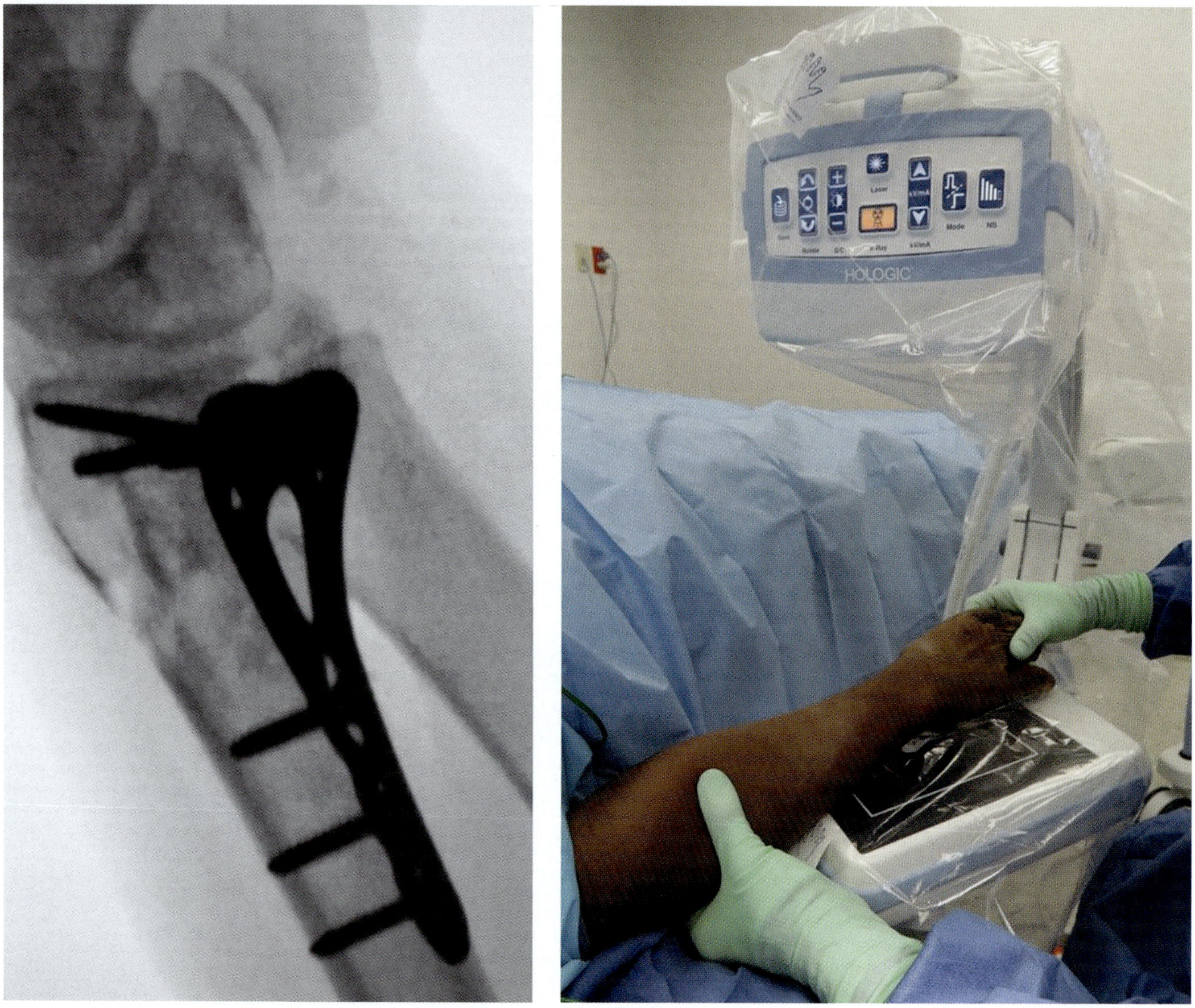

Figure 11-6 | Oblique images can be helpful for assessing screw lengths.

- **Lateral tilt view**
  - Taken by directing fluoroscopy beam 25 to 30 degrees from distal to proximal (Fig. 11-8).
  - Provides better visualization of the distal radius articular surfaces, especially the scaphoid and lunate facets, as the articular surface has approximately 23 degrees of radial inclination.
  - Necessary after volar locked plating to examine articular congruency of both the scaphoid and lunate facets, restoration of volar tilt, and subchondral placement of distal locking screws or pegs.
- **Dorsal horizon view**
  - This newly described dorsal tangential view provides a more complete visualization of the triangular distal radius cortex, particularly at Lister's tubercle, allowing for a more accurate assessment of screw protrusion (Fig. 11-9).[5–8]
  - Obtained by supinating the forearm, hyperflexing the wrist, and aiming the beam of the image intensifier along the long axis of the radius.
- **Advanced imaging (CT)**
  - Helpful for further evaluation of comminution, intra-articular involvement, and lunate facet congruity.
  - Can also identify dorsal shear fragments and centrally impacted fractures.

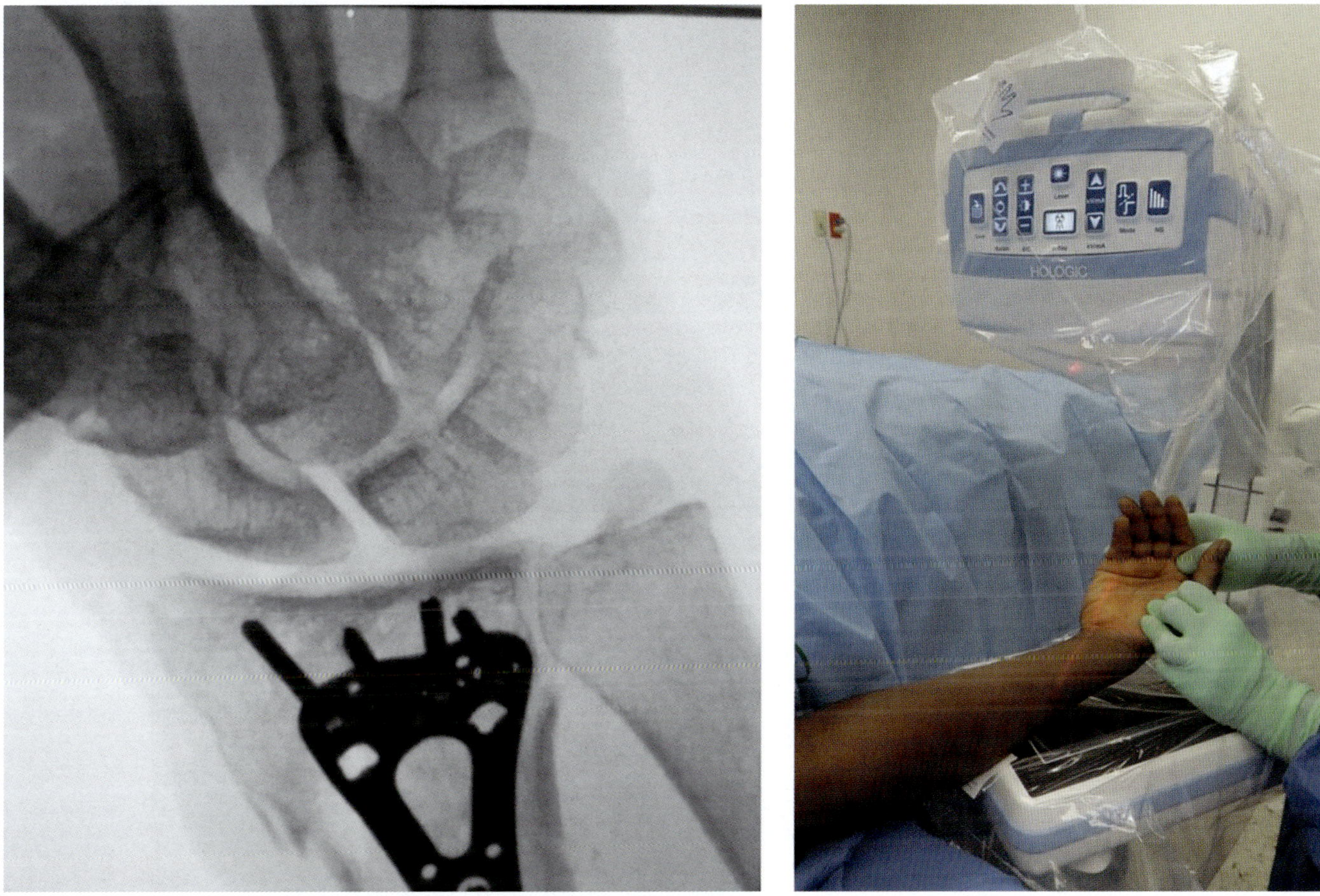

Figure 11-7 | PA tilt view demonstrating subchondral distal screw placement.

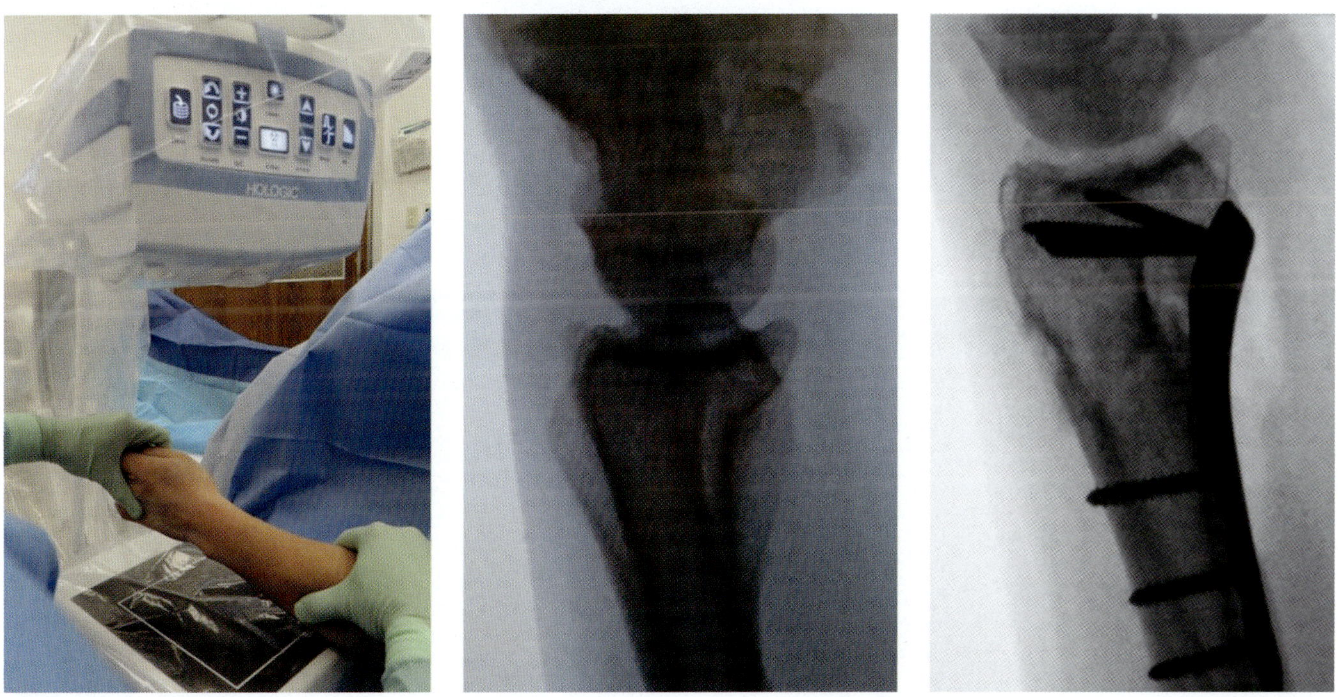

Figure 11-8 | Lateral tilt view.

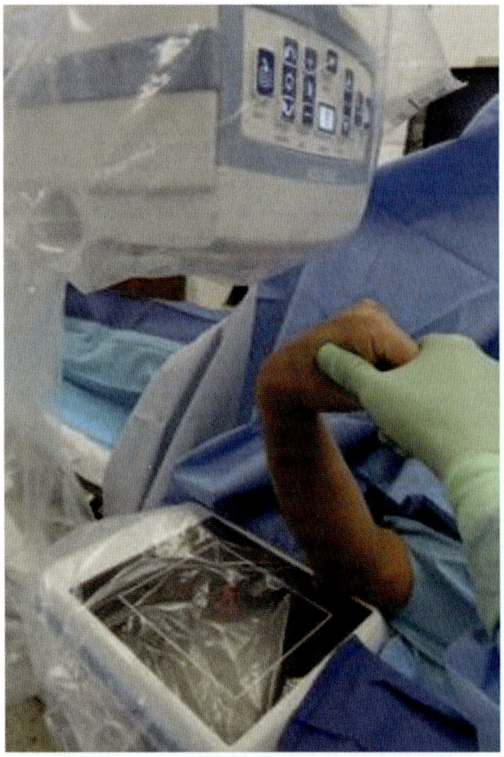

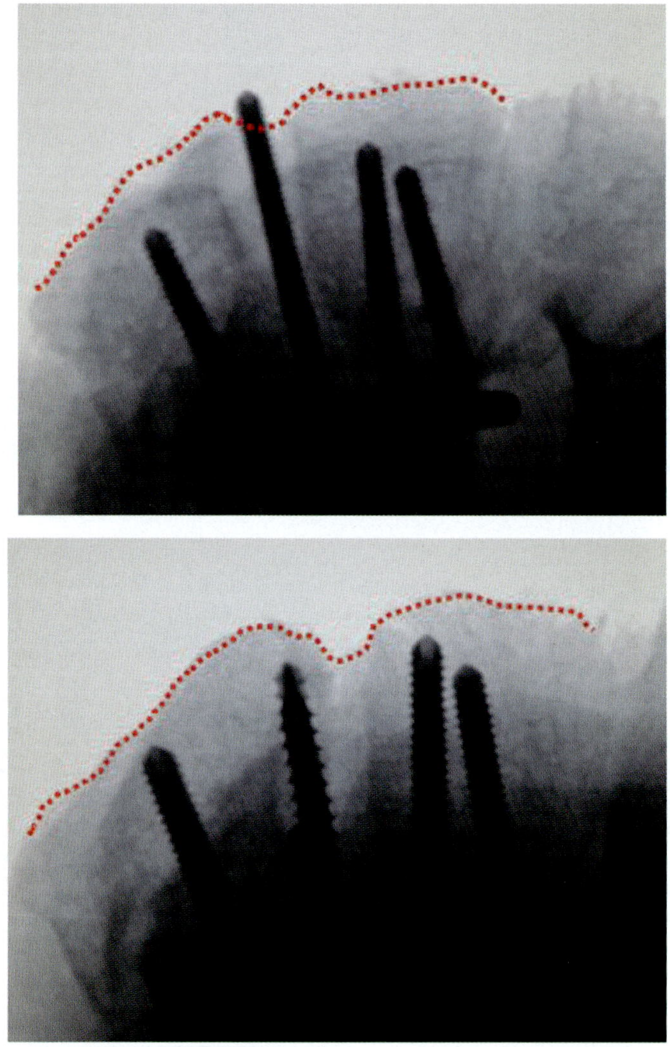

Figure 11-9 | Dorsal horizon view showing dorsal cortex screw penetration just ulnar to Lister's tubercle, which may be missed on lateral fluoroscopic images.

- Intra-articular involvement on plain films will many times warrant obtaining a CT scan for preoperative fracture fixation planning (Fig. 11-10).

- **Advanced imaging (MRI)**
  - Although not commonly used, this modality can be employed to investigate concomitant soft tissue injuries such as SL/LT ligament disruption or TFCC tears.

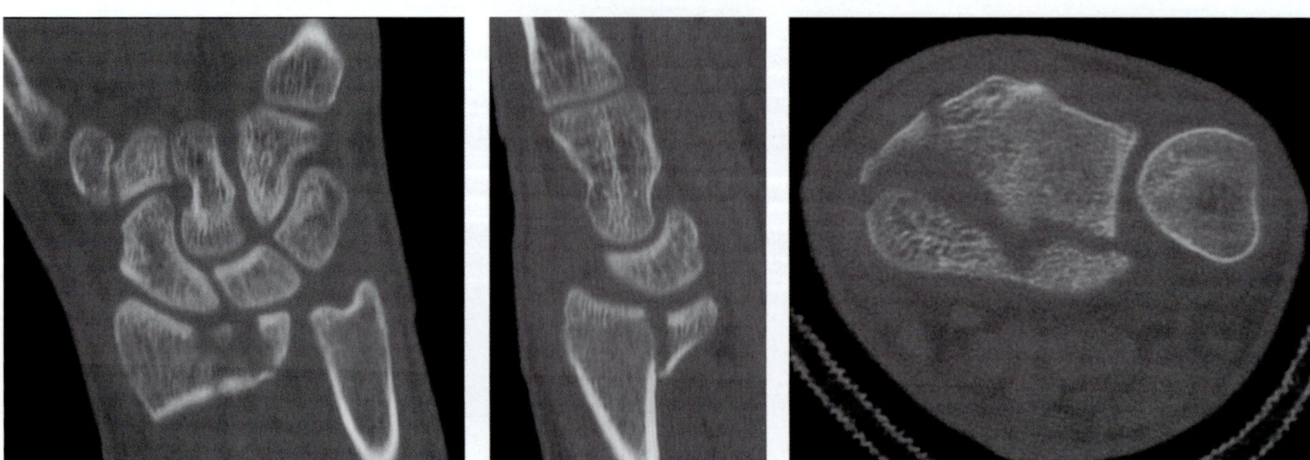

Figure 11-10 | CT scan showing displacement of volar lunar facet with volar radiocarpal subluxation.

Preoperative Imaging

- Appropriate preoperative x-rays of the wrist are critical in accurate characterization of distal radius fractures.
- Radiographic examination should include at minimum PA, lateral, and oblique views. Tilt views and advanced imaging can further elucidate the nature of comminuted fractures.
- Forearm/elbow/hand/scaphoid views should be taken as well if there is any concern for concomitant injuries.
- The radiographic indications for operative management are based on severity of radial shortening/angulation, comminution, displacement, and intra-articular involvement.
- Indications for reduction and of fracture instability, requiring operative fixation, are shown in Tables 11-1 and 11-2.

Intraoperative Positioning

- Percutaneous pinning, external fixation, and open reduction internal fixation (ORIF) are all surgical options for treating distal radius fractures. External fixation may be combined with percutaneous pinning
- Options for ORIF include volar or dorsal plating, fragment specific fixation, as well as bridge plate fixation.
- For all operative treatments of distal radius fractures, the patient will be positioned supine on the operating table with the operative extremity placed on a radiolucent hand table.
- A mini C-arm provides adequate images, involves less radiation exposure, and does not require an x-ray technician to operate. However, a traditional C-arm can be utilized.

1. Supine Positioning

- The injured arm should be abducted 90 degrees and placed on an armboard that is at the same height as the operating table.
- A radiolucent armboard is used to facilitate intraoperative fluoroscopy.
- The C-arm may be brought in on the ipsilateral side, or parallel to the patient and operating room table. The operative extremity can be then positioned on the flat portion of the mini C-arm. Images can be obtained by manipulating the injured wrist so that the beam can be aimed either horizontally or vertically (Fig. 11-11).
- The C-arm can be brought in and out of the surgical field as needed to obtain desired images of the reduction and fixation.
- Before beginning the surgical procedure, a detailed fluoroscopic examination should be performed to confirm the nature of the fracture. This may include traction views.

Table 11-1 | Indications for Reduction of Distal Radius Fractures

Indications for Fracture Reduction	
Dorsal tilt	>10 degrees
Articular step-off	>2 mm
Loss of radial height	>5 mm
Radial inclination	<15 degrees

Table 11-2 | Indication of Fracture Instability Requiring Operative Fixation

Indications of Fracture Instability
>10 degrees loss of volar tilt
>5 mm of radial shortening
>2 mm of articular step-off
Comminution of dorsal and palmar cortices
Irreducible fracture
Loss of fracture reduction at follow-up

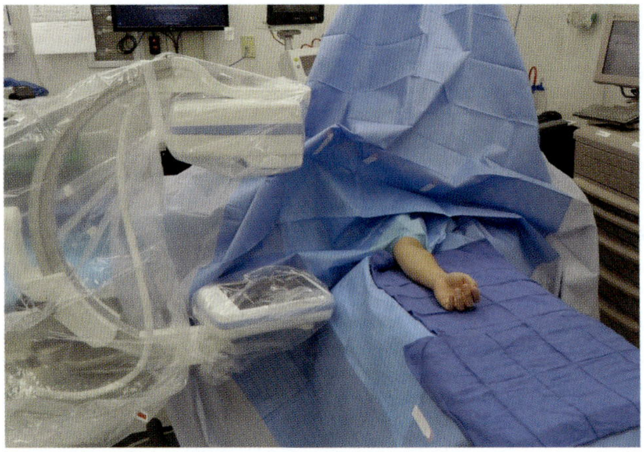

Figure 11-11 | Vertical mini C-arm positioning allows the intensifier to be used as an extension of the hand table. The injured arm can be manipulated to obtain oblique or tilt views as needed.

2. ORIF Tips

- ORIF is the most common method of surgical fixation for distal radius fractures.
- Volar plating has become increasingly popular, as it provides stable internal fixation while avoiding extensor tendon irritation commonly seen with dorsal plates. However, care must be taken to avoid dorsal screw penetration with volar plating, which can also result in extensor tendon irritation and rupture.[9]
- Reduction is of paramount importance during distal radius fixation. Fracture displacement, comminution, and intra-articular involvement help determine the definitive operative technique. Nonetheless, strategically placed percutaneous K-wires can assist in restoring coronal radial length and inclination prior to plate fixation (Fig. 11-12) or suffice as a reduction aid for sagittal volar tilt before final fixation (Fig. 11-13).
- After surgical approach and visualization of the fracture, AP and lateral fluoro views should first be used to assess proper plate positioning on the radius prior to any screw insertion. The plate must be positioned so that distal screws support the subchondral bone but do not violate the articular surface. The plate should be centered on the radius—if too radial, it may be palpable beneath the skin, and if too ulnar, the screws may violate the DRUJ.
- The plate should be provisionally held with K-wires. The distal K-wires can be a visual guide for expected screw trajectory, though variable angle locking plates do allow some adjustment to screw trajectory for maximal purchase in fracture fragments while avoiding the articular surface. Once the plate is positioned correctly, screw fixation to the radius is performed.

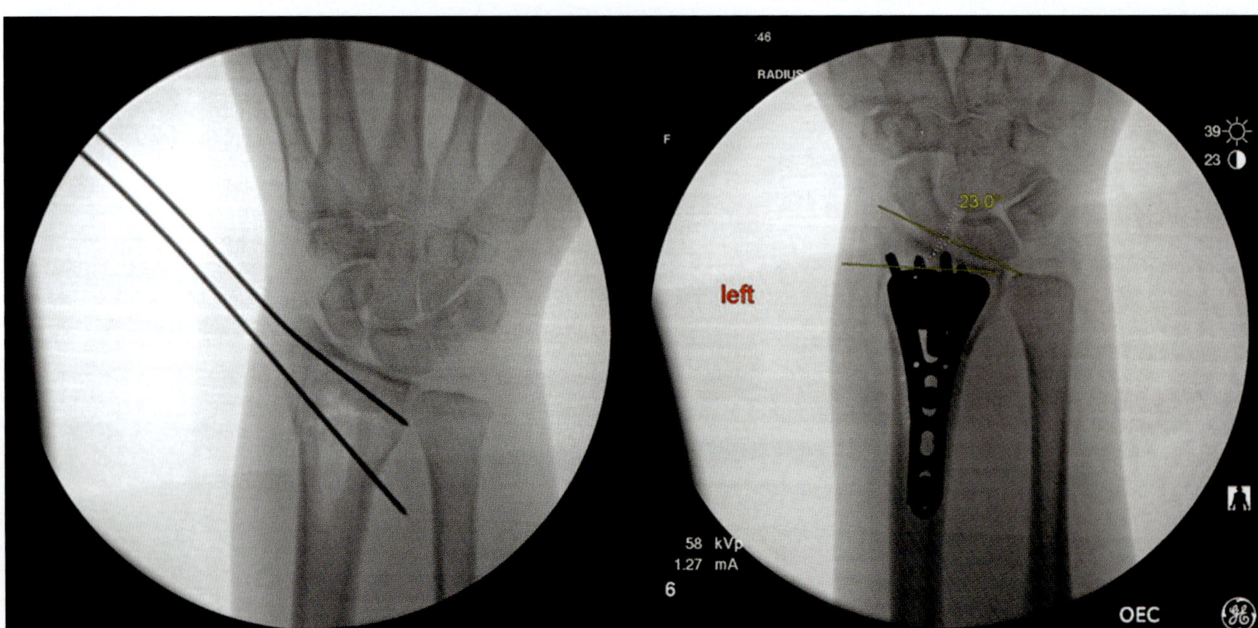

Figure 11-12 | Distal K-wire is used as reduction joystick to restore radial length and inclination prior to temporizing distal wire fixation and eventual plating.

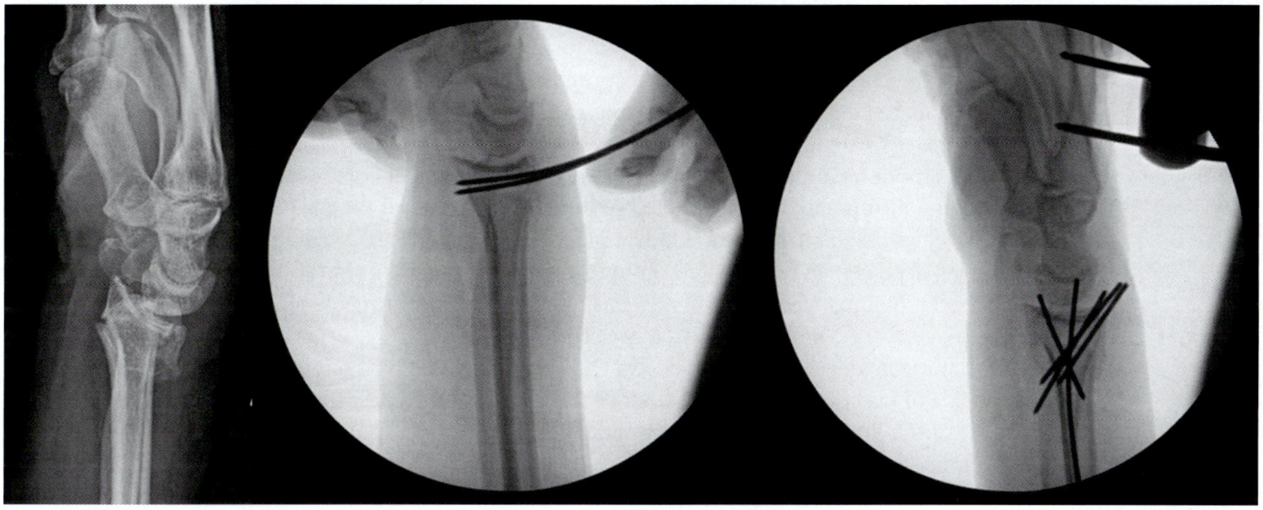

Figure 11-13 | This extreme, comminuted distal radius fracture with significant dorsal tilt was restored with subchondral joystick reduction K-wires followed by numerous fixation K-wires and spanning external fixation.

- The contour of the volar plate can be used to aid in restoring volar tilt if distal locking screws are placed first, followed by cortical screws in the shaft. Note that numerous distal screws are placed first with the plate purposely off the radial shaft. Proximal screws then compress the plate to the volar radial cortex resulting in a mechanical restoration of the sagittal volar tilt. Care must be taken that the plate is properly positioned (with temporary K-wires) before utilizing this maneuver in order to avoid a malreduction or improper plate placement in the coronal plane (Fig. 11-14).

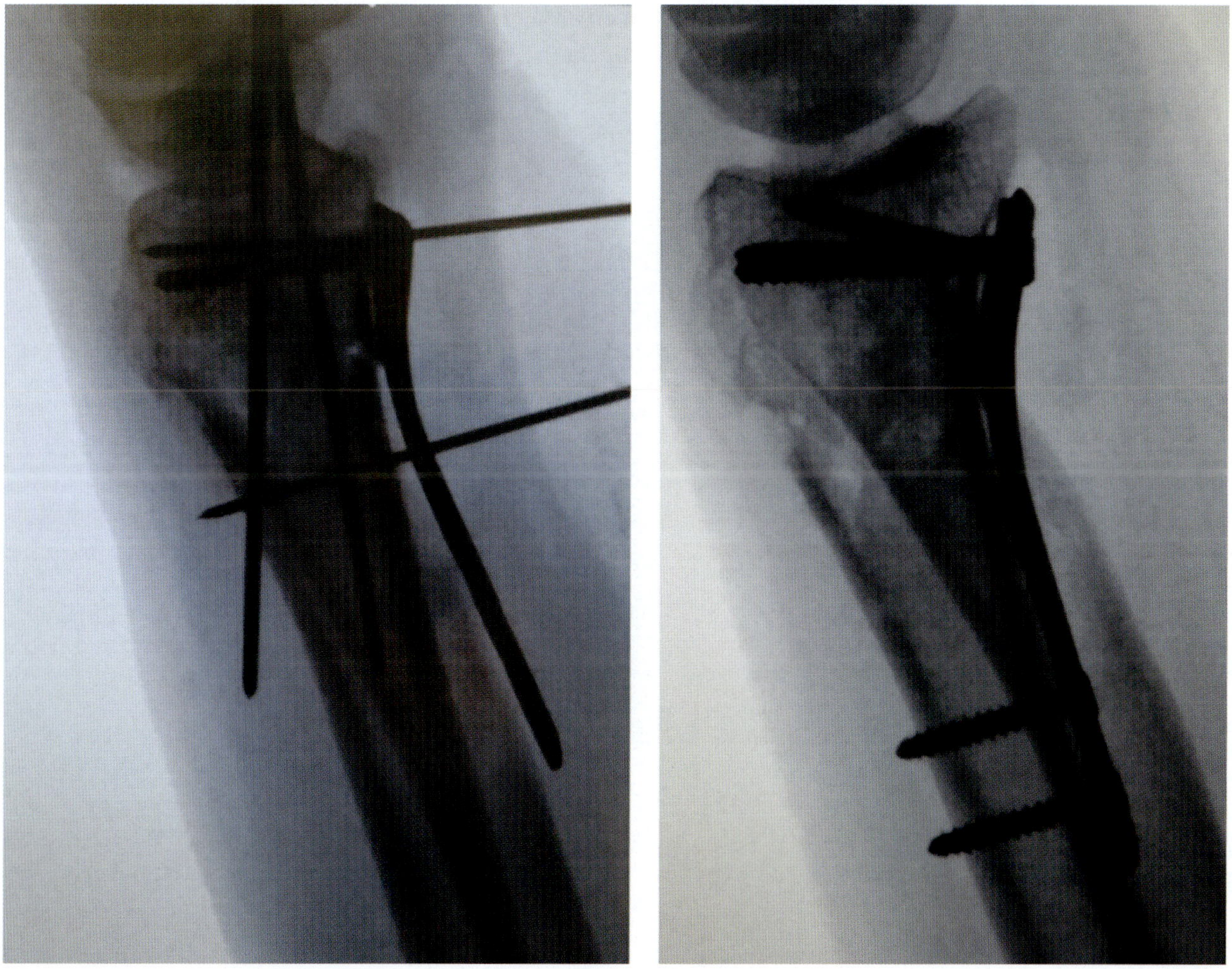

Figure 11-14 | Demonstrates technique using plate to aid reduction, restoring volar tilt.

- When using volar locking plates, the screws will engage the plate and the subchondral bone of the distal radius. There is no need to engage the dorsal cortex, and this should be avoided given close proximity of the extensor tendons. It is recommended that screw lengths be 2 to 4 mm short of the dorsal cortex on a lateral view. Past-pointing should be avoided, as even the leading screw threads can irritate extensor tendons.
- Multiple fluoro views are needed to adequately assess for dorsal cortex screw penetration, including lateral, supinated and pronated oblique, PA tilt, lateral tilt, and dorsal horizon views.[10]
- Lateral tilt views can confirm subchondral placement of radial styloid screws.
- For volarly placed screws, a pronated oblique view can show penetration into the radiocarpal joint. However, even oblique views can be misleading, and so many surgeons also rely on live rotational fluoroscopy views to detect intra-articular screw placement.[11]
- The dorsal horizon view is recommended to ensure there is no dorsal screw penetration, particularly on the ulnar side of Lister's tubercle at the floor of the third dorsal compartment, shown in Figure 11-9.[8]
- The depth of the lunate, as measured on plain lateral radiographs, can be used to predict safe screw lengths.[12]
- Always assess DRUJ stability with the forearm in neural and supination. It is helpful to assess the contralateral uninjured DRUJ preoperatively for comparison.

3. Additional Tips for Intraoperative Fluoroscopy of the Hand and Wrist

- Scaphoid long axis can be well visualized on a PA view by ulnarly deviating the wrist (Fig. 11-15).
- When fixing a Bennett's fracture dislocation, the base of the thumb metacarpal and the CMC joint are best visualized with the wrist in slight flexion and also slightly ulnarly deviated, as pictured (Fig. 11-16).
- When evaluating alignment of the metacarpals and CMC joint congruency, the bases of the index and long metacarpals are best seen on a perfect lateral view of the hand (Fig. 11-17).

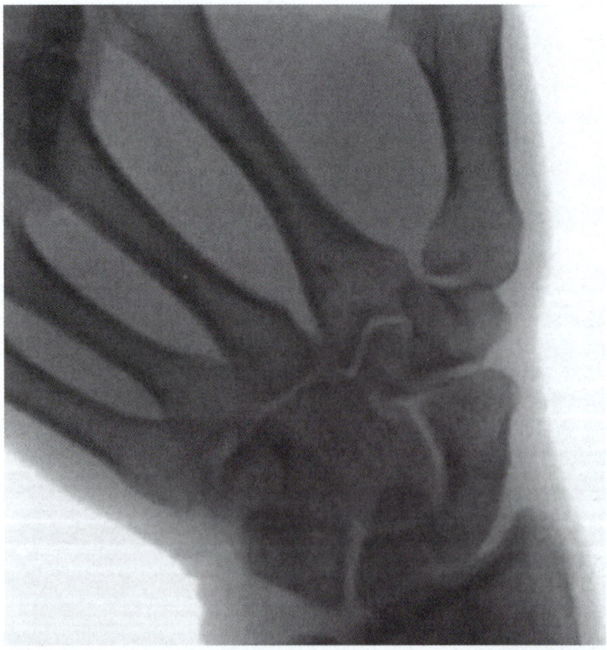

Figure 11-15 | PA ulnar deviated view gives an excellent view of the scaphoid long axis.

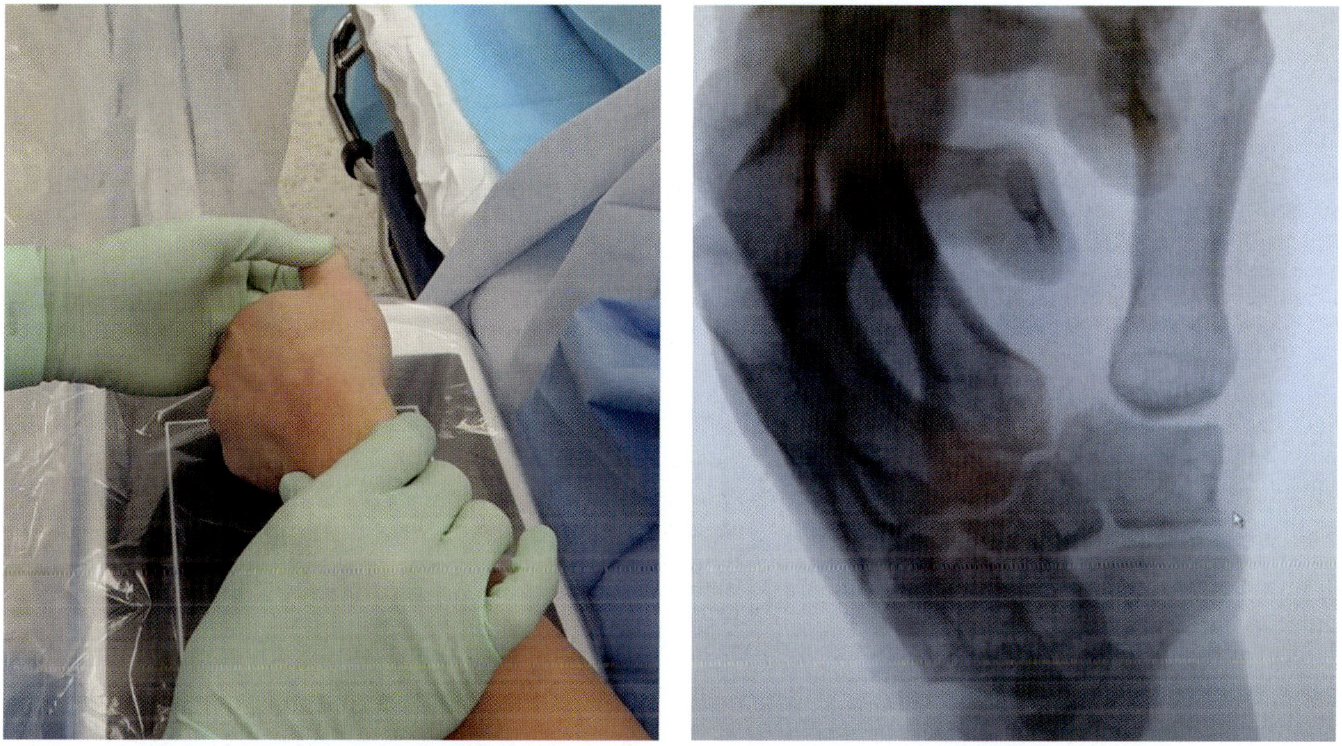

Figure 11-16 | PA view of trapeziometacarpal joint is best seen with wrist in slight flexion and ulnar deviation.

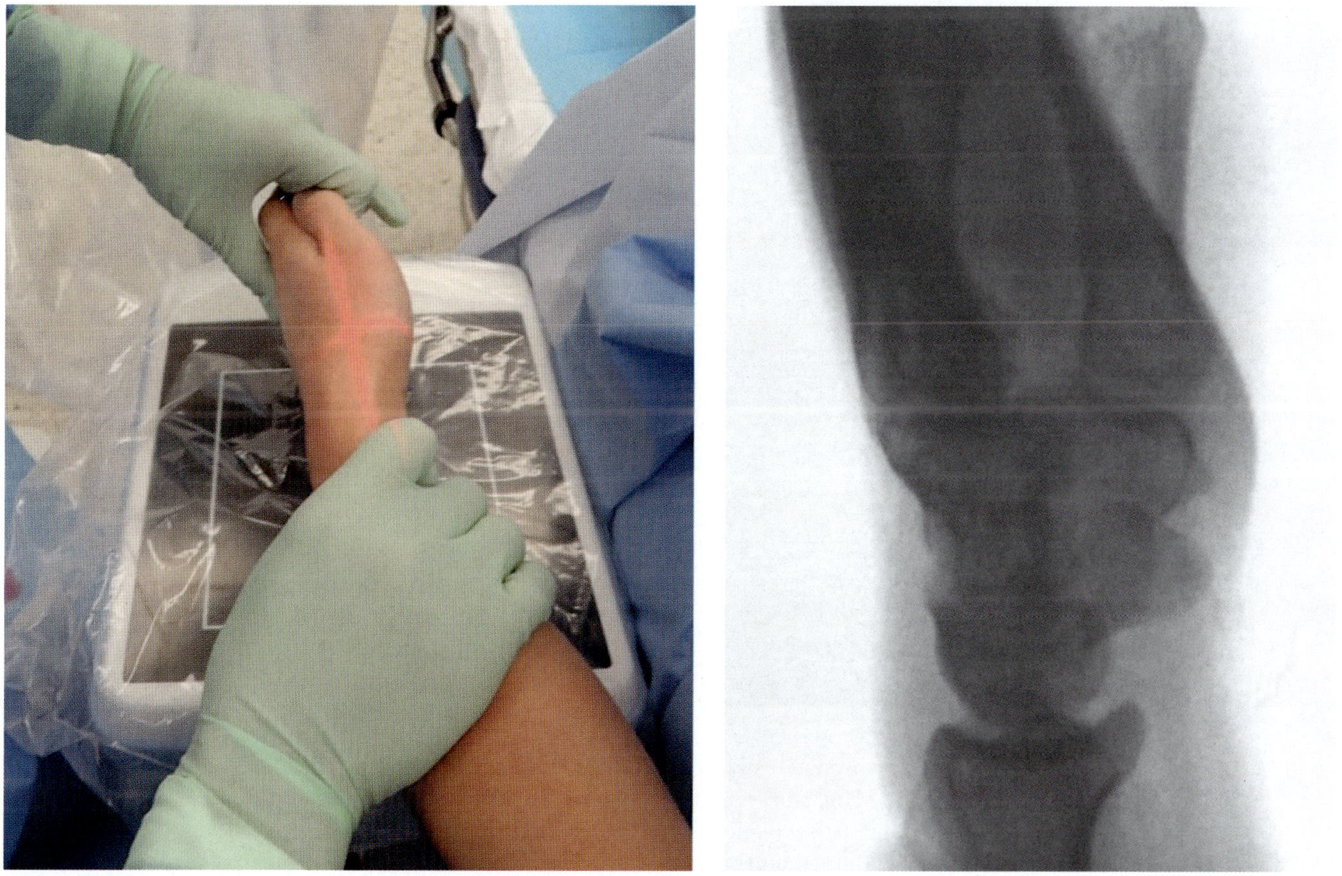

Figure 11-17 | Lining up the index and long finger metacarpal bases will give a perfect lateral of the wrist.

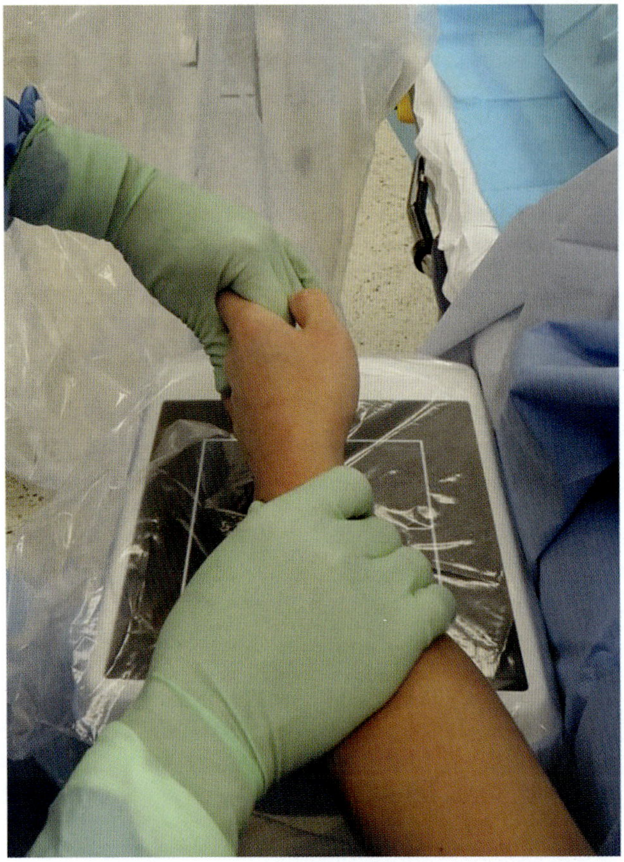

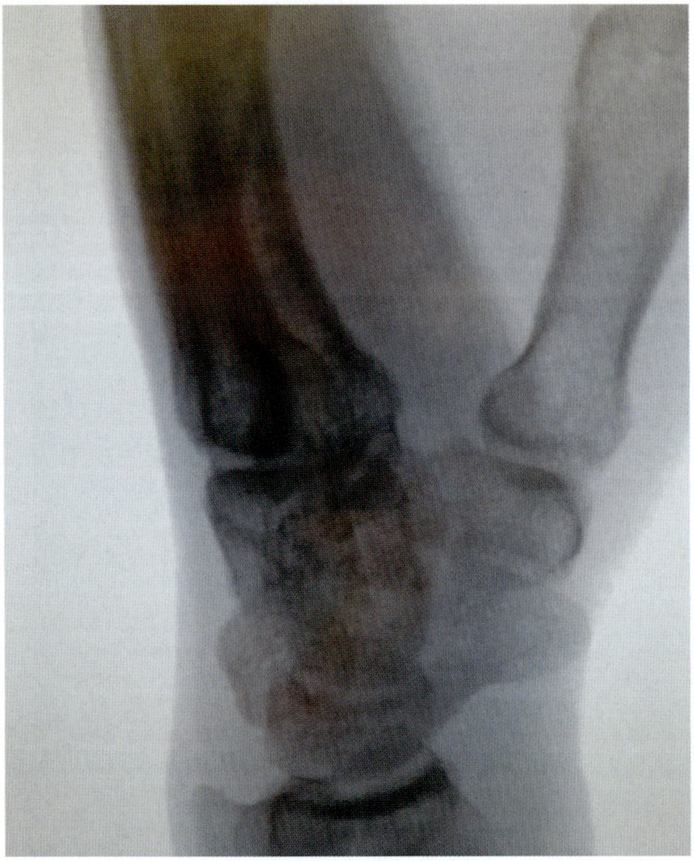

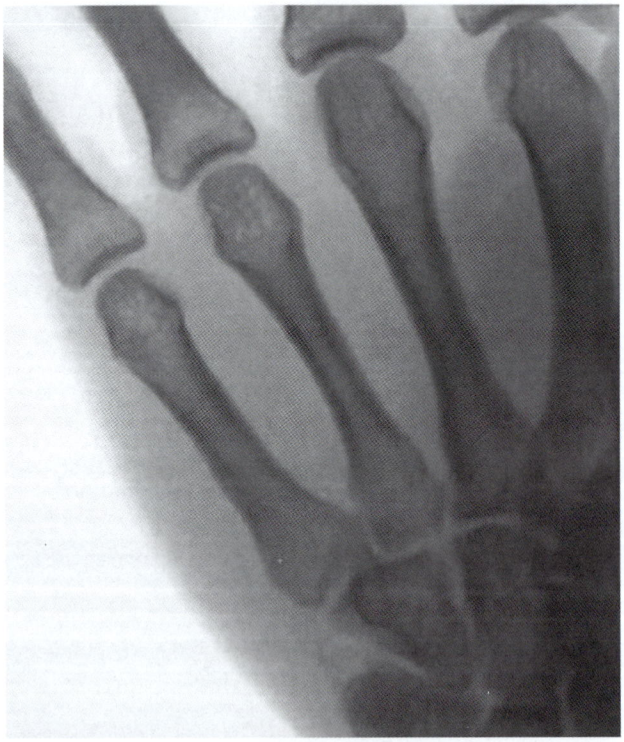

Figure 11-18 | By lining up the ring and small finger metacarpal bases, the articulation of the fourth and fifth CMC joint can be seen. With the hand supinated, an AP view of the articular surface of the ring and small finger metacarpal bases with the hamate can be seen well.

- The hand must be pronated slightly in order to visualize the base of the fourth and fifth metacarpals. The hamate is seen in profile with the hand slightly pronated, and the base of the 4th and 5th metacarpals will align with the hamate when congruently reduced, as pictured below. On an AP view with the hand supinated, the base of the 4th and 5th metacarpals will align with the hamate (Fig. 11-18).

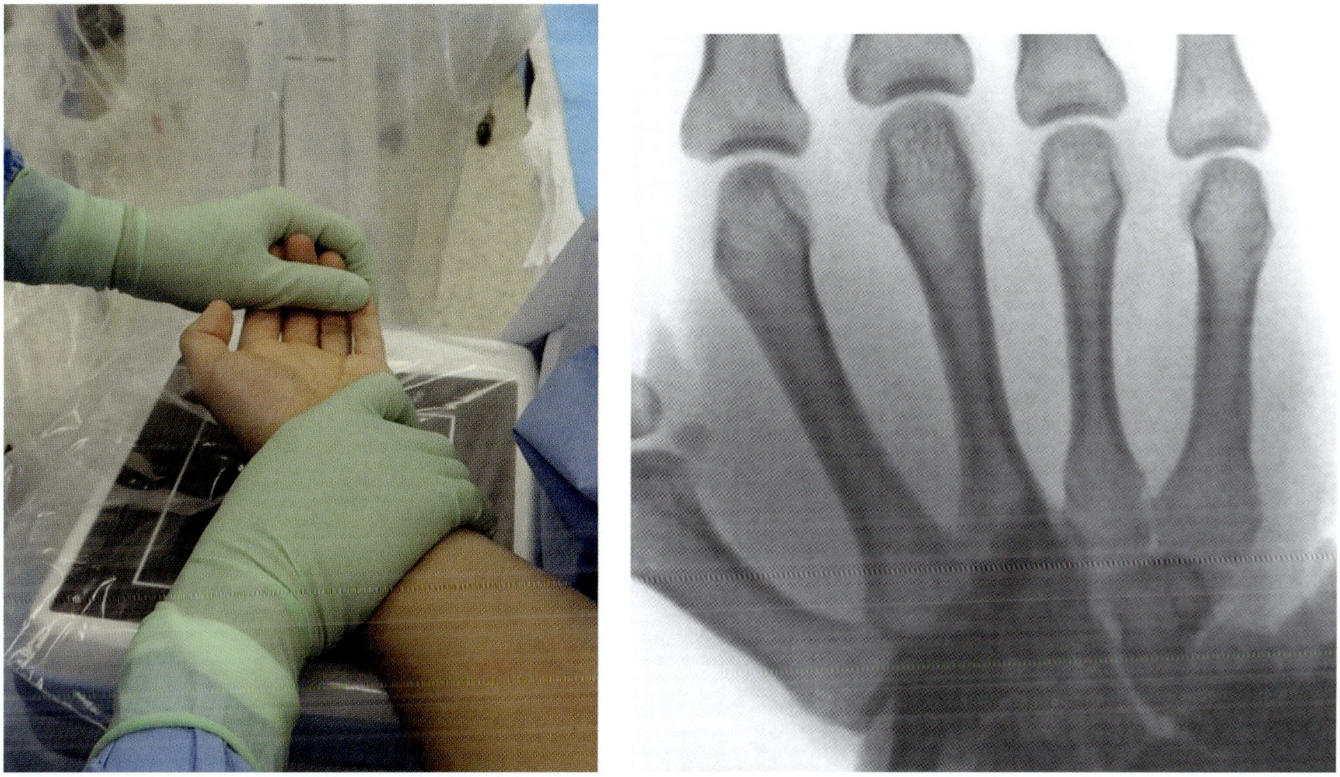

Figure 11-19 | Brewerton view showing articular surfaces of the MCP joints in the coronal plane.

- The MCP joints and metacarpal head fractures are well visualized on a Brewerton view, obtained with the MCP joints flexed and beam angled 15 degrees from the ulnar side of the hand (Fig. 11-19).

References

1. Goldfarb CA, Yin Y, Gilula LA, et al. Wrist fractures: what the clinician wants to know. *Radiology.* 2001;219(1):11–28.
2. Medoff RJ. Essential radiographic evaluation for distal radius fractures. *Hand Clin.* 2005;21(3):279–88.
3. Smith DW, Henry MH. The 45 degrees pronated oblique view for volar fixed-angle plating of distal radius fractures. *J Hand Surg Am.* 2004;29(4):703–706.
4. Soong M, Got C, Katarincic J, et al. Fluoroscopic evaluation of intra-articular screw placement during locked volar plating of the distal radius: a cadaveric study. *J Hand Surg Am.* 2008;33(10):1720–1723.
5. Joseph SJ, Harvey JN. The dorsal horizon view: detecting screw protrusion at the distal radius. *J Hand Surg Am.* 2011;36(10):1691–1693.
6. Haug LC, Glodny B, Deml C, et al. A new radiological method to detect dorsally penetrating screws when using volar locking plates in distal radial fractures. The dorsal horizon view. *Bone Joint J.* 2013;95-B(8):1101–1105.
7. Ozer K, Toker S. Dorsal tangential view of the wrist to detect screw penetration to the dorsal cortex of the distal radius after volar fixed-angle plating. *Hand (NY).* 2011;6(2):190–193.
8. Ozer K, Wolf JM, Watkins B, et al. Comparison of 4 fluoroscopic views for dorsal cortex screw penetration after volar plating of the distal radius. *J Hand Surg Am.* 2012;37(5):963–967.
9. Sugun TS, Karabay N, Gürbüz Y, et al. Screw prominences related to palmar locking plating of distal radius. *J Hand Surg Eur Vol.* 2011;36(4):320–324.
10. Hill BW, Shakir I, Cannada LK. Dorsal screw penetration with the use of volar plating of distal radius fractures: how can you best detect? *J Orthop Trauma.* 2015;29(10):e408–e413.
11. Tweet ML, Calfee RP, Stern PJ. Rotational fluoroscopy assists in detection of intra-articular screw penetration during volar plating of the distal radius. *J Hand Surg Am.* 2010;35(4):619–627.
12. Ljungquist KL, Agnew SP, Huang JI. Predicting a safe screw length for volar plate fixation of distal radius fractures: lunate depth as a marker for distal radius depth. *J Hand Surg Am.* 2015;40(5):940–944.

Chapter 12
Iliosacral Screws

GEOFFREY S. MARECEK

Bony Anatomy

- The pelvis is composed of two innominate bones and the sacrum. The innominate bone and sacrum are joined at the sacroiliac joint. The joint has complex geometry, and multiple views are required to confirm appropriate reduction and safe implant position.
- The sacrum is roughly trapezoidal in the axial plane with the widest point anteriorly and inverted-triangular in the coronal plane with the base at the lumbosacral articulation. In the sagittal plane, the sacrum may be straight or markedly curved but is usually linear through the upper sacral segments.
- The sacrum is perforated with tunnels for the sacral nerve roots. The tunnels slope caudally and laterally from the spinal canal to their exit points.

Radiographic Anatomy

AP

- In a true AP view, the tip of the coccyx will be aligned with the superior border of the pubic symphysis. This ensures appropriate rotation and pelvic tilt. The pelvic brim gently curves from the symphysis to the sacroiliac joint where it meets the anterior border of the sacrum.
- Asymmetry in the AP pelvis will provide information about the displacement of the hemipelvis (Figs. 12-1 and 12-2).

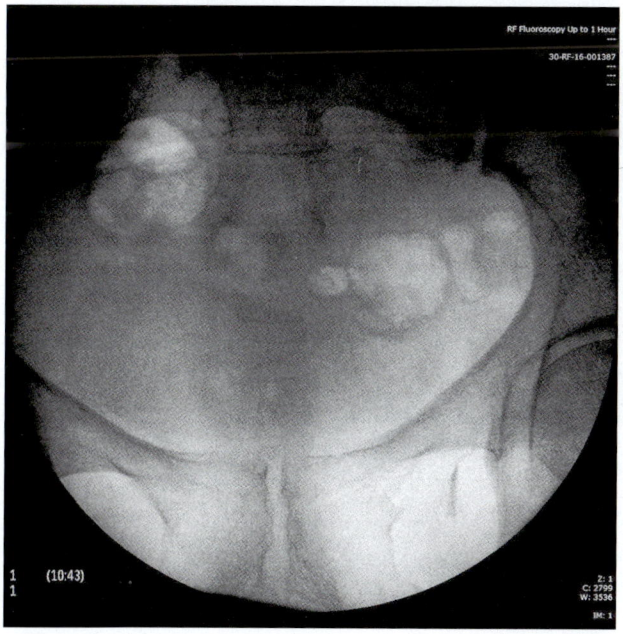

Figure 12-1 AP fluoroscopic view of the pelvis. Note the tip of the coccyx is at the superior aspect of the pubic symphysis.

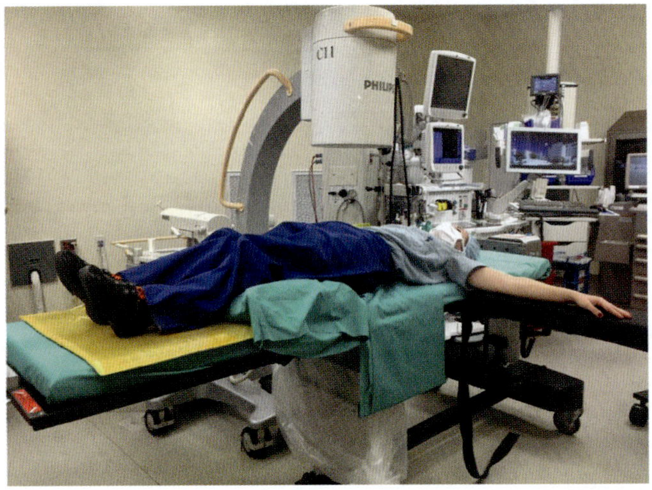

Figure 12-2 | Patient and C-arm positioning for AP fluoroscopic view of the pelvis.

Inlet

- The inlet view provides information and detail about anteroposterior displacement and rotational deformity of the hemipelvis.
- A true inlet view is parallel to the anterior cortex of the sacral segment of interest. An estimate of the orientation of the beam can be obtained from the sagittal reformat on the preoperative CT scan.
- The indentations formed by the alar slope are easily seen on this view and are the anterior limit of safe screw position in the 1st sacral segment. These indentations may be particularly pronounced with sacral dysmorphism (Figs. 12-3 and 12-4).

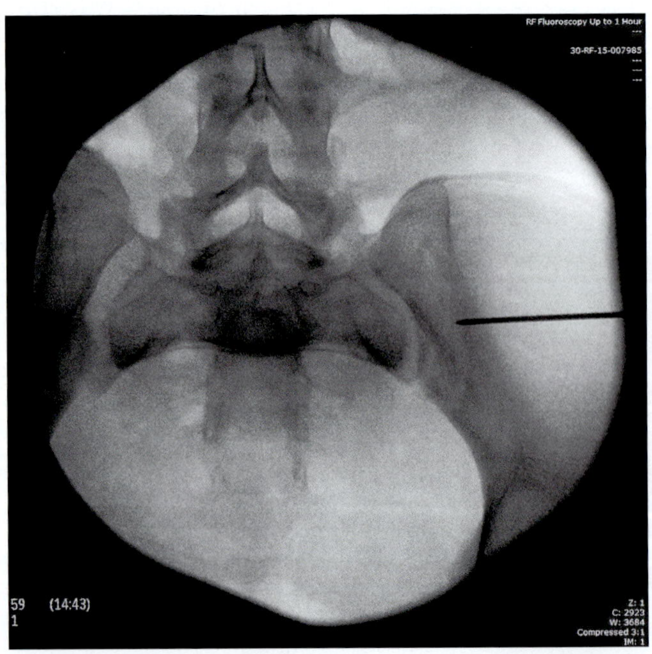

Figure 12-3 | Inlet fluoroscopic view of the posterior pelvic ring. The sacral promonotory and upper segment are collinear.

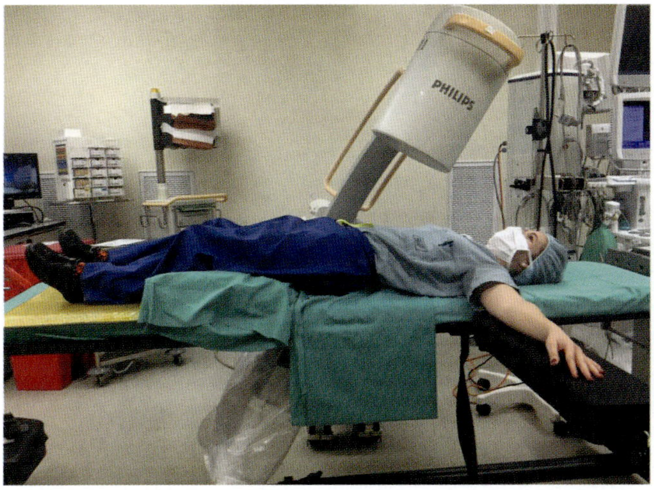

Figure 12-4 | Patient and C-arm positioning for inlet fluoroscopic view of the pelvis.

Outlet

- The outlet view provides information about craniocaudal displacement of the hemipelvis. Information about flexion-extension can also be gleaned by observing differences in the shapes of the obturator foramina.
- A true outlet view provides an *en face* view of the sacral nerve tunnel exits at the sacral segment desired. Appropriate rotation is achieved when the spinous processes are in line with the pubic symphysis. An estimate of the orientation of the beam can be obtained from the sagittal reformat on the preoperative CT scan.
- The lateral borders of the nerve root tunnels are best visualized on the outlet view. A sacral lateral view should be obtained when the drill bit or wire reaches the lateral border of the tunnel (Figs. 12-5 and 12-6).

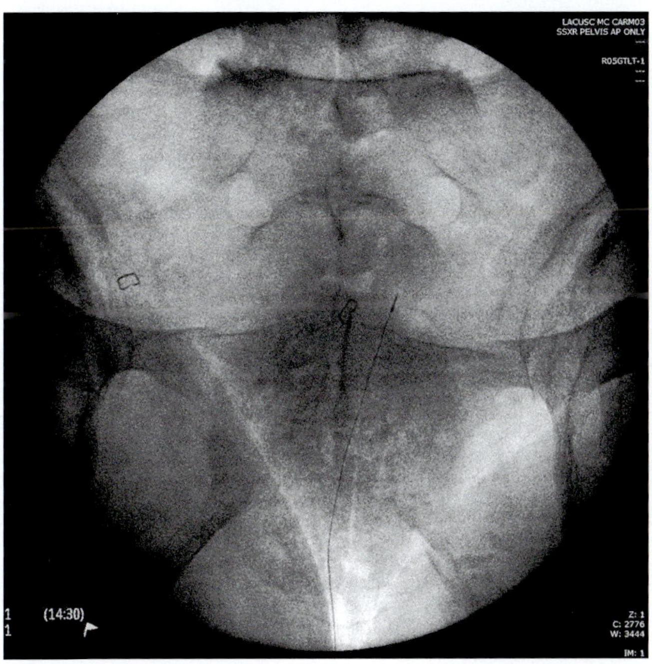

Figure 12-5 | Outlet fluoroscopic view of the pelvis. Note the lateral border of the sacral tunnels sloping toward the tunnel exit.

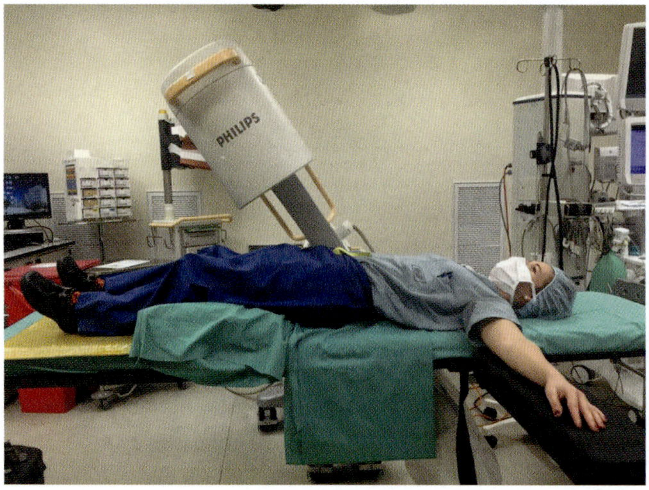

Figure 12-6 | Patient and C-arm positioning for outlet fluoroscopic views of the pelvis.

Lateral

- A true lateral view is critical during iliosacral screw placement to accurately determine the position of the drill prior to passing through the narrowest point of the osseous fixation pathway.
- A sacral lateral is defined by superimposition of the greater sciatic notches (white arrow). The drill tip should reside within the safe zone defined by the sacral ala superiorly, anterior cortex of the sacrum anteriorly, and roof of the 1st sacral nerve root tunnel posterocaudally (black arrowheads) (Figs. 12-7 and 12-8).

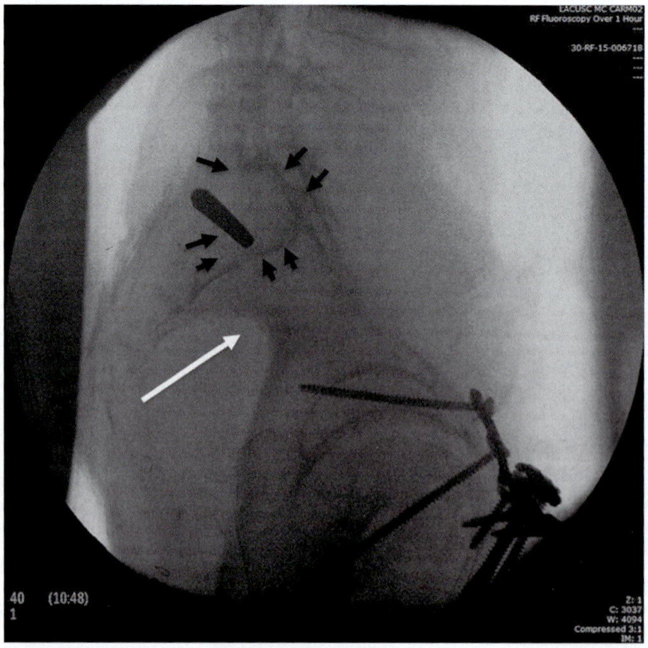

Figure 12-7 | True lateral view of the sacrum. Note overlap of the greater sciatic notch (*white arrow*). The iliac cortical densities overlap at the superior border of the safe zone (*black arrows*).

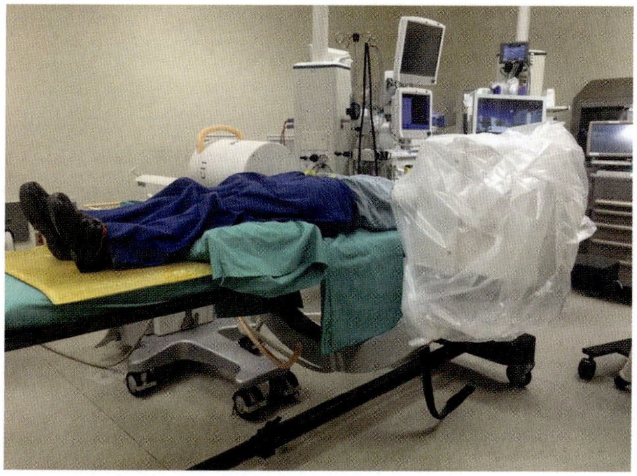

Figure 12-8 | Patient and C-arm positioning for a true lateral view of the sacrum.

"Rollover"

- A "rollover" or "rollback" view is taken tangential to the outer table of the ilium and is typically approximately 15 degrees from the vertical beam position. This view can provide valuable information about when a washer or screw head is flush to the ilium or when a drill or wire has perforated the far ilium. It is also useful during measurement to ensure the depth gauge or subtraction wire is appropriately positioned (Figs. 12-9 and 12-10).

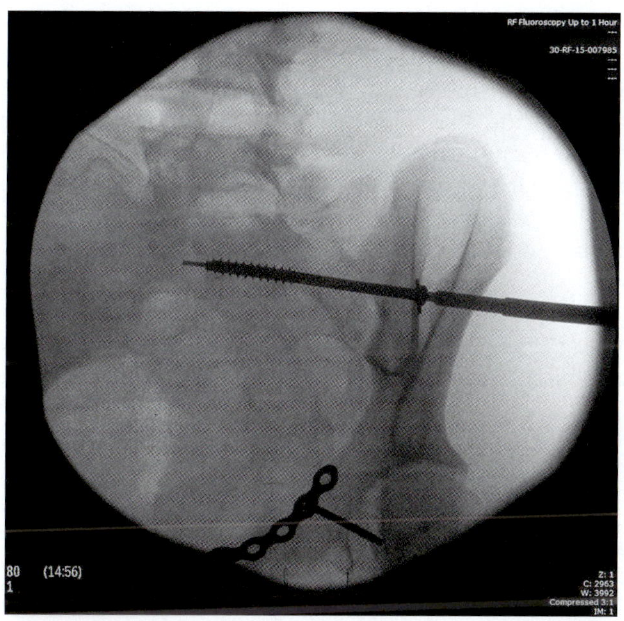

Figure 12-9 | A "rollover" view of the left hemipelvis. The washer is flush with the outer cortex of the ilium.

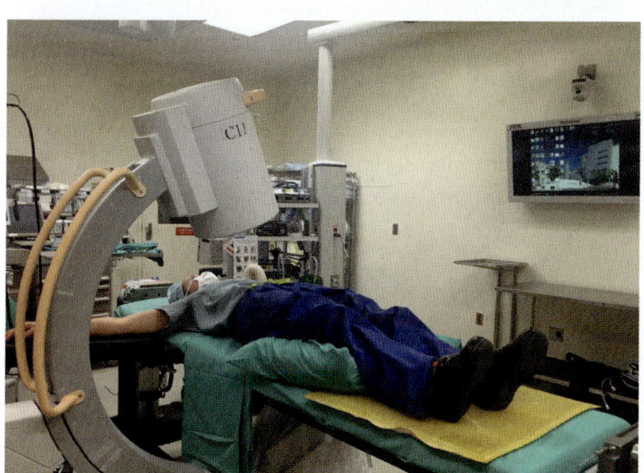

Figure 12-10 | Patient and C-arm positioning for a "rollback" view of the right hemipelvis. This view is useful for identifying screw engagement in the contralateral ilium.

Preoperative Imaging

Radiographs

- AP, inlet, and outlet radiographs are essential for identifying the components of the pelvic ring injury, understanding deformity of the hemipelvis, and planning surgical reduction.
- Additional useful information may be obtained from Judet (iliac and obturator oblique) views.
- Traditionally, inlet and outlet radiographs have been performed with the beam tilted 45 degrees caudally or cranially, respectively, to allow for orthogonal radiographs. More accurate representations can be obtained with 25 degrees inlet tilt and 60 degrees outlet tilt.[1]
- Alternately, plain radiographs representing all five views may be reformatted from the CT scan without loss of accuracy.[2]

CT

- A CT scan is critical for evaluation of pelvic ring injuries. Axial images with coronal and sagittal reformats should be obtained.
- Preoperative assessment of the safe space available for iliosacral screw placement and anticipated screw lengths as well as templating of inlet, outlet, and rollover tilt should be performed.
- The axial CT images may underestimate the volume available for safe screw placement unless the CT is reformatted in the plane of the sacrum.

Sacral Dysmorphism

- Sacral dysmorphism is a failure of segmentation at the lumbosacral junction and may be unilateral or bilateral.
- The characteristic features of dysmorphic sacra are best visualized on the outlet view: irregularly shaped sacral nerve tunnel exits, a residual intervertebral disk between the upper and second sacral segments, the presence of mammillary processes, and the upper sacral segment endplate being collinear with the top of the iliac crests. The axial CT cuts may reveal a tongue-in-groove sacroiliac articulation.[3]
- In dysmorphic sacra, the sacral ala have a steep slope from cranial to caudal, posterior to anterior, and medial to lateral.
- The starting point and trajectory of sacroiliac-style screws will need to be altered for safe placement in the upper sacral segment. Sacral-style screws cannot be safely placed in the upper sacral segment, but a larger volume exists in the second sacral segment for safe screw placement.

Intraoperative Positioning

- The choice of surgical positioning depends on the fracture pattern, associated injuries, anticipated procedure, and surgeon preference.
- A full radiolucent table without central support (e.g., OSI/Jackson) should be used to allow full mobility of the fluoroscopy unit.

Supine

- Supine positioning is commonly used when concomitant open reduction internal fixation of the anterior ring or sacroiliac joint, placement of an anterior external fixator, or percutaneous medullary ramus screw (particularly retrograde) is anticipated.
- Supine positioning may be easier in the setting of polytrauma.
- A soft lumbosacral support should be placed beneath the sacrum, centered at the patient's midline. Folded OR blankets or commercially available ramps can be used.
- The armboards should be placed as cranial as possible with the arms fully extended at 90 degrees as they may prevent proximal translation or caudal tilt of the C-arm (Fig. 12-11).

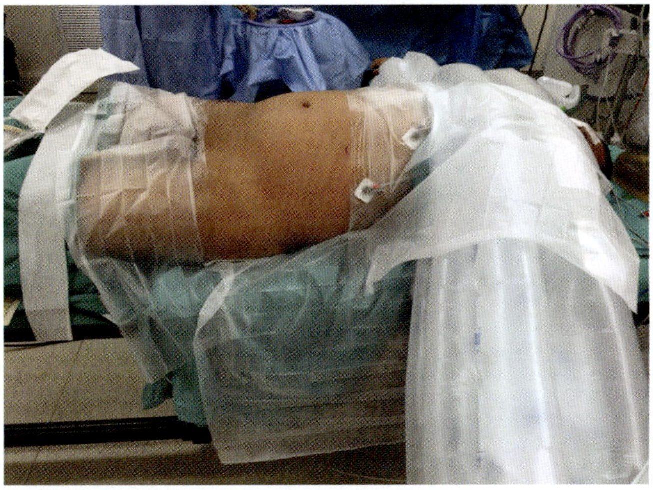

Figure 12-11 | Patient positioing for supine iliosacral screw fixation of the pelvis. The abdomen is prepped from just above the genitalia to the xiphoid process.

Prone

- Prone positioning is commonly used when an open reduction of the posterior ring is planned or when lumbopelvic fixation will be performed.
- The patient should be placed on radiolucent chest rolls. Ensure that the ASIS and iliac crest hang free of the chest rolls to allow manipulation of the hemipelvis.
- The knees and lower extremities must be well padded and the arms should be placed in a comfortable resting position that avoids tension on the brachial plexus (Fig. 12-12).

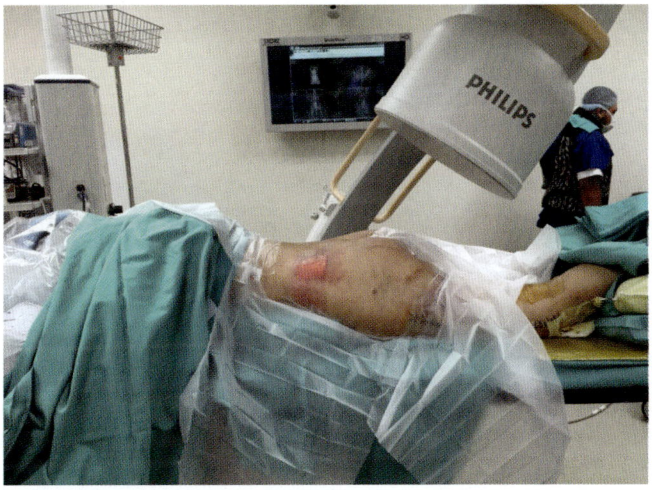

Figure 12-12 | Prone positioing for iliosacral screw fixation of the pelvis. The entire back and flank are prepped in. The intergluteal cleft is excluded.

Additional Tips

- Nitrous oxide anesthetic should be avoided as the gas will enhance the bowel and potentially obscure important bony detail.
- Reproducible quality fluoroscopic views are critical. Ask the fluoroscopist to mark the position of the C-arm beam and the wheels on the floor for the inlet and outlet views.

References

1. Ricci WM, Mamczak C, Tynan M, et al. Pelvic inlet and outlet radiographs redefined. *J Bone Joint Surg Am.* 2010;92(10):1947–1953.
2. Bishop JA, Rao AJ, Pouliot MA, et al. Conventional versus virtual radiographs of the injured pelvis and acetabulum. *Skeletal Radiol.* 2015;44(9):1303–1308.
3. Miller AN, Routt ML Jr. Variations in sacral morphology and implications for iliosacral screw fixation. *J Am Acad Orthop Surg.* 2012;20(1):8–16.

Chapter 13
Superior Medullary Ramus Screw

RAYMOND D. WRIGHT JR
JASON L. SHEWMAKER

Bony Anatomy

- The superior medullary ramus is an irregularly shaped bone that constitutes the anterior portion of the pubic region of the innominate bone.
- The anterior surface of the superior ramus is asymmetrical and provides the origin for several hip adduction muscles that may contribute deforming forces.
- The posterior surface is smooth but concave and forms the anterior border of the true pelvis (Fig. 13-1).
- The superior surface has an undulating contour that begins medially with the pubic tubercle (rectus attachment) near the midline. The pectineus recess is present just lateral to the pubic tubercle and represents a narrow corridor with the femoral neurovascular bundle just above (red arrow with vessels and nerves below). As the ramus precedes cranial, lateral, and posterior, the ramus becomes wider on its superior surface. The iliopectineal eminence is present as the anterior portion of the acetabular anterior wall and lies just medial to the iliopsoas gutter. Lateral to this is another narrow corridor adjacent to the acetabular dome (red arrow) (Fig. 13-2).
- Although 3D reconstruction CT remodeling has been advocated to determine the safe zones of the superior medullary ramus, it is important to note that the corridor is determined by the safe placement of a screw utilizing intraoperative fluoroscopy and that female gender and fracture patterns may limit acceptable screw diameter, length, and angulation.

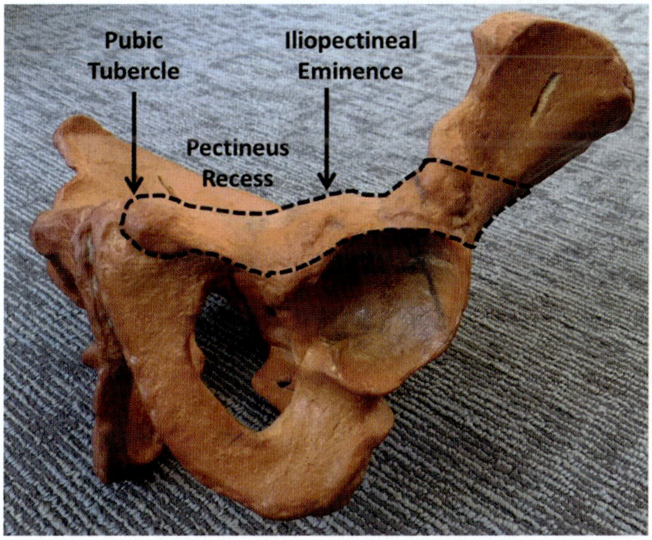

Figure 13-1 | Oblique view of a synthetic bone pelvic model demonstrating the region of the superior medullary ramus.

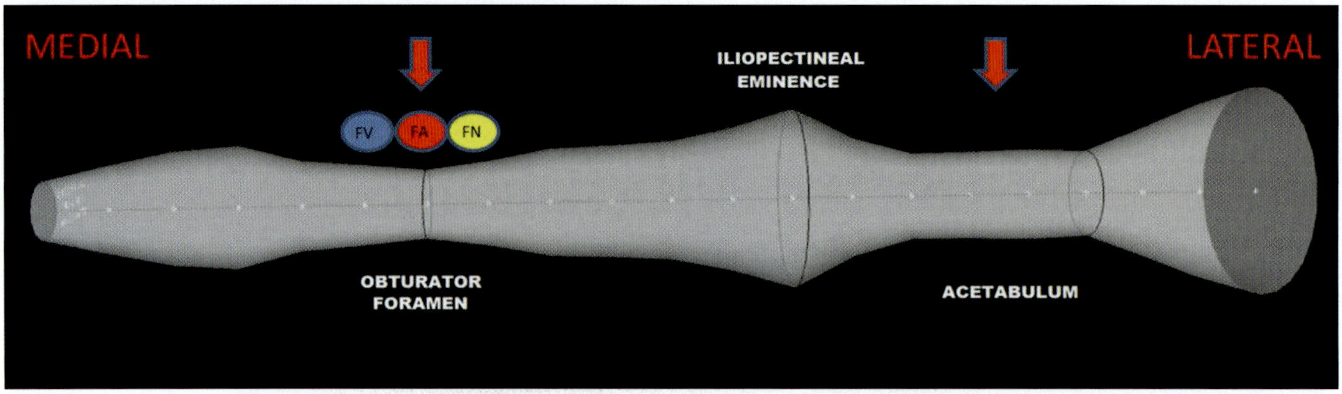

Figure 13-2 | A linear extrapolation of the superior medullary ramus. The variance in available osseous volume for medullary screw containment is demonstrated.

Preoperative Imaging

AP View

- Screening study—essential for all patients with pelvic fracture.
- Should include the entire pelvis.
- Symphysis pubis should be centered on film and be aligned with coccyx and lumbar spinous processes (Fig. 13-3).

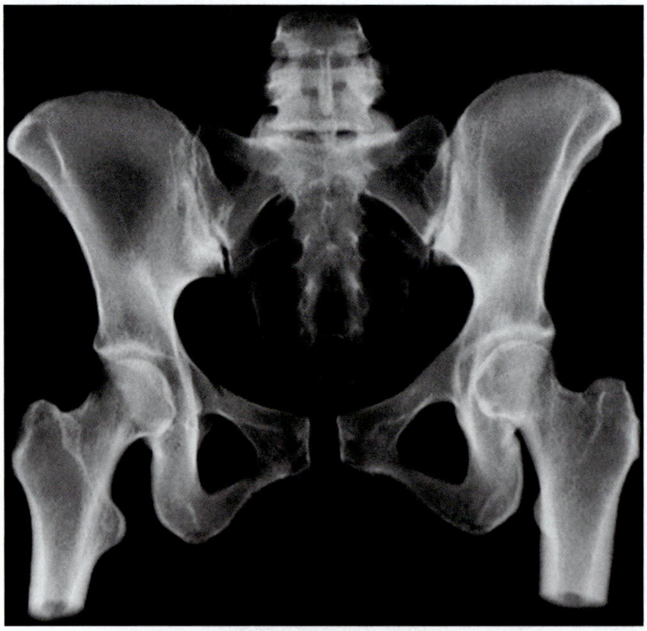

Figure 13-3 | AP pelvis radiograph.

Inlet/40- to 45-Degree Caudal View

- Variable inlet tilt—depends on patient's degree of lumbosacral lordosis.
- Upper and second sacral segments should overlap.
- Allows provider to inspect anteroposterior displacement as well as lateral displacement of osseous pelvic structures (Fig. 13-4).

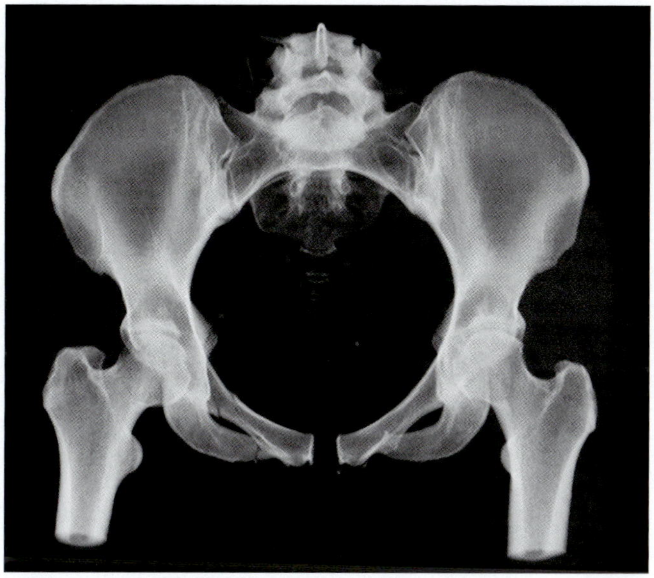

Figure 13-4 | Inlet pelvis view.

Outlet/15- to 40-Degree Cranial View

- Variable outlet tilt—depends on the patient's degree of lumbosacral lordosis
- Ideally centers upper portion of symphysis at second sacral segment or slightly lower
- Allows practitioner to inspect craniocaudal displacement as well as lateral displacement of osseous pelvic structures (Fig. 13-5).

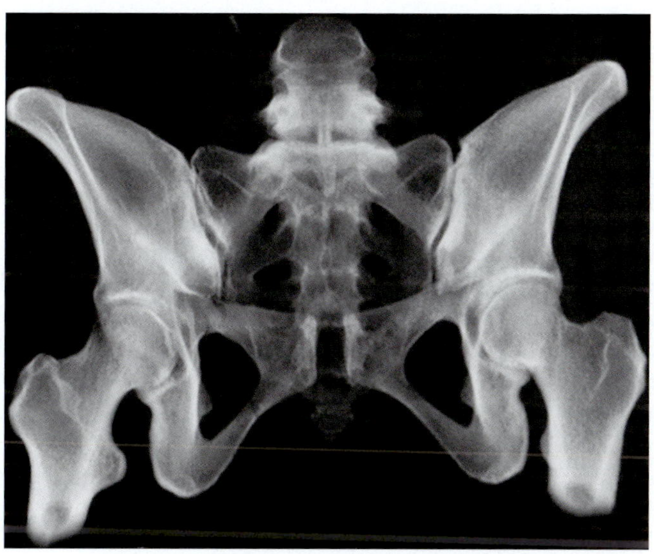

Figure 13-5 | Outlet pelvis view.

Judet Oblique View (Obturator Oblique)

- Allows for preoperative planning—determining if the superior ramus will accept and contain a medullary superior ramus screw.
- This view provides for understanding cranial or caudal displacement of the superior ramus at the pubic root.
- Acetabular fractures (if any) can be evaluated best on this view (Fig. 13-6).

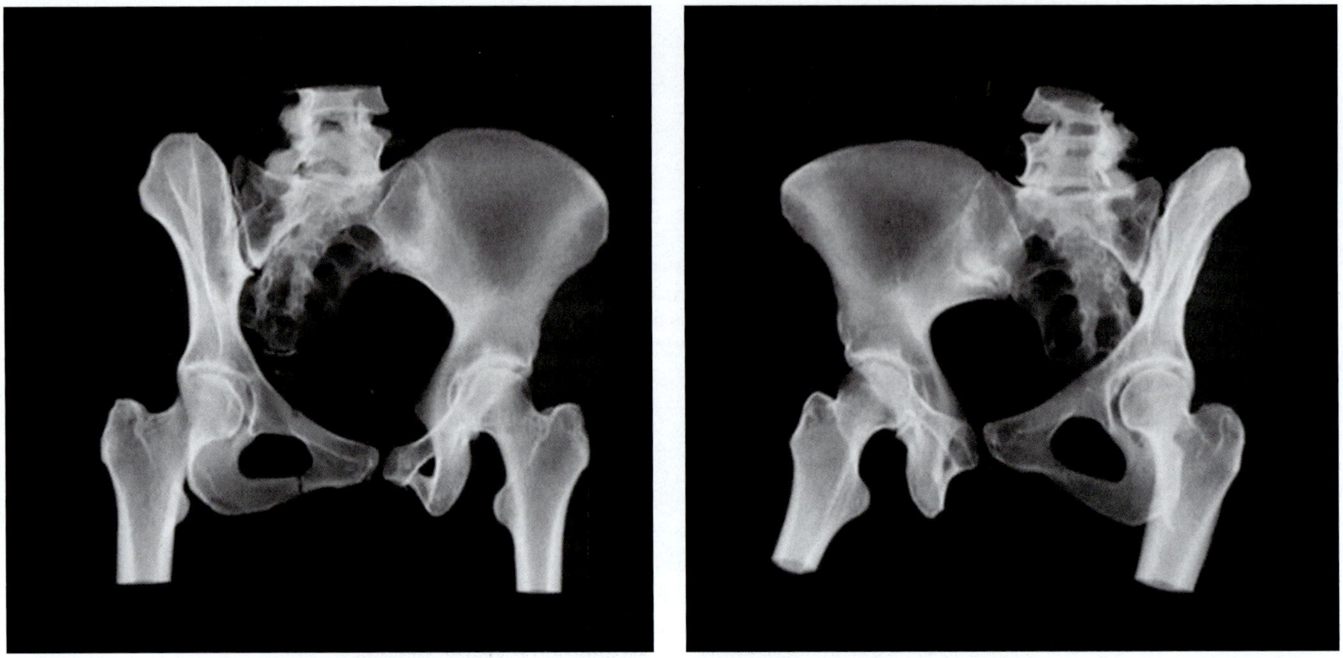

Figure 13-6 | Judet oblique views of the pelvis.

Intraoperative Positioning

1. Supine Position

- The patient is placed supine on a radiolucent table. A midline lumbosacral bump is placed to elevate the pelvis and extend the hips.
- Both antegrade and retrograde insertion of superior ramus screws are possible in the supine position (Fig. 13-7).[1]

Two views are required to safely place medullary superior ramus screws: an inlet view and an obturator-outlet oblique view.

- Fluoroscopic guidance for a superior screw requires accuracy and reproducibility on the part of the fluoroscope operator. The C-arm is generally set up on the unaffected side.
- The **inlet view** is obtained by tilting the C-arm 15 to 25 degrees cephalad.
  - Appropriate tilt is achieved when the superior and inferior rami create a minimally visible obturator foramen.
  - The superior and inferior rami should not be superimposed (Fig. 13-8).
  - The field of view should include a hemipelvis with the affected side ASIS at approximately 1 o'clock on the left hemipelvis and the ASIS at 11 o'clock for the right hemipelvis.
  - The contralateral portion of the pubic symphysis should just be visible on screen (Fig. 13-9A and B).

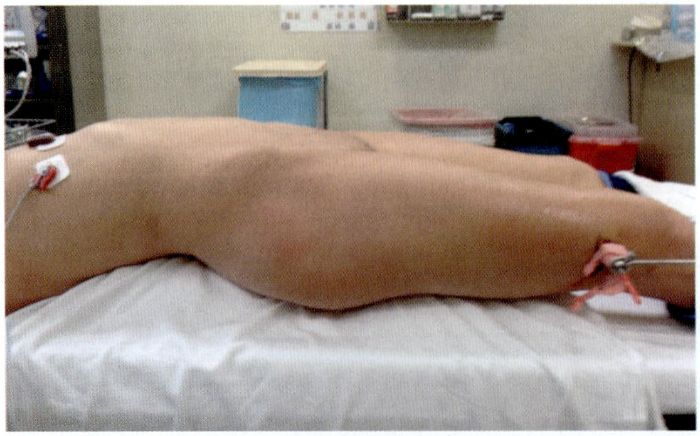

Figure 13-7 | A patient is placed supine on a radiolucent table in preparation for medullary ramus screw. A lumbosacral bump is placed in the patient's midline to elevate the pelvis from the table and extend the patient's hips.

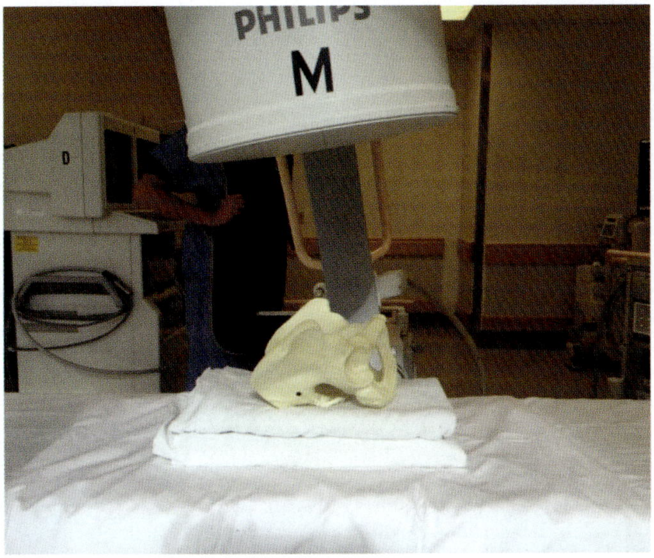

Figure 13-8 | Inlet view in the supine position. The inlet tilt should be adjusted such that the superior and inferior rami are not superimposed. This amount of inlet tilt varies based on the patient's lumbosacral lordosis.

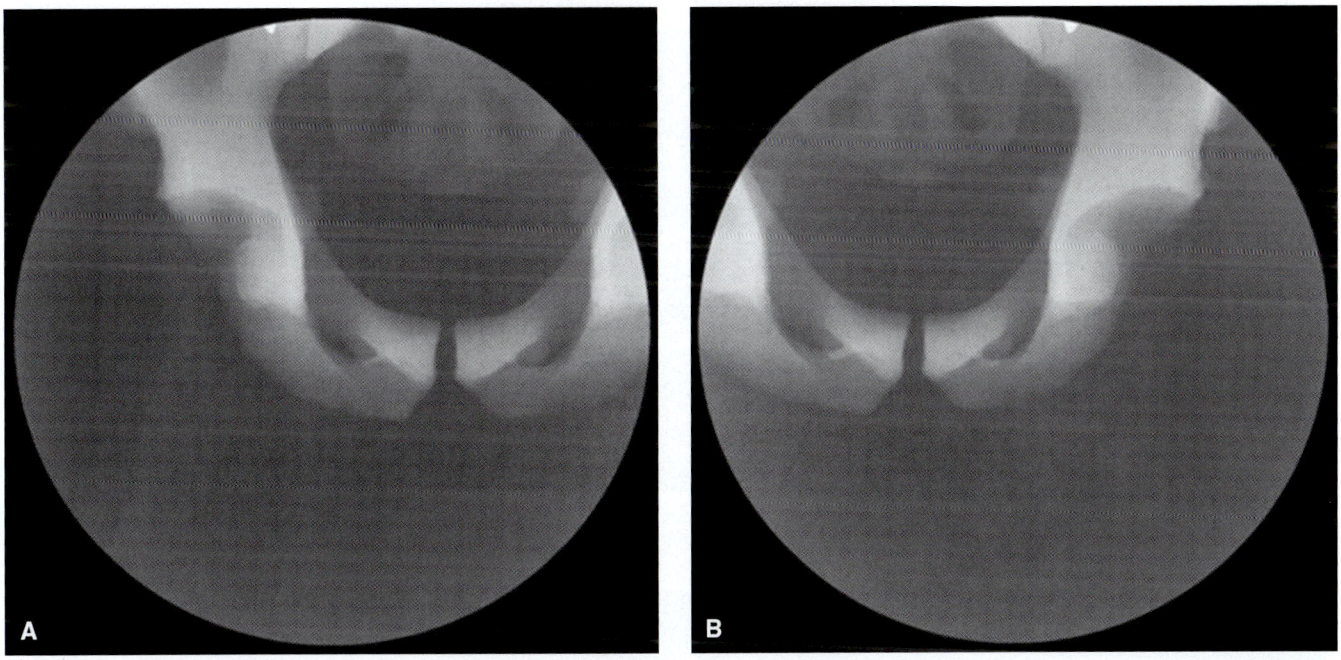

Figure 13-9 | Inlet image of right hemipelvis **(A)** and left hemipelvis **(B)**. The inlet tilt has been adjusted such that the superior and inferior rami are not superimposed and that the obturator canal imparts a small amount of separation of the rami. The ASIS is at 11 o'clock on the right and 1 o'clock on the left.

  - The superior ramus centering should be equal on both views in order to prevent overpenetration.
  - In order to achieve diagnostic quality, the image intensifier should be as close to the patient as possible and accurate centering will allow for consistent collimation.
- The second view is an **obturator-outlet oblique**.
- This combined view gives an image of the superior ramus in profile.
- The outlet tilt is achieved by angling the x-ray tube caudally 25 to 35 degrees and arcing the machine toward the affected hemipelvis approximately 25 degrees (Fig. 13-10A and B).
- In the case of the example in Figure 13-10, the fluoroscopist is imaging the right hemipelvis.
- Obturator-outlet oblique view of the contralateral hemipelvis can be obtained by rolling the C-arm back toward the C-arm operator (Fig. 13-11A and B).
- The obturator-outlet oblique images should be adjusted such that the obturator canal is maximally in profile. The exact amount of outlet tilt and appropriate roll will vary from patient to patient. The superior ramus should be centered to achieve optimal imaging quality (Fig. 13-12).

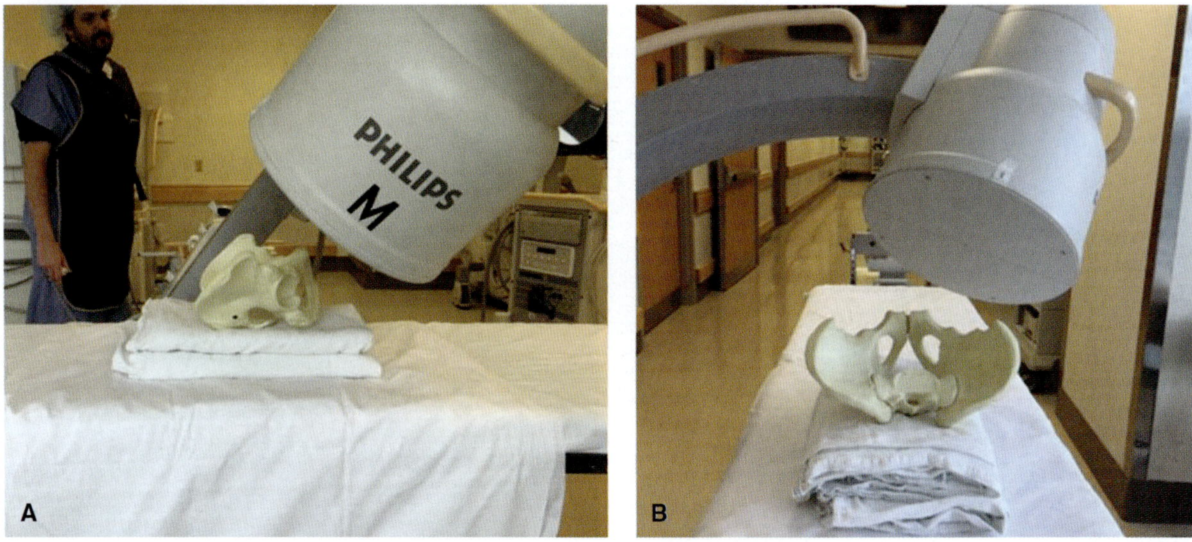

Figure 13-10 I An obturator-outlet oblique is obtained of the right superior ramus. The image intensifier is positioned as closely to the patient as possible **(A)**. The position of the image intensifier is perpendicular to the obturator canal **(B)**.

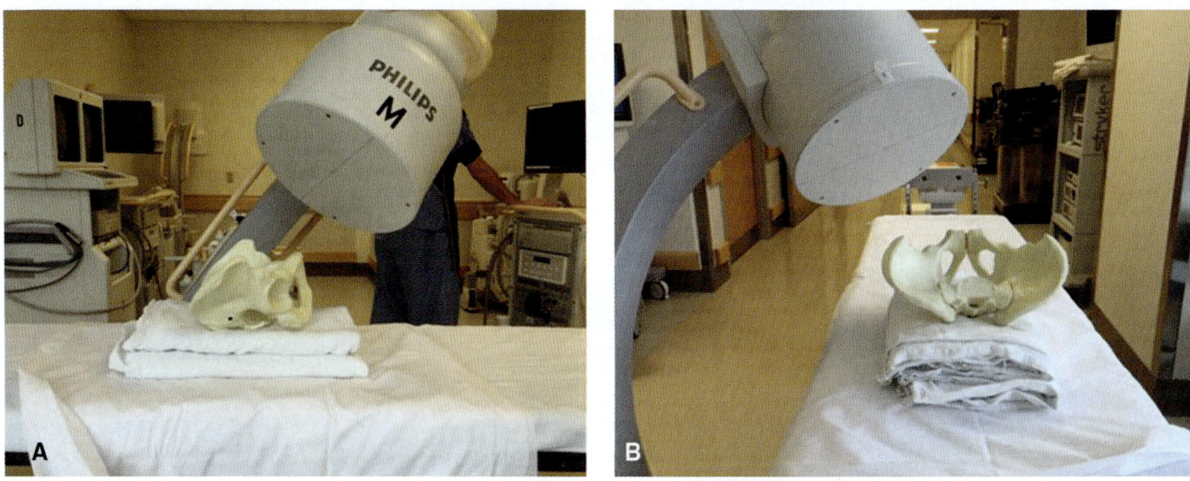

Figure 13-11 I An obturator-outlet oblique is obtained of the left superior ramus. The image intensifier is positioned as closely to the patient as possible **(A)**. The position of the image intensifier is perpendicular to the obturator canal **(B)**.

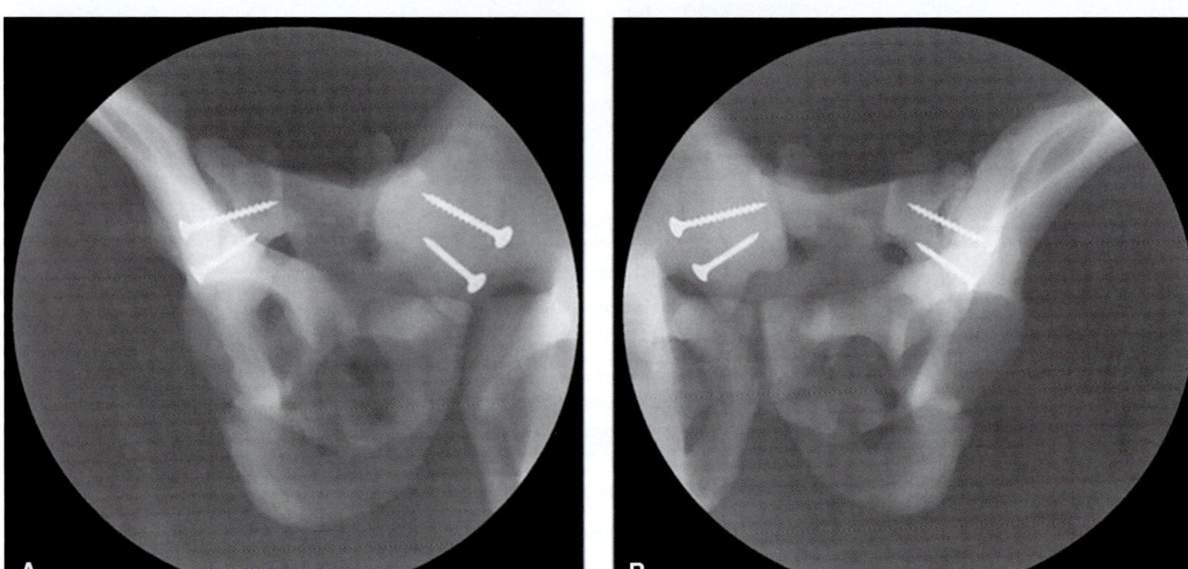

Figure 13-12 I The obturator-outlet oblique view is obtained of the right **(A)** and left **(B)** hemipelvis. The superior ramus is centered on each image and the obturator canal is on profile. This view demonstrates the cranial and caudal extents of safety for medullary ramus screw insertion.

- For antegrade ramus screw insertion, the surgeon sits or stands on the ipsilateral side of the ramus being instrumented. The C-arm is brought in from the opposite side of the surgeon to allow for simultaneous image acquisition and instrumentation (Fig. 13-13). When a ramus is being instrumented in retrograde fashion, the surgeon stands contralateral to the injured ramus. The C-arm can be positioned ipsilateral or contralateral to the surgeon depending on what other injuries are present in the pelvic ring and what instrumentation is planned (Figs. 13-14 and 13-15).
- Once the positions on the C-arm are established to obtain inlet and obturator-outlet views, the fluoroscopist can record them. This is easily done by placing strips of tape on the C-arm and on the floor to mark degrees of tilt and roll as well as the position of the C-arm in the room. When the two views can be quickly and reliably obtained, insertion of the medullary ramus screws can be most efficiently inserted.

The sequence of images for a safe **retrograde medullary ramus screw** is detailed in the figures below (Fig. 13-16A–F).[2] First, a 2.0-mm guidewire is placed in percutaneous fashion. On the inlet view, the wire is placed on the anteromedial corner of the superior ramus adjacent to the symphysis pubis.

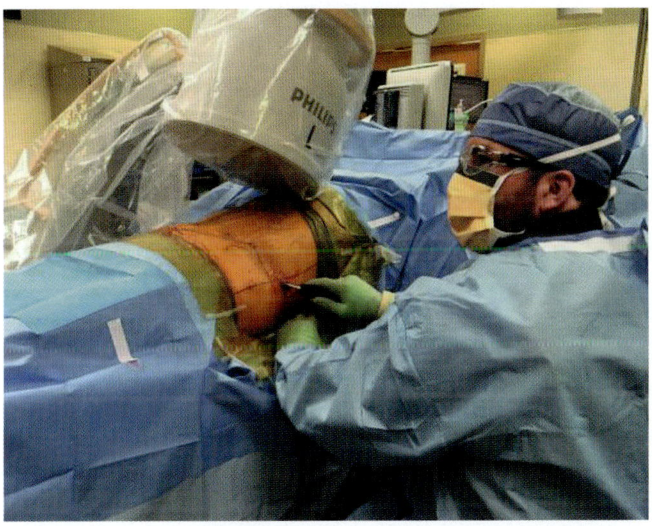

Figure 13-13 | An antegrade screw is being placed on the patient's left side. The C-arm is positioned on the opposite side of the surgeon.

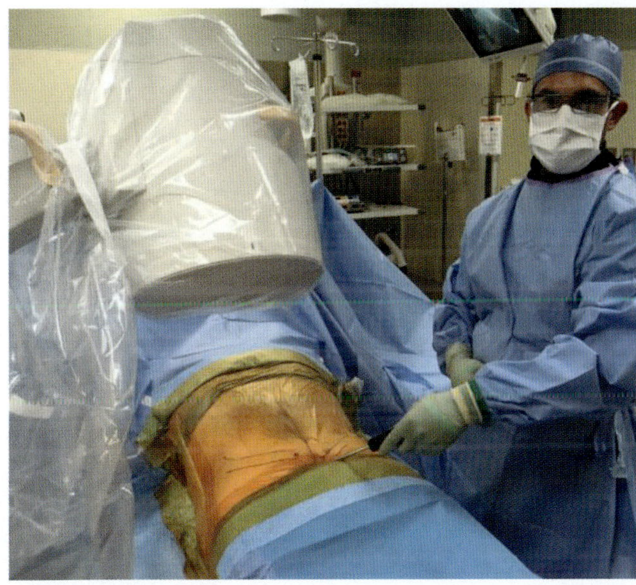

Figure 13-14 | A retrograde screw is being placed on the patient's right side. The C-arm is being brought in from the side opposite the surgeon.

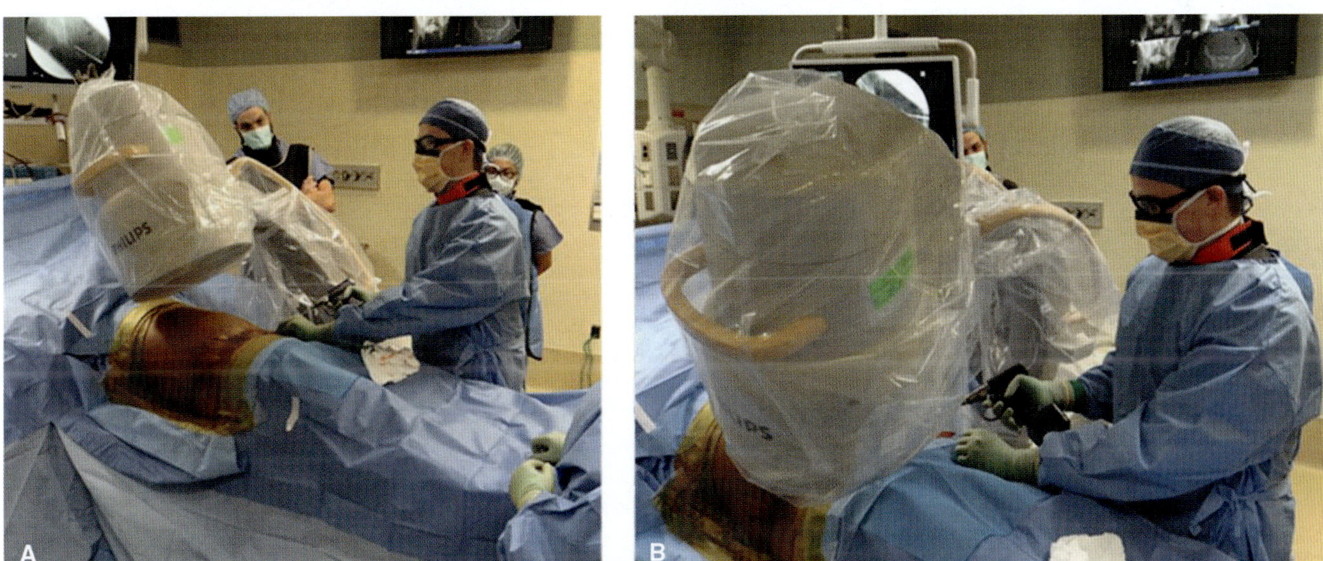

Figure 13-15 | The surgeon is instrumenting the right superior ramus in retrograde fashion. The surgeon stands on the opposite side of the instrumented ramus. The C-arm is positioned on the ipsilateral side of the surgeon to accommodate the instrumentation of a concomitant right sacral fracture. The inlet **(A)** and obturator-outlet oblique **(B)** views are easily obtained.

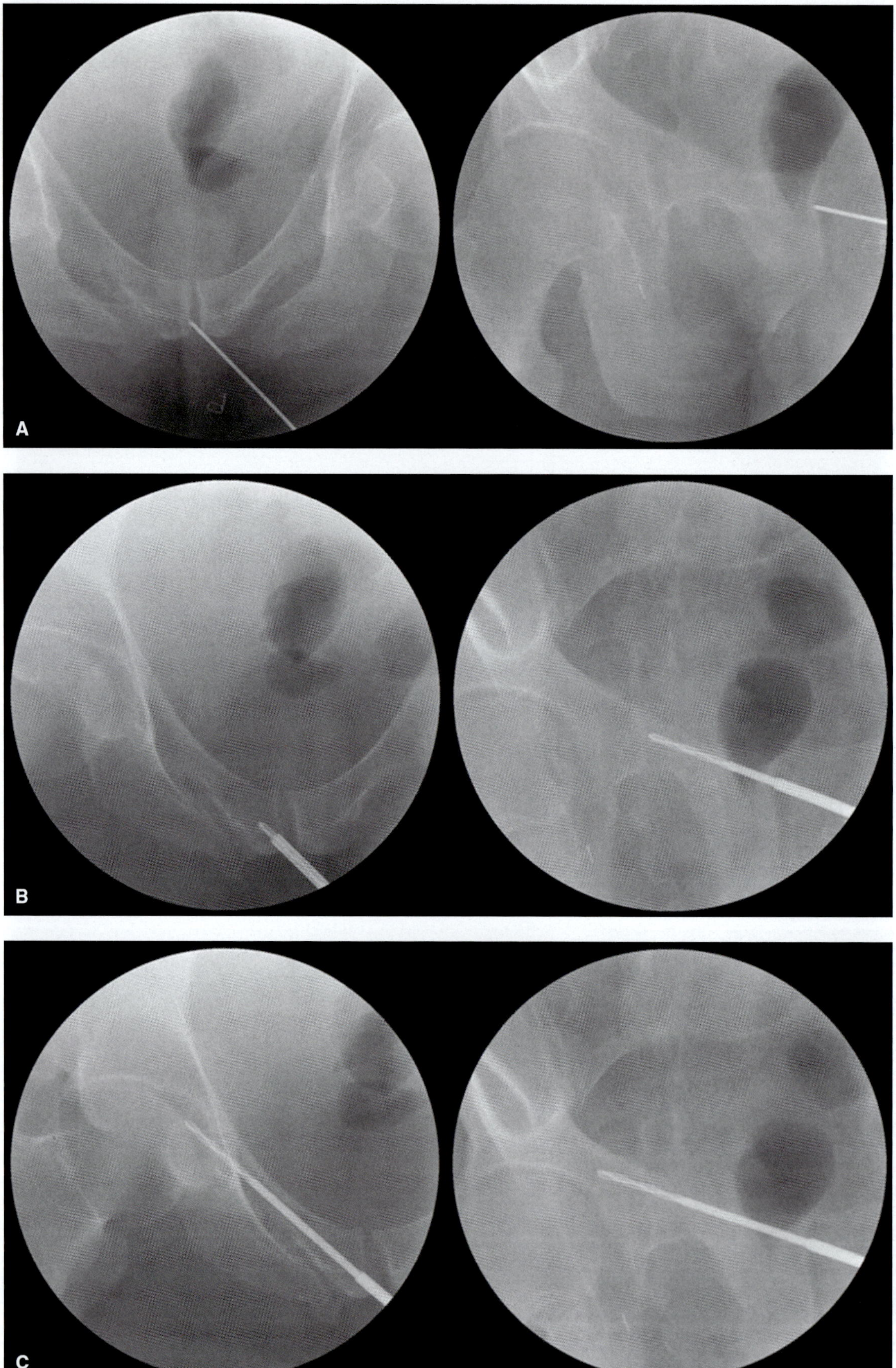

Figure 13-16 | A: 2.0-mm guidewire is placed percutaneously. **B:** The guidewire is exchanged for a 3.5-mm drill through a 3.5-mm drill sleeve. **C:** The 3.5-mm drill is advanced retrograde in order to establish trajectory.

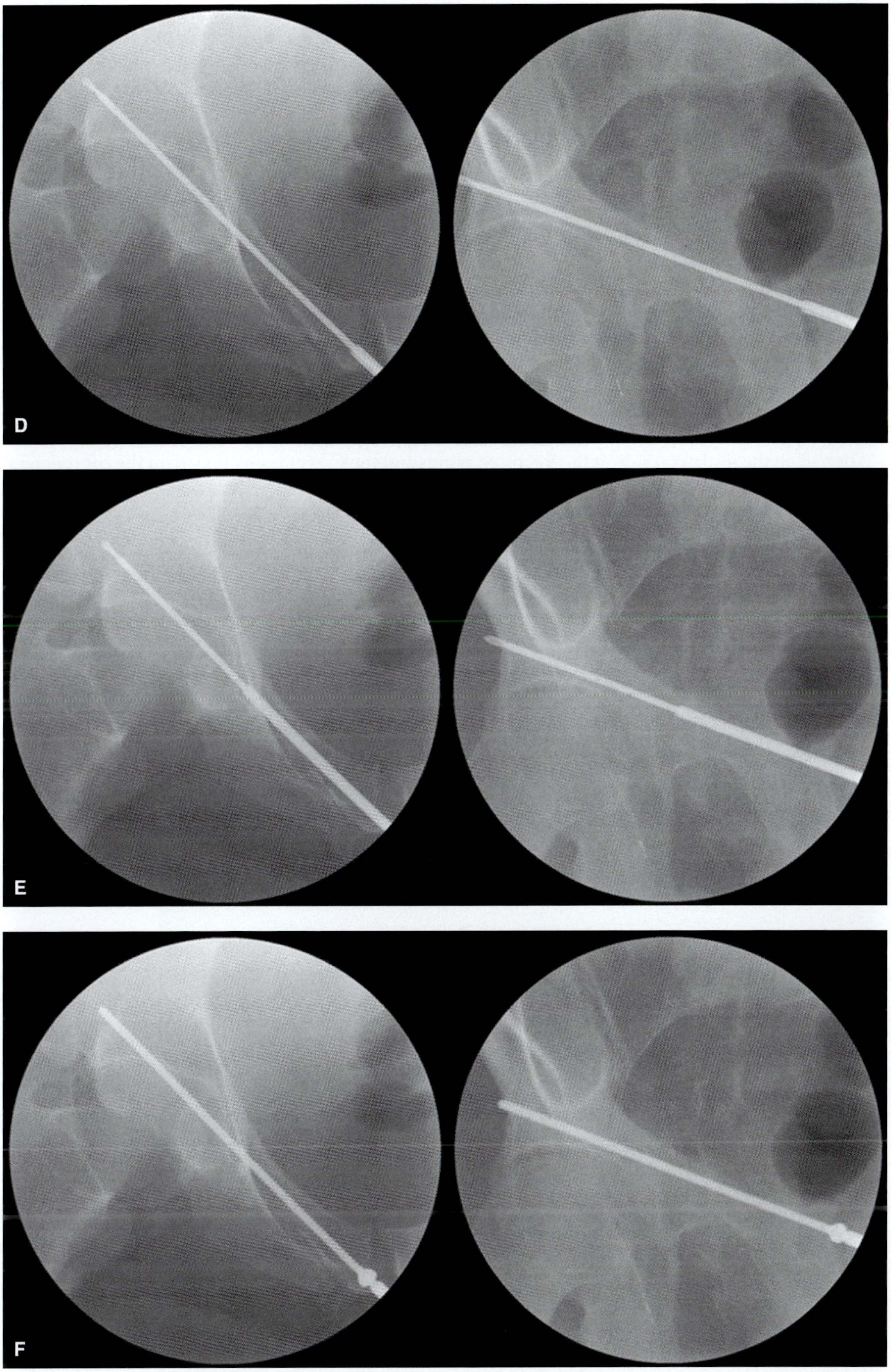

Figure 13-16 | *(Continued)* **D:** The 3.5-mm drill is exchanged for a 2.8-mm guide pin with a drill bit tip. **E:** The guide pin is overdrilled with a 5.0-mm cannulated drill. **F:** A 4.5-mm blunt-tip screw is placed in retrograde fashion.

On the outlet view, the wire is positioned to create a start point that will allow a drill trajectory to proceed safely above the acetabulum but below the cranial extent of the superior ramus.

Next, a small incision is created around the 2.0-mm guidewire, and a 3.5-mm drill sleeve of 110 mm in length is placed over the wire and inserted to the bone (inner drill sleeve from Synthes Triple Guide for femoral distractor half pins; the robust length and rigidity of this sleeve allow the surgeon to control drill trajectory minimizing risk of drill bit fracture within the medullary canal). The 2.0-mm wire is withdrawn, and a 3.5-mm drill is inserted.

The 3.5-mm drill is inserted to its maximal depth through the 3.5-mm drill sleeve. Placement of the 3.5-mm drill allows the surgeon to establish a safe trajectory for the screw.

The 3.5-mm drill is withdrawn, and a 2.8-mm drill bit–tipped guide pin is inserted and drilled to the final insertion depth of the screw. Note that the 2.8-mm guide pin cannot change the trajectory established by the 3.5-mm drill. If the surgeon wishes to change the trajectory, it must be done with the 3.5-mm drill.

The depth of the guide pin is measured and the guide pin is overdrilled with a 5.0-mm cannulated drill just beyond the fracture site. This creates a pilot hole for a 4.5-mm screw. Note that larger diameter cannulated screws may be used if accommodated by the intramedullary canal.

Finally, the 2.8-mm guide pin is withdrawn and the 3.5-mm sleeve removed. A 4.5-mm blunt-tipped screw is inserted by hand to stabilize the ramus fracture.

Antegrade screw placement follows a similar sequence (Fig. 13-17A–E). The surgeon is positioned on the ipsilateral side of the fractured ramus and the C-arm is positioned on the contralateral

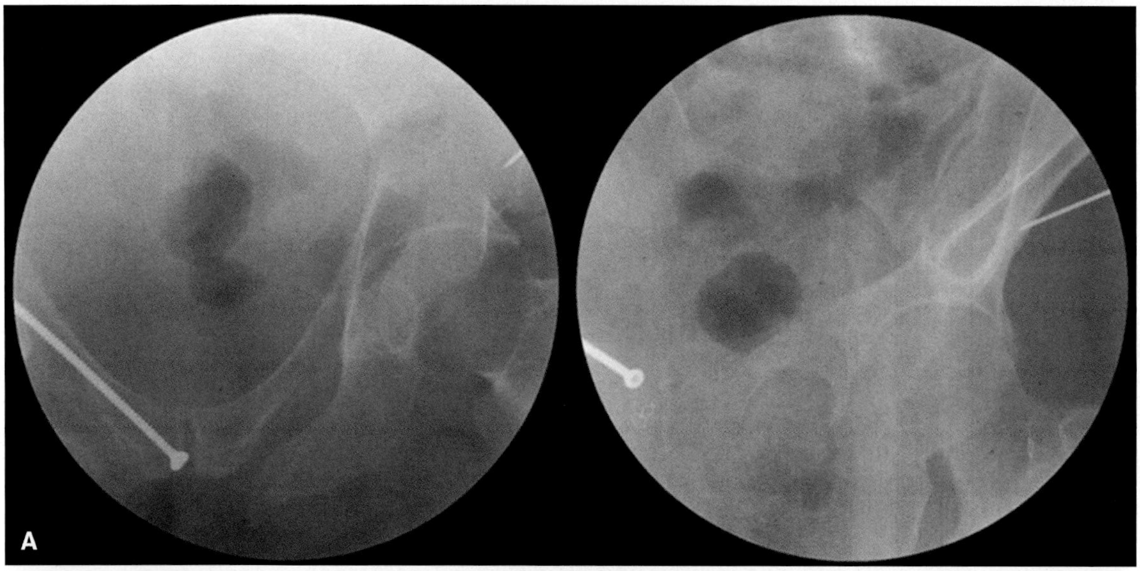

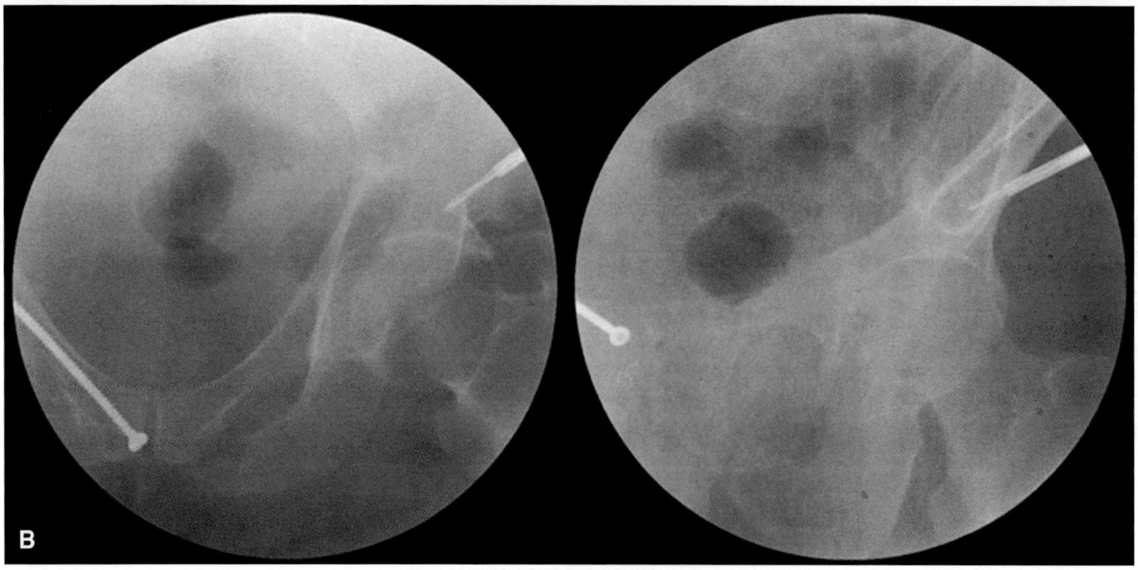

Figure 13-17 | A: Inlet and obturator-outlet views of the left superior ramus. **B:** The 2.0-mm wire is withdrawn and exchanged for a 3.5-mm drill.

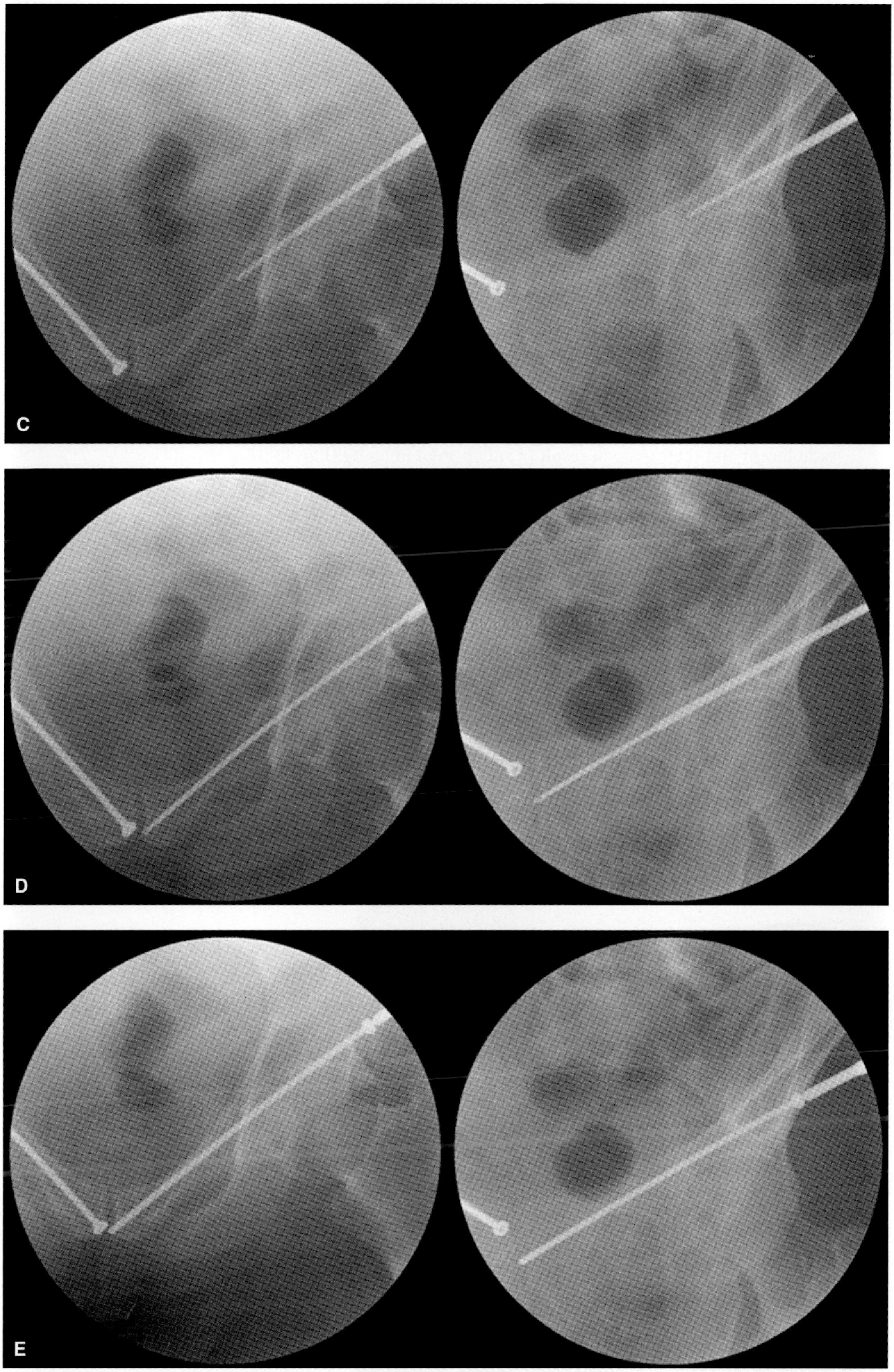

Figure 13-17 | *(Continued)* **C:** The 3.5-mm drill is used to set trajectory and advanced as far as the 3.5-mm drill sleeve will allow. **D:** The 3.5-mm drill is exchanged for a 2.8-mm guide pin and advanced to the pubic tubercle. A 5.0-mm drill is advanced over the guide pin just beyond the fracture site. **E:** The 4.5-mm screw is fully inserted.

side. The inlet and obturator-outlet oblique views are used to obtain a start point above the acetabulum on the obturator-outlet oblique view and positioned on the inlet view to maximize screw length within the osseous superior ramus. The start point is obtained in percutaneous fashion with a 2.0-mm wire.

The 2.0-mm wire is withdrawn, and a 3.5-mm drill is inserted. The drill is inserted to its maximal depth to set strategic trajectory.

Once the trajectory is set, a 2.8-mm drill bit–tipped guide pin is inserted to the maximal safe depth. A depth gauge is then used to ascertain screw length. Once screw length is determined, a 5.0-mm cannulated drill is passed over the guide pin, just beyond the fracture.

The guide pin is removed, and a 4.5-mm screw is inserted to stabilize the ramus fracture.

2. Prone Position

- Medullary ramus screw may be placed in the prone position. *Only antegrade insertion is possible while the patient is prone.* The medullary ramus screw may be used to secure acetabular fracture fixation or pelvic ring fixation.
- The patient is placed prone on laminectomy rolls made of two rolled blankets each. Manufactured laminectomy rolls made of plastic of jelly-like substance should not be used as they are not radiolucent and their use will result in suboptimal imaging (Fig. 13-18).
- The perineum is isolated from the sterile prep. The ipsilateral lower extremity is circumferentially prepped in addition to the pelvic region (Figs. 13-19 and 13-20).

The clinical example above is a patient who is being treated for a transverse posterior wall acetabulum fracture that is being exposed via a prone Kocher-Langenbeck approach (Fig. 13-21).

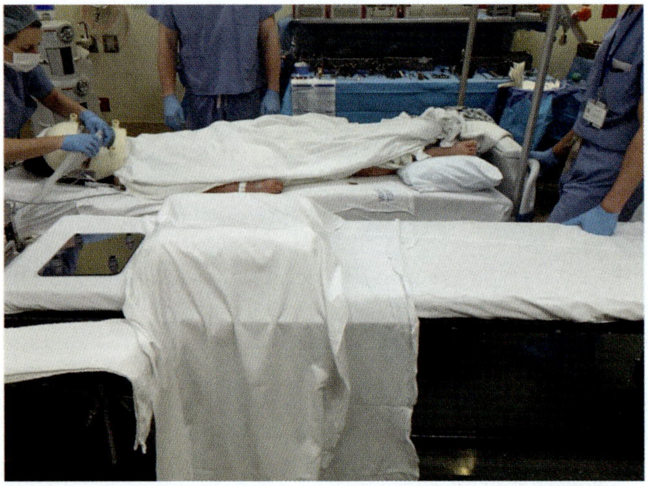

Figure 13-18 I Laminectomy rolls are made of rolled blankets and can be custom made to the patient's size.

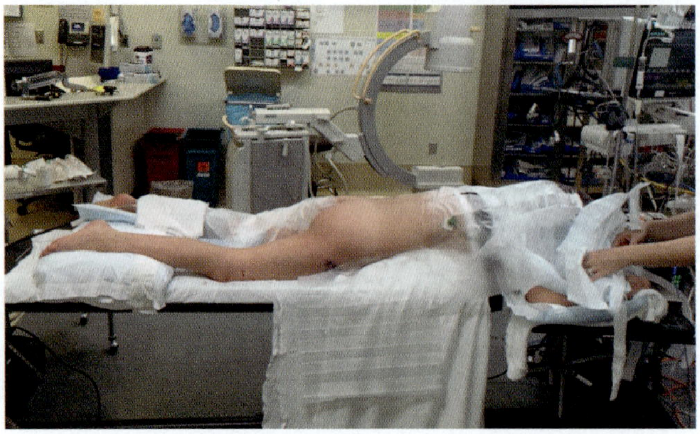

Figure 13-19 I The patient is positioned prone, and care is taken to pad all bony prominences well. The patient is placed level on the table, and the perineum is isolated from the sterile prep.

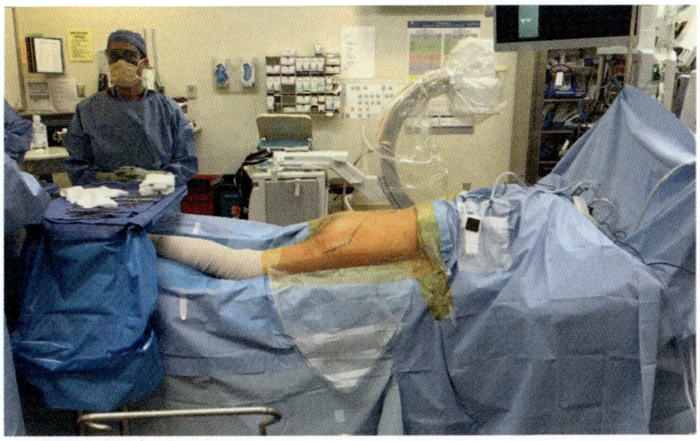

Figure 13-20 | The right lower extremity is circumferentially prepped. Prep of the pelvic region can include bilateral flanks if necessary.

The transverse portion of the fracture has been clamped through the Kocher-Langenbeck and the anterior portion of the transverse fracture is instrumented with a medullary ramus screw placed in antegrade fashion (Fig. 13-22).

Inlet and obturator-outlet views are again used to guide drill and screw placement. *Note that the position of the C-arm is reversed to obtain the correct images on a prone patient.* The surgeon is positioned in the patient's axilla. Notice that the medullary ramus screw and drills to prepare its path are placed in a small incision separate from the Kocher-Langenbeck exposure (Fig. 13-23).

The final construct includes a medullary ramus screw and a posterior plate (Fig. 13-24).

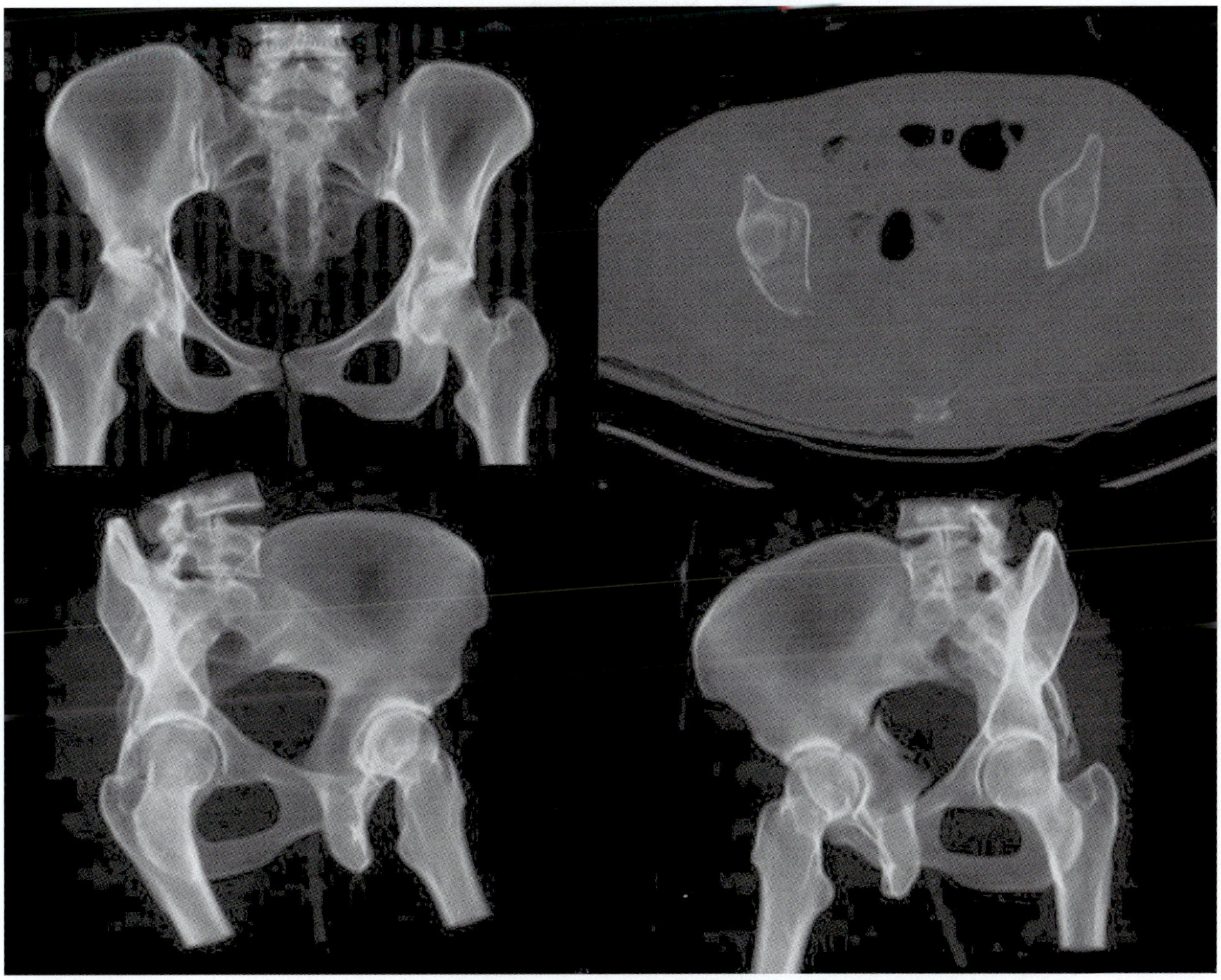

Figure 13-21 | Plan films and representative CT scan image of a transverse posterior wall acetabulum fracture.

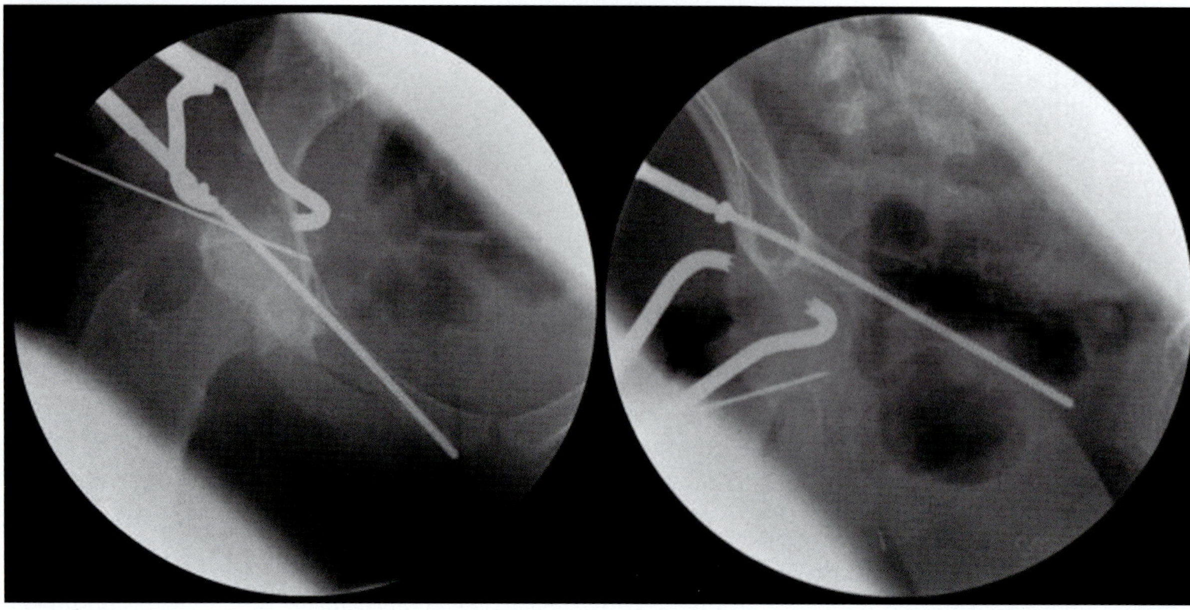

Figure 13-22 | The transverse fracture has been reduced and clamped. The posterior wall fracture has also been reduced and is being provisionally stabilized with a K-wire. An antegrade medullary ramus screw has been placed under fluoroscopic guidance to stabilize the anterior portion of the transverse fracture.

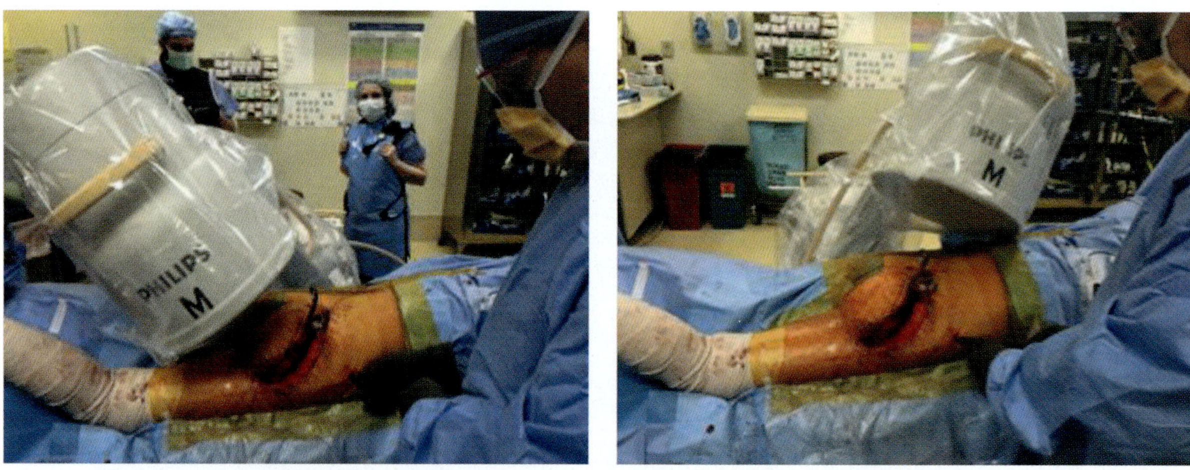

Figure 13-23 | Inlet **(left)** and obturator-outlet **(right)** positions for antegrade medullary ramus screw insertion in the prone position. The medullary screw is inserted in a small incision remote from the Kocher-Langenbeck exposure to facilitate proper trajectory.

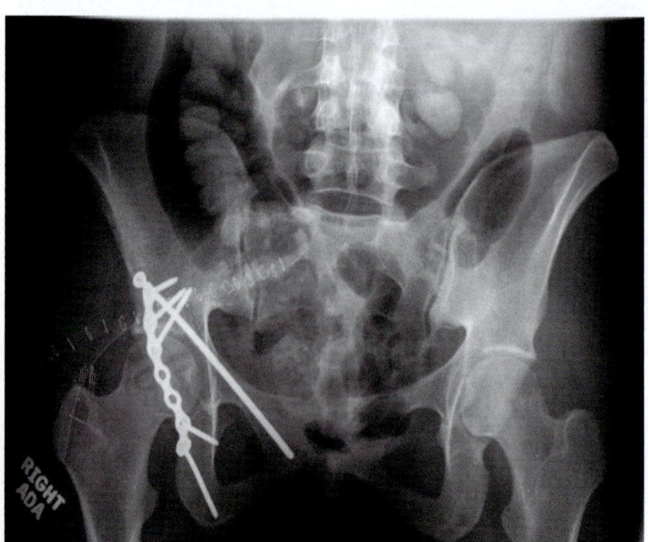

Figure 13-24 | AP radiograph of the transverse posterior wall fracture after ORIF.

Additional Positioning Tips

- Ensure that the patient is level on the radiolucent table prior to prepping and draping. This will simplify acquisition of symmetric images.
- The supine lumbosacral bump and prone laminectomy rolls should be made of blankets or sheets. This will provide a reliably radiolucent surface.
- Secure all free tubes and wires in a manner such that the lower portion of the C-arm can move freely. Urinary catheters and chest tubes may create clutter on the floor around the operating room table and can be positioned strategically.

References

1. Routt ML Jr, Nork SE, Mills WJ. Percutaneous fixation of pelvic ring disruptions. *Clin Orthop Relat Res.* 2000;(375):15–29.
2. Routt ML, Jr, Simonian PT, Grujic L. The retrograde medullary superior pubic ramus screw for the treatment of anterior pelvic ring disruptions: a new technique. *J Orthop Trauma.* 1995;9(1):35–44.

Chapter 14
Placement of Posterior Column Screws for Acetabular Fractures

JOSHUA L. GARY

Bony Anatomy

- The acetabulum is a concave socket formed at the confluence of the ilium, ischium, and pubis. It has been described as an inverted "Y" formed as the anterior and posterior columns join at the dome of the acetabulum and transition into the iliac wing proximally.
- The posterior column (PC) of bone includes the greater and lesser sciatic notches and the ischium and has much less surface area than the anterior column. The bone about the greater sciatic notch is normally the densest bone of the human skeleton.
- The bony corridor for screw placement runs from the iliac bone of the pelvic brim just anterior and lateral to the sacroiliac joint cranially to the ischium caudally.
- It is bordered medially by the quadrilateral surface and laterally by the ischial bone to the greater and lesser sciatic notches. These notches and the ischial spine define the posterior border with the articular surface of the acetabulum constraining the anterior limit of the corridor.

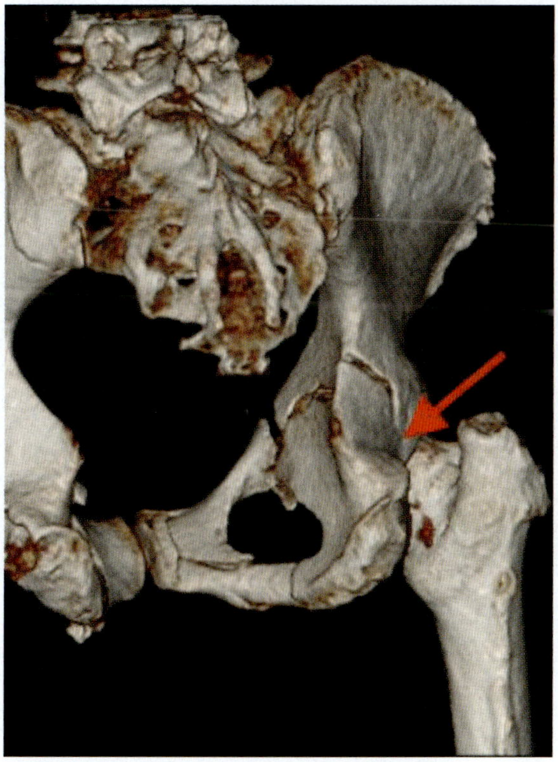

Figure 14-1 3D surface-rendered image of posterior acetabulum demonstrating concavity and isthmus of the posterior column corridor near the lesser sciatic notch (*red arrow*).

- The undulation of the lateral border with a concavity just anterior to the lesser sciatic notch and cranial to the ischial tuberosity must be taken into account to prevent placement of an "in-out-in" screw (Fig. 14-1). This concavity (red arrow below) serves as the isthmus of the bony corridor for columnar fixation of the posterior column.

Radiographic Anatomy

- Disruption and displacement of the posterior column are represented by an interruption in the ilioischial line on the anteroposterior (AP) view of the pelvis (Fig. 14-2A).

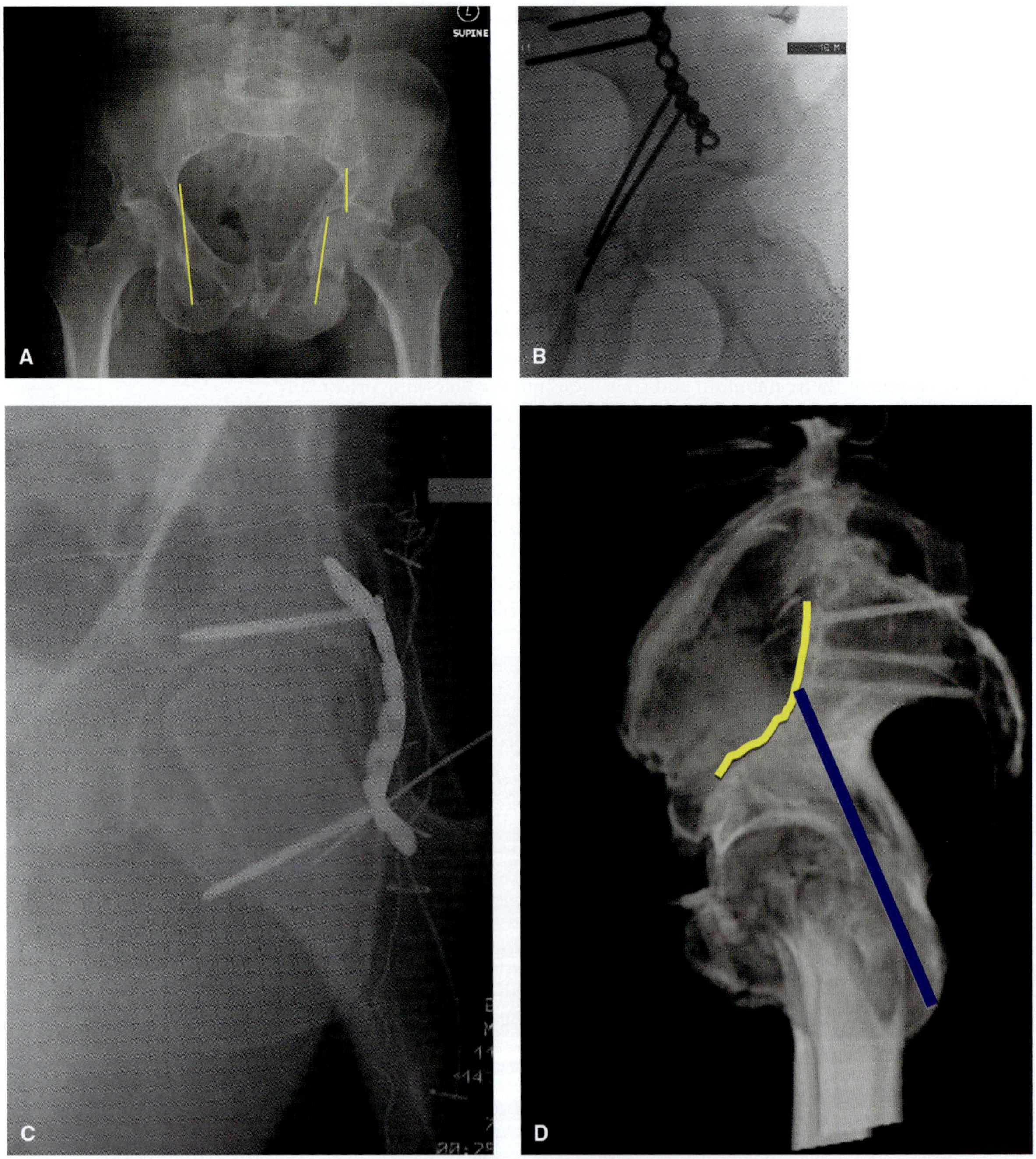

Figure 14-2 | A: AP pelvis of a displaced left anterior column with posterior hemitransverse acetabulum fracture with displacement of the posterior column. The intact (*right*) and disrupted (*left*) ilioischial lines are outlined in *yellow*. **B:** Fluoroscopic iliac oblique view with two antegrade posterior column screws through a pelvic brim plate stabilizing the posterior column component of an associated fracture of the acetabulum. **C:** Fluoroscopic obturator oblique view of a buttress plate stabilizing a posterior wall acetabular fracture. **D:** Postoperative lateral view of the pelvis. The *yellow line* represents a plate applied to the pelvic brim and cranial limit of the corridor. The *blue line* represents the path of a posterior column screw from the ischial tuberosity to the pelvic brim.

- The ilioischial line on the AP view represents the medial border of the PC corridor. The AP view also demonstrates the quality of reduction in the coronal plane, with excellent reduction denoted by restoration of a contiguous ilioischial line.
- The iliac oblique view brings the greater sciatic notch, ischial spine, and lesser sciatic notch into profile and provides excellent visualization of the anterior and posterior limits of the PC corridor (Fig. 14-2B). Fracture lines involving the posterior column are usually best seen with this radiographic view. The iliac oblique view allows for judgment of reduction quality in the sagittal plane and for caudal displacement of the ischial segment.
- The obturator oblique view provides excellent visualization of the lateral border of the PC corridor and its undulation; the plate contour used to buttress a posterior wall fragment provides an excellent visual representation of the lateral border (Fig. 14-2C).
- The lateral sacral or lateral pelvic view is also useful, especially with retrograde screw placement. The iliac cortical density represents the pelvic brim, and screws terminating cranial to this line may protrude into the iliacus muscle (Fig. 14-2D).
- The iliac and obturator oblique views, or Judet views, are generally obtained rolling the patients with wedges or bumps under each hemipelvis. An iliac oblique view of the left hemipelvis is an obturator oblique view of the right hemipelvis and vice versa.
- When a fluoroscope is used, the patient usually remains stationary on the operative table, and the C-arm is rotated over and back to obtain Judet view. The fluoroscopy machine should generally enter contralateral to the operative extremity.
- The iliac oblique is obtained in the supine position by rolling the C-arm approximately 30 degrees away from the acetabulum (Fig. 14-3A).
- The obturator oblique view is obtained in the supine position by rolling approximately 30 degrees toward the acetabulum and surgeon (Fig. 14-3B).
- When in the prone position, the direction of rotation of the C-arm is reversed for all imaging sequences.

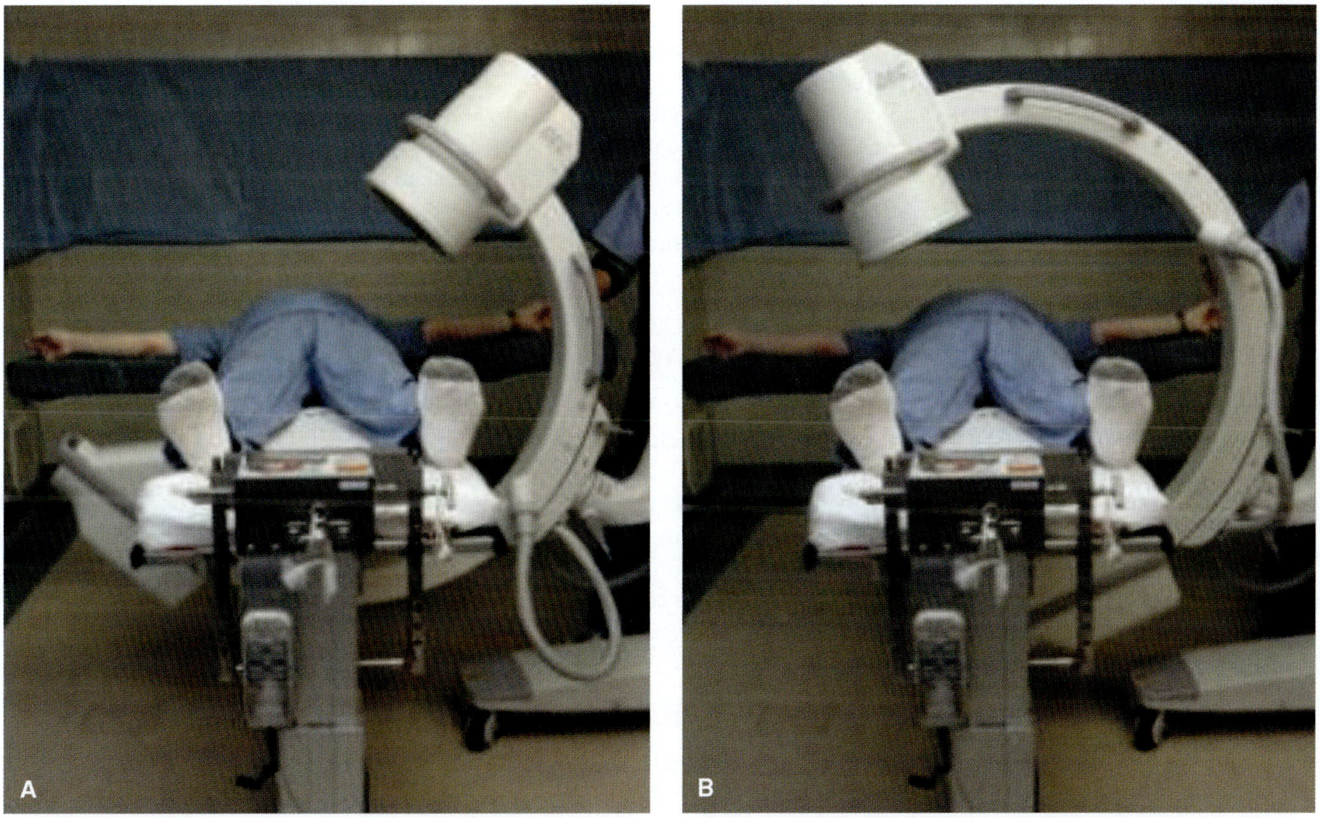

Figure 14-3 | A: Clinical photo of an intraoperative iliac oblique view (right acetabulum) in the supine position. The surgeon and operative hemipelvis are opposite the C-arm. From Bates et al. *The Percutaneous Treatment of Pelvic and Acetabular Fractures* (with permission). **B:** Clinical photo of an intraoperative obturator oblique view (right acetabulum) in the supine position. The surgeon and operative hemipelvis are opposite the C-arm. From Bates et al. *The Percutaneous Treatment of Pelvic and Acetabular Fractures* (with permission).

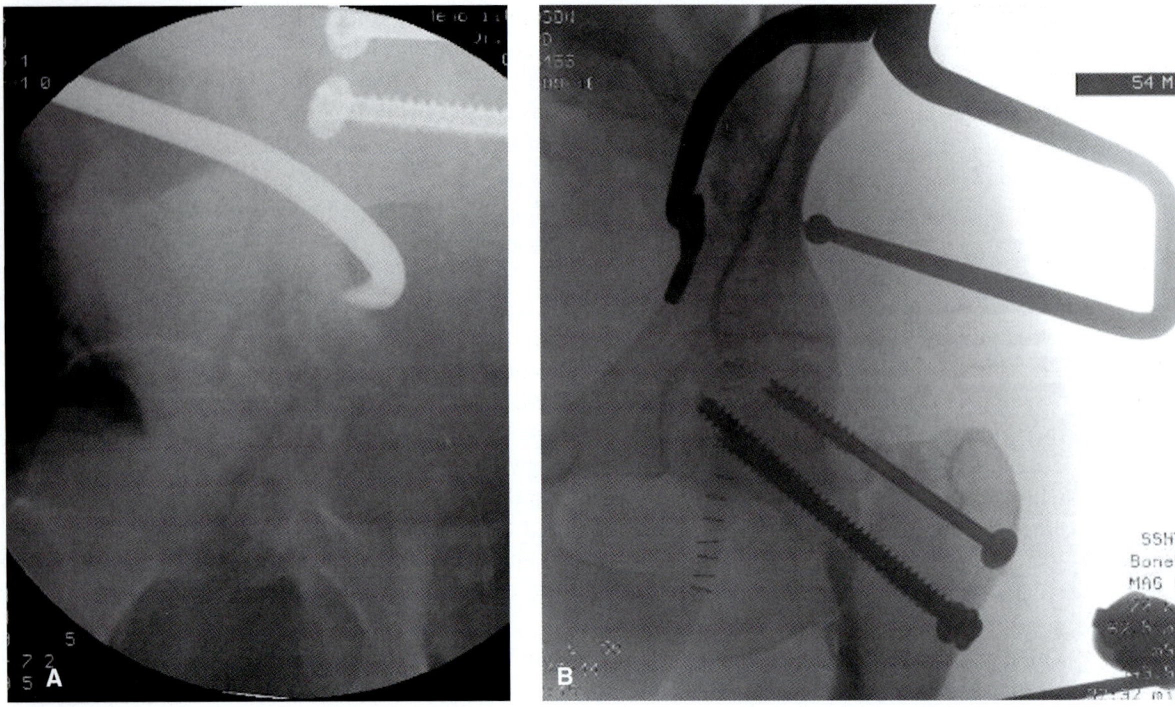

Figure 14-4 | A: Fluoroscopic iliac oblique view of a collinear clamp docked in the true pelvis just anterior to the greater sciatic notch. **B:** Fluoroscopic obturator oblique view of a Reinert clamp placed to reduce a transverse acetabular fracture through a limited portion of the lateral window of the ilioinguinal approach.

- The articular reduction of the acetabulum is usually evaluated indirectly with fluoroscopy during operative fixation. Note that open approaches typically involve indirect extracortical reads of the articular reduction, in which the reduction of the cartilaginous surface is rarely visualized directly.
- Fluoroscopy is commonly used to place and guide reduction clamps without direct visualization of one or more of the cortical surfaces.
- The lateral window of the ilioinguinal approach provides indirect access to the quadrilateral surface and greater and lesser sciatic notches. Collinear (Fig. 14-4A) or modified offset (Reinert) pelvic reduction clamps (Fig. 14-4B) may be placed through a lateral window into the true pelvis. Remaining subperiosteal and using fluoroscopic guidance allows for safest placement of the clamps without direct visualization of at-risk neurovascular structures in the true pelvis.

Preoperative Planning

- An AP view of the pelvis is diagnostic for displaced acetabular fractures and allows for proper classification of a majority of fractures. Judet views provide further details of fracture pattern and displacement.
- Rollover Judet views (the patient placed on wedges) allow for an assessment of dynamic instability.
- Fine-cut computed tomography scanning with 2-mm slices allows for detailed understanding of the bony injury, including marginal impaction and intra-articular debris.
- 3D surface-rendered reconstructions can be made with modern software and are helpful in diagnosis and operative planning of reduction clamp and implant applications.

Intraoperative Positioning

- Antegrade posterior column screws are usually placed in a supine position. A radiolucent table is mandatory. The ipsilateral hindquarter should be included in the surgical preparation and draping.
- The lateral window of the ilioinguinal approach is required to place the screw(s).
- Flexing the ipsilateral hip and knee with a radiolucent triangle or bump relaxes the iliopsoas and femoral nerve.

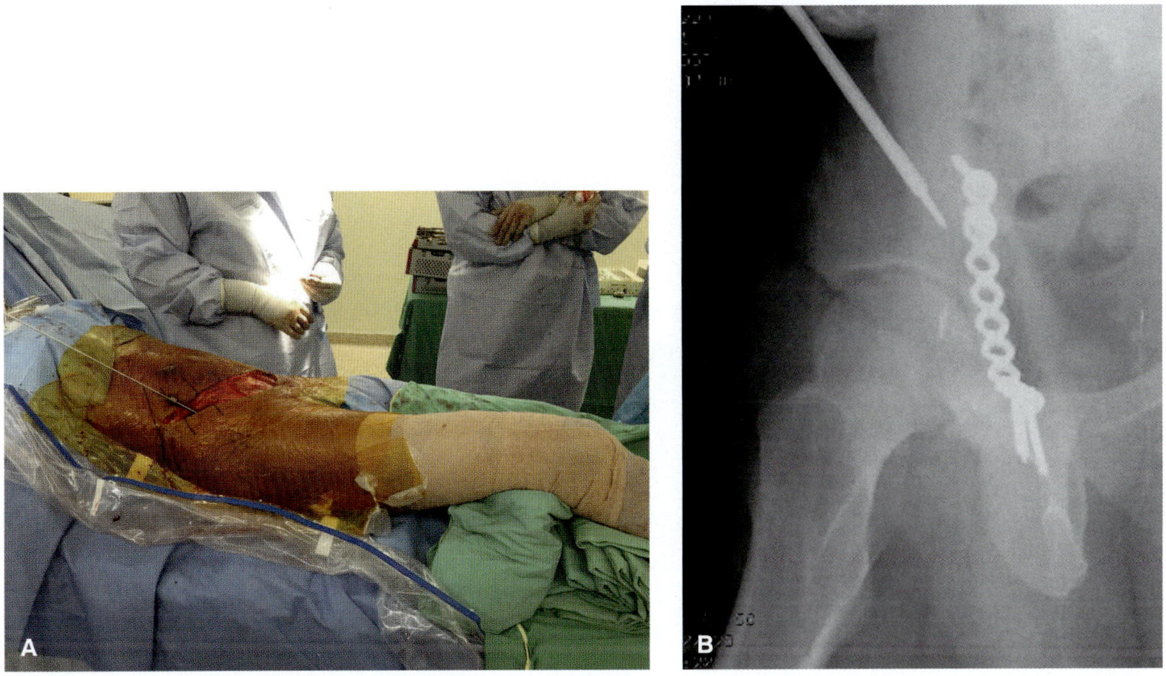

Figure 14-5 | A: Intraoperative photo of a guidewire for an antegrade posterior column screw. The chest wall limits aiming further anteriorly. **B:** Intraoperative fluoroscopic iliac oblique view showing the aim of the wire toward the ischial spine. The chest wall prevents frequent precludes placement of a screw to the ischial tuberosity.

- Antegrade screws are difficult to pass beyond the lesser sciatic notch because the rib cage and chest wall prevent the surgeon from aiming further anterior toward the ischial tuberosity (Fig. 14-5A and B).
- Limited portions of the lateral window can be used for more minimally invasive screw placement (Fig. 14-6).

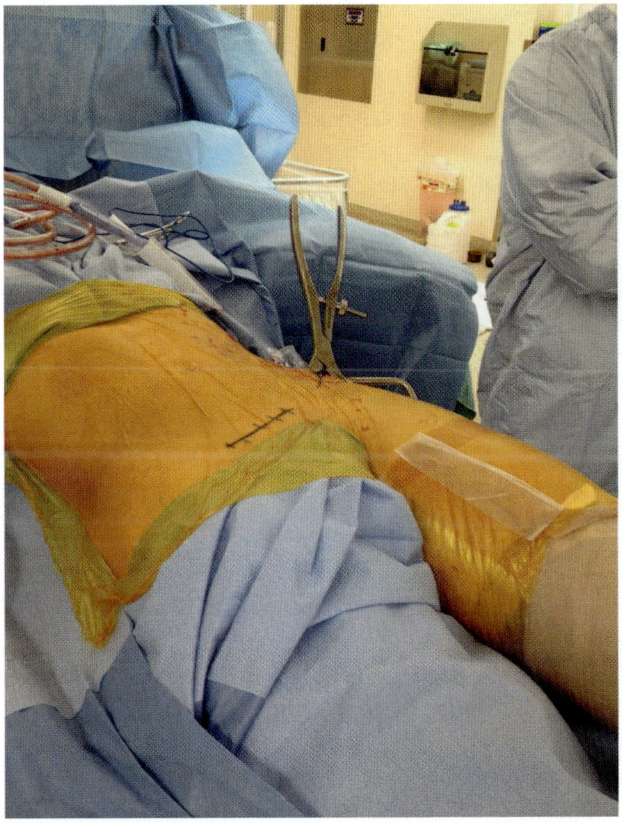

Figure 14-6 | Clinical photo of placement of a modified offset (Reinert) pelvic reduction clamp through a limited portion of the lateral window of the ilioinguinal approach.

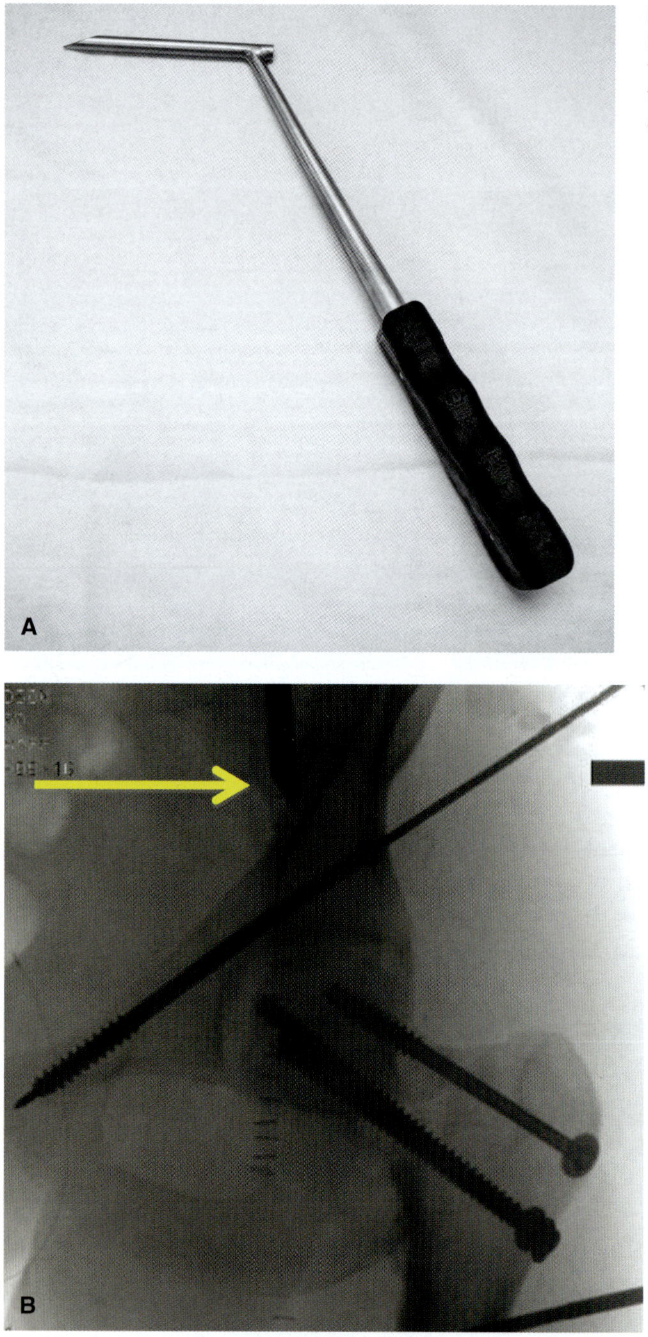

Figure 14-7 | A: Photo of an offset "pigsticker." **B:** Intraoperative obturator oblique image of the offset pigsticker (*yellow arrow*) being used to obtain an excellent starting point for an antegrade posterior column screw.

- An offset "pigsticker" is very helpful for gaining an accurate starting point, allowing fluoroscopic imaging, and preventing soft tissues from creating tension and misdirection of a narrow wire or drill bit (Fig. 14-7A and B).
- The C-arm is brought in usually brought in from the contralateral side opposite the surgeon. Standard AP, iliac oblique, and obturator oblique images are used to correctly position the screw. Some surgeons use an outlet view to guide screw placement in the coronal plane, ensuring that the wire/drill/screw are placed just lateral to the ilioischial line.
- Retrograde posterior column screws may be placed with the patient supine or prone. A radiolucent table is mandatory. The ipsilateral hindquarter should be included in the surgical preparation and draping.
- For supine positioning, a central sacral bump is very helpful. The bump is made from two standard sheets folded into thirds. Elevating the patient slightly from the bed allows the surgeon to aim further anterior if need. A seated position is helpful for the surgeon.
- An assistant is required to flex the ipsilateral hip and knee to 90 degrees to allow palpation of the ischial tuberosity and place screw (Fig. 14-8A–D).

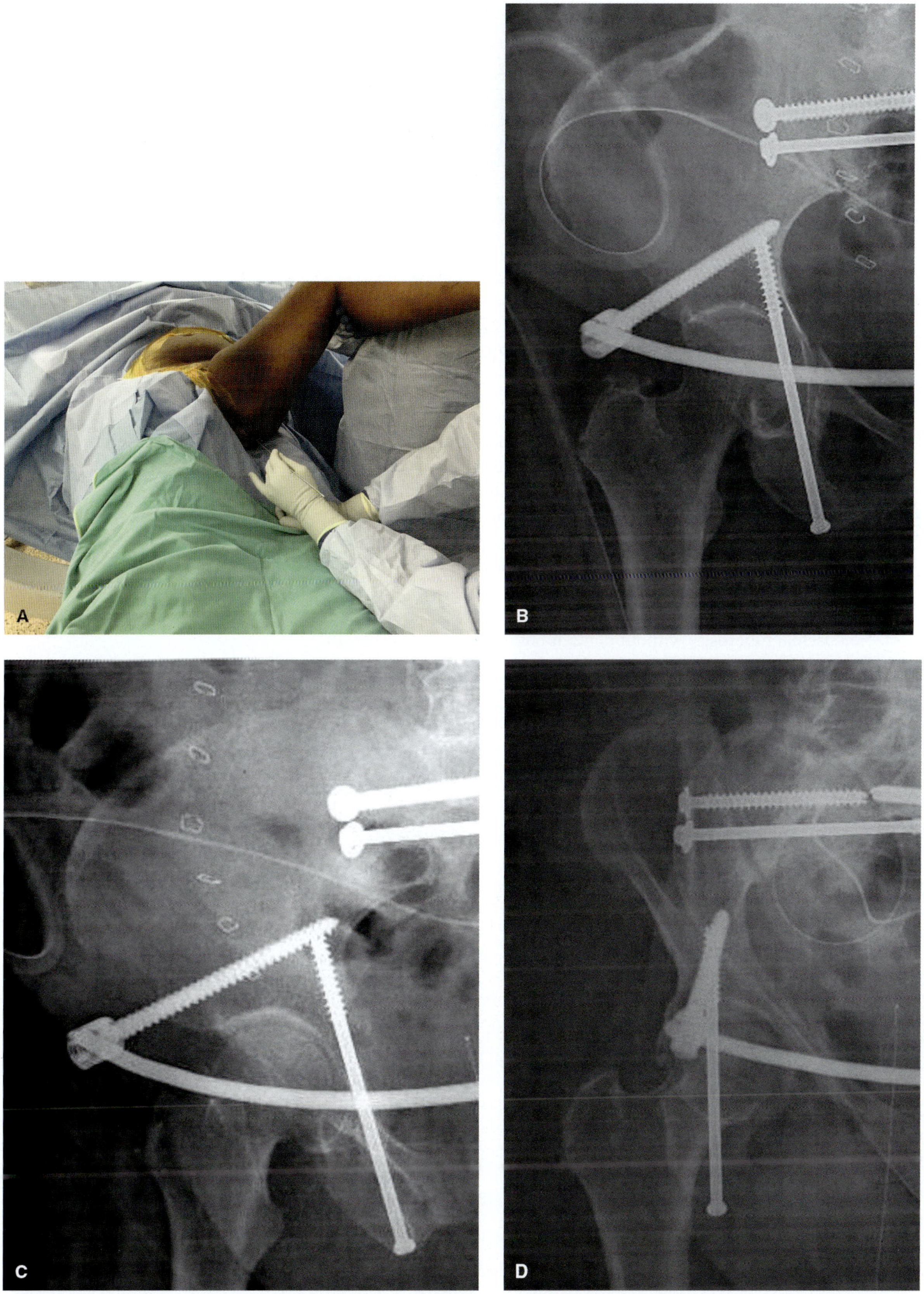

Figure 14-8 | A: Intraoperative photo of flexion of the ipsilateral hip and knee to palpate the ischial tuberosity and obtain a starting point for a retrograde posterior column screw. **B:** Postoperative AP view of a retrograde posterior column screw. The screw begins at the ischial tuberosity and is just lateral to the ilioischial line. **C:** Postoperative iliac oblique view demonstrates screw placement anterior to the greater and lesser sciatic notches and the ischial spine and posterior to the acetabulum. **D:** Postoperative obturator oblique view demonstrates screw placement lateral to the obturator ring and medial to the undulating lateral border of the corridor.

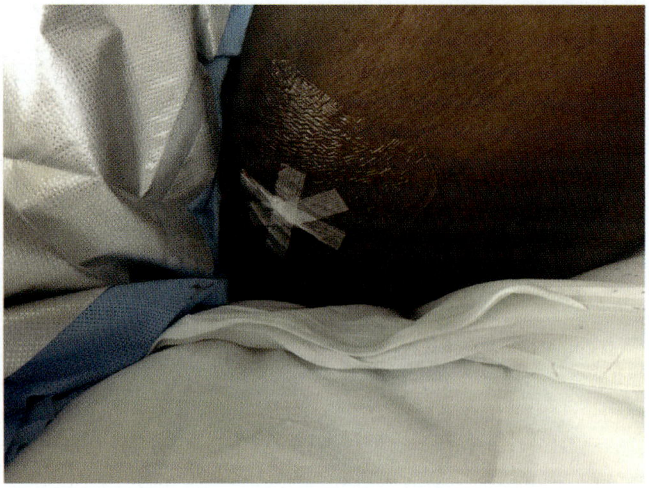

Figure 14-9 | Clinical photo of an occlusive dressing has been placed with multiple steristrips and a tegaderm to prevent contamination from the perineum.

- Careful detail to surgical preparation and draping must be paid to ensure the anus is not included in the field and that the ischial tuberosity can be accessed. An occlusive dressing is placed postoperatively due to the proximity to the perineum (Fig. 14-9).
- Supine positioning allows for the placement of reduction clamps through the lateral window of the ilioinguinal approach.
- Prone positioning is done in standard fashion on a radiolucent table with chest rolls and careful protection of the head and neck.
- Careful attention must be paid to surgical preparation and draping to ensure there is access to the ischial tuberosity without contamination from the perineum.
- A prone position allows for a simultaneous posterior approach to the hip if needed.
- The C-arm must be brought in from the contralateral side and standard AP, iliac oblique, and obturator oblique images are used for screw placement.

Chapter 15
Acetabular Fractures

ANNA N. MILLER
TIMOTHY S. ACHOR

Bony Anatomy

- The acetabulum is a hemispherical portion of the bony pelvis. The pelvis itself is made up of the sacrum and two innominate bones, joined at the sacroiliac joints and symphysis pubis.
- Each innominate bone consists of the iliac wing, from the posterior superior iliac spine posteriorly to the anterior superior iliac spine anteriorly, and extending inferiorly to the greater sciatic notch.
- Anterior to the greater sciatic notch and inferoposterior to the anterior inferior iliac spine is the acetabulum, bounded medially by the quadrilateral surface.
- The ischial tuberosity extends distal below the acetabulum.
- The acetabulum has various degrees of tilt and retroversion depending on the patient's bony anatomy and possible dysplasia (Figs. 15-1 and 15-2).

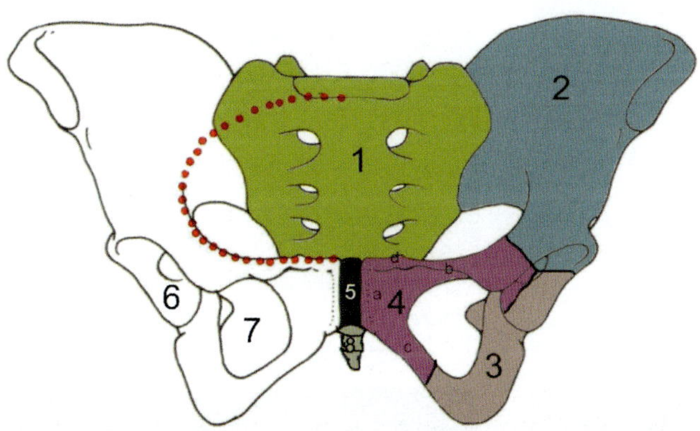

Figure 15-1

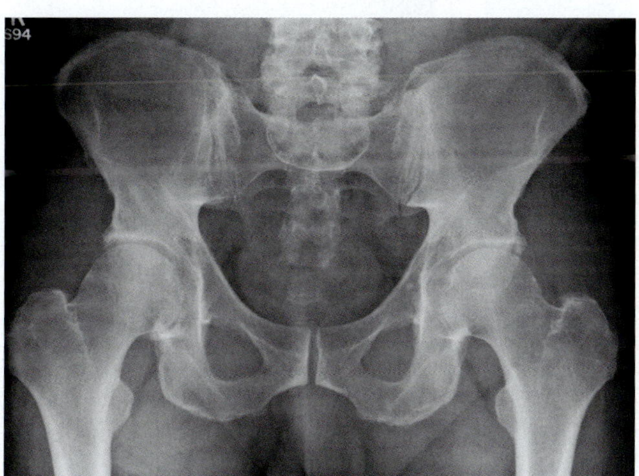

Figure 15-2

Radiographic Anatomy

- The commonly assessed views for the acetabulum are AP and Judet views.
- A good AP view should have the spinous processes in line with the symphysis pubis. The coccyx should be at the level of the superior portion of the symphysis pubis (Fig. 15-3).
- Judet views consist of tilting the patient to the right or left (or digitally manipulating the image instead) such that the AP view is rotated to the point where the coccyx overlaps with the femoral head.
- The two Judet views are "obturator oblique" and "iliac oblique."
- On the obturator oblique view, the obturator foramen of the side of interest is tilted anteriorly, and the anterior column and posterior wall of the acetabulum are more visible (Fig. 15-4).
- On the iliac oblique view, the greater and lesser sciatic notches and ischial spine of the side of interest are visible as the obturator foramen is tilted posteriorly. This view is better for evaluating the posterior column (Fig. 15-5).
- The six lines of Judet and Letournel are the anterior wall (red), posterior wall (white), ilioischial line (posterior column; orange), iliopectineal line (anterior column; blue), sourcil (dome; yellow), and teardrop (medial wall; light green) (Fig. 15-6).
- Advanced imaging (CT) is recommended for further delineation of fracture pattern, including articular fragments and marginal impaction.

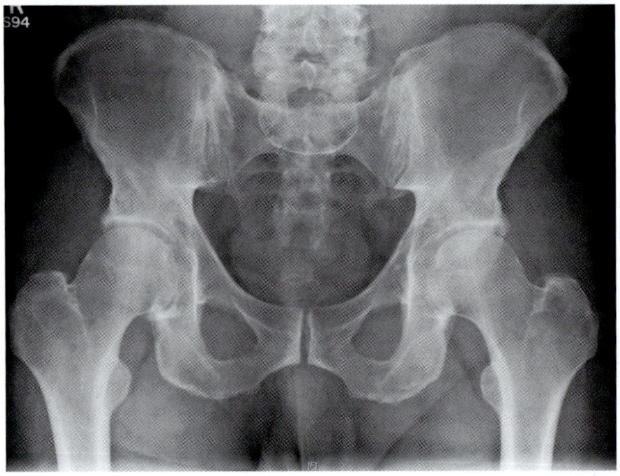

Figure 15-3 |

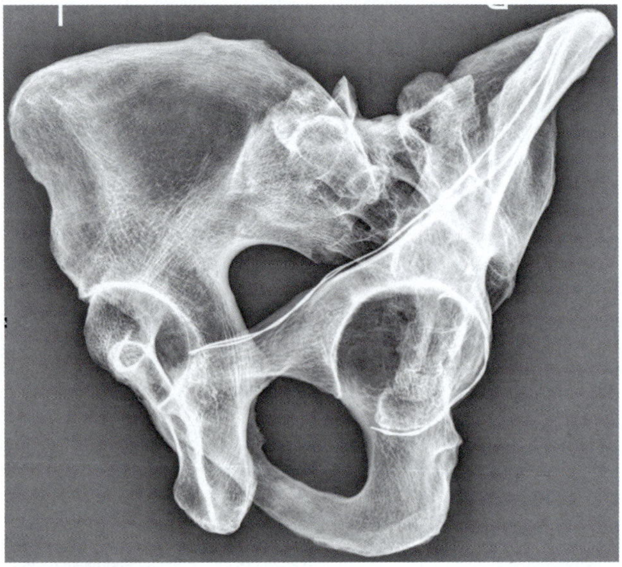

Figure 15-4 |

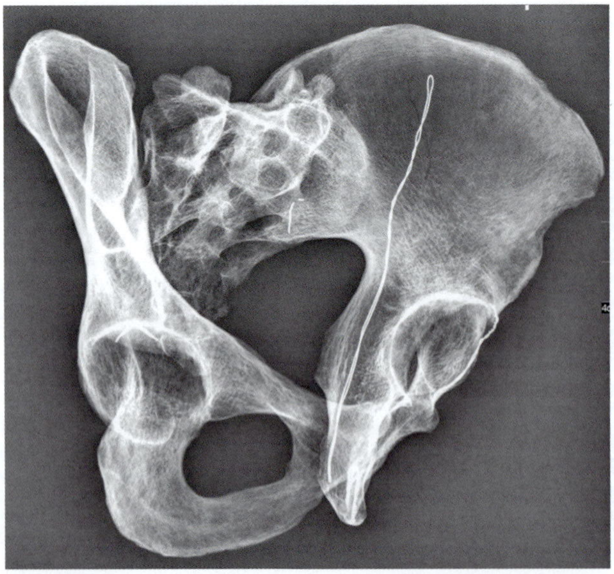

Figure 15-5 |

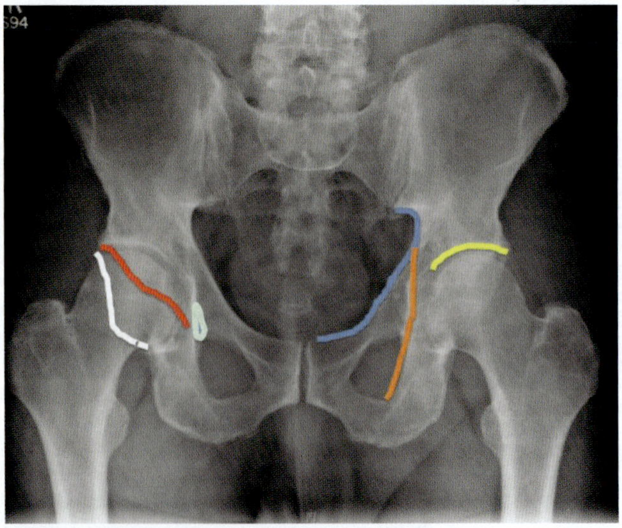

Figure 15-6 |

Intraoperative Imaging

- For both anterior and posterior approaches to the acetabulum, intraoperative views are similar to those discussed above (AP and Judet).
- The obturator oblique outlet view is also helpful specifically to delineate the superior pubic ramus for interosseous screw fixation from a prone or supine position (Fig. 15-7).
- Obturator outlet (Fig. 15-8)
- Inlet (Fig. 15-9)
- Obturator outlet with drill (Fig. 15-10)

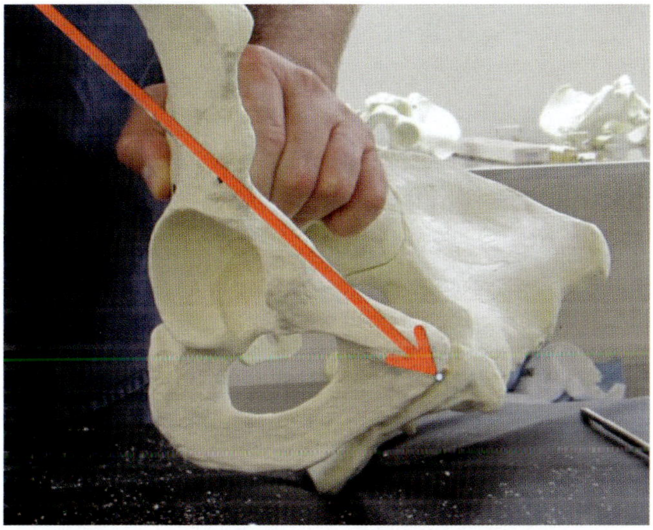

Figure 15-7 |

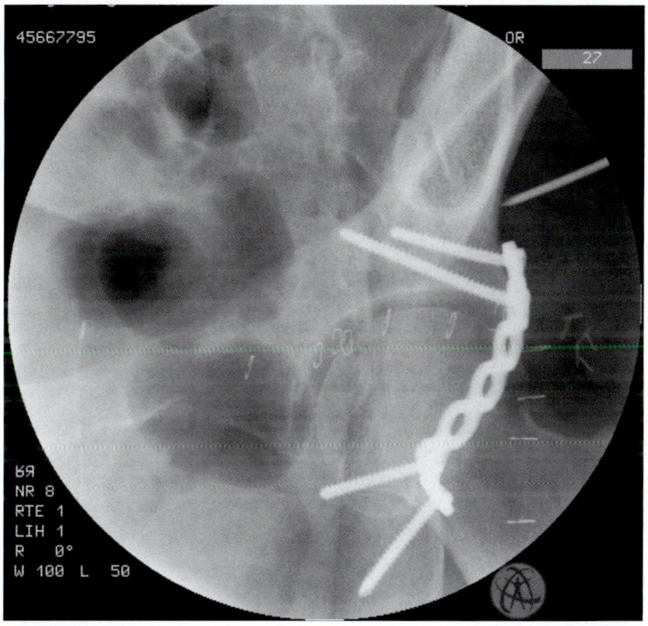

Figure 15-8 |

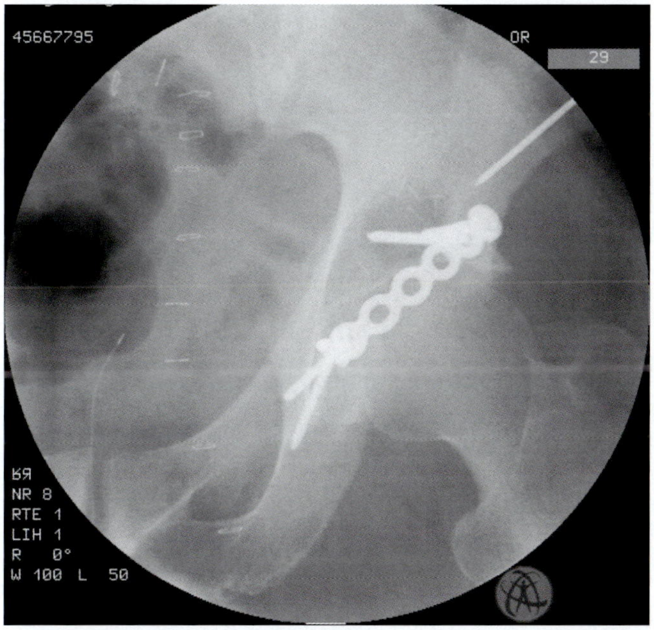

Figure 15-9 |

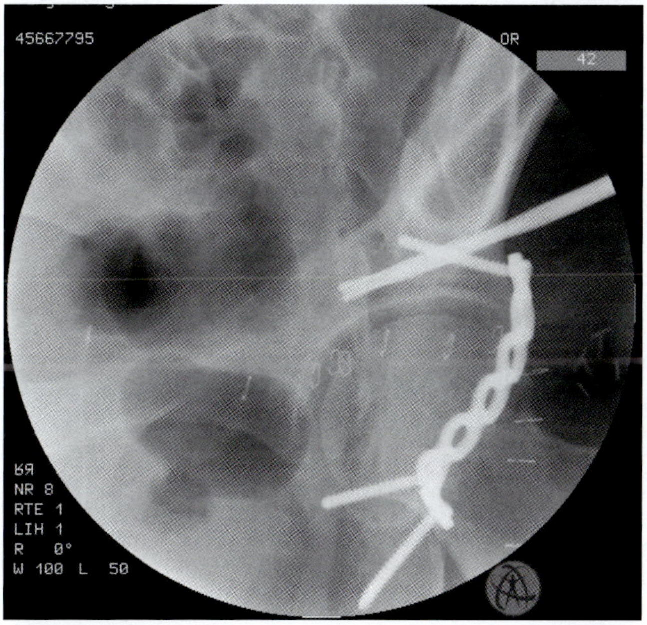

Figure 15-10 |

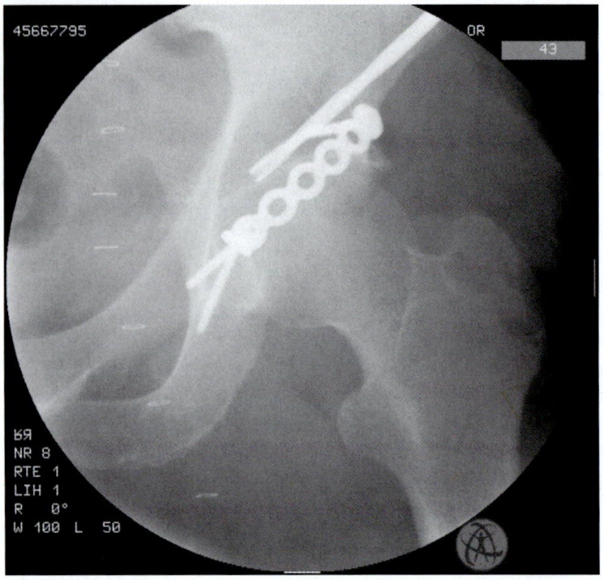

Figure 15-11

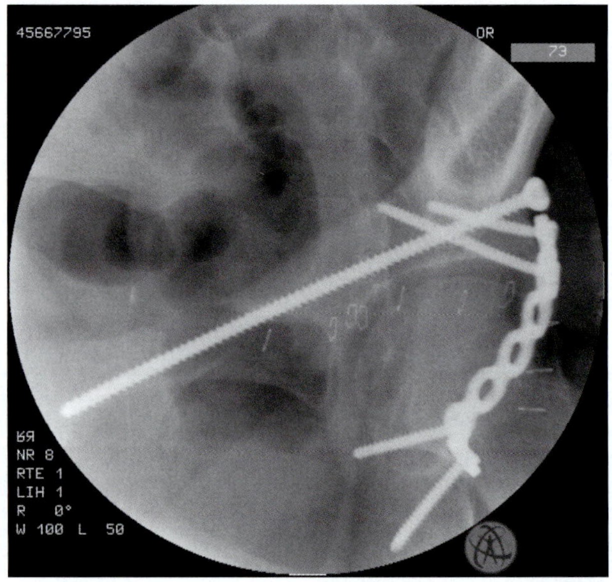

Figure 15-12

- Inlet with drill (Fig. 15-11)
- Final obturator outlet with screw (Fig. 15-12)
- Final inlet with screw (Fig. 15-13)
- Beware of getting tricked with "in-out-in" ramus screw that can appear "in" on both views. This can be avoided with a screw trajectory along the medial corridor of the anterior column on the inlet view and superior corridor on the obturator outlet view (Fig. 15-14).

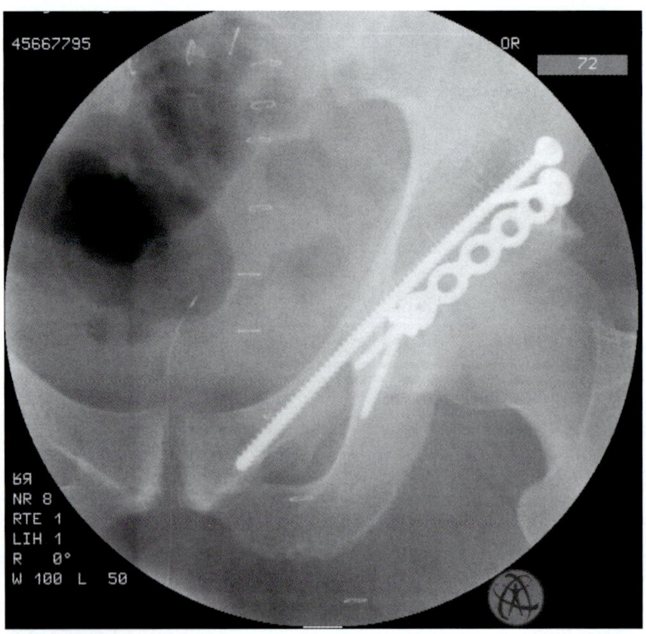

Figure 15-13

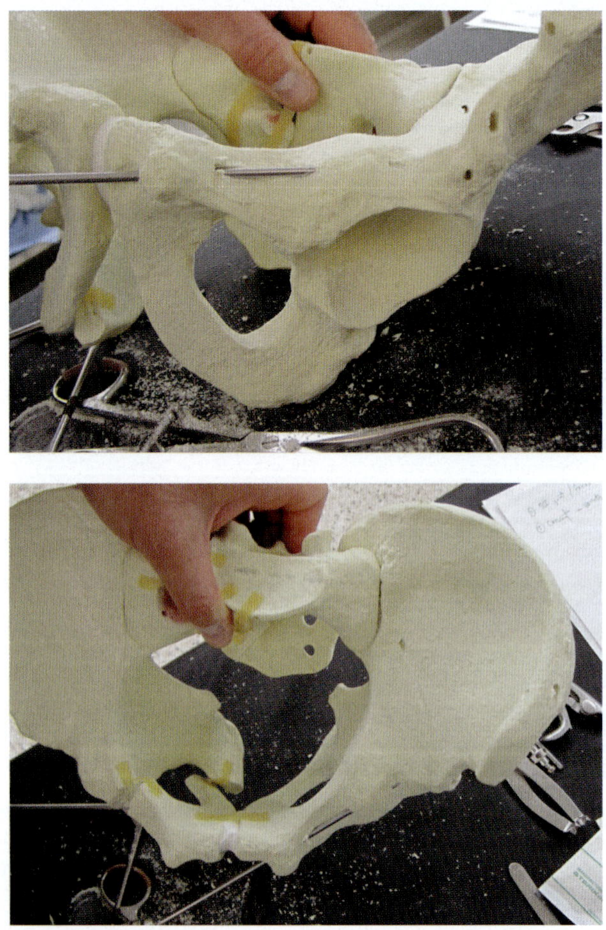
Figure 15-14

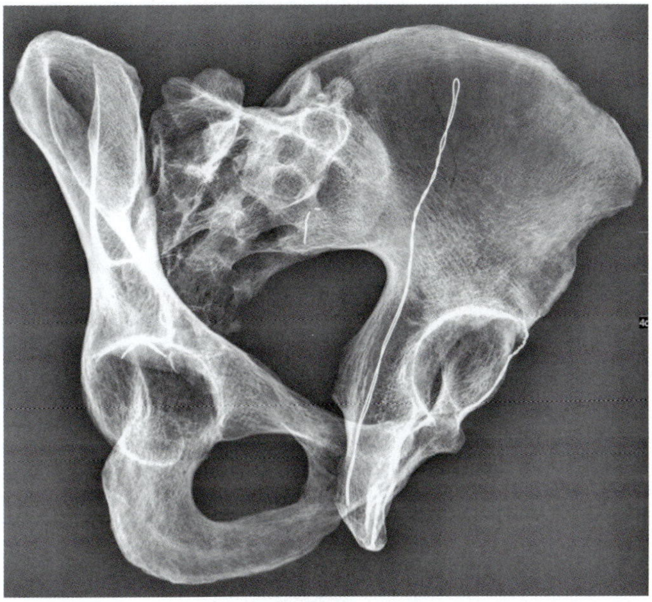

Figure 15-15 |

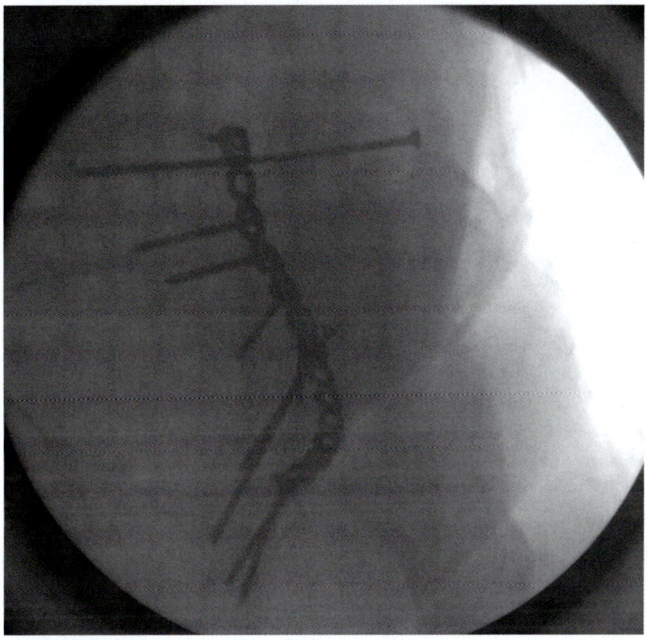

Figure 15-16 |

- Posterior column screws can be placed from antegrade or retrograde trajectory. Iliac oblique view best visualizes posterior column (Figs. 15-15–15-17).
- With all approaches, it is important to avoid screw penetration into the acetabulum, which can be confirmed with a combination of the views above. The surgeon should remember that due to its concavity, any single view can confirm that a screw is out of the acetabulum, even when appearing to penetrate on other views.
- Anterior column screw appears in the acetabulum in Figure 15-18.

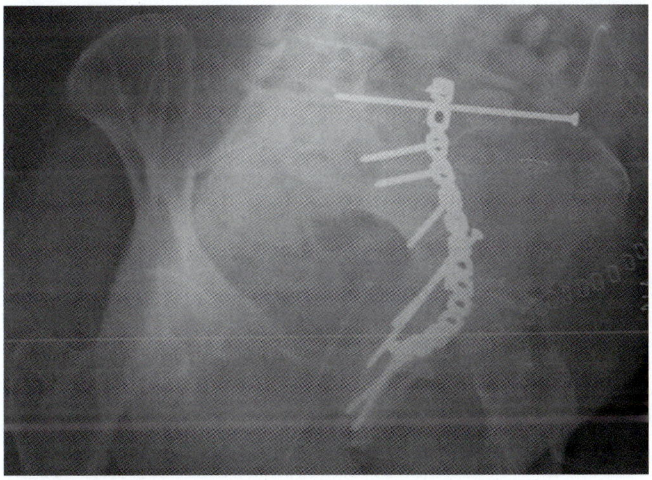

Figure 15-17 |

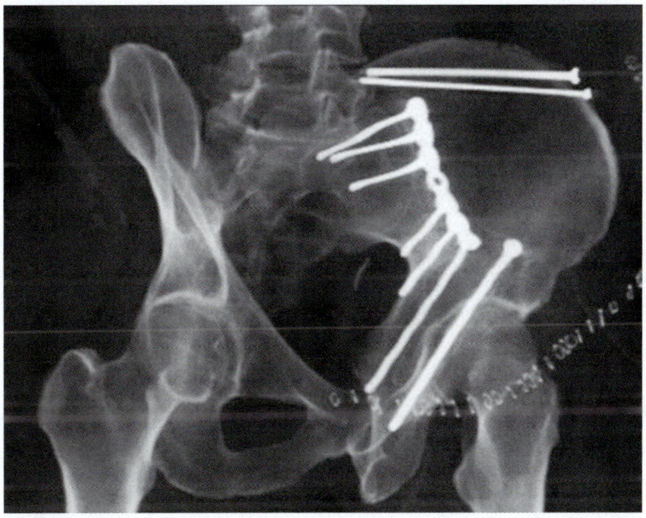

Figure 15-18 |

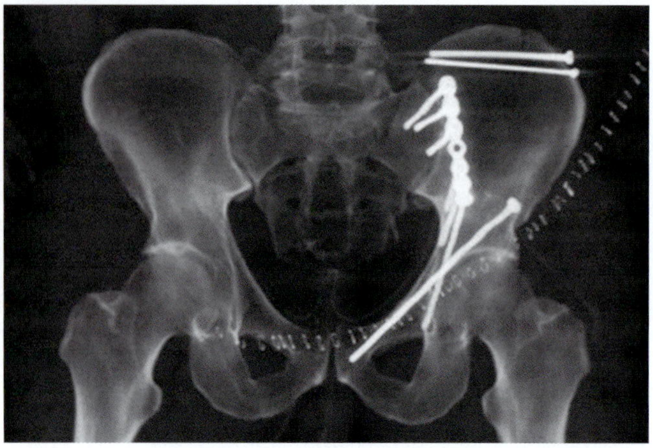

Figure 15-19 |

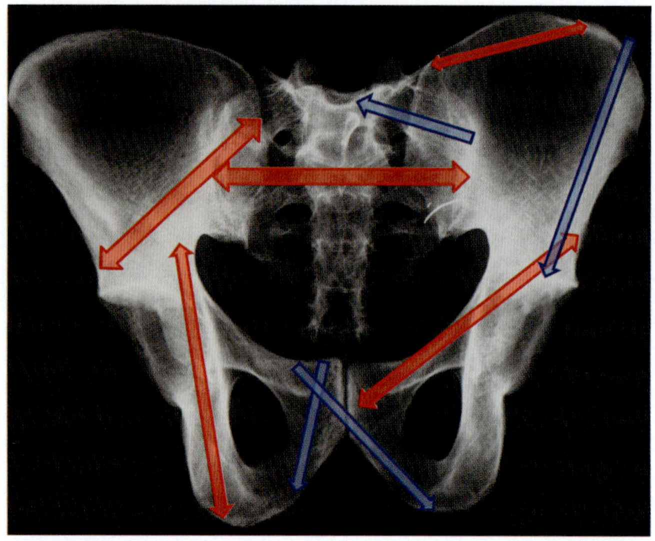

Figure 15-20 |

- Same screw appears out of the acetabulum in Figure 15-19.
- Safe locations for acetabular plating from an anterior (ilioinguinal or Stoppa) approach include the iliac wing, brim of the true pelvis above the quadrilateral surface, and along the anterior column past the psoas gutter to the superior pubic ramus.[1] Potential percutaneous screw corridors are shown in Figure 15-20.
- Safe locations for acetabular plating from a posterior (Kocher-Langenbeck) approach include the posterior column from the greater sciatic notch down to the ischial tuberosity (Fig. 15-21).
- Examples of pre– and post–posterior column screw placement (Figs. 15-22–15-26)

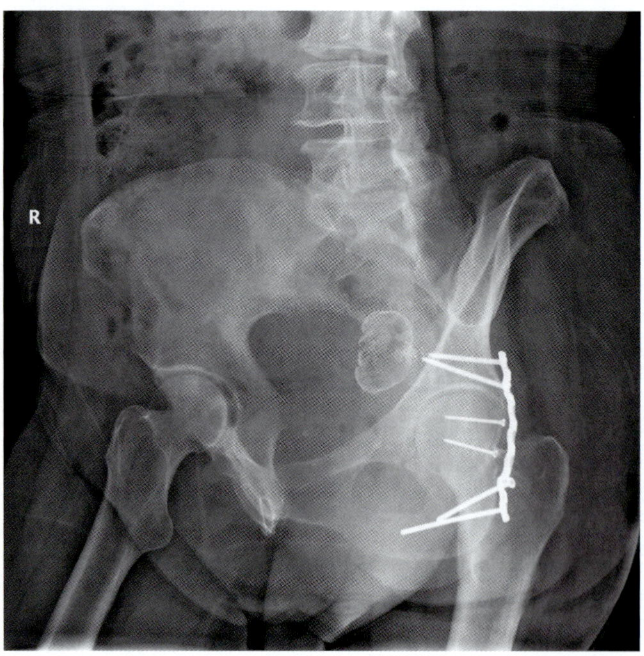

Figure 15-21 |

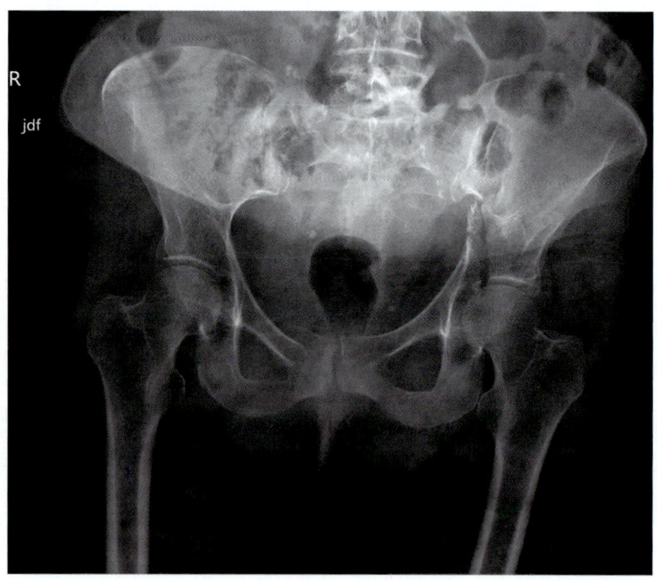

Figure 15-22 |

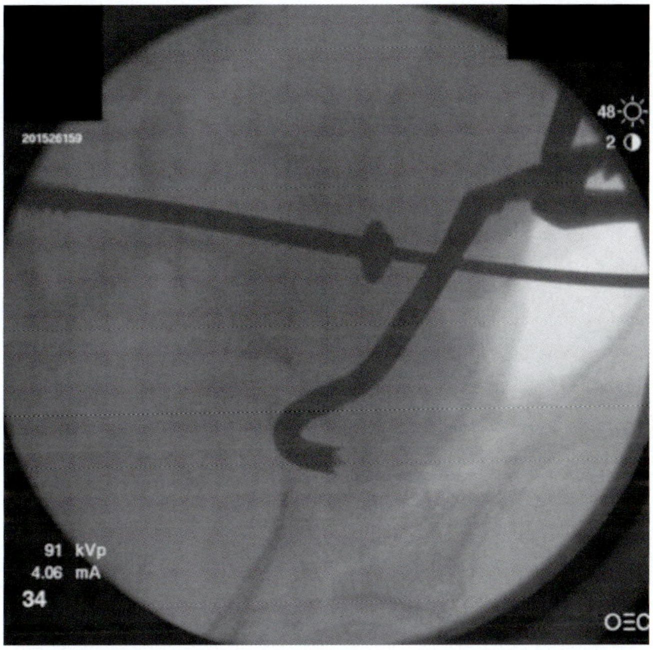

Figure 15-23 |

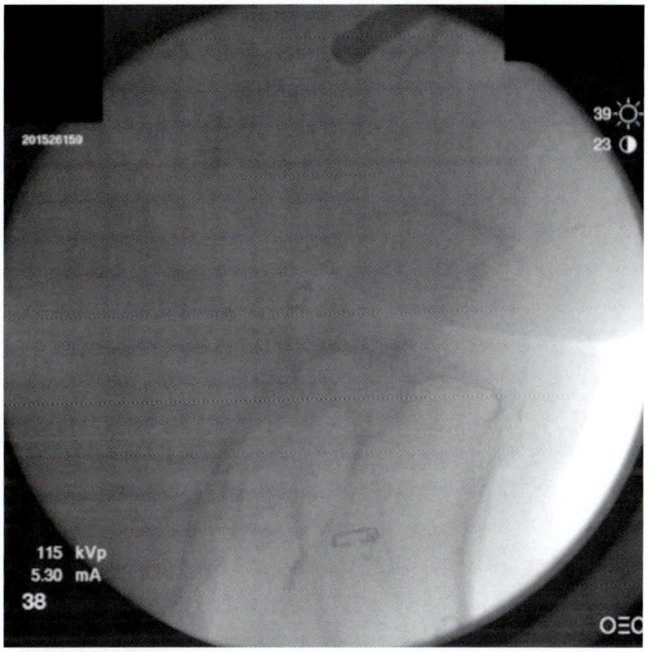

Figure 15-24 |

- Placement of clamp through lateral/middle windows of ilioinguinal approach (Fig. 15-23)
- Reduction with clamp in place (Fig. 15-24)
- Screw placement, iliac oblique view (Fig. 15-25)
- Final (Fig. 15-26)
- Pre– and post–anterior column screw placement (Figs. 15-27–15-30)
- Reduction with clamp, obturator outlet (patient in prone position) (Fig. 15-28)
- Inlet view (from prone position) (Figs. 15-29 and 15-30)

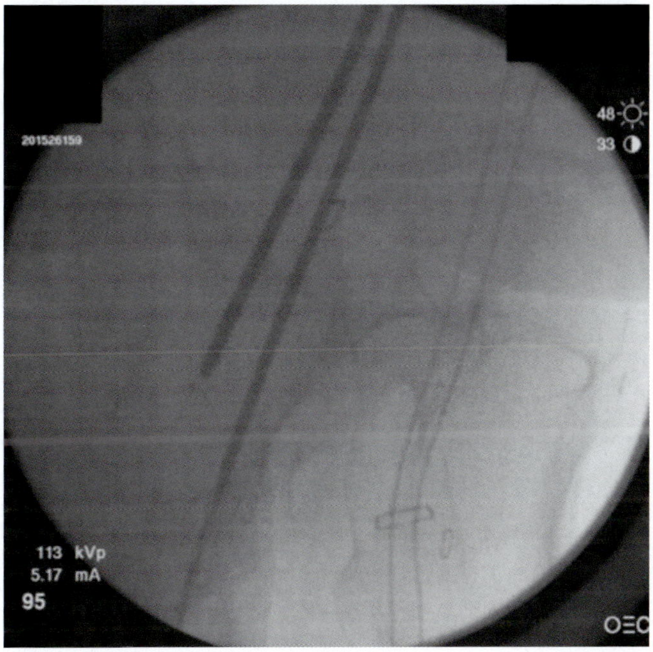

Figure 15-25 |

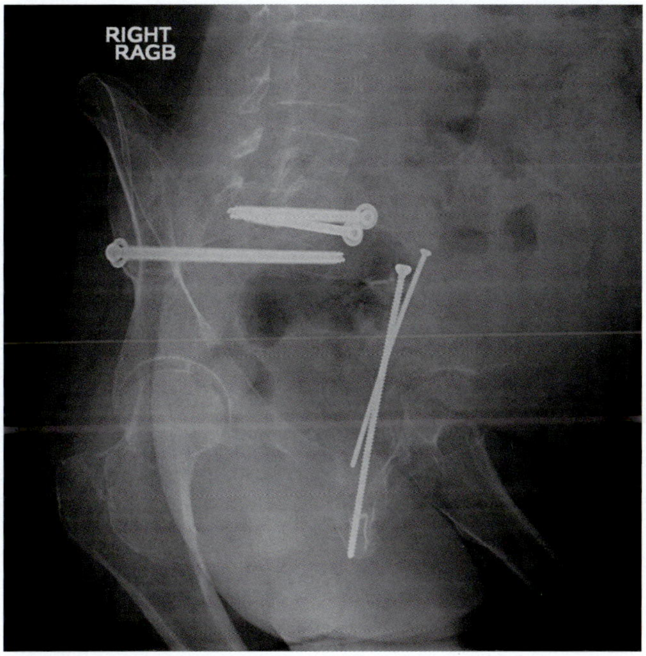

Figure 15-26 |

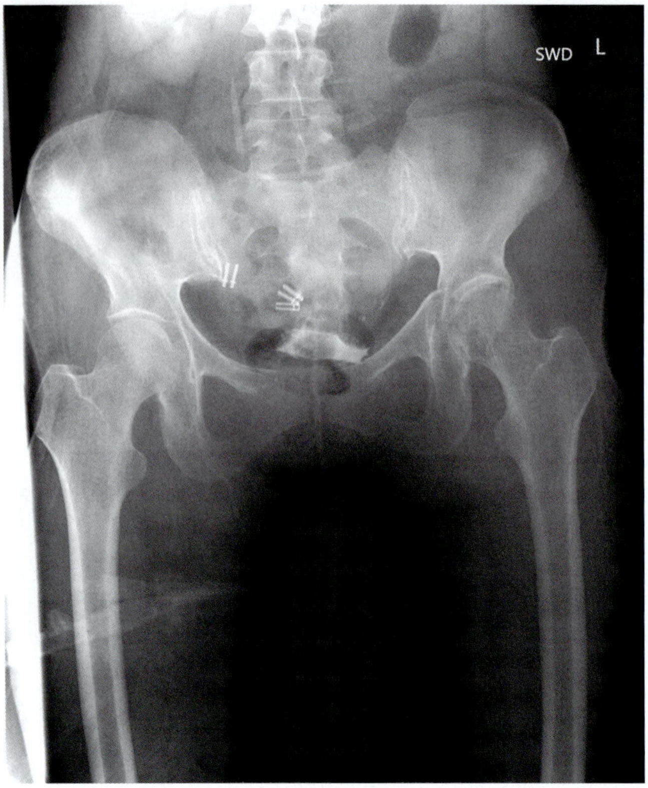

Figure 15-27 |

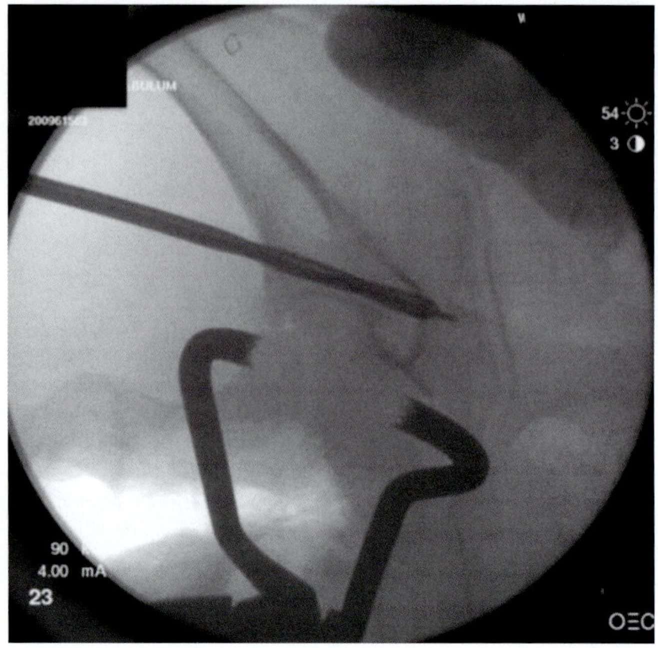

Figure 15-28 |

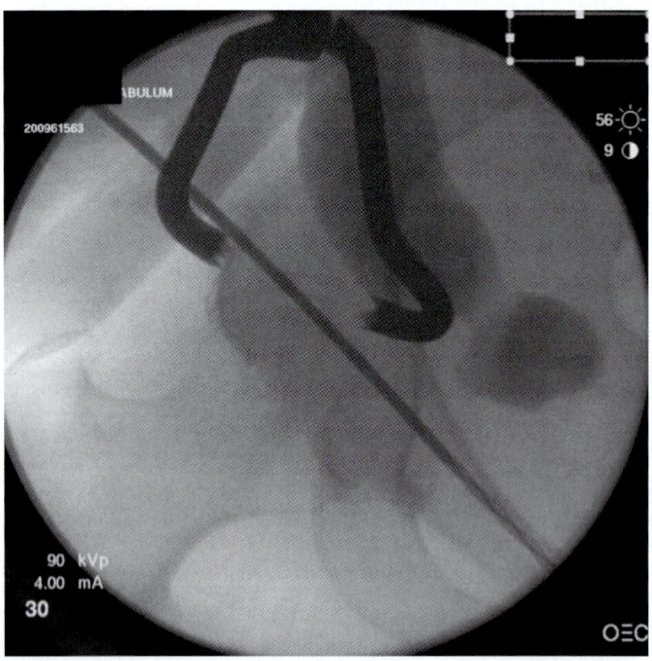

Figure 15-29 |

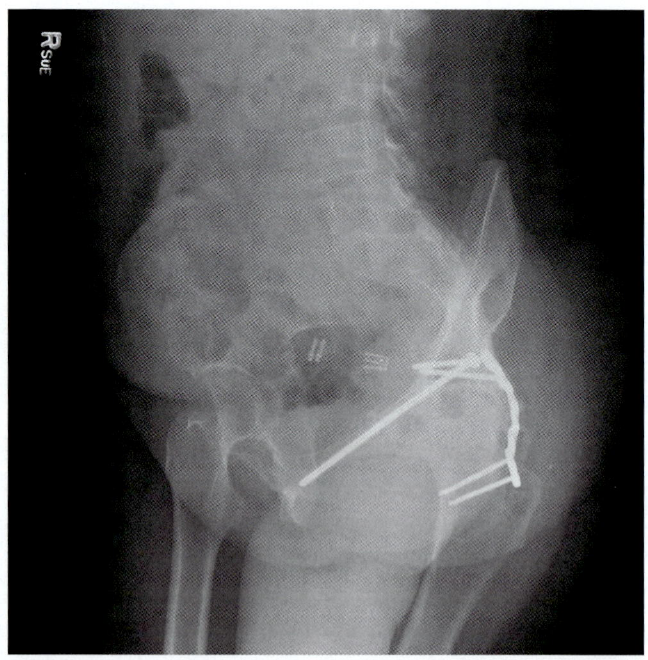

Figure 15-30 |

Intraoperative Positioning

- To perform a stress view of a posterior wall acetabular fracture, an obturator oblique view is used; the C-arm should be positioned on the same side of the table as the injured leg, so that the patient's knee does not contact the C-arm with flexion and internal rotation of the hip (Fig. 15-31).
- Supine positioning: a Jackson table is used to allow for free motion of the C-arm and full visualization. It is important to avoid any free-hanging wires or tubing (such as catheters or compression devices) to avoid getting caught on the C-arm. In addition, the arms should be at 90 degrees on both sides in a cruciform position to avoid collision with the C-arm. A small, centrally placed bump under the sacrum can elevate the pelvis to allow for any potential percutaneous screw fixation. Care should be taken to allow for exposure above the iliac wing as needed for any ilioinguinal approach. Any extremities that are not included in draping should be well padded and secured. The C-arm should be on the opposite side of the table from the injured extremity; however, this may need to move if the surgeon switches sides for visualization during an anterior intrapelvic (modified Stoppa) approach (Figs. 15-32 to 15-35).

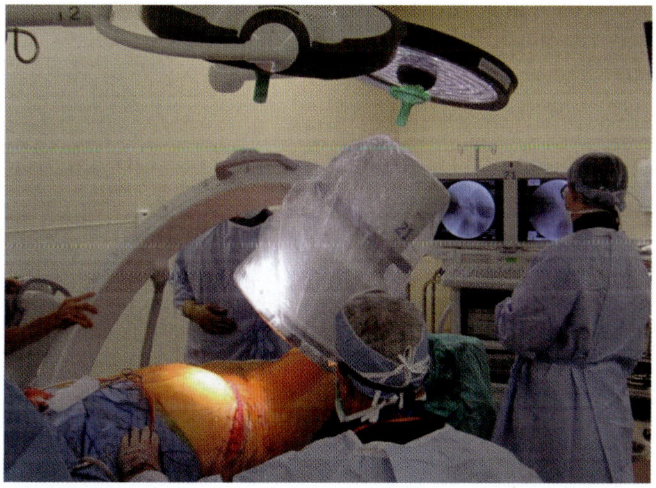

Figure 15-31 |

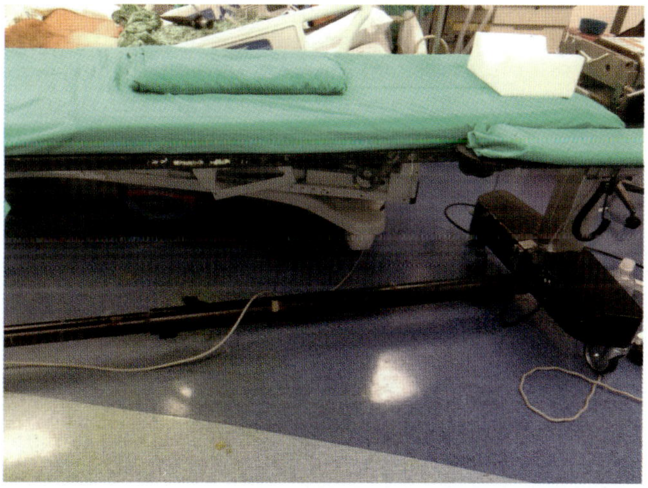

Figure 15-32 |

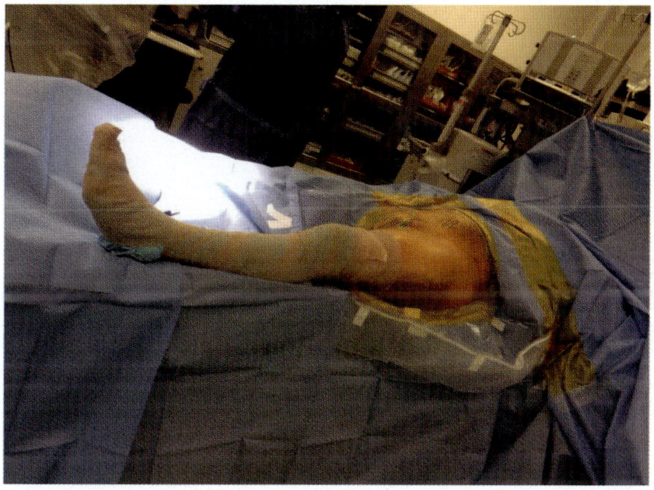

Figure 15-33 |

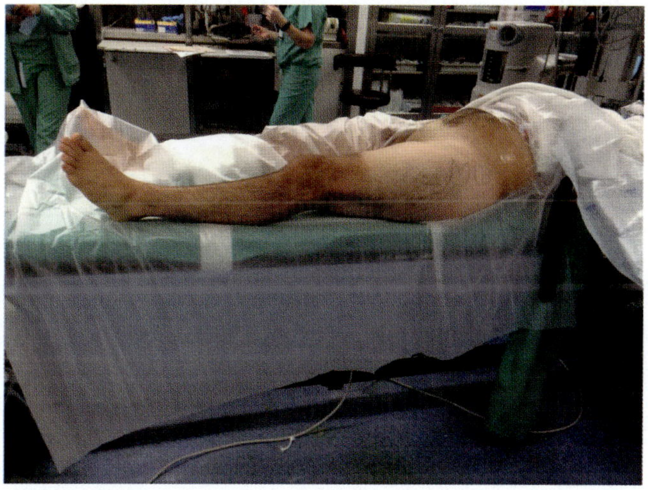

Figure 15-34 |

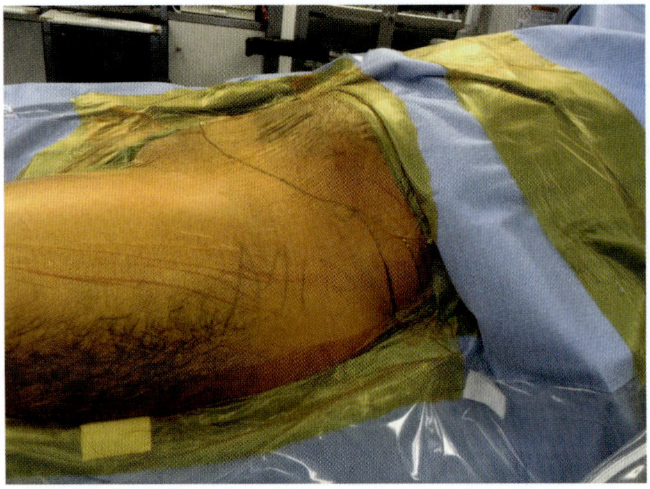

Figure 15-35 |

- Prone positioning: a Jackson table is used to allow for free motion of the C-arm and full visualization. It is important to avoid any free-hanging wires or tubing (such as catheters or compression devices) to avoid getting caught on the C-arm. Gel rolls should be placed under the torso to allow the abdomen to hang free and avoid any pressure on the brachial plexus. In addition, the arms should be flexed on arm holders (taking care to avoid hyperextension at the shoulder) to avoid collision with the C-arm. Care should be taken to allow for exposure anterior to the greater trochanter as needed for the Kocher-Langenbeck approach. Any extremities that are not included in draping should be well padded and secured.
- Lateral positioning: a Jackson table is used to allow for free motion of the C-arm and full visualization. It is important to avoid any free-hanging wires or tubing (such as catheters or compression devices) to avoid getting caught on the C-arm. A vacuum-pressure beanbag should be placed under the torso with an axillary roll to avoid pressure on the brachial plexus. Care should be taken to avoid placing the beanbag too distally, which may interfere with fluoroscopic visualization. Care should be taken to allow for exposure anterior to the iliac crest and greater trochanter as needed for the Kocher-Langenbeck approach. Any extremities that are not included in draping should be well padded and secured.

Reference

1. Bishop JA, Routt ML Jr. Osseous fixation pathways in pelvic and acetabular fracture surgery: osteology, radiology, and clinical applications. *J Trauma Acute Care Surg.* 2012;72(6):1502–1509. doi:10.1097/TA.0b013e318246efe5

Chapter 16
Pelvic Ring Injuries: External Fixation and INFIX

CHRISTIAAN N. MAMCZAK

Bony Anatomy

- The pelvis is a complex, three-dimensional ring structure with many irregular topographic surfaces that are not clearly defined by tangential imaging.
- The bony pelvis is composed of the right and left ilium, which articulate posteriorly with the sacrum (sacroiliac/SI joint) and become confluent with the right and left pubic bones for the anterior symphyseal joint.
- Pelvic ring fracture patterns and/or symphyseal and SI joint dislocations are dependent upon the mechanism of injury, the imparted force, the direction of that force, and the degree of bony resiliency (with a spectrum from pediatric to geriatric patients).
- The anterior symphyseal joint between left and right pubic bodies is fairly linear and easily assessed for abnormal widening (>2 cm) on standard AP pelvic imaging.
- The posterior sacroiliac joints have greater anatomic variability with an oblique orientation to the coronal, sagittal, and axial planes. Standard AP imaging offers some diagnostic clues to widening or displacement, but specialized views (i.e., inlet, outlet, and obturator-inlet) better delineate this joint.
- Sacral dysmorphism of the superior sacral segment may be present in up to 40% of cases with the following radiographic markers: (1) upper sacral segment collinear with the level of the iliac crests (AP and outlet views), (2) irregular, noncircular superior sacral segment foramina (outlet view), (3) underdeveloped transverse processes (a.k.a. mammillary bodies) (AP and outlet views), and (4) residual upper sacral segment disks (AP and outlet views) and tongue-in-groove SI joint contour as seen on CT imaging.[1]
- The ilium is most commonly used for external fixation and pelvic INFIX frames. Traditionally, iliac crest fixation occurs 3 to 4 cm posterior to the ASIS at the gluteus medius pillar with pins aimed between the iliac inner and outer tables. Supra-acetabular frame or INFIX fixation utilizes a large corridor of bone beginning anterolaterally at the AIIS and traversing posteromedially toward the PSIS. Due to its location near the equator of the bony pelvis, supra-acetabular fixation constructs yield the greatest power and control of hemipelvic displacements.

Radiographic Anatomy

AP View

- The AP pelvic view is an excellent initial diagnostic tool for the assessment of acute trauma patients with a suspected pelvic ring injury. Note that static images with pelvic sheeting or binders may misrepresent the actual degree of pelvic ring instability (Fig. 16-1).
- Although an excellent initial diagnostic tool, the AP pelvic view alone is insufficient to accurately assess the complex anatomy. A refined knowledge of specific pelvic radiographic views is imperative to assure that adequate reduction and safe instrumentation have been achieved.
- "Open book" (APC) injuries will display various degrees of symphyseal widening (with or without rami fractures), as well as posterior pelvic sacroiliac widening/dislocation or sacral fractures (Fig. 16-2).

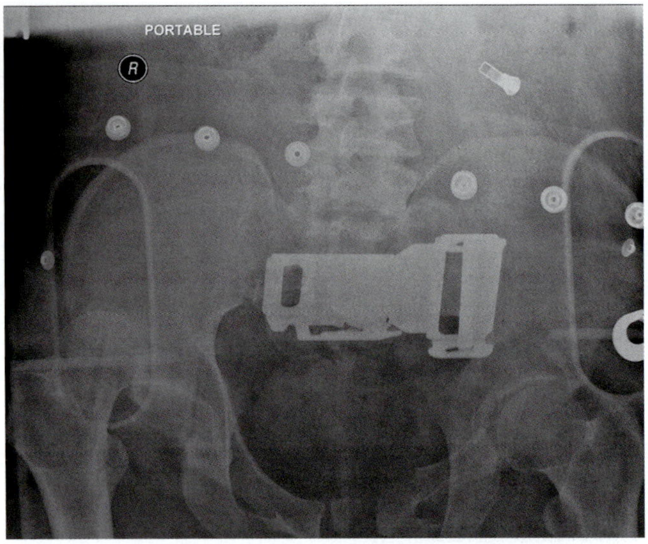

Figure 16-1 | A screening AP pelvic radiograph demonstrates symphyseal widening and concern for a left hemipelvic rotational deformity. The backboard buckle obscures the posterior pelvic anatomy. Note that the right hip is posteriorly dislocated.

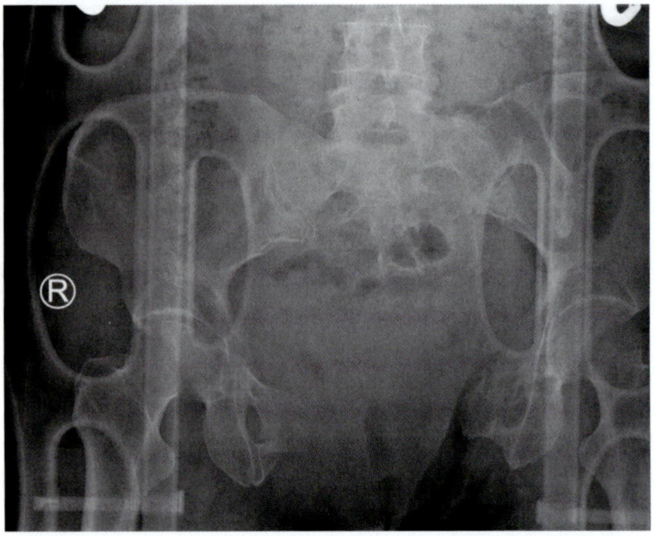

Figure 16-2 | This trauma AP radiograph depicts significant widening of the anterior and posterior pelvis (open book injury). This patient is at risk for hemodynamic shock and requires emergent reduction of the pelvic ring.

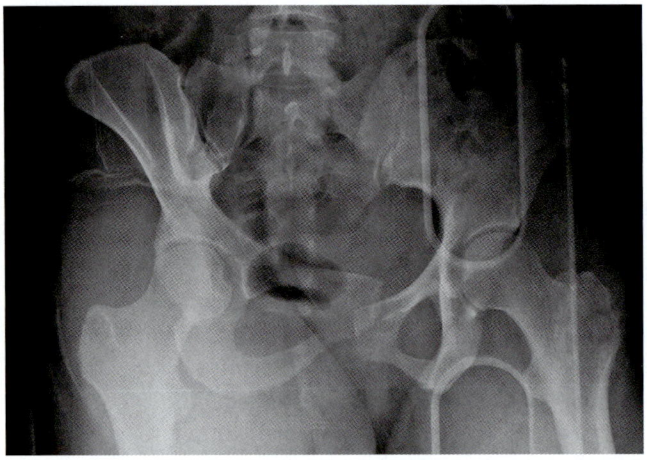

Figure 16-3 | This AP pelvic radiograph demonstrates a lateral compression injury to the right hemipelvis with considerable internal rotation deformity. Note the difference in obturator ring projections.

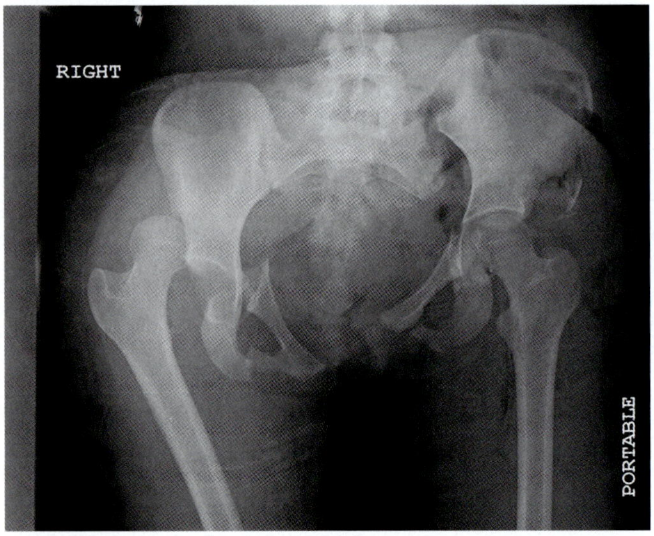

Figure 16-4 | This AP pelvic view shows a combined pelvic ring and acetabular injury pattern globally disrupting the normal anatomy: the left hemipelvis has a vertical translation with complete anterior and posterior instability. This patient requires reduction of the dislocated right hip, left lower extremity skeletal traction and a binder.

- Lateral compression injuries may show laterality of ramus and sacral fractures with degrees of internal rotation and occasionally contralateral hemipelvic windswept deformities (Fig. 16-3).
- Vertical shear injuries display affected hemipelvic vertical instability of the anterior and posterior pelvis structures (Fig. 16-4).

Inlet View

- Although traditional techniques describe a 45-degree inlet view, posterior pelvic screening assessment in the average patient is generally best illustrated with a 20-degree cranial-to-caudal tilt.[2] The actual degree of necessary intraoperative fluoroscopy angle is dependent upon patient positioning, individual natural pelvic obliquity, or posterior pelvic displacement from injury but can be estimated from the sacral sagittal CT (Fig. 16-5).[3]
- Posterior pelvic sacroiliac dislocation/widening and crescent fractures are well visualized with this view, including the degree of anterior or posterior displacement of the SI joint. Anterior pelvic translation and rotational (internal or external) deformities are also well visualized (Figs. 16-6 and 16-7).

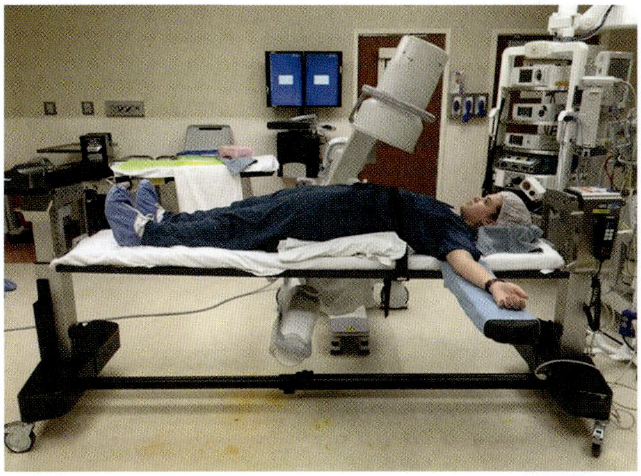

Figure 16-5 | Clinical demonstration of a pelvic inlet view with the patient in a supine position.

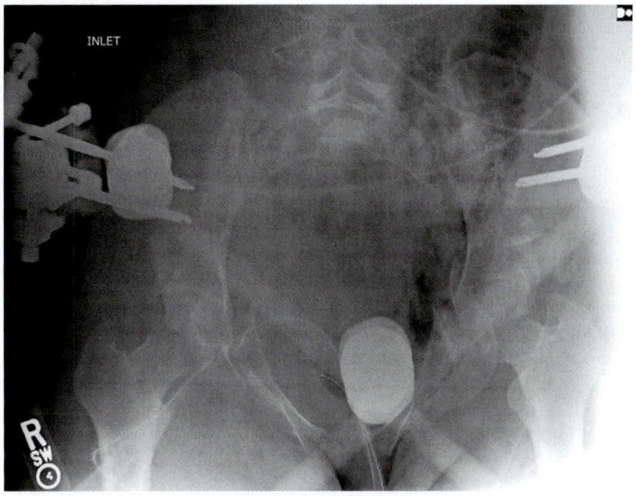

Figure 16-6 | This pelvic inlet view depicts left hemipelvic posterior translation and anterior symphyseal widening. External fixation has dramatically improved the ring anatomy from the original deformity (Fig. 16-4).

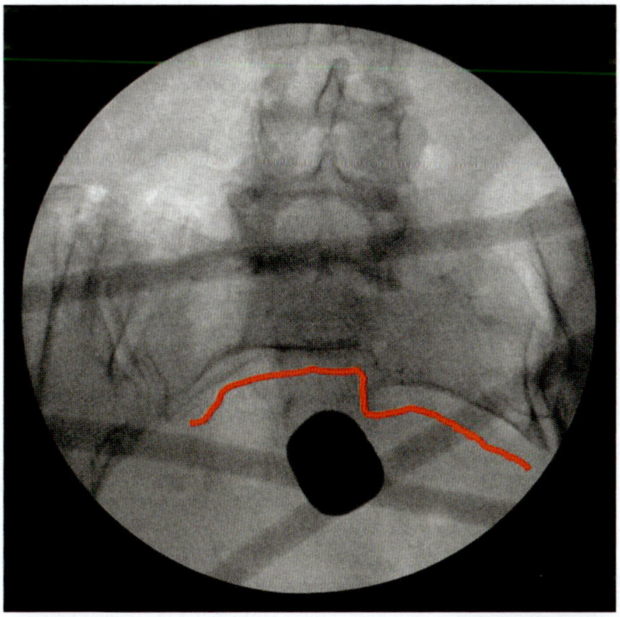

Figure 16-7 | This inlet fluoro view demonstrates the anterior displacement of this left zone 2 sacral fracture relative to the right hemipelvis.

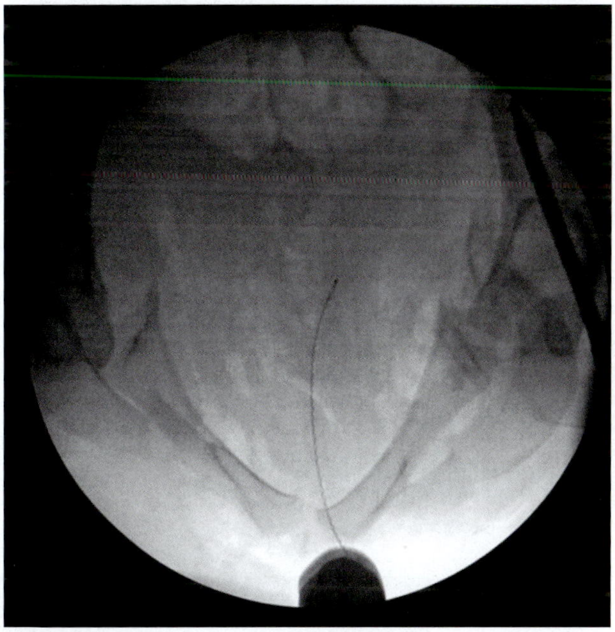

Figure 16-8 | This inlet fluoro view demonstrates improved reduction of the anterior pelvic widening. Bilateral pubic root fractures with symphyseal disruption represent a challenging injury pattern.

- A hyperinlet (>45 degree) of the anterior pelvis can display the degree of symphyseal or ramus fracture displacement, widening, and malrotation (internal or external). Increasing inlet tilt is performed until the superior and inferior rami overlap. Postreduction inlet images should demonstrate an acceptable posterior and anterior reduction (Figs. 16-8 and 16-9).

Outlet View

- Although traditional radiographic techniques describe a 45-degree outlet view, screening radiographs for posterior pelvic injury are generally best illustrated with a 55-degree caudal-to-cranial tilt in the average patient (Fig. 16-10).[2]
- Craniocaudal hemipelvic displacement and flexion deformities of the anterior and posterior pelvis are well visualized on the outlet view. Again, the actual degree of necessary intraoperative fluoroscopy angle is dependent upon patient positioning, individual natural pelvic obliquity, or posterior pelvic displacement from injury but can be estimated from the lateral sacral CT (Figs. 16-11 and 16-12).[3]

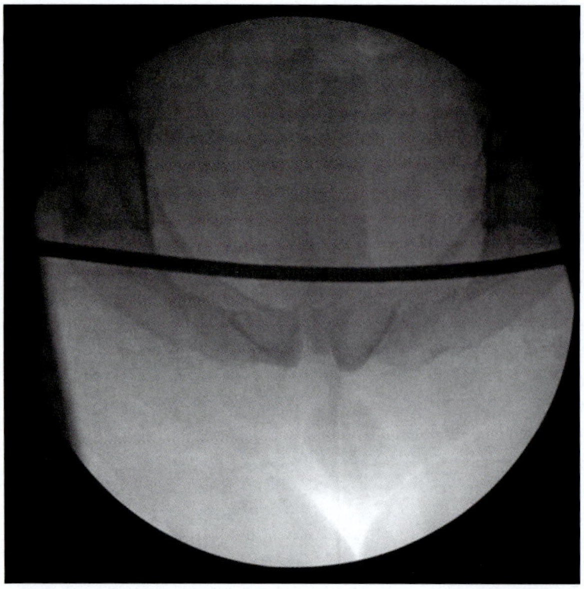

Figure 16-9 | This hyperinlet fluoro view confirms adequate reduction of the anterior symphysis in a ring injury where a pelvic INFIX was utilized.

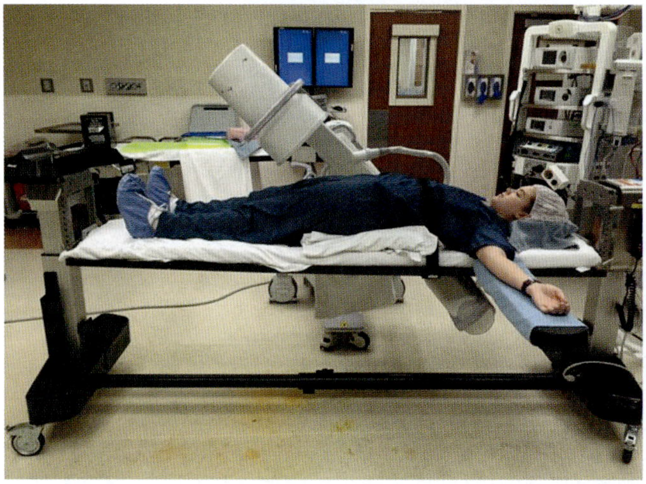

Figure 16-10 | Clinical demonstration of a pelvic outlet view with the patient in a supine position.

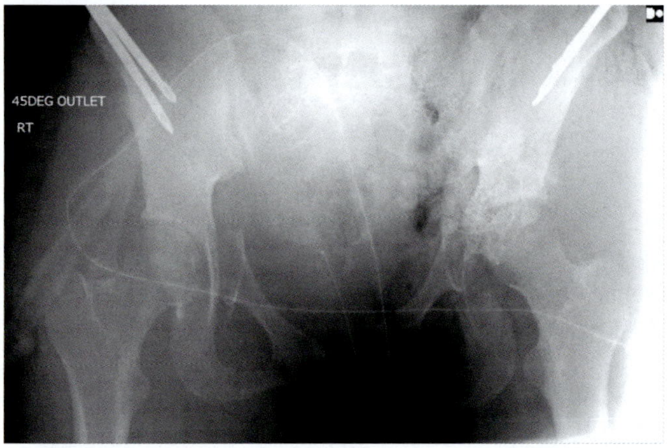

Figure 16-11 | This pelvic outlet view depicts a subtle left hemipelvic vertical translation and flexion moment. External fixation has dramatically improved the ring anatomy from the original deformity (Fig. 16-4).

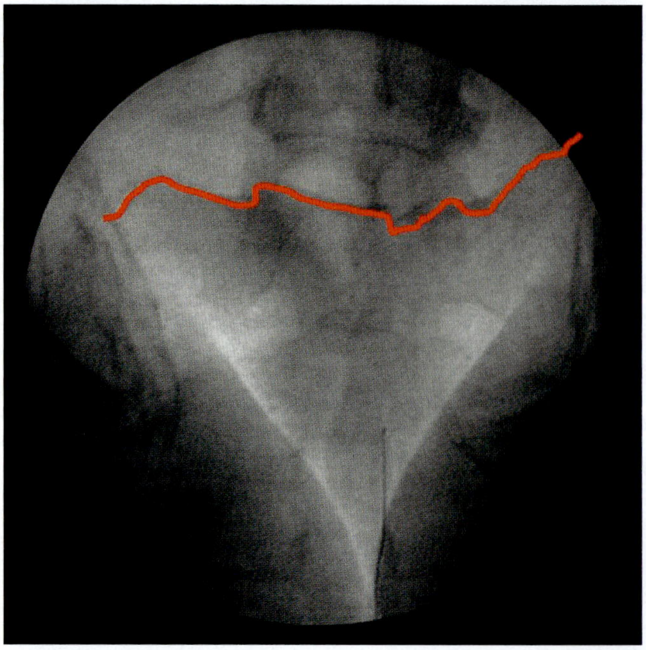

Figure 16-12 | This outlet fluoro view depicts vertical displacement of the left zone 2 sacral fracture relative to the right hemipelvis.

Preoperative Imaging

- Standard AP with inlet and outlet views should be obtained on all pelvic ring injuries in order to assess the degree of instability and displacement. Judet views should be added for associated ring and acetabular patterns.
- Static pelvic images (radiographs or fluoroscopy) do not necessarily correlate with the degree of pelvic ring instability (i.e., open book injury temporized with pelvic binder).
- Dynamic stress fluoroscopy of the injured pelvis (in a controlled operative environment under anesthesia) can be an instrumental part of understanding the degree of instability and the treatment algorithm for various fracture patterns.[4]
- Two-dimensional CT imaging and three-dimensional CT imaging have been shown to be a useful preoperative planning adjunct to diagnostic pelvic radiographs. Recently, the value of customized pelvic CT images has been described for accessing fracture pattern displacement and bony corridor safe zones.[2,3]

Intraoperative Positioning

- Surgical fixation of pelvic ring injuries is dependent on the patient's hemodynamic stability, the fracture pattern(s), surgical approach, definitive fixation preference (i.e., formal ORIF vs. percutaneous fixation), and surgeon preference or experience.
- Patients in extremis or demonstrating borderline signs and symptoms of hemodynamic shock are best treated with damage control temporizing pelvic stabilization: pelvic binder, antishock pelvic sheeting, pelvic C-clamp, or external fixation + skeletal traction.
- Although anterior subcutaneous fixation (INFIX) is an additional anterior pelvic fixation construct, it has select indications and associated risk/benefits that should not be employed as an immediate fixation construct in a highly unstable patient (due to the differences in operative time versus temporizing external fixation).[5,6]
- A fully radiolucent table (i.e., OSI/Jackson) permits the most degrees of freedom for fluoroscopic imaging of the pelvis (Fig. 16-13).
- The patient should be positioned supine on a midline sacral bump or commercially available Bone Foam device in order to facilitate percutaneous posterior pelvic fixation (if indicated).
- Arms should be abducted 90 degrees (at the shoulder) on armboards to prevent interference with the surgical area and fluoroscopy machine (Fig. 16-14).

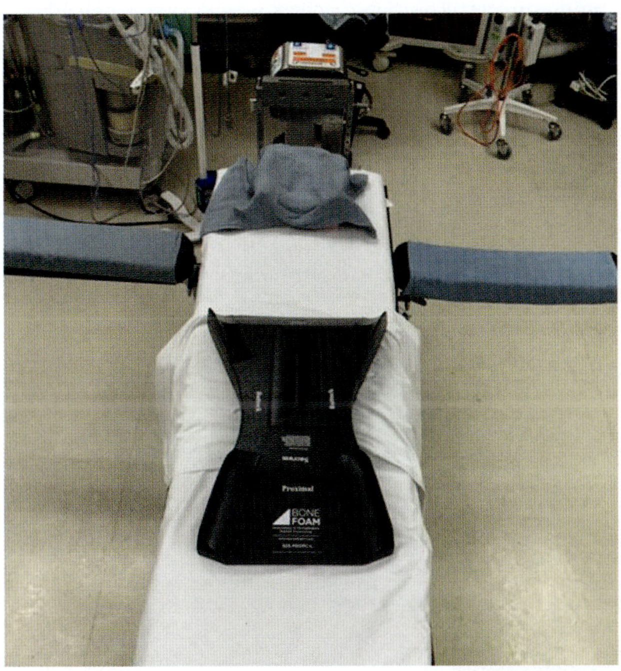

Figure 16-13 | This radiolucent Jackson operating table allows for unobstructed fluoroscopic imaging of the pelvis. Elevation of the pelvis with a Bone Foam sacral positioner allows access to the gluteal regions for sacroiliac screw fixation of a supine patient.

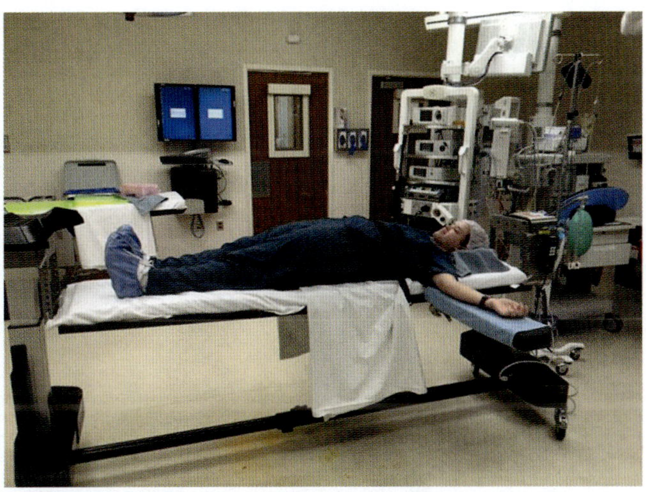

Figure 16-14 | Clinical demonstration of a supine patient on a Jackson table with a sacral foam positioner.

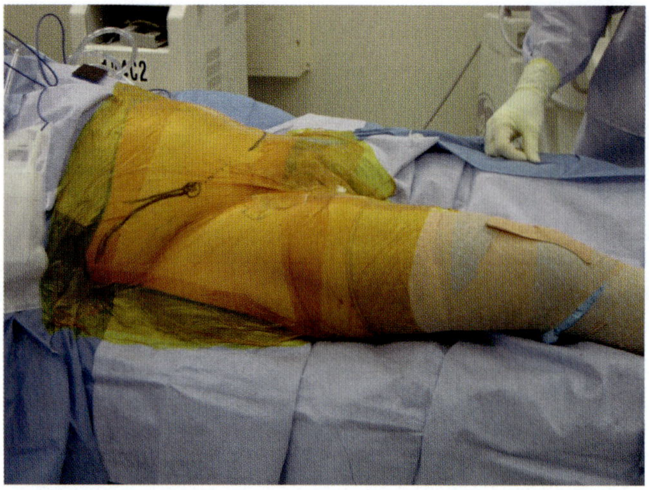

Figure 16-15 | Clinical demonstration of a widely draped pelvis and affected right lower extremity.

- Widely drape the anterior pelvis and gluteal areas from above the umbilicus to the perineal region including an affected lower extremity if necessary (vertical shear injury with skeletal traction) (Fig. 16-15).
- The C-arm should approach the table orthogonally from the side of the least complicated pelvic injury. Note that the surgeon will need to perform anterior pelvic external fixation or INFIX instrumentation from both sides. If possible, dual C-arms facilitate less surgeon interference with the fluoroscopy unit.

Iliac Crest External Fixation Imaging Techniques

- Iliac crest pins should be placed approximately 3 to 4 cm posterior to the anterior superior iliac spine (ASIS) and directed between the inner and outer tables of the ilium for depths as long as possible without penetration of the tables or acetabulum. It is customary to place at least two 5-mm Schanz pins per side through a small open incision to assure greater stability if one pin is poorly orientated. Right and left pin-to-bar constructs are secured anteriorly over the symphysis after reduction of pelvic volume. Multiplanar bars can be added for stability.
- A common mistake is to place pins too vertically where they quickly penetrate the outer table with minimal bony purchase and risk impinging on the abdomen or chest wall. K-wires placed along the inner and outer tables help delineate the trajectory intraoperatively (slightly anterior and medial closely following the slope of the inner table) (Fig. 16-16).

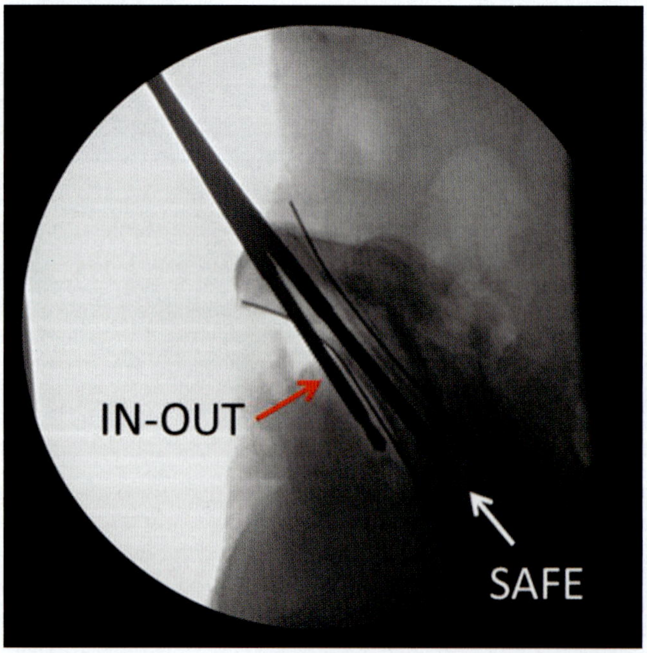

Figure 16-16 | This obturator-outlet fluoro view depicts a Schanz pin safely placed within the iliac tables and one with a vertical trajectory that leads to early outer table penetration and failure to engage the iliac crest with the working length of the pin.

- Another common fault is failure to advance the pins within the iliac crest thereby resulting in a less powerful pin-bone interface for fracture reduction and stabilization; this yields a risk for pin loosening or iliac fracture. These fluoro images demonstrate shallow pin advancement in the iliac oblique view and an attempt looking "down" the pins through a modified obturator view (Figs. 16-17 and 16-18).
- The ideal fluoroscopic image for iliac crest pin placement is the obturator-outlet view, which involves a combination of C-arm movements to efface the inner and outer tables of the ilium from a profile view (Fig. 16-19).[7]
- Although the obturator-inlet view may "look down" a pin within the ilium, it does not yield any information about the pin working length within the bone (Fig. 16-20).

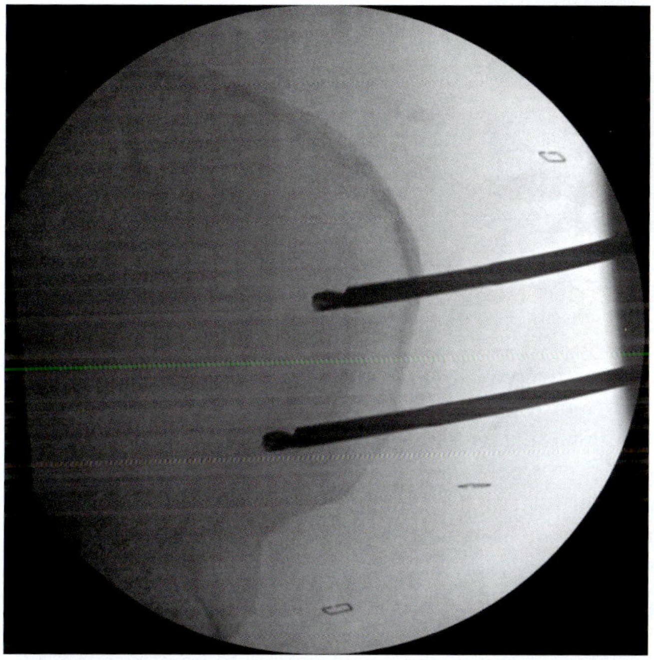

Figure 16-17 I This iliac fluoro view shows a very short working length for pelvic external fixation pins.

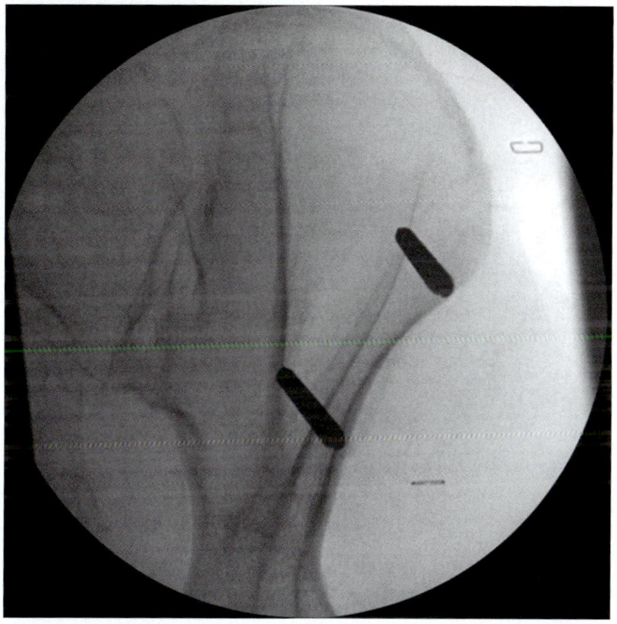

Figure 16-18 I This obturator-inlet fluoro view shoots down the short pins providing only proof that the pins have been placed into the iliac crest but offers no confirmation of the working length or penetration of the inner or outer table.

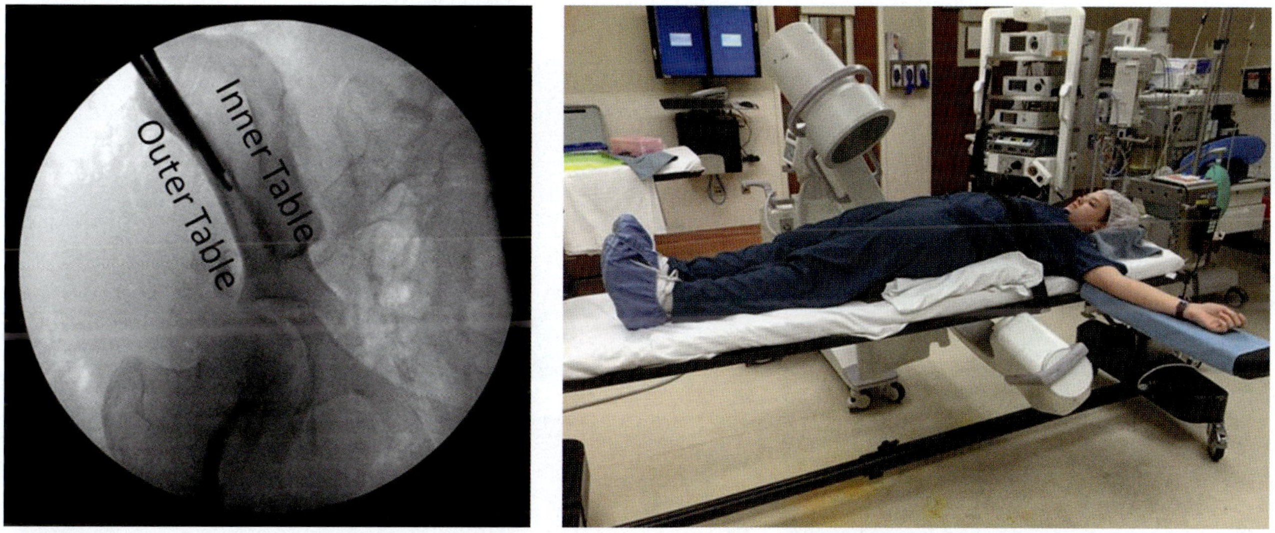

Figure 16-19 I This obturator-outlet fluoro view depicts the safe placement of two iliac crest pins within the tables for a desired working length. A clinical demonstration of a right obturator-outlet view is shown.

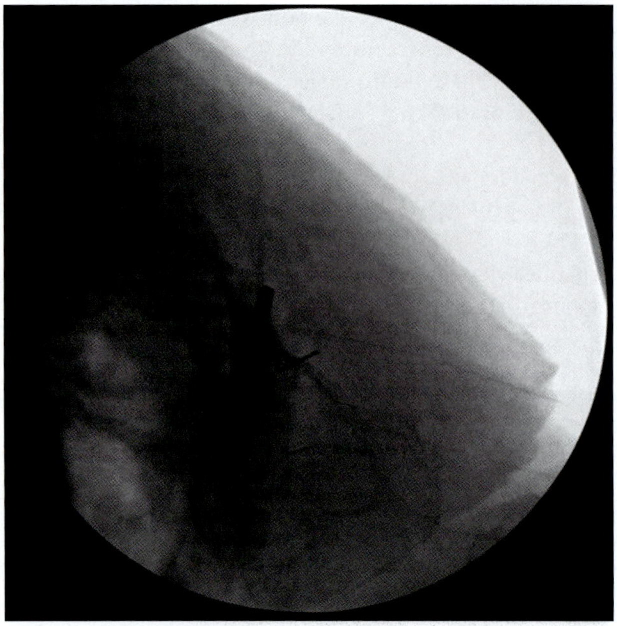

Figure 16-20 | This obturator-inlet fluoro view only depicts a proper starting point on the iliac crest (note the K-wires outlining the inner and outer tables).

Supra-acetabular/AIIS External Fixation and INFIX Imaging Techniques

- A sizable bony corridor is available just above the pelvic brim and extends within each ilium from the ASIS to the PSIS. External fixation pins and/or pedicle screws for the subcutaneous INFIX system placed within this location give commanding hemipelvic control to use as reduction aids or definitive fixation.
- The obturator-outlet view effaces the AIIS starting point (green highlight) for this bony corridor. Note that pelvic ring injuries (i.e., open book) may have external rotational displacement that exceeds the C-arm capability to get this perfect view necessitating an iliac oblique view to delineate the starting point (Fig. 16-21).
- The iliac oblique view involves C-arm roll to visualize the ilium in profile; this depicts a sagittal view of the AIIS start point and trajectory of pins/screws aimed within ilium to point just above the sciatic notch. Note that pins or INFIX pedicle screws should be >5 mm above the acetabulum to remain extracapsular and decrease the risk of joint sepsis. The trajectory for pins/screws is from cranial to caudal to the dense bone just above the greater sciatic notch (without cortical penetration to avoid risk to the superior gluteal vessels) (Fig. 16-22).

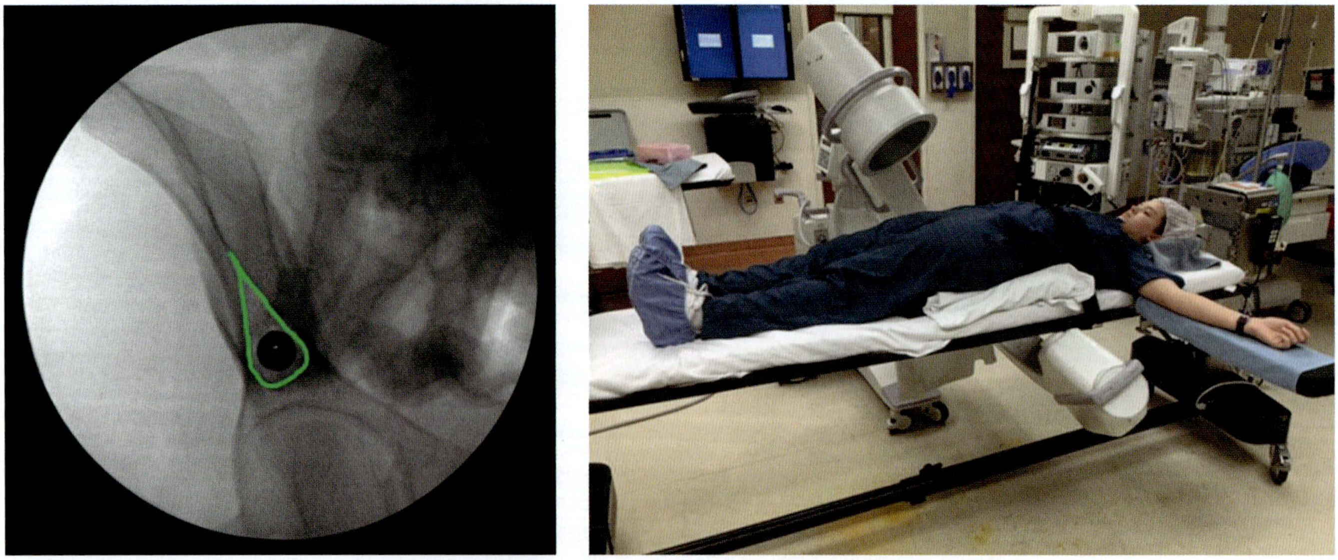

Figure 16-21 | This obturator-outlet fluoro view shows the "teepee" radiographic outline of the AIIS when visualized straight on, denoting the proper starting point for supra-acetabular fixation. A clinical demonstration of a right obturator-outlet view is shown.

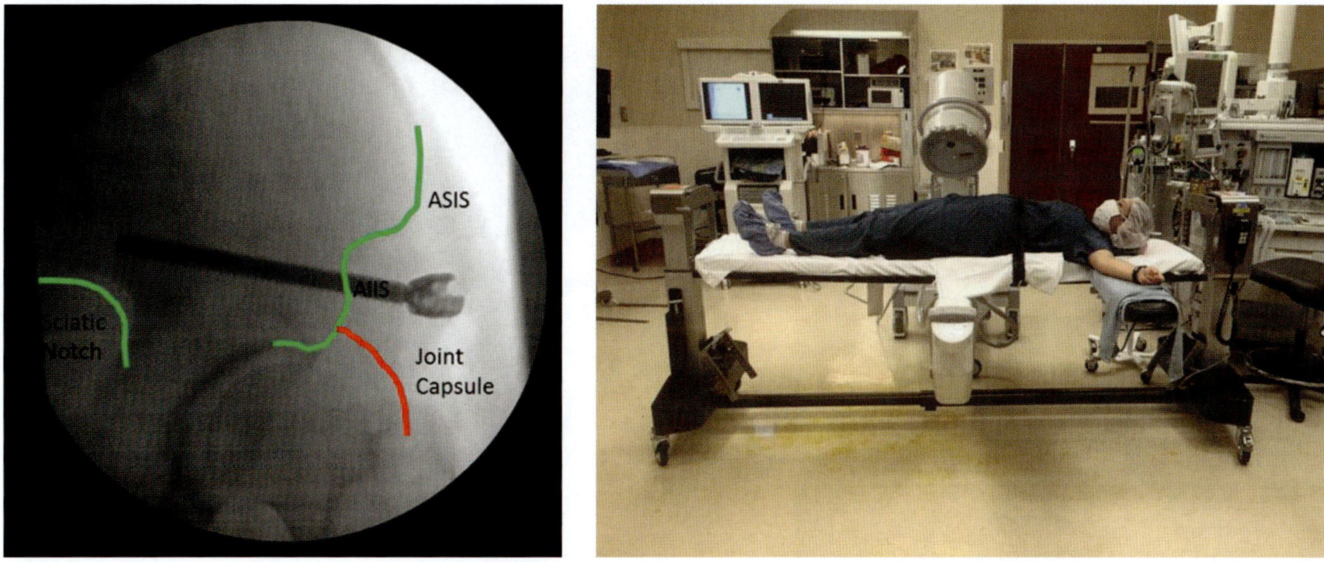

Figure 16-22 | This iliac oblique fluoro view depicts a safely placed INFIX pedicle screw with an optimal AIIS starting point away from the joint capsule. A clinical demonstration of a left iliac oblique view is shown.

- The obturator-inlet view involves a combination of C-arm movements within two planes to view down the ilium and can clearly demonstrate the bony corridor between the inner and outer tables from the AIIS to the PSIS. The trajectory for pin/screw placement usually involves a lateral to medial vector as depicted below, and a cranial-to-caudal vector as verified by the iliac oblique view (above) (Fig. 16-23).
- Lateral sacral view is an additional supplementary view that may be used during iliosacral screw placement. Care should be made to adjust table height and C-arm roll and wag to perfectly overlap the greater sciatic notches, as this represents a true lateral view. Supra-acetabular pin/screw fixation is assessed to assure placement just above the sciatic notch without cortical penetration (Fig. 16-24).
- The following fluoroscopy sequences demonstrate pelvic INFIX pedicle screw placement utilizing the obturator-outlet, obturator-inlet, iliac, and lateral sacral views (as described above) (Fig. 16-25).
- Below is an anatomic model of pelvic INFIX instrumentation as viewed from the AP, inlet, outlet, and lateral vantage points. Note the anterior curvature of the connecting (subcutaneous) rod in the inlet image and superior reflection in the lateral view (Fig. 16-26).

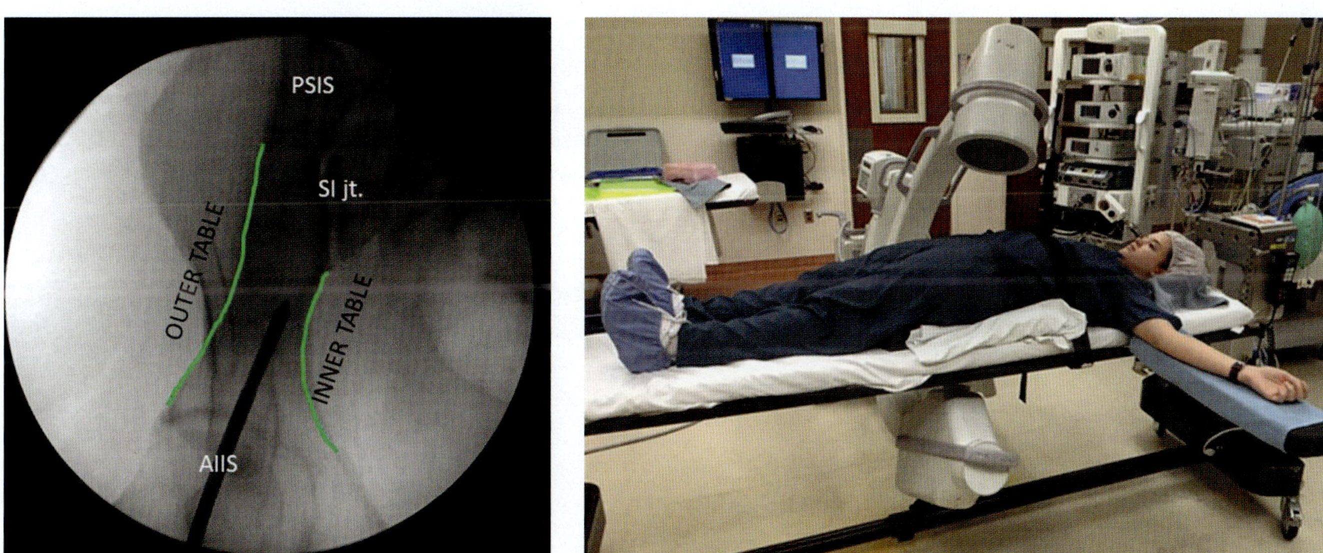

Figure 16-23 | This obturator-inlet fluoro view shows a safely placed supra-acetabular Schanz pin within the iliac corridor; note that it stops short of the trajectory for an iliosacral screw. A clinical demonstration of a right obturator-inlet view is shown.

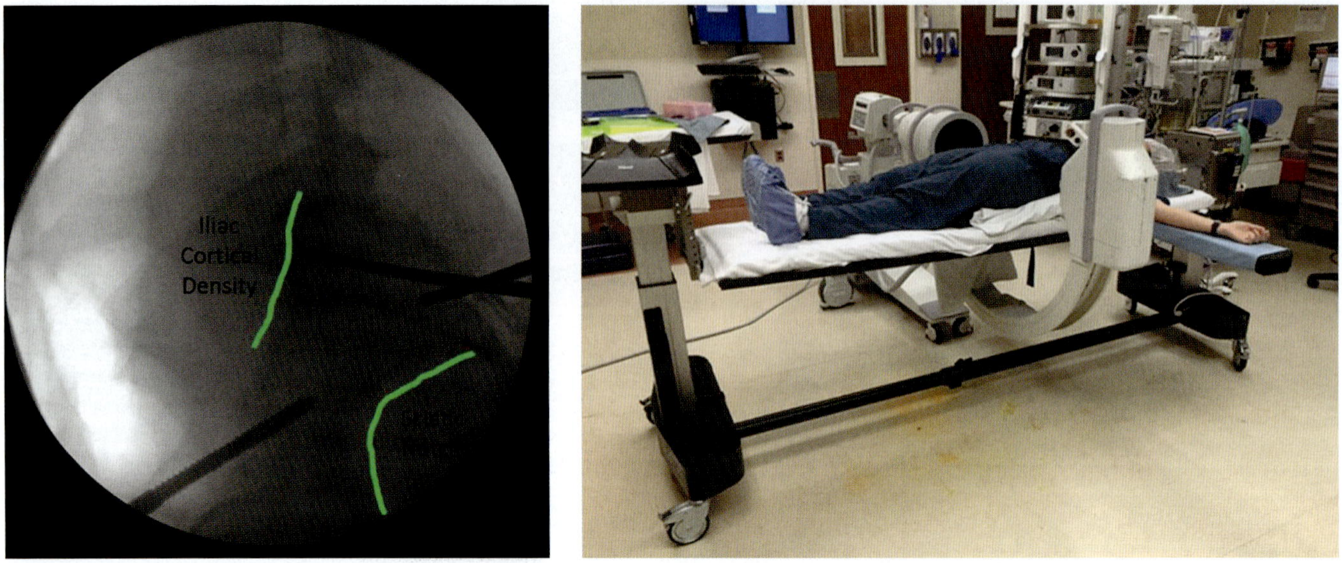

Figure 16-24 | This sagittal sacral fluoro view depicts an S-1 guide wire appropriately placed below the iliac cortical density and the proper starting point for an S-2 guide wire. A clinical demonstration of a lateral sacral view is shown.

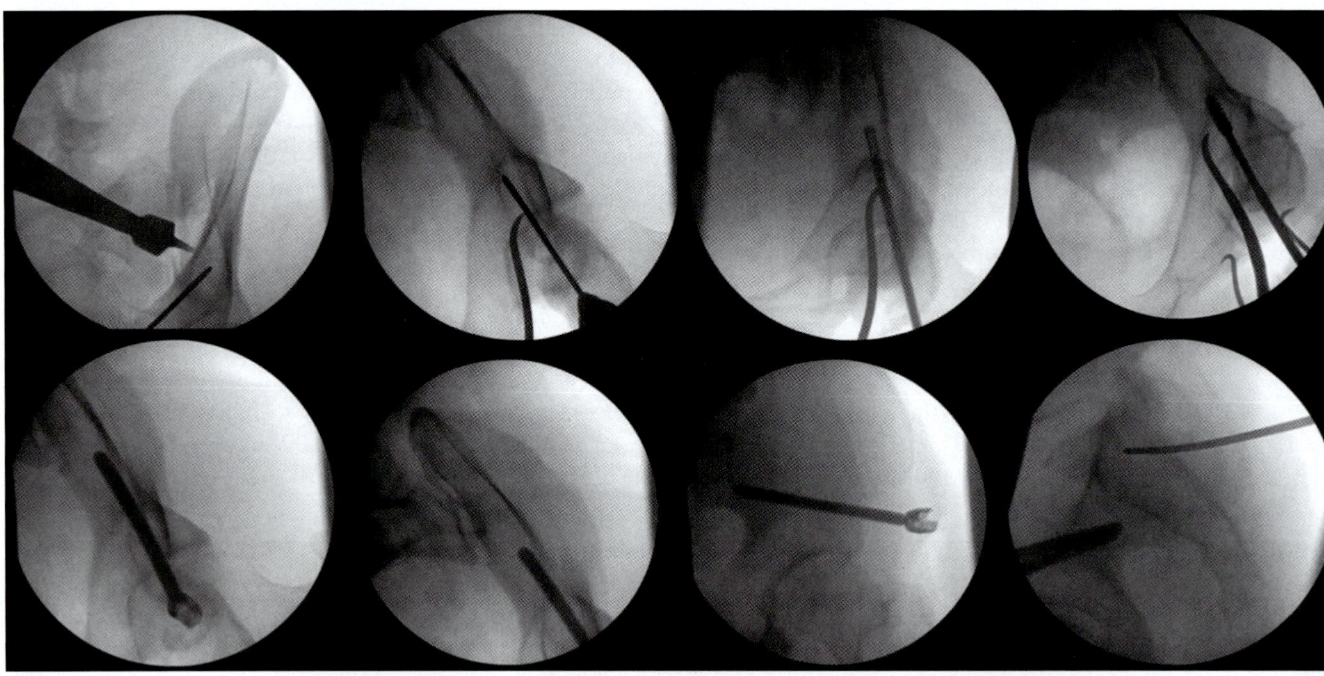

Figure 16-25 | This fluoro sequence demonstrates the proper AIIS "teepee" starting point (obturator-outlet) and the safe placement of an INFIX pedicle screw on obturator-inlet, iliac, and sagittal sacral views.

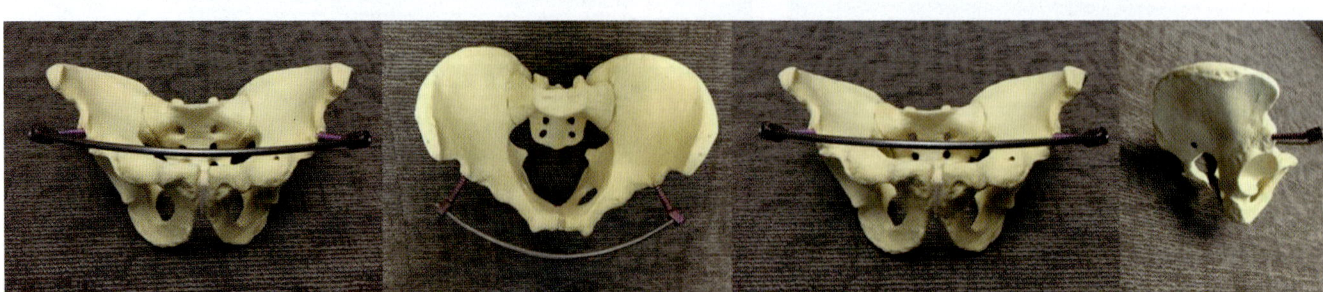

Figure 16-26 | Anatomic model demonstrating a pelvic INFIX system viewed from the AP, inlet, outlet, and sagittal vantage points.

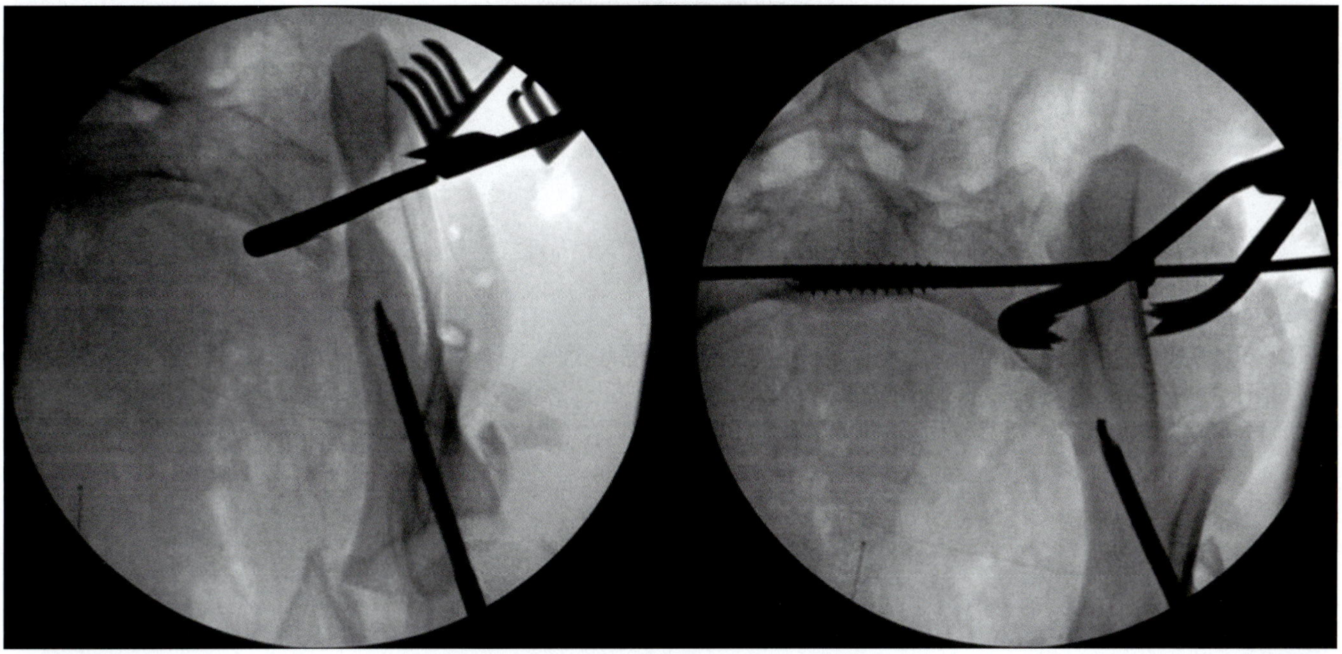

Figure 16-27 | Obturator-inlet views demonstrate AIIS Schanz pin used as accessory reduction aid for open SI joint reduction and iliosacral screw fixation. Note that the anterior pin stops short of the SI joint in order to facilitate unobstructed SI screw placement.

- Supra-acetabular Schanz pins or INFIX pedicle screws are valuable for posterior pelvic reduction aids and capable of controlling rotation, flexion, and translational displacements (Figs. 16-27 and 16-28).
- In all cases, final AP, inlet, and outlet fluoro views of the anterior and posterior pelvis should demonstrate acceptable symphyseal and sacral/SI reduction (Figs. 16-29 and 16-30).

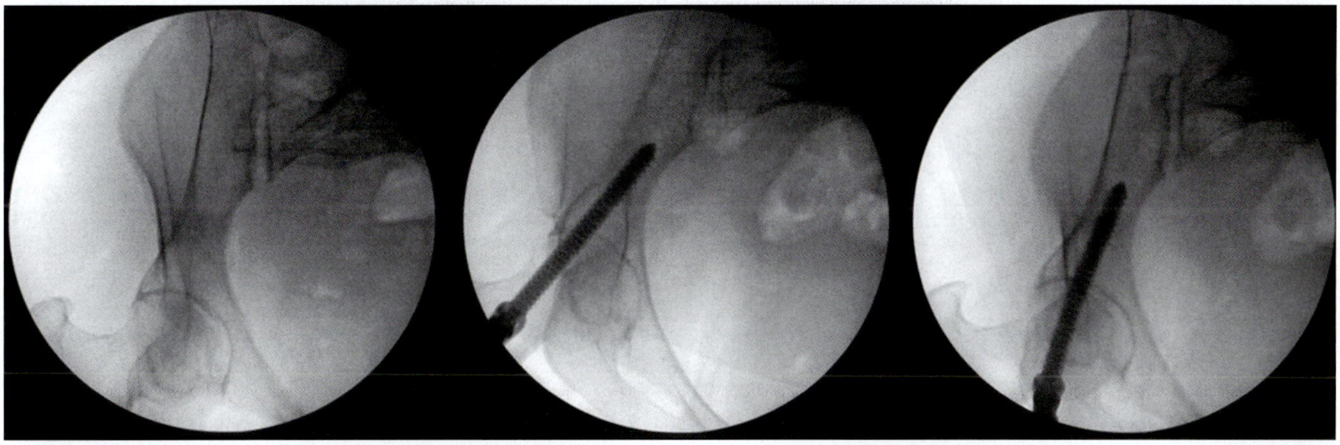

Figure 16-28 | Obturator-inlet view shows INFIX screw used for stress examination of SI joint instability (intraoperative finding during fixation of contralateral posterior ring injury demonstrating LC-3 type windswept deformity). Note the last image demonstrating reduction of the SI joint.

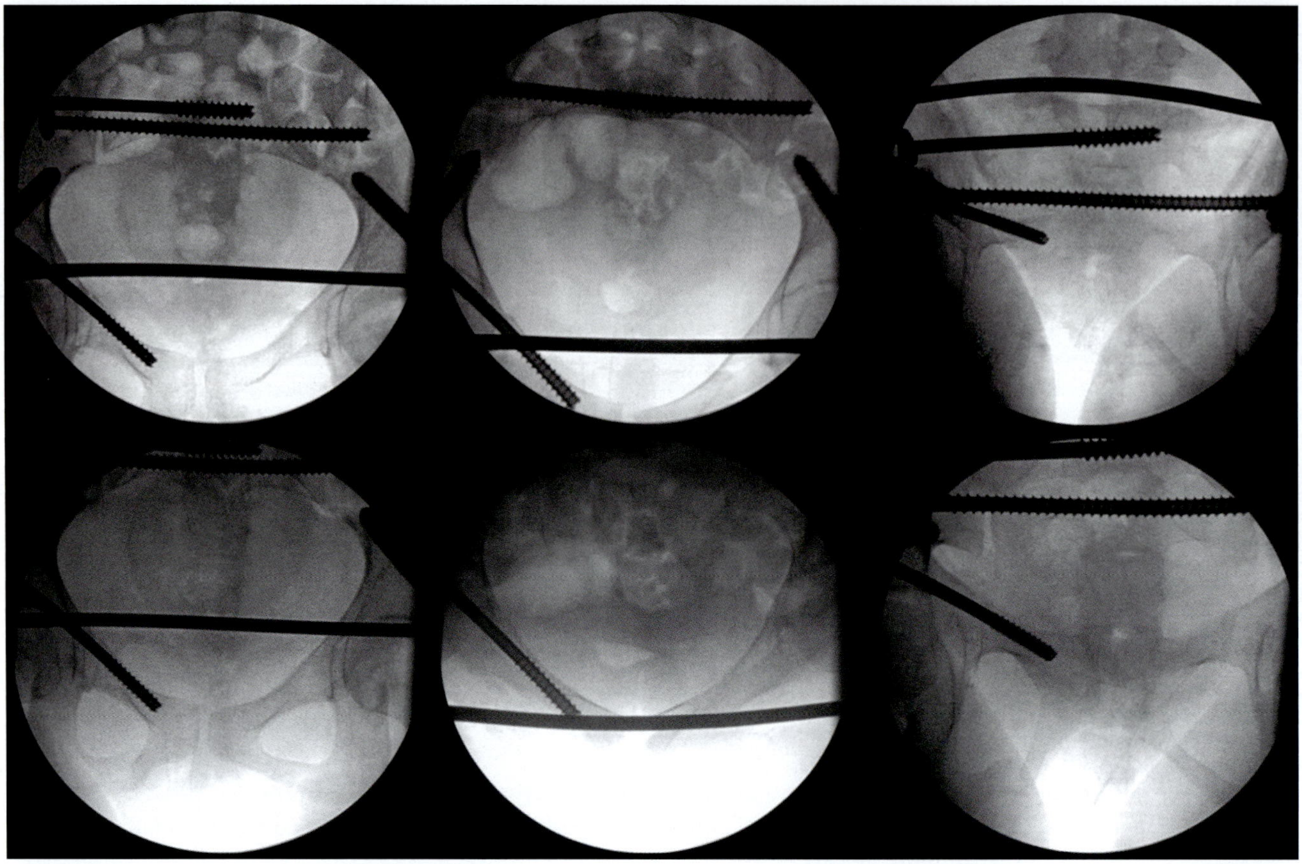

Figure 16-29 | Case example of final intraoperative fluoro images depicting anterior and posterior pelvic ring stability with safe instrumentation in AP, inlet, outlet views.

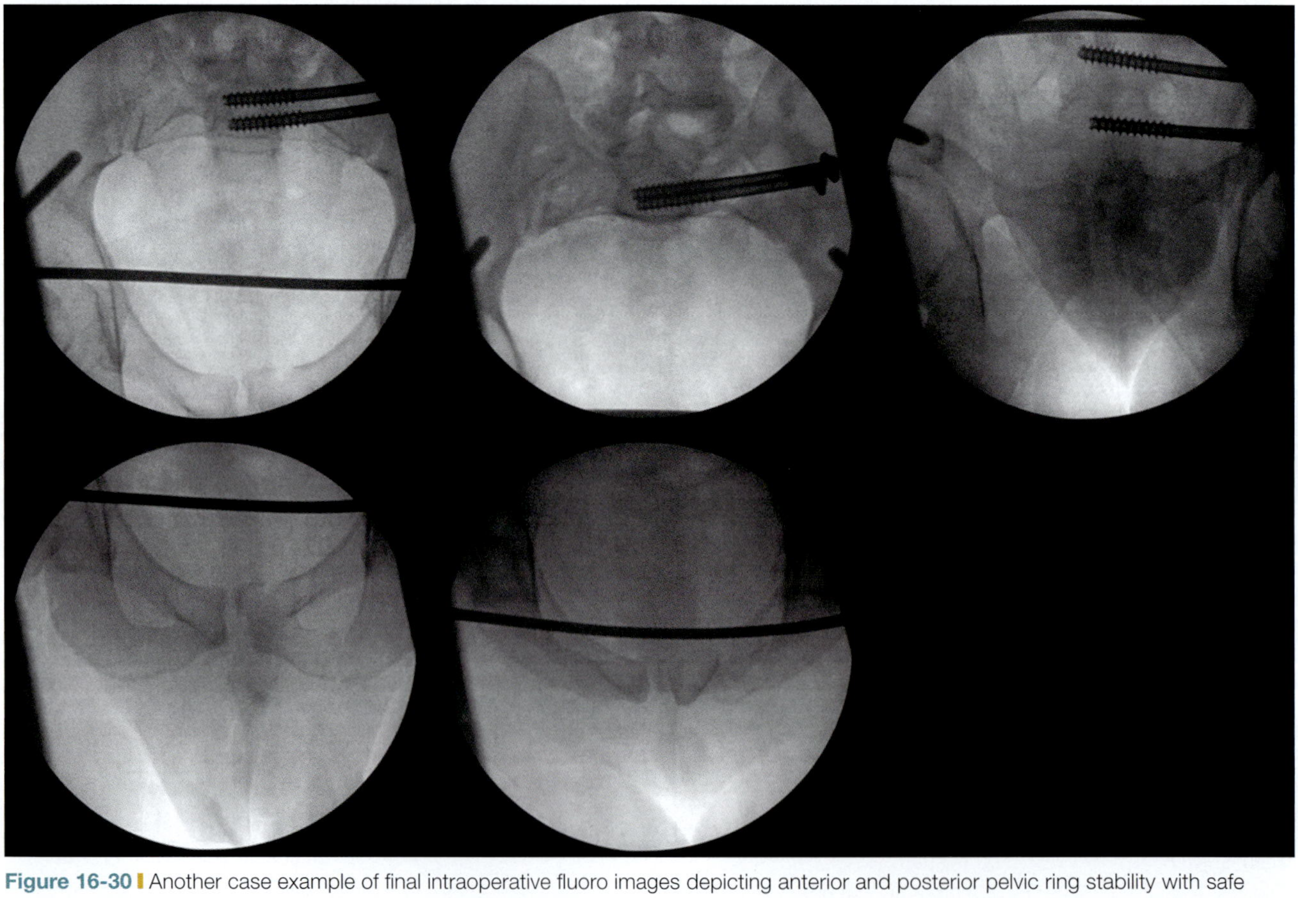

Figure 16-30 | Another case example of final intraoperative fluoro images depicting anterior and posterior pelvic ring stability with safe instrumentation in AP, inlet, outlet views.

References

1. Miller AN, Routt ML. Variations in sacral morphology and implications for iliosacral screw fixation. *J Am Acad Orthop Surg.* 2012;20:8–16.
2. Ricci WM, Mamczak CM, Tynan M, et al. Pelvic inlet and outlet radiographs redefined. *J Bone Joint Surg Am.* 2010;92:1947–1953.
3. McAndrew CM, Merriman DJ, Gardner MJ, et al. Standardized posterior pelvic imaging: use of CT inlet and outlet for evaluation and management of pelvic ring injuries. *J Orthop Trauma.* 2014;28:665–673.
4. Sagi HC, Coniglione FM, Stanford JH. Examination under anesthesia for occult pelvic ring instability. *J Orthop Trauma.* 2011;25:529–537.
5. Vaidya R, Colen R, Vigdorchik J, et al. Treatment of unstable pelvic ring injuries with an internal anterior fixation and posterior fixation: initial clinical series. *J Orthop Trauma.* 2012;26:1–8.
6. Gardner MJ, Mehta S, Mirza A, et al. Anterior pelvic reduction and fixation using a subcutaneous internal fixator. *J Orthop Trauma.* 2012;26:314–321.
7. Tucker MC, Nork SE, Simonian PT, et al. Simple anterior pelvic external fixation. *J Trauma.* 2000;49:989–994.

Chapter 17
Intraoperative Imaging of Proximal Femur Fractures

WILLIAM W. CROSS III
IAN P. MCALISTER

Introduction

- Clear visualization of the femoral neck with intraoperative fluoroscopy is vital in the treatment of femoral neck fractures and proximal femur fractures.
- Implant malposition and poor reductions secondary to inadequate imaging are common and may lead to early clinical failures.
- The proximal femur is highly intolerant to varus malalignment, and every effort should be made to ensure adequate imaging ensues to identify subtle angular deficiencies.
- Failure to appropriately position implants in the femoral head and neck has led to early failures. Optimal visualization around the spherical femoral head is critical to avoid these complications.

Bony Anatomy Appreciated on Intraoperative Imaging

- The spherical femoral head requires (at least) orthogonal imaging sequences to assure that implants are safely placed within the subchondral bone and do not penetrate the convex articular surface.
  - Thus, a screw is "safe" if it appears within the femoral head on every image. If it appears to penetrate the femoral head on any image, that screw must be revised to a shorter length or direction.
- The angle of inclination, also referred to as the neck-shaft angle, and neck version are the most clinically relevant angular measurements when managing fractures of the femoral neck, intertrochanteric, and subtrochanteric regions.
- Angle familiarity can assist with intraoperative fluoroscopy management.
- The neck-shaft angle for adults, irrespective of sex, is 129 degrees (±6 degrees) on average.[1]
- Male femoral neck anteversion with respect to the shaft is 7.0 degrees ± 6.8 degrees.
- Female femoral neck anteversion with respect to the shaft is 8.0 degrees ± 10.0 degrees.[2]
- The insertion of the short external rotators (posterior trochanteric ridge), the hip abductors (greater trochanter), and the psoas muscle (lesser trochanter) all provide deforming forces for fractures in this region and must be addressed with fracture surgery.
- The word calcar is derived from the Latin word *calcaria*, which means a spur or spur-like projection, such as one found on the base of a petal or on the wing or leg of a bird.
  - The calcar femorale is a dense vertical plate of bone within the proximal femur (yellow line in Figs. 17-1 and 17-2).[3]
  - It originates in the posteromedial aspect of the femoral shaft, under the lesser trochanter, and radiates laterally through the cancellous bone toward the greater trochanter.
  - Clinically, this area of thickened bone helps resist medial compressive loads.
  - Involvement of the calcar is important in distinguishing stable versus unstable fracture patterns.
  - It is this area where implants engage the bone with the most resistance to deformation.

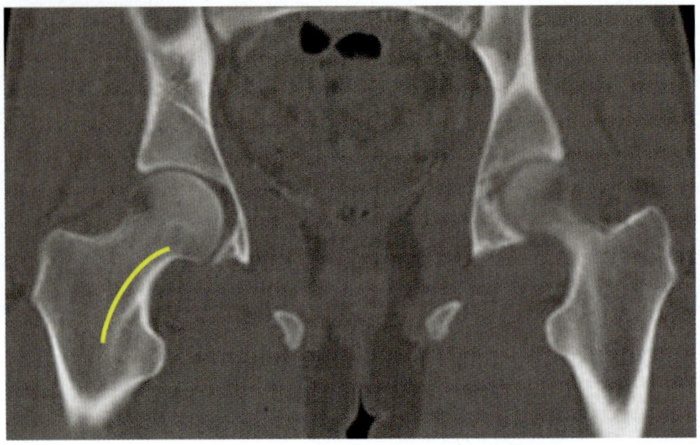

Figure 17-1 |

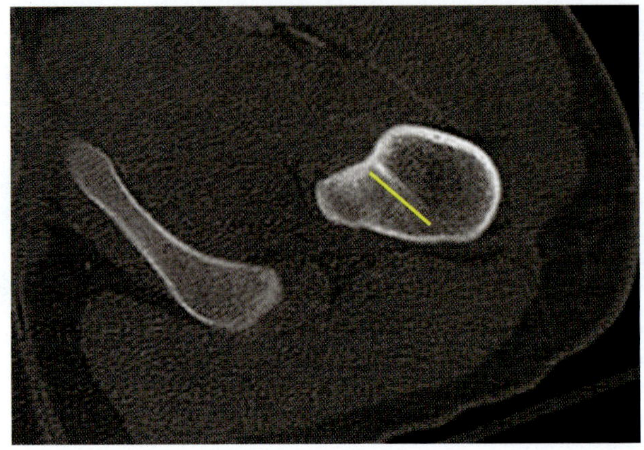

Figure 17-2 |

Intraoperative Positioning and Associated Imaging for Proximal Femoral Trauma

- There are inherent pros and cons of supine versus lateral positioning. This includes advantages or limitations with intraoperative fluoroscopy. Each must be considered when preoperatively planning for positioning and imaging needs.
  - Supine on standard or specialized fracture table
  - Supine on radiolucent table (free-legged)
  - Lateral on radiolucent table (free-legged)
  - Lateral on a fracture table
  - Two C-arm technique for proximal femur surgery

1. Supine Position on Fracture Table

- Imaging is easiest in this position.
  - Rollover lateral imaging places the shaft, neck, and head in colinear alignment allowing the surgeon to see subtle malreductions in the sagittal plane. Further, placement of the implant into the femoral neck and head can be well visualized (Fig. 17-3).
- **AP pelvis and hip views:**
  - Anteroposterior pelvic (AP pelvis) radiograph may be taken in the surgical suite to compare injured and uninjured sides. Further, AP pelvis imaging is important for the assessment of version with direct anterior total hip replacement for displaced femoral neck fractures.
  - In a true AP pelvis, the obturator foramina should appear symmetric.
  - The tip of the coccyx should lie approximately 1 to 3 cm directly superior to the symphysis pubis.
  - The spinous processes should be midline within the vertebrae. The lumbar pedicles should be symmetric but may be challenging to see intraoperatively on the same image as the symphysis on routine AP imaging. This is different for inlet and outlet imaging (Fig. 17-4).

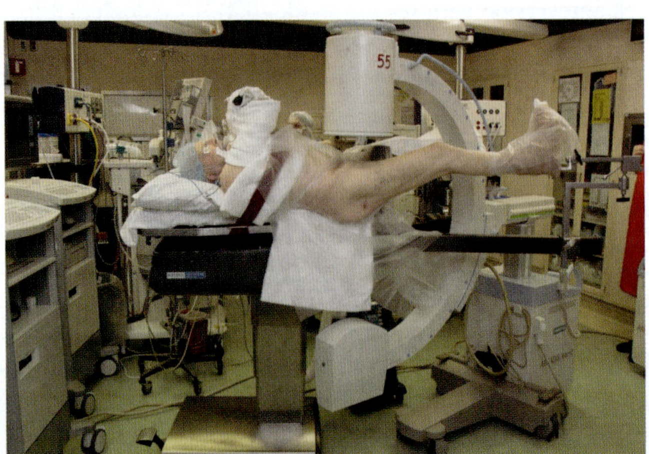

Figure 17-3 |

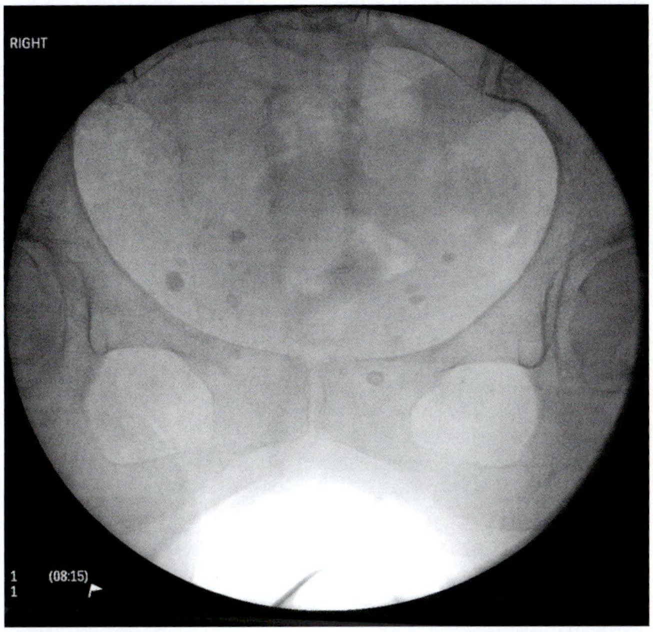

Figure 17-4 |

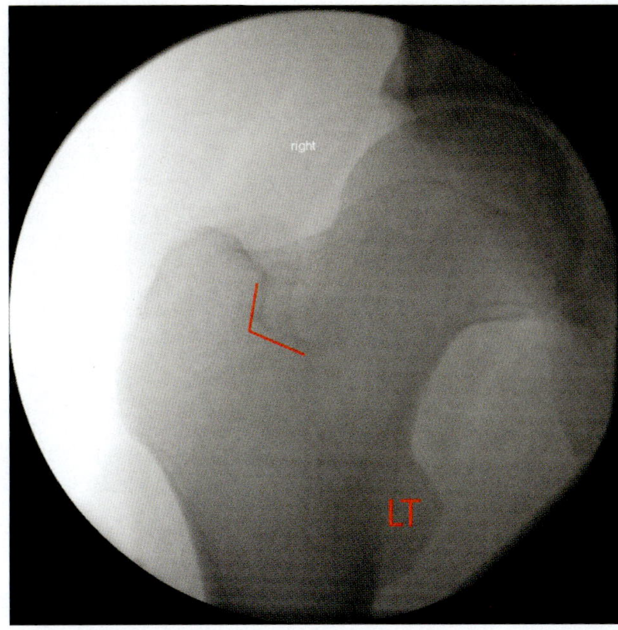

Figure 17-5 |

- AP hip view should include the lesser trochanter, and in many cases, the outline of the piriformis fossa can be detailed (red markings) (Fig. 17-5).

- **Lateral imaging:**
  - Standard lateral (parallel to floor lateral)
    - Best for viewing calcar region reduction. Can be challenging to optimize perfect implant positioning into the femoral head.
    - Should be used in conjunction with the rollover lateral. It may lack the accuracy to detect subtle deformities in the sagittal plane (Fig. 17-6).
  - Rollover lateral (inline lateral): places the shaft, neck, and head in colinear alignment allowing the surgeon to see subtle malreductions in the sagittal plane. Further, placement of the implant into the femoral neck and head can be well visualized. Best used for positioning of implant into femoral head. Calcar region not well visualized here. Should be in conjunction with standard lateral (Fig. 17-7).

Case Example: Cannulated screw fixation of femoral neck fracture. Preoperative fluoro imaging sequences demonstrate stable slightly valgus impacted femoral neck fracture with minimal inferior neck comminution and no sagittal plane step-off or angulation (Fig. 17-8).

Postoperative images demonstrate safely placed cannulated screws compressing the fracture with a widely spaced inverted fixation pattern (Fig. 17-9).

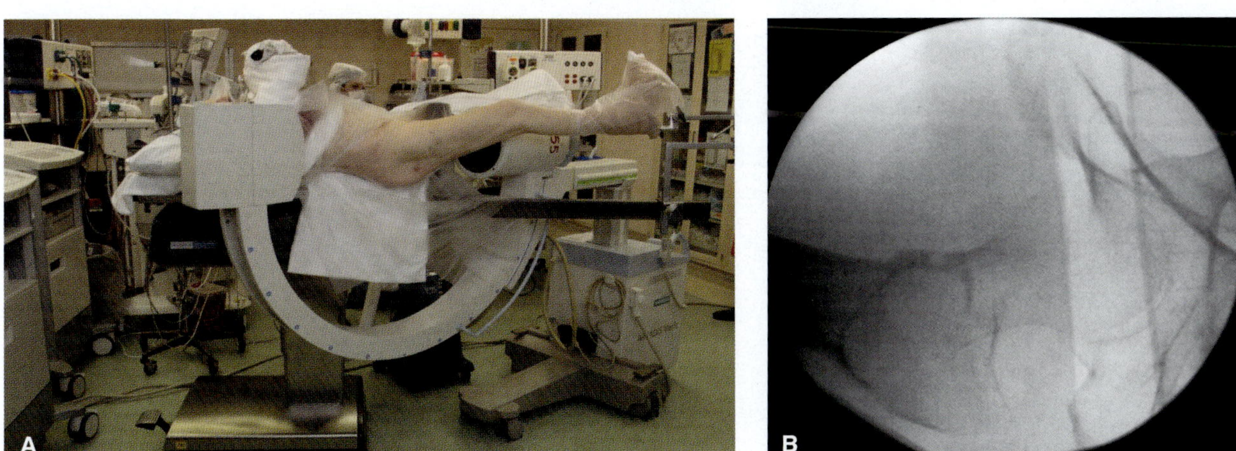

Figure 17-6 |

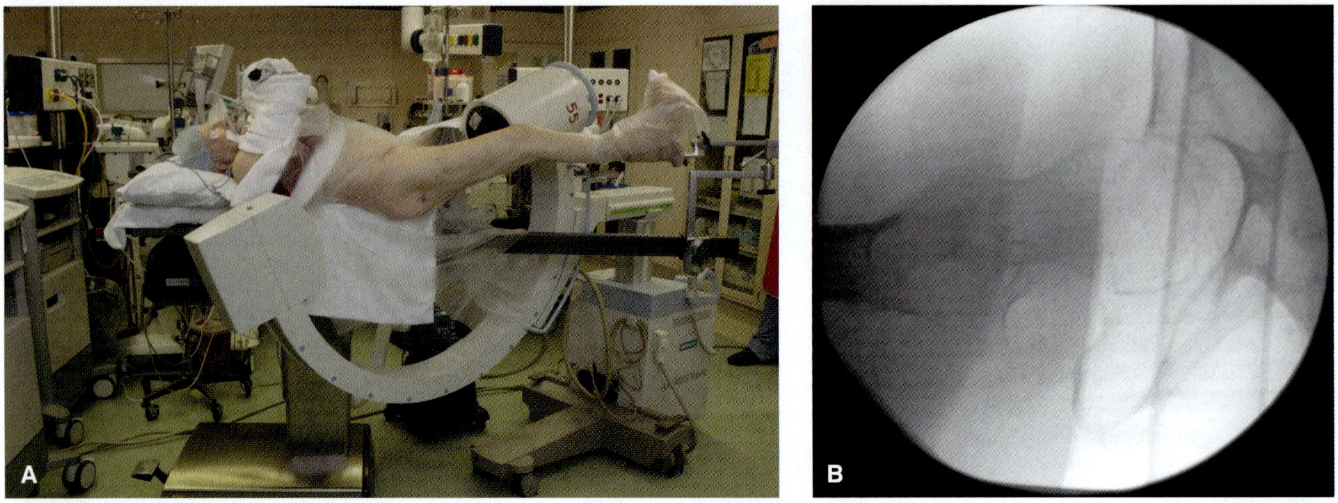

Figure 17-7 |

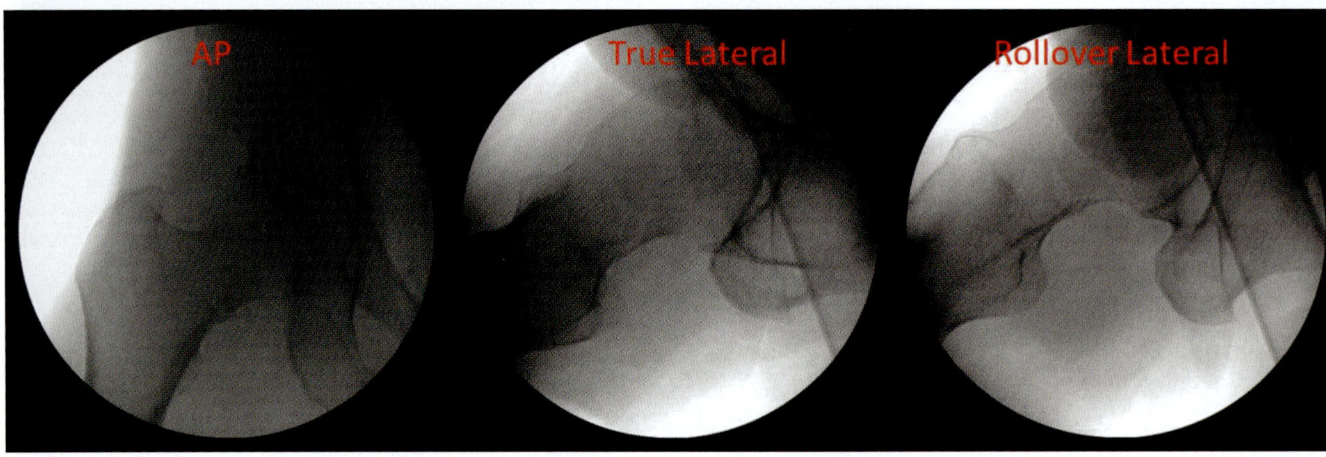

Figure 17-8 |

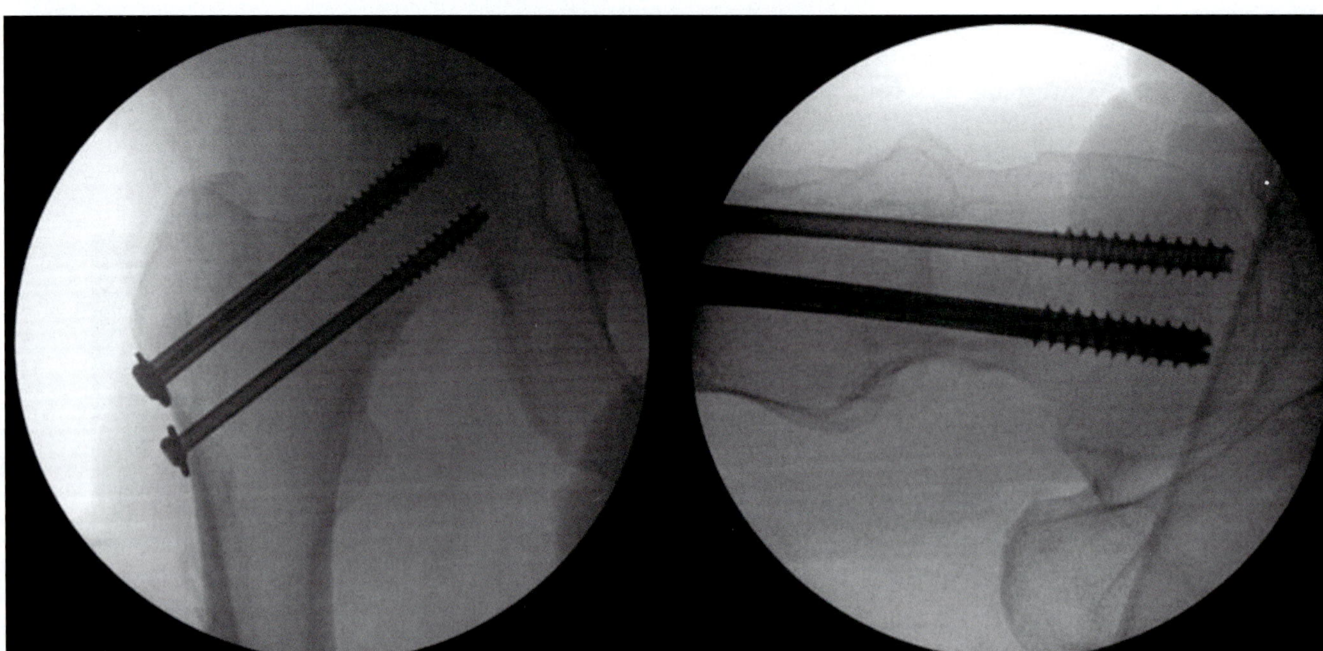

Figure 17-9 |

2. Supine Positioning on Radiolucent Table (Free-Legged)

- **AP imaging**
  - Accurate AP imaging must incorporate the tilt of the patient from their positioning on the radiolucent table (a wedge or bump is typically placed under the thorax and gluteal origin) (Figs. 17-10 and 17-11).
  - Various internal and external views may be obtained to better visualize the femoral neck and proximal femur. These views may help identify minimally displaced fracture lines (Fig. 17-12).
  - Note that the leg can be significantly adducted to aid in achieving appropriate starting point in reference to axially straight pelvis.

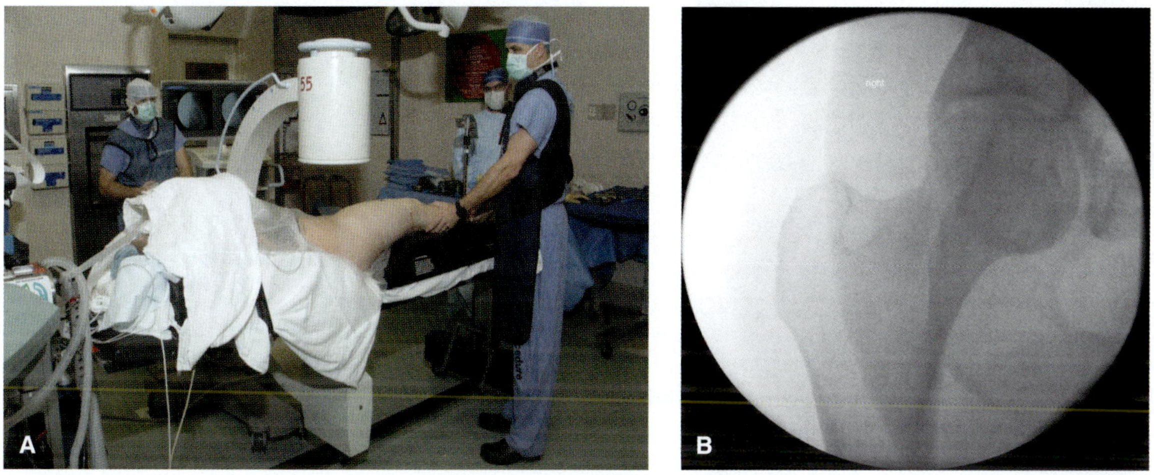

Figure 17-10 |

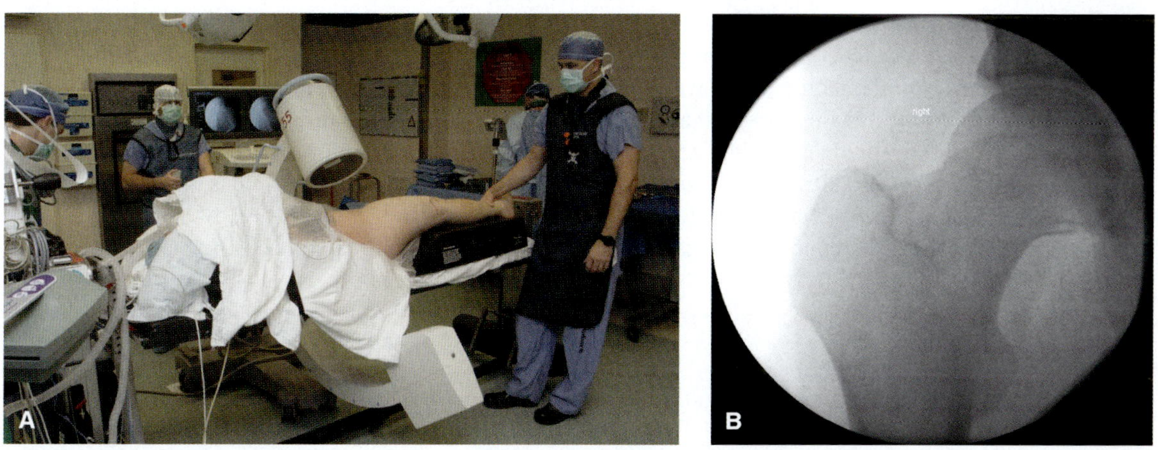

Figure 17-11 |

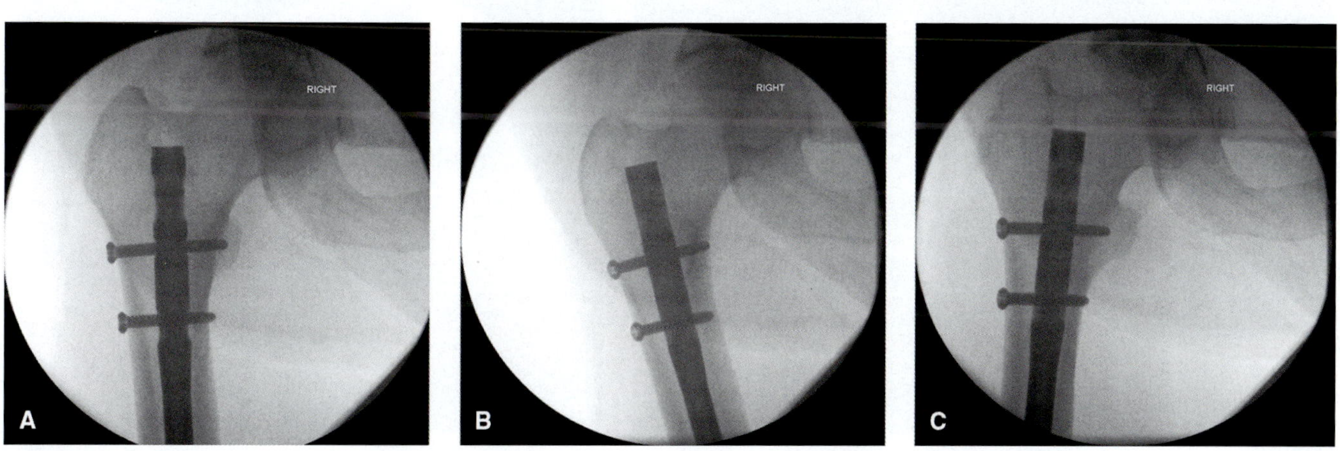

Figure 17-12 |

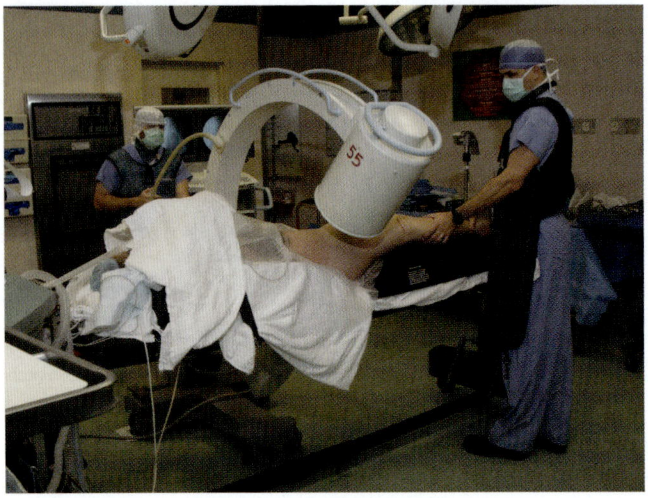

Figure 17-13 |

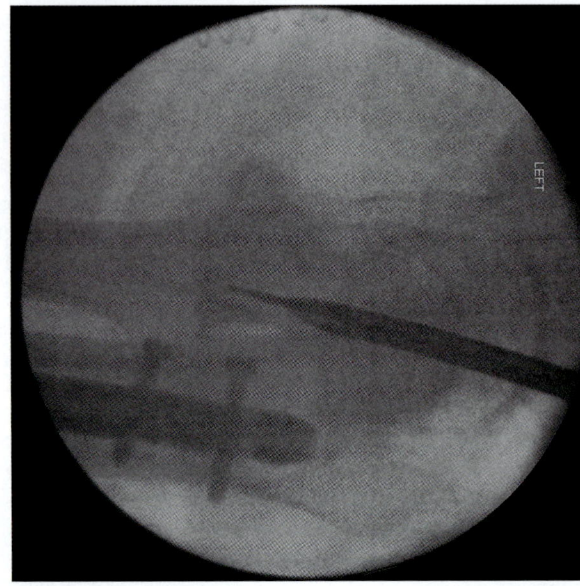

Figure 17-14 |

- **Lateral imaging**
  - Lateral imaging may be an (1) extreme rollover, (2) standard lateral, and (3) semifrog leg lateral. Lateral imaging may be challenging in this position, and *care must be taken not to displace a tenuous fracture reduction* (Fig. 17-13).
  - Extreme lateral rollover imaging requires the surgeon to be familiar with fluoroscope image intensifier positioning. In this case, the intensifier is above the patient making the operative hip appear smaller than the nonoperative hip. This is true as the operative side is farther from image emission. Once this differentiation is clear, the surgery may be performed with ease (Fig. 17-14).
  - Standard lateral imaging may have challenges seeing the proximal femur due to (1) abdominal girth, (2) poor imaging directionality, (3) contralateral thigh size, and (4) inadequate operative side elevation (preoperatively placed wedge or "bump" under thorax and hip) (Fig. 17-15).
  - Semi–frog leg lateral can be utilized if the fracture reduction is stable. There is always risk of displacement of the starting position or fracture reduction with this method. However, the imaging quality with this form of lateral exceeds the previous two methods (Fig. 17-16).

3. Lateral Decubitus Positioning on Radiolucent Table (Free Legged)

- This position is preferred by the authors for plate fixation of proximal femur trauma as well as extensile approaches to the femur (Figs. 17-17 and 17-18).

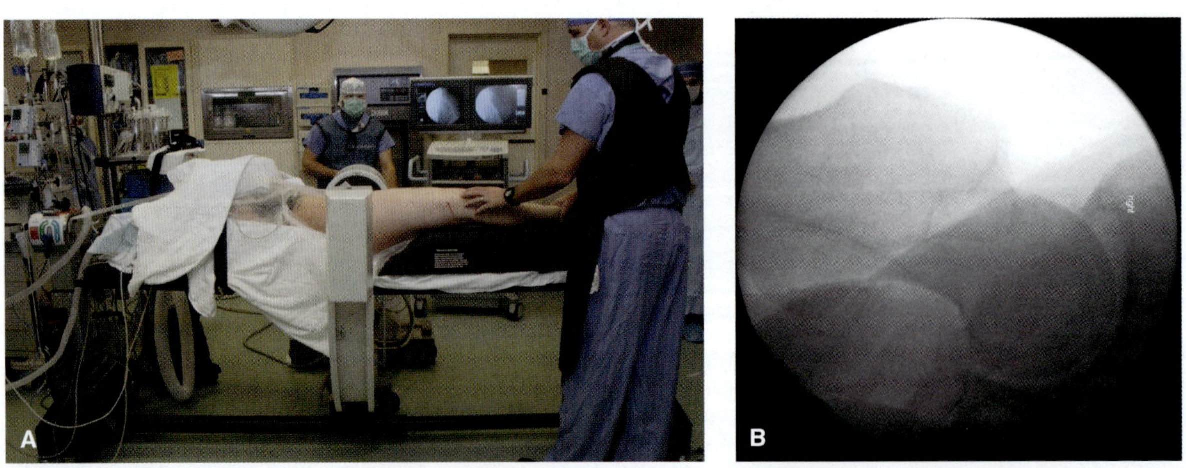

Figure 17-15 |

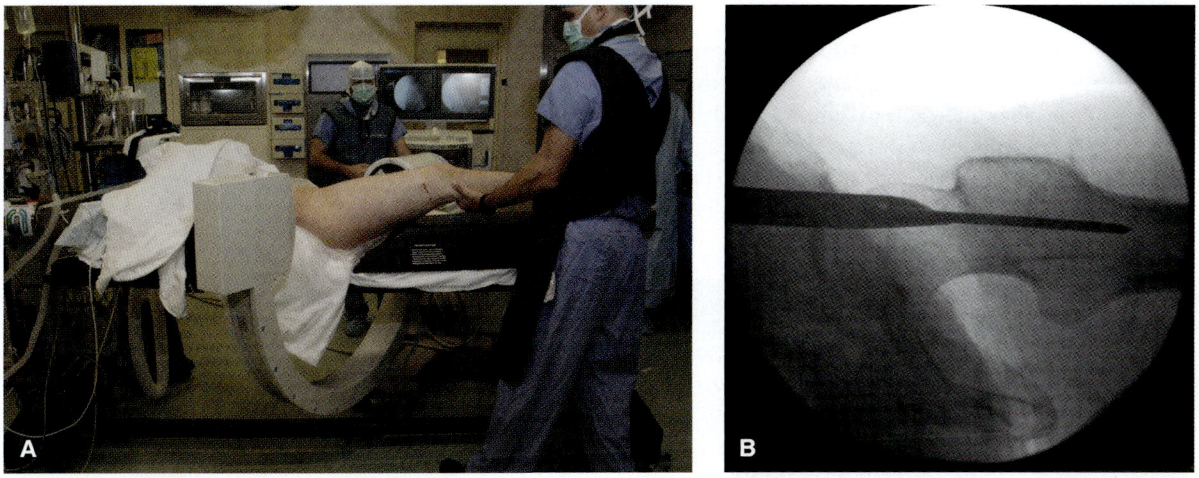

Figure 17-16

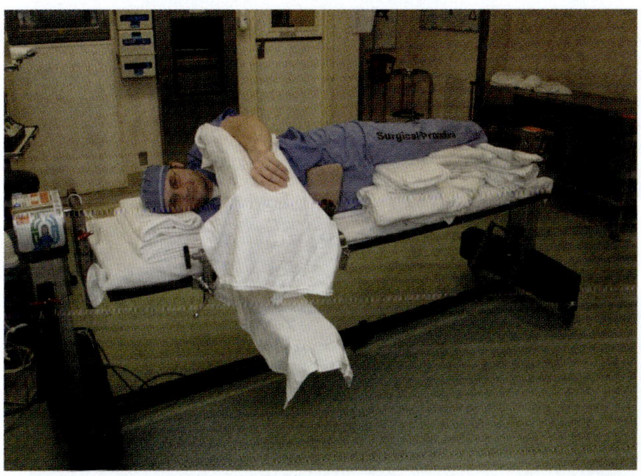

Figure 17-17

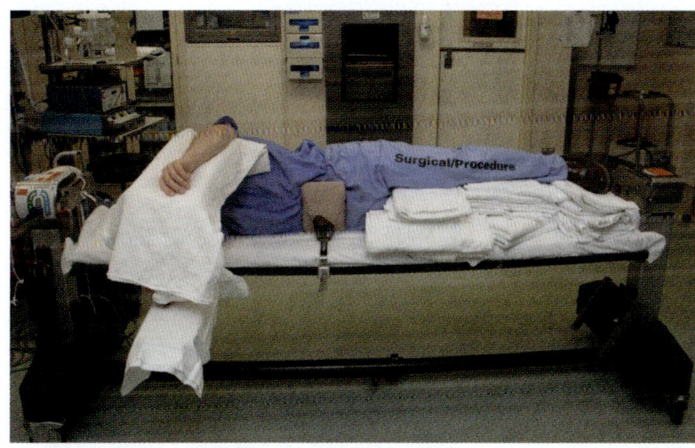

Figure 17-18

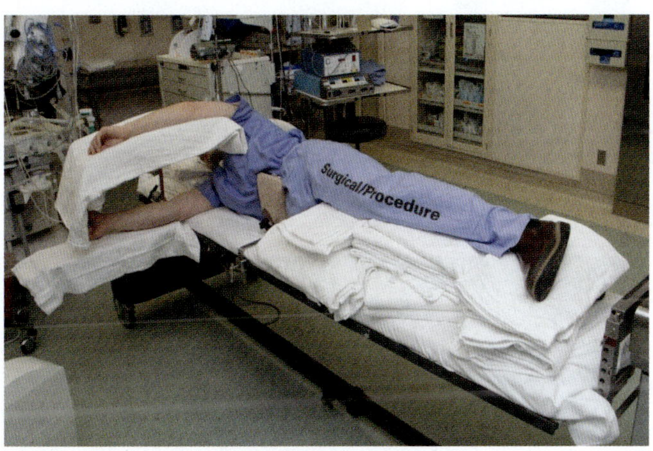

Figure 17-19

- Positioning aids can help with neutral femur positioning. The authors typically use several folded blankets given their radiolucent nature and ease of minor adjustments to fine-tune femoral and hip positioning (Fig. 17-19).
- **AP imaging**
  - Standard cross-table imaging for AP views can be used here. Matching the flexion of the femur is easy to do with adjustment of the C-arm's wag component (Fig. 17-20).

- **Lateral imaging**
  - May be confusing due to the contralateral hip overlying the operative side. Further, preexisting contralateral implants may further confuse imaging. This can easily be differentiated by paying close attention to femoral head size (Figs. 17-21 and 17-22).
  - As shown in intraoperative imaging below, the femoral head closest to the image intensifier (farthest from beam emission) appears smaller and contains the implant. Conversely, the femoral head closest to beam emission is the largest by a significant margin (Fig. 17-23).

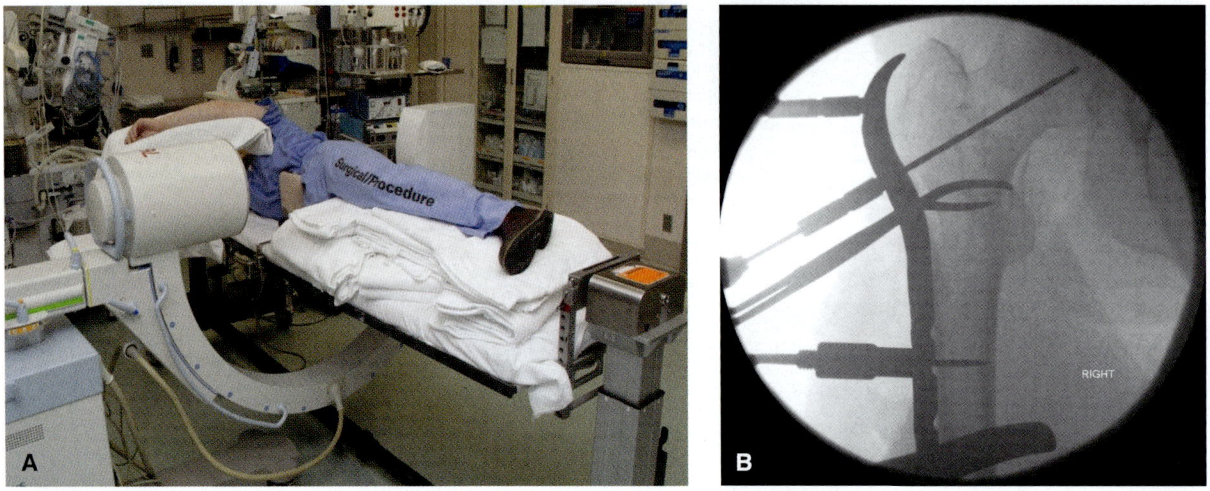

Figure 17-20 |

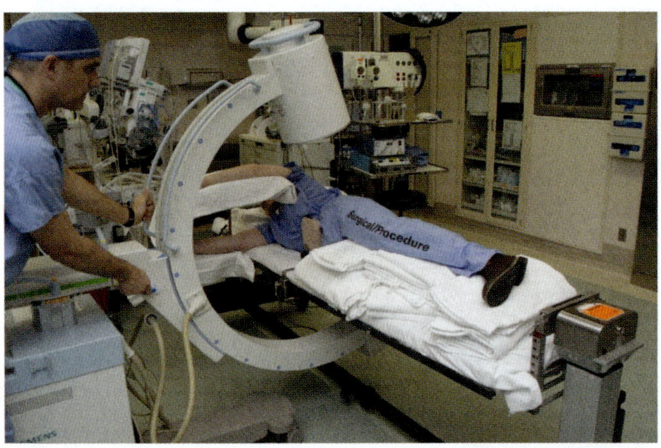

Figure 17-21 |

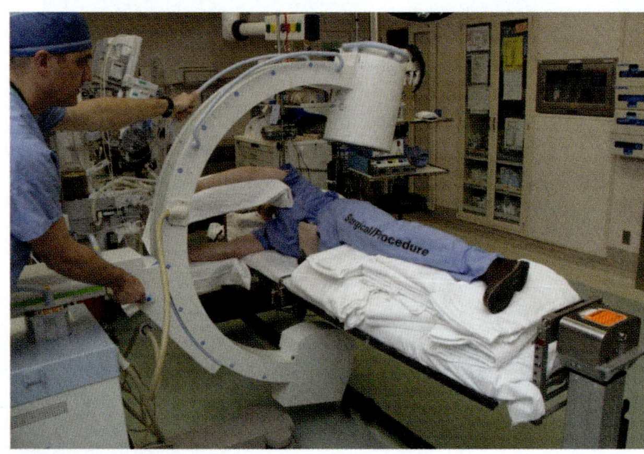

Figure 17-22 |

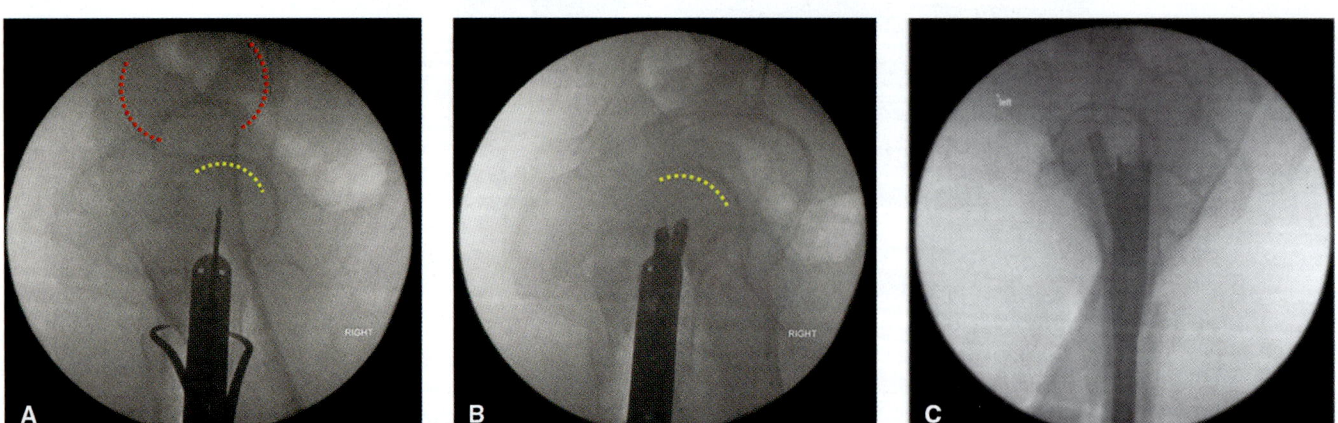

Figure 17-23 |

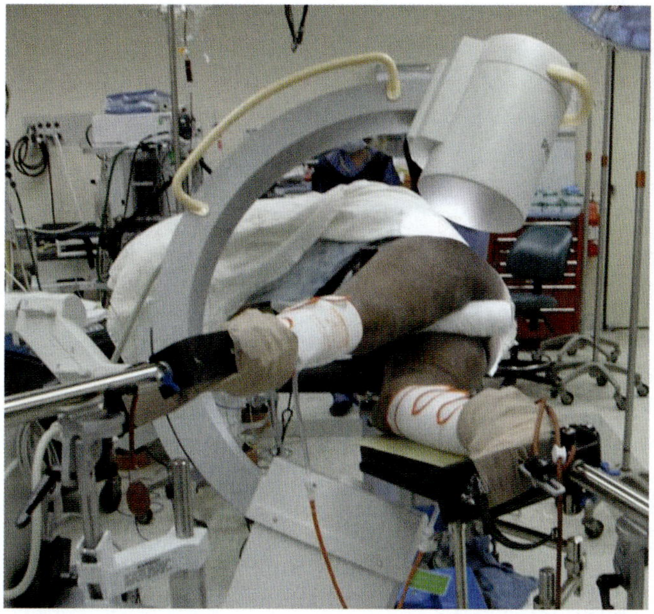

Figure 17-24 |

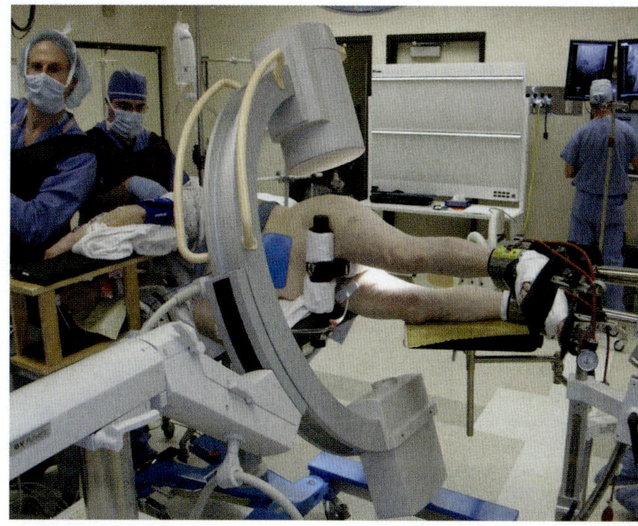

Figure 17-25 |

4. Lateral Decubitus Positioning on Fracture Table

- This position is especially advantageous for the following situations:
  - Morbid obese patients
  - Subtrochanteric femur fractures with significant flexion deformity (Figs. 17-24 and 17-25)
- An often quoted challenge with positioning a patient in the lateral position is the setup and time to position. This need not be so.
  - Trick: Elevate patient transport gurney to level or fracture table.
    - Place patient in the lateral position on gurney.
    - Slide patient over to fracture table while already in the lateral position.
- **AP imaging**
  - Standard cross-table AP imaging is easily managed in this position.
  - Following the flexion of the femur, to ensure an accurate image, is managed by modifying the angle or "wag" of the fluoroscopy unit.
- **Lateral imaging**
  - Can be tailored to visualize the calcar and sagittal alignment based the degree of C-arm "tilt" over the patient (Fig. 17-26).

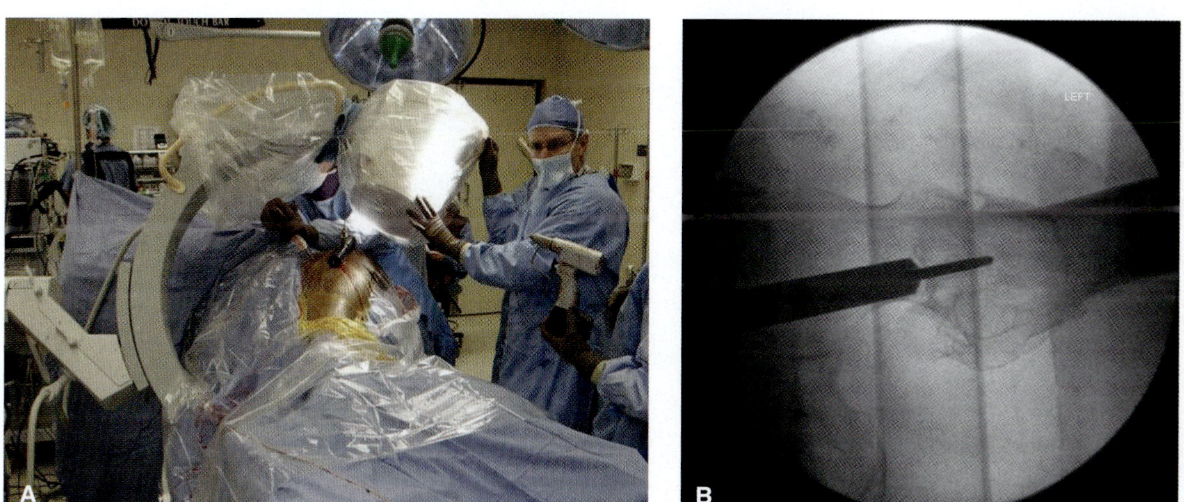

Figure 17-26 |

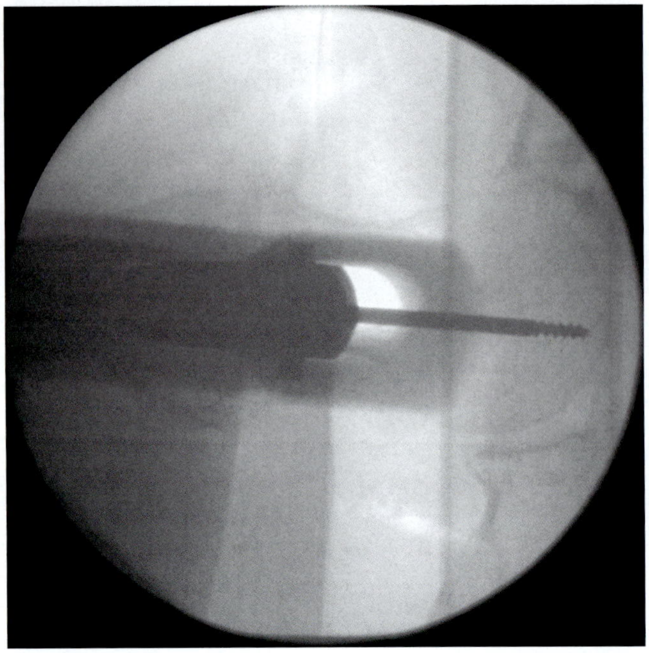

Figure 17-27

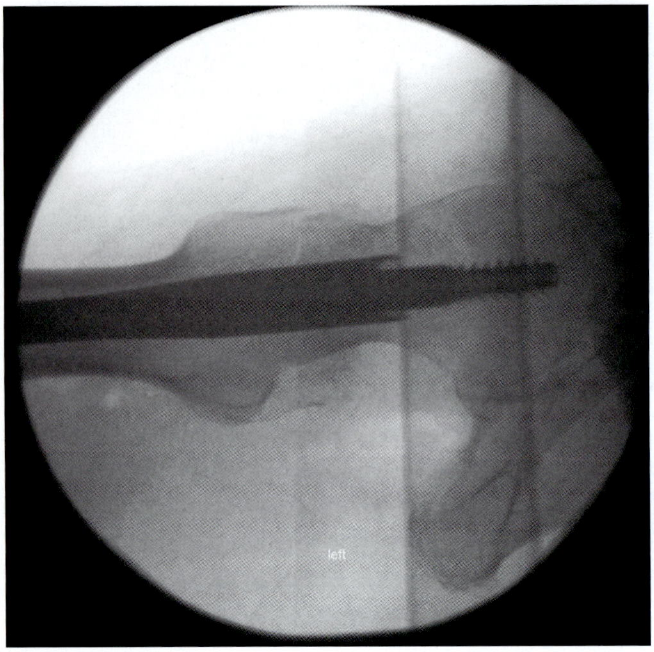

Figure 17-28

- A highlight of this position is the ease of visualization of the cephalic component of fixation in the femoral head and neck region. This may be the best view of this region from any of the mentioned positions in this section (Figs. 17-27 and 17-28).

5. Two C-Arm Technique for Proximal Femur Surgery

- Two C-arms may be used for some proximal femur surgery.
  - Cannulated screw fixation of femoral neck fractures
  - Short cephalomedullary implants
  - Sliding hip screw constructs (Fig. 17-29)
- Standard AP and lateral imaging is used as noted above in Section 1 (Supine Position on Fracture Table).
- Preoperative imaging is required before skin preparation to ensure adequate imaging is possible. Anything more than subtle imaging modifications may be challenging in this setup (Fig. 17-30).
- The lateral view may be manipulated during or at the end of the case to ensure safe implant placement and that accurate calcar visualization and sagittal alignment is restored.
- This technique may save operative time, but it is clear that additional time is spent with patient preparation for surgery (Fig. 17-31).

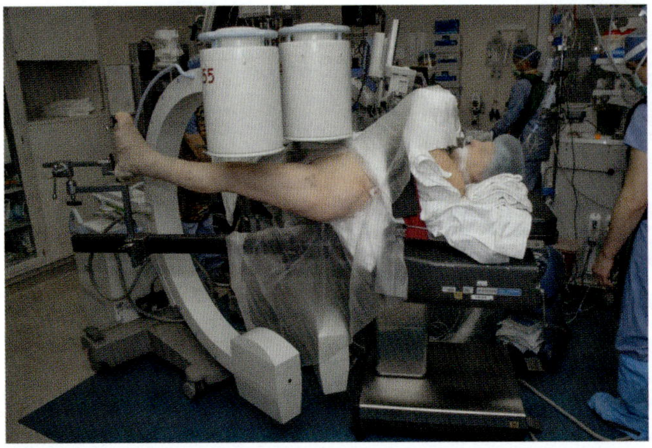

Figure 17-29

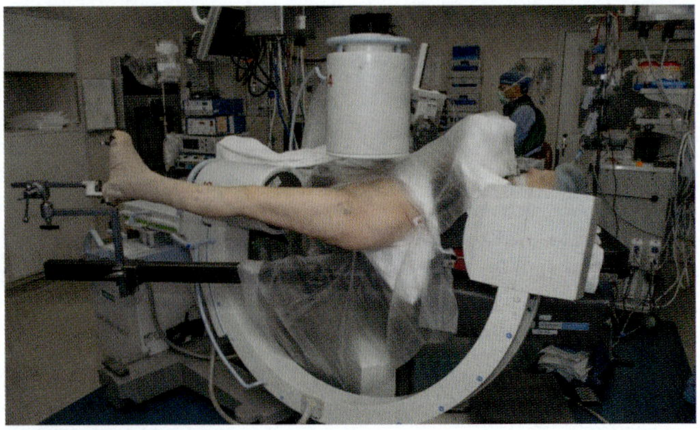

Figure 17-30

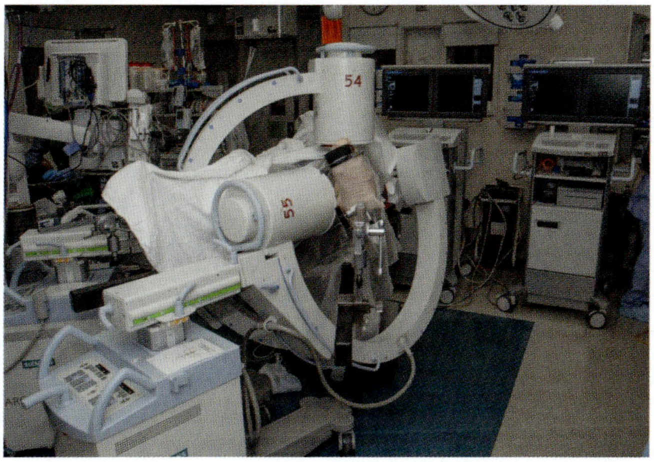

Figure 17-31 |

References

1. Toogood PA, Skalak A, Cooperman DR. Proximal femoral anatomy in the normal human population. *Clin Orthop Relat Res.* 2009;467(4):876–885.
2. Yoshioka Y, Siu D, Cooke TD. The anatomy and functional axes of the femur. *J Bone Joint Surg Am.* 1987;69(6):873–880.
3. Griffin JB. The calcar femorale redefined. *Clin Orthop Relat Res.* 1982;164:211–214.

Chapter 18
Intertrochanteric Fractures

ADAM G. COTA
GREGORY D. DIKOS

Most intertrochanteric fractures occur in patients older than 65 years of age as the result of low-energy falls. The vast majority of these fractures are treated surgically to decrease complications associated with prolonged immobility such as respiratory infection, venous thromboembolism, decubiti, and generalized deconditioning. Appropriate implant selection, adequate fracture reduction, and proper implant placement are critical to reduce postoperative complications. These surgeon-controlled factors can be optimized with quality preoperative and intraoperative imaging, along with a thorough understanding of the radiographic anatomy of the proximal femur.

Applied Anatomy

- The hip joint capsule inserts at the intertrochanteric line anteriorly and the base of the femoral neck posteriorly. The intertrochanteric region of the proximal femur is extracapsular and has a robust blood supply. Therefore, intertrochanteric fractures have much better healing potential than do intracapsular femoral neck fractures.
- The proximal femur is the insertion site for a number of opposing muscle groups. Forces exerted by these muscles result in shortening, varus angulation, and external rotation typical of intertrochanteric fracture. These forces must be understood to obtain acceptable fracture reduction.
- The gluteus medius inserts on the tip of the greater trochanter and abducts the head and neck fracture fragment. The adductor muscle group inserts on the medial proximal femoral shaft. These two opposing muscle forces result in the typical varus alignment of the fracture.
- The gluteus medius internally rotates the head and neck fracture fragment. In contrast, the forces generated by the gluteus maximus and gluteus minimus externally rotate the proximal femoral shaft. Depending on the fracture anatomy, the short external rotators remain attached to and act on either the head and neck fragment or the femoral shaft fragment.
- The rectus femoris and hamstrings cross the intertrochanteric zone of injury and result in axial shortening of the fracture.
- The iliopsoas flexes, adducts, and externally rotates the fracture fragment in continuity with the lesser trochanter. With comminution of the posteromedial cortex, forces on the head and neck fragment generated by the abductors will be unopposed by the iliopsoas.

Radiographic Anatomy

AP Hip Radiograph

- The femoral neck is anteverted 10 to 15 degrees relative to the femoral condyles.
- A true AP image of the hip is taken with the lower extremity internally rotated 10 to 15 degrees to account for femoral anteversion.
- The neck-shaft angle is the angle between the long axis of the femur and the axis of the femoral neck. A normal neck-shaft angle is 120 to 135 degrees. A neck-shaft angle >135 degrees indicates valgus alignment, while a neck-shaft angle <120 degrees indicates varus alignment (Fig. 18-1).

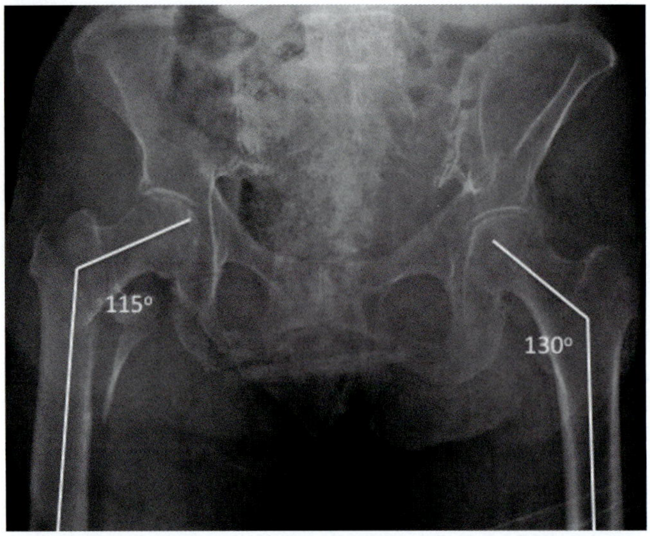

Figure 18-1 | The normal neck-shaft angle is 120 to 135 degrees. The typical deformity of an intertrochanteric fracture is varus or a neck-shaft angle <120 degrees.

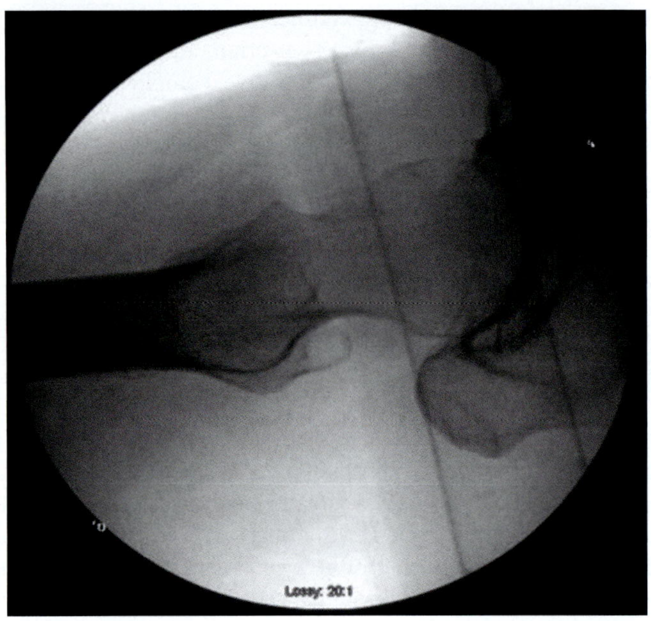

Figure 18-2 | The femoral neck is anterior to the axis of the femur, and the greater trochanter overhangs the femur posteriorly.

Lateral Hip Radiograph

- A lateral image is obtained with the affected hip internally rotated 15 degrees. The x-ray beam is oriented parallel to the table and angled 45 degrees cephalad relative to the long axis of the patient's body to orient the x-ray beam perpendicular to the axis of the femoral neck (Fig. 18-2).
- When viewed on the lateral image, the femoral neck lies anterior to the axis of the femur.
- The greater trochanter is a posterior structure. When viewed on a lateral image, the greater trochanter overhangs the femoral shaft posteriorly.

Preoperative Imaging

AP Pelvis Radiograph

- The AP radiograph is used to assess the fracture pattern, comminution, coronal plane alignment, and bone quality.
- Stable intertrochanteric fractures are those with intact lateral and posteromedial cortices. Once reduced, stable fracture patterns are able to share compressive forces with internal fixation devices (Fig. 18-3).

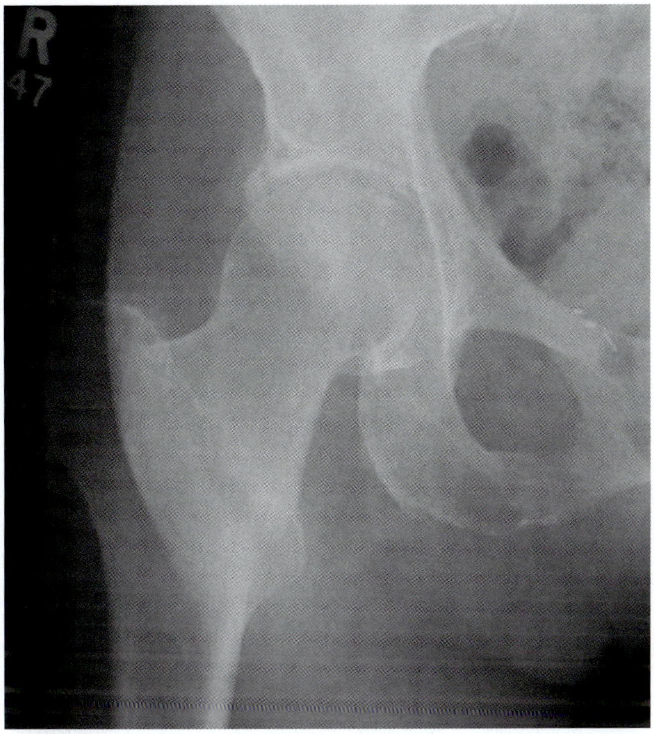

Figure 18-3 | Stable intertrochanteric fracture pattern.

- Unstable intertrochanteric fractures involve the lateral cortex or have posteromedial comminution and are unable to share physiologic loads with internal fixation devices. The unstable patterns are reverse obliquity fractures, transtrochanteric fractures, fractures with posteromedial comminution, fractures with lateral wall involvement, and fractures with subtrochanteric extension.[1] Identification of these fracture patterns is imperative for appropriate implant selection (Fig. 18-4A–D).

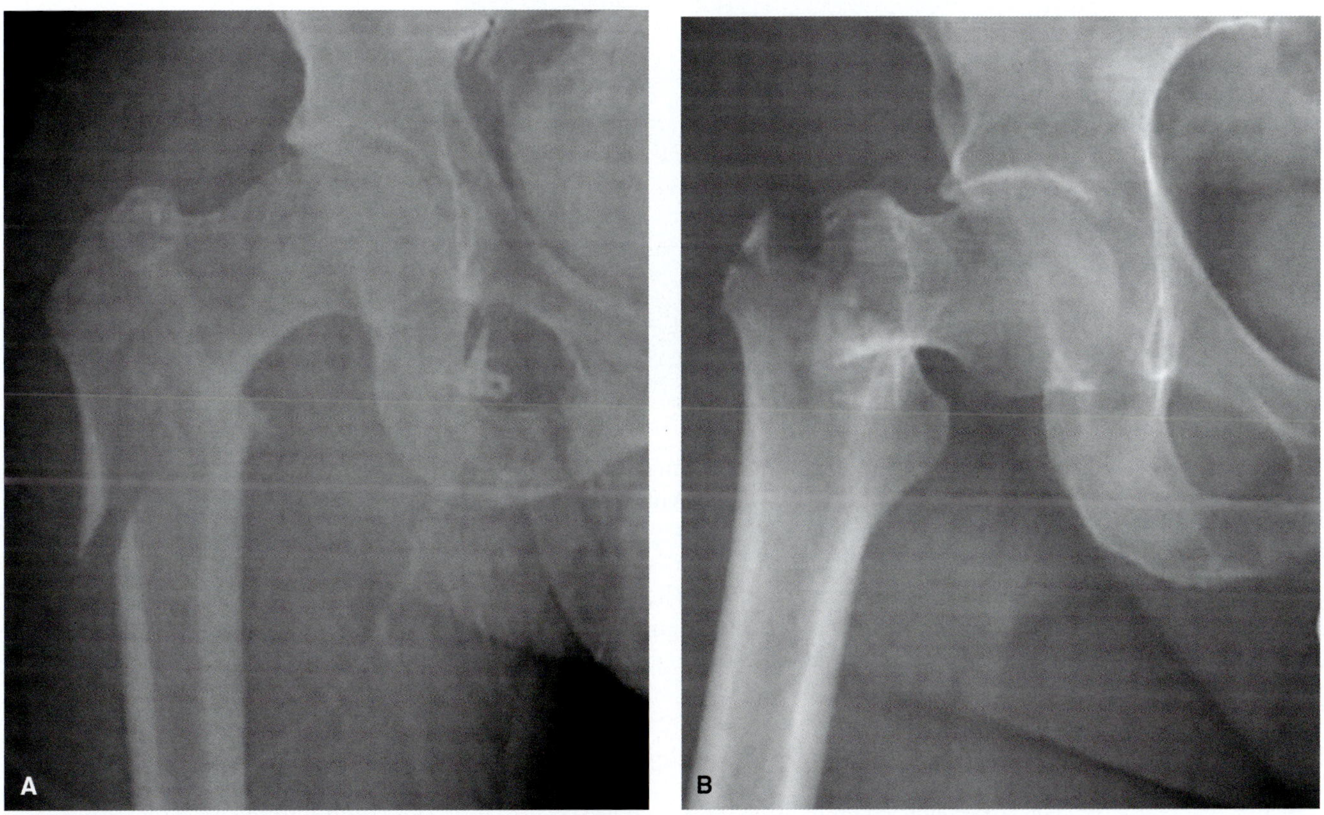

Figure 18-4 | Examples of unstable intertrochanteric fracture patterns. **A:** Reverse obliquity fracture. **B:** Transtrochanteric fracture.

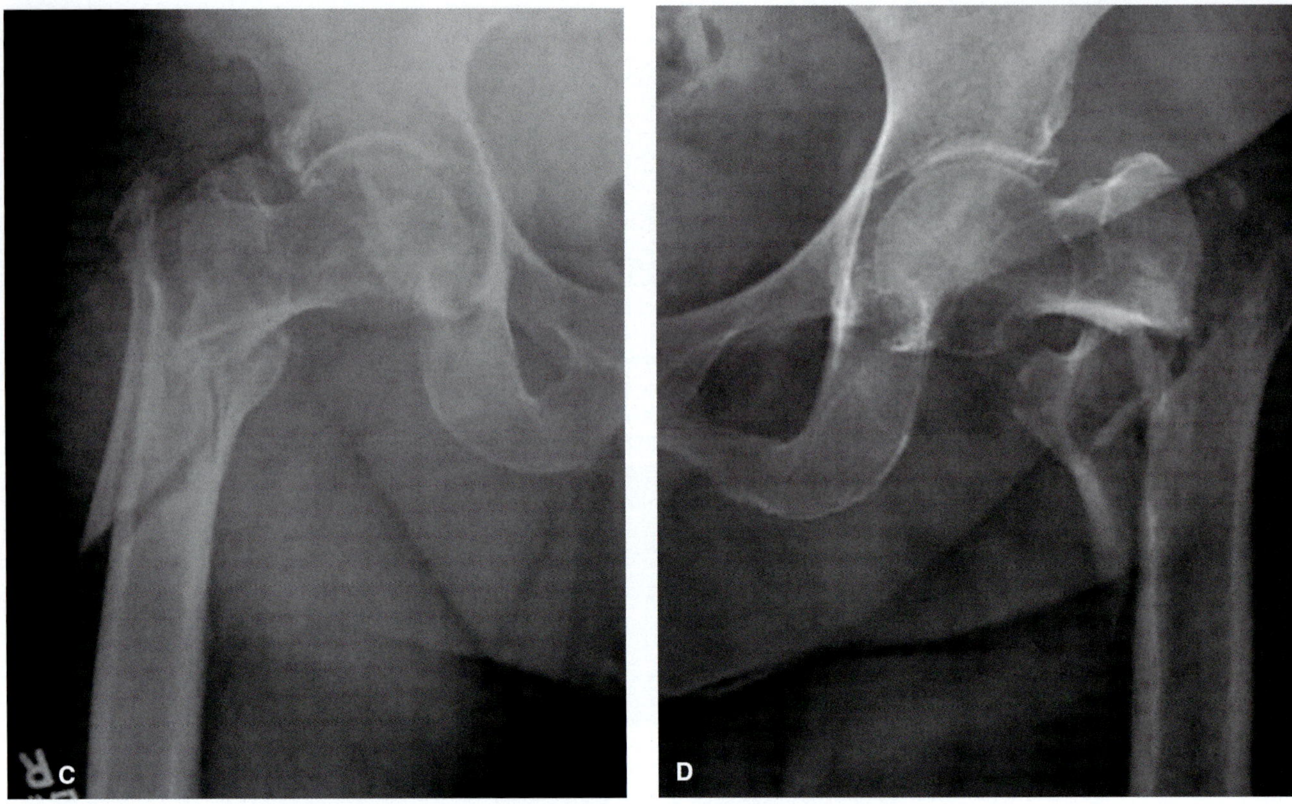

Figure 18-4 | *(Continued)* **C:** Subtrochanteric extension. **D:** Posteromedial comminution.

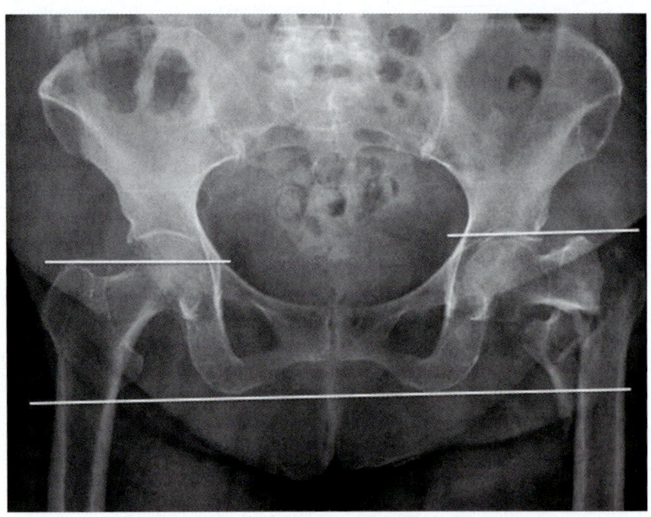

Figure 18-5 | The tip of the greater trochanter should be coplanar with the center of the femoral head.

- On the AP pelvis radiograph, the patient's normal neck-shaft angle should be measured from the contralateral, uninjured hip. This normal neck-shaft angle is used intraoperatively to assess the reduction of the fracture.
- Coronal plane alignment can also be assessed using the tip of the greater trochanter as a radiographic landmark (Fig. 18-5). The tip of the greater trochanter should be coplanar with center of the femoral head. Varus alignment will cause the tip of the trochanter to be cephalad to the center of the femoral head. Valgus alignment will result in the tip of the trochanter being caudal to the center of the head.[1]

Cross-Table Lateral Radiographs

- The cross-table lateral radiograph is used to visualize posterior comminution, anterior cortical overlap, and sagittal plane alignment (Fig. 18-6).

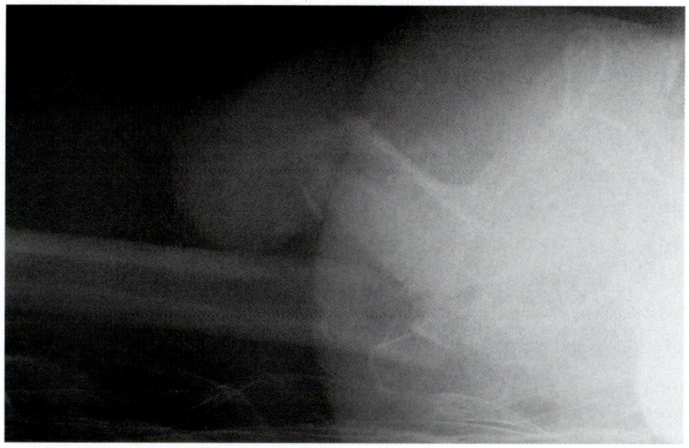

Figure 18-6 | The lateral radiograph of the hip reveals sagittal plane displacement and alignment.

Femur Radiographs

- When planning for a long cephalomedullary implant, full-length femur radiographs are indicated to evaluate for shaft deformities and previous implants that may preclude the use of the intended fracture implant.
- Anterior femoral bow and canal diameter should be assessed to ensure appropriate implant selection.

Traction Radiographs

- A traction AP radiograph of the injured hip is performed with gentle traction and internal rotation of the affected lower extremity.
- When there is significant shortening through the fracture, traction radiographs are helpful in defining the fracture pattern.

CT Imaging

- Although not routinely indicated, CT imaging can be used to evaluate complex, multifragmentary patterns to assist with implant selection and reduction strategy.

MRI

- MRI is more accurate than is CT imaging in the detection of occult intertrochanteric fractures (Fig. 18-7).[2]

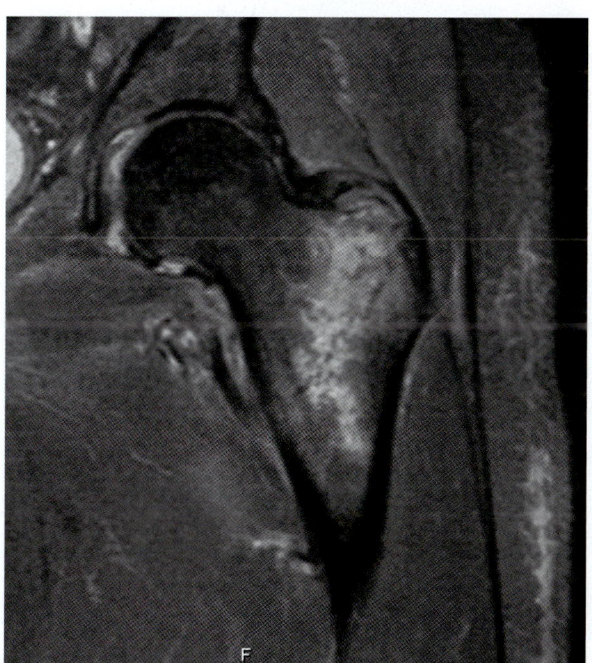

Figure 18-7 | MRI revealing an occult intertrochanteric fracture.

Intraoperative Patient Positioning

- Reduction and fixation of intertrochanteric fractures is generally performed with the patient in the supine position.
- Although any flat, radiolucent table can be used, a fracture table facilitates intraoperative imaging and reduces the reliance on a surgical assistant.
- The image intensifier is positioned opposite the surgeon with the monitor at the foot of the bed.
- Shifting the patient's torso away from the operative side with adduction of the injured extremity can improve access to the starting point for cephalomedullary implants.
- The arm on the side of the fracture is padded and secured across the patient's chest.
- The pannus of obese patients can be elevated and taped out of the surgical and radiographic fields.

Positioning of the Uninjured Lower Extremity

1. Hemilithotomy Position

- The uninjured lower extremity is positioned with the hip flexed, abducted, and externally rotated. The knee is flexed, and the extremity is secured in a padded leg holder (Fig. 18-8).
- Care must be taken to ensure that there is no compression on the common peroneal nerve.
- The image intensifier is positioned between the patient's thighs and angled 45 degrees cephalad relative to the long axis of the patient's body.

2. Abduction Position

- The uninjured lower extremity is positioned with the hip extended and abducted. The knee is extended, and the foot is secured with a padded boot (Fig. 18-9).

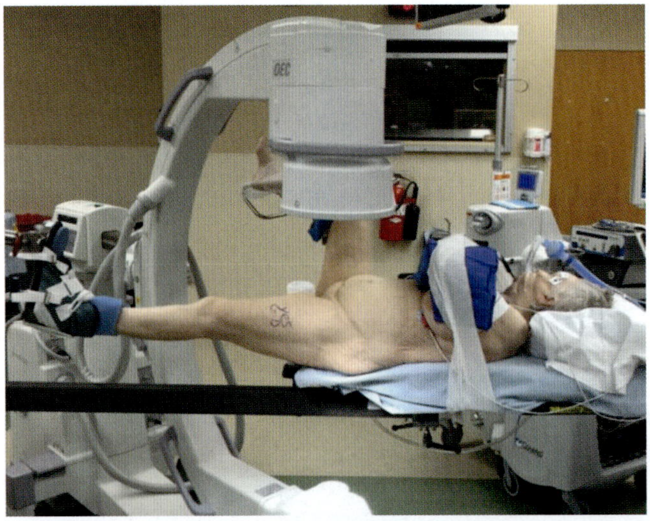

Figure 18-8 | Uninjured extremity in the hemilithotomy position.

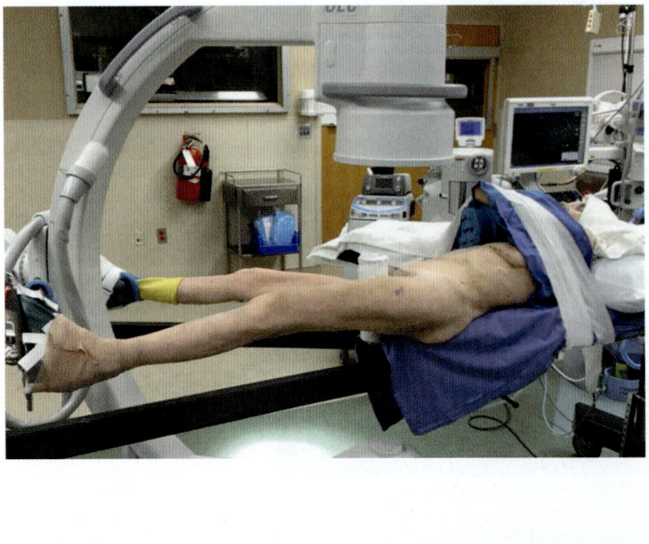

Figure 18-9 | Uninjured extremity in abduction.

- The image intensifier is positioned between the patient's thighs and angled 45 degrees cephalad relative to the long axis of the patient's body.
- The abduction position may make lateral imaging of the distal thigh for insertion of distal interlocking screws difficult.

3. Scissor Position

- The uninjured lower extremity is positioned with knee and hip extended below the plane of the injured extremity (Fig. 18-10).
- The image intensifier is positioned lateral to the uninjured lower extremity and angled 45 degrees cephalad relative to the long axis of the patient's body.
- The scissor position is ideal for patients with restricted hip or knee range of motion.
- The scissor position facilitates positioning of the image intensifier for lateral imaging of the thigh for insertion of distal interlocking screws.

Draping

- Prior to prepping and draping, fluoroscopic images should be taken to ensure adequate reduction and unobstructed biplanar visualization of all osseous landmarks.
- Ensure the prepped area and drapes extend proximally to include the entry site and working area for an intramedullary implant.
- A drape that extends to the floor can serve as the sterile cover for the image intensifier as it is positioned for lateral imaging (Fig. 18-11).

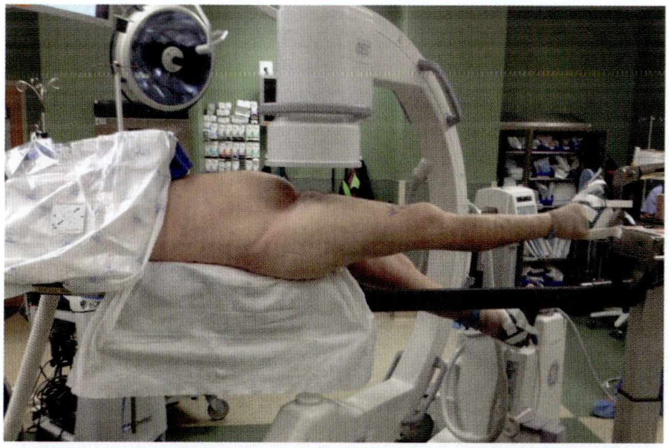

Figure 18-10 | Uninjured extremity in the scissor position.

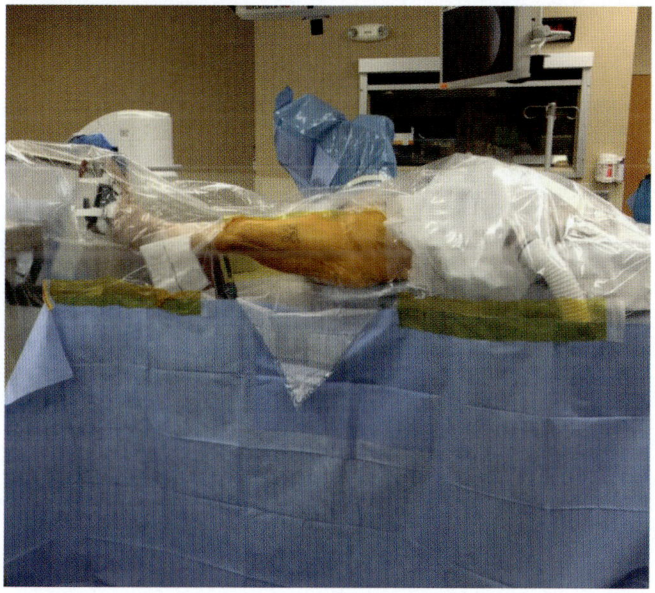

Figure 18-11 | Sterile draping for fixation of an intertrochanteric fracture.

Intraoperative Fluoroscopic Imaging

AP Fluoroscopic Image

- The AP view is used to assess reduction of the medial calcar buttress. Residual overlap of the proximal and distal fragments is visualized as a double density along the intertrochanteric line.
- Reference indices measured preoperatively such as the patient's uninjured neck-shaft angle and the normal relationship of the tip of the trochanter to the center of the femoral head can be used to assess coronal plane alignment (Fig. 18-12).
- The fluoroscopic projection will influence the apparent neck-shaft angle (Fig. 18-13). A true AP image of the proximal femur will have the most varus neck–shaft angle. As the lower extremity or the image intensifier is rotated, the neck-shaft angle will appear to increase. The true lateral image demonstrates the maximum apparent valgus. A fluoroscopic projection will never result in more varus alignment than the true AP. If the fluoroscopic image indicates excessive varus alignment, the fracture is malreduced.

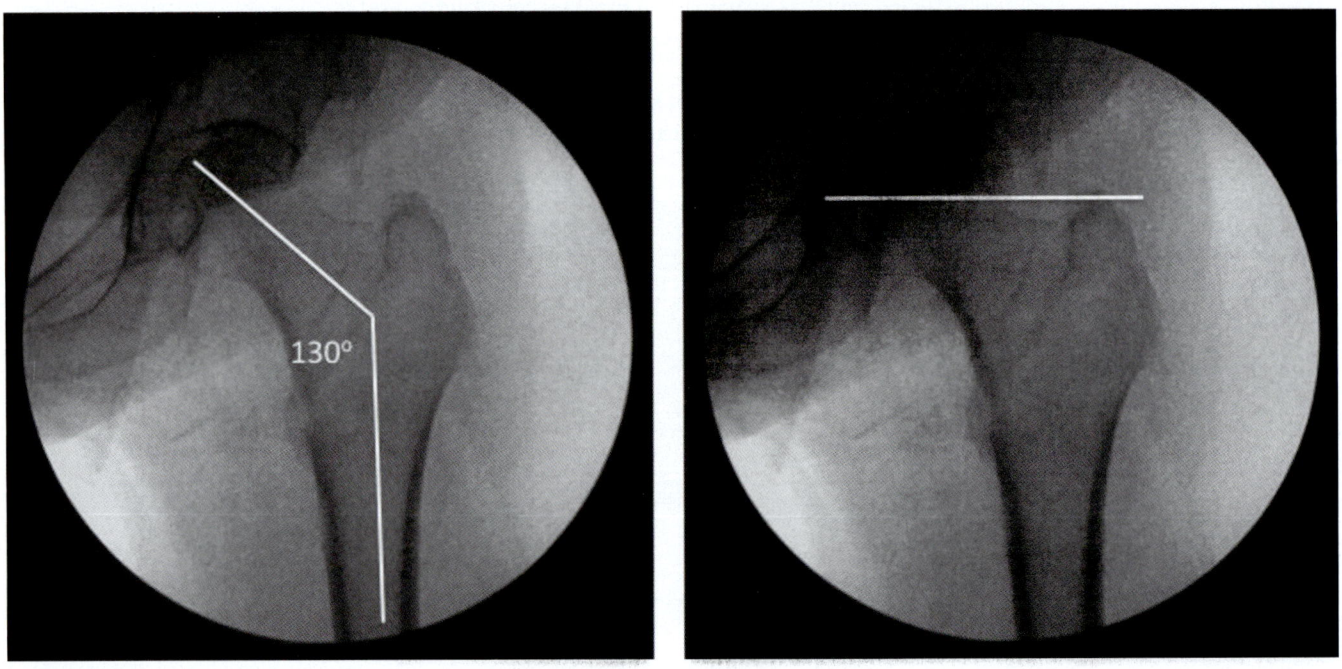

Figure 18-12 | Intraoperative assessment of fracture reduction.

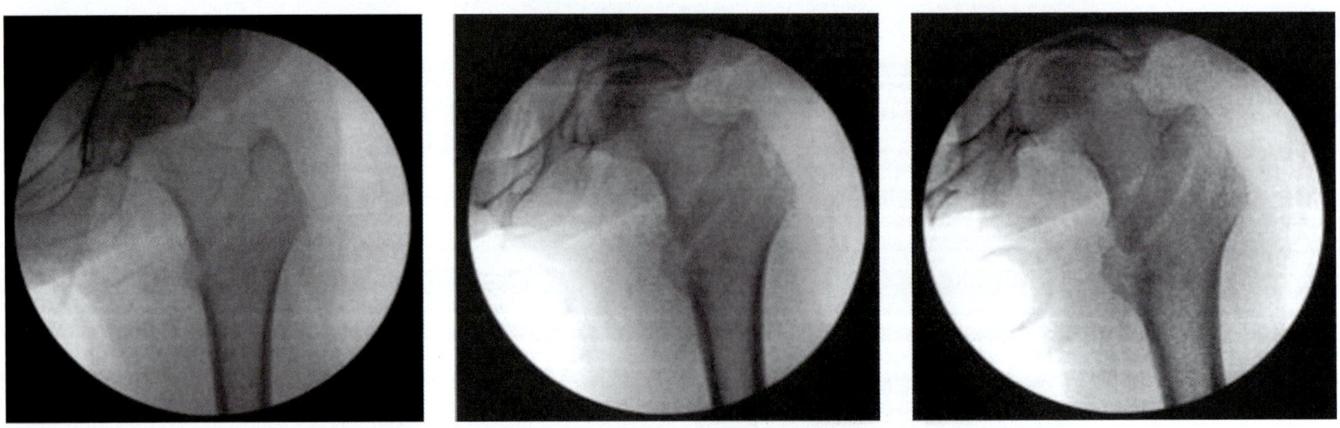

Figure 18-13 | Apparent valgus increases as the extremity or the image intensifier is rotated.

Lateral Fluoroscopic Imaging

- The reduction must be critically assessed on the lateral image for any residual sagittal plane displacement or angulation. The presence of anterior cortical overlap or step-off indicates residual neck-shaft overlap.
- Intertrochanteric fractures will commonly have an apex posterior sagittal plane deformity. This needs to be identified and corrected prior to fixation.[3]
- Angling the image intensifier 10 to 15 degrees from horizontal will account for femoral anteversion and a true lateral image of the femoral neck is produced (Fig. 18-14A and B).

Lateral Fluoroscopic Image of the Femur

- The accentuated anterior femoral bow in geriatric patients increases the potential for anterior cortical penetration during insertion of a long cephalomedullary implant with a large radius of curvature. If resistance is encountered during nail insertion, a lateral view of the distal femur should be obtained to confirm intramedullary placement of the tip of the nail.[1]

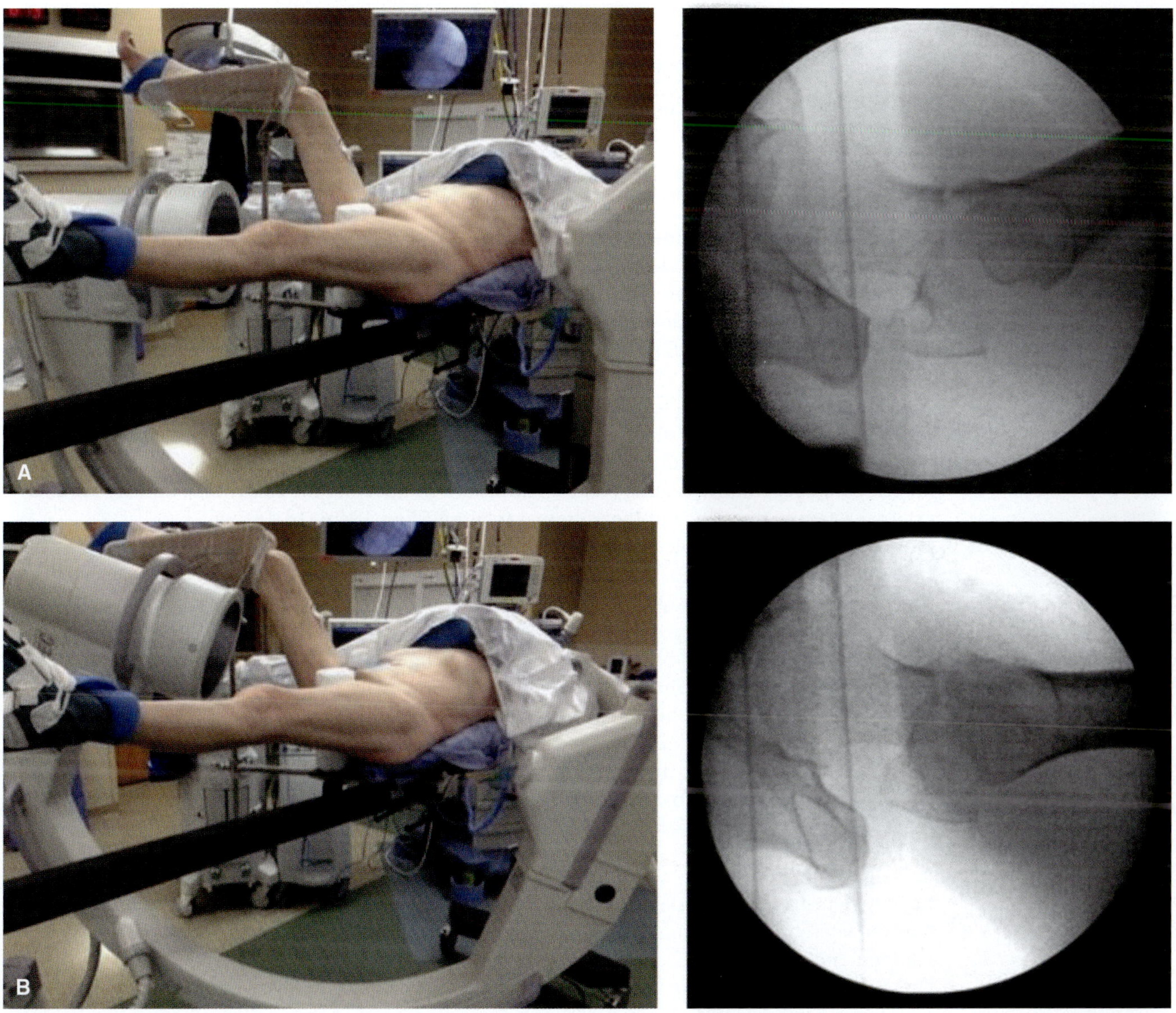

Figure 18-14 | Lateral fluoroscopic imaging. **A:** A lateral image of the hip demonstrates femoral anteversion. **B:** A true lateral of the femoral neck is produced by rotating the image intensifier 10 to 15 degrees from horizontal.

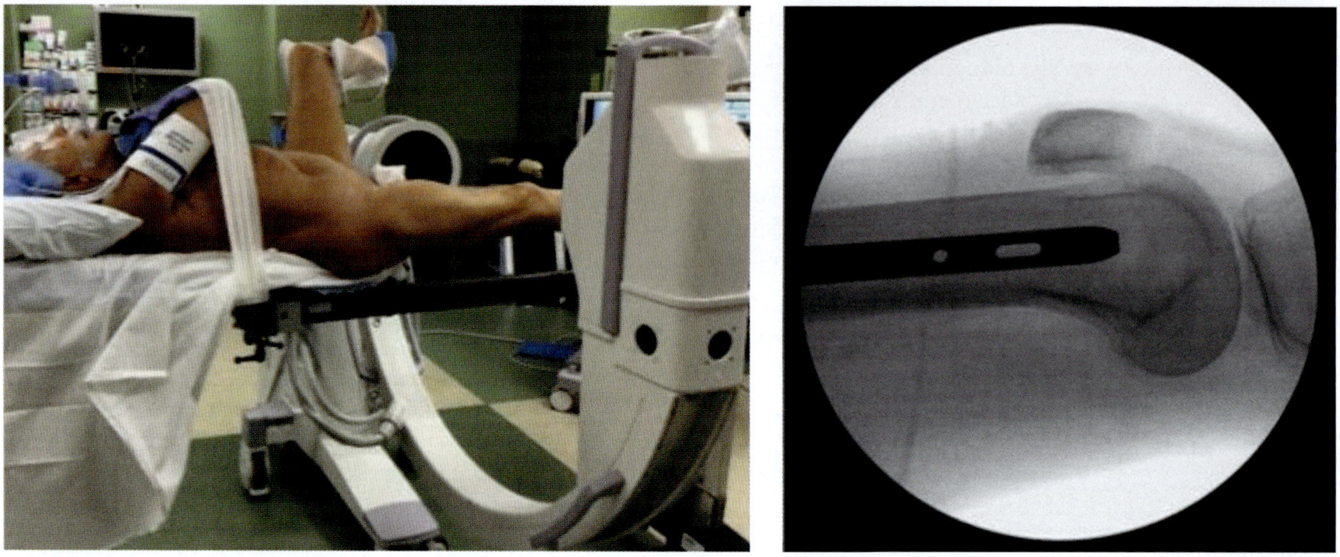

Figure 18-15 | Lateral fluoroscopic imaging of the distal femur.

- A good lateral fluoroscopic image of the distal femur is necessary for placement of distal interlocking screws in a long cephalomedullary implant (Fig. 18-15).

Fracture Reduction

- The fracture must be anatomically aligned prior to reaming and insertion of implants. The recommended implants are designed to generate compression across the fracture. However, because of the large metaphysis of the proximal femur and the poor bone quality typical of hip fracture patients, implants do not realign the fracture, nor should they be used to manipulate the fragments. The implants will simply maintain the reduction achieved by the surgeon prior to their insertion.
- A gentle closed reduction is frequently successful. Applying longitudinal traction typically restores length and coronal plane alignment. The external rotation deformity is then corrected by internally rotating the femur to align it with the head and neck fragment. Finally, elevating or lowering the foot restores sagittal plane alignment. Disimpacting the calcar may initially require external rotation, traction, and then internal rotation (Figs. 18-16–18-18).
- Occasionally, an acceptable reduction cannot be attained by closed means alone. Instruments such as clamps, bone hooks, spiked pushers, or Schanz pins can be inserted percutaneously to manipulate the fracture fragments without significant soft tissue disruption (Fig. 18-19).
- Once attained, reduction must be maintained during fixation. Unstable fractures may require provisional fixation with clamps or percutaneously placed pins (Fig. 18-20). Provisional fixation must be placed wisely so as not to interfere with insertion of definitive fixation.
- AP and lateral fluoroscopic images must be critically assessed to confirm restoration of length and alignment in both the coronal and sagittal planes.

Starting Point for Cephalomedullary Implants

- Repetitive instrumentation of the nail insertion site at the tip of the greater trochanter tends to lateralize the starting point. Excessive lateralization of the nail will result in a varus malreduction.
- On the AP view, the starting point for a cephalomedullary nail should be slightly medial to tip of greater trochanter (Fig. 18-21).[1]

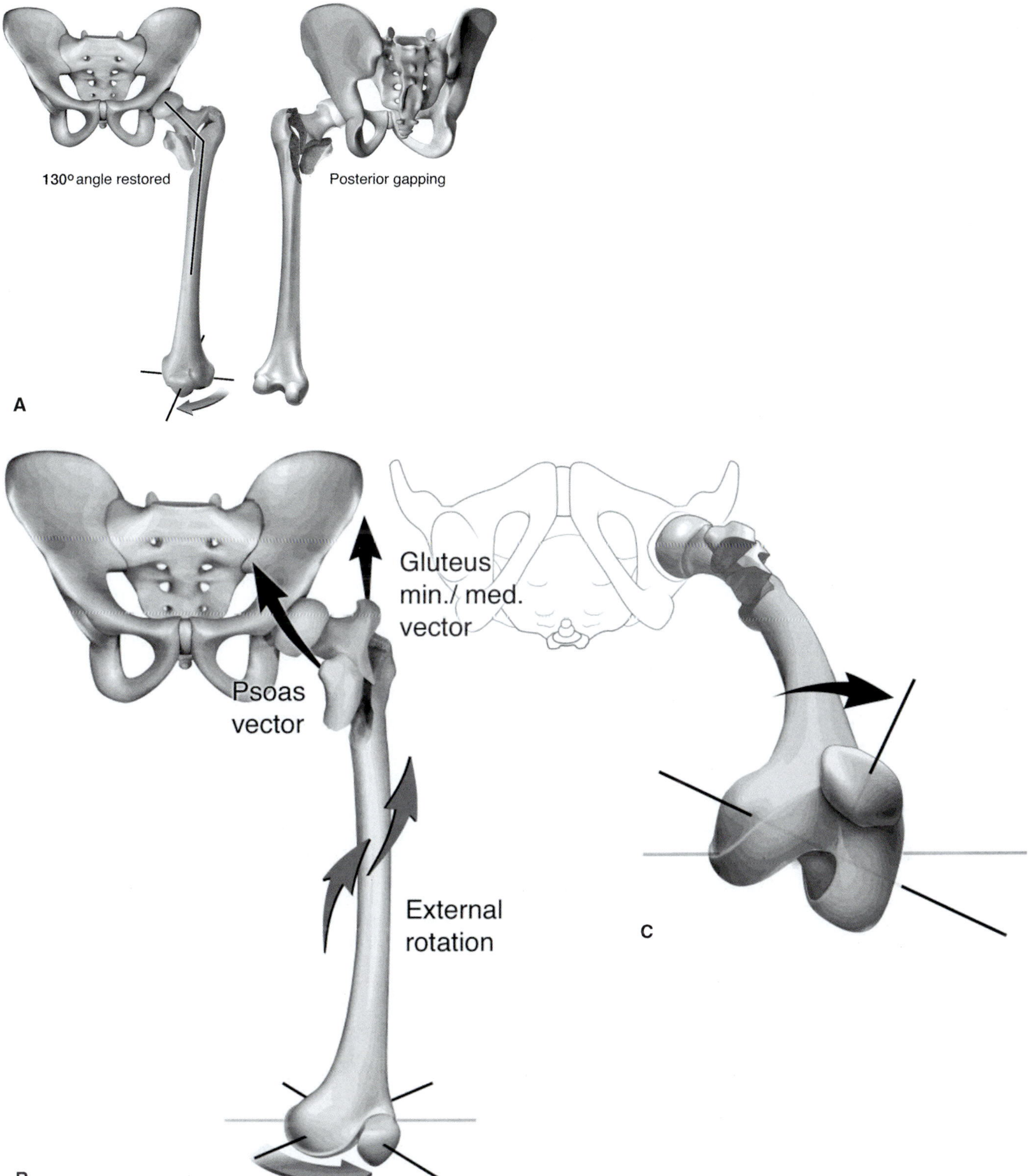

Figure 18-16 | Classically, intertrochanteric hip fractures present with clinical leg length shortening and external rotation. However, complex three to four-part fracture patterns are more prone to deforming muscle forces acting upon the separate fracture fragments. These injury illustrations demonstrate typical fracture deformity with loss of the normal femoral neck-shaft angle, displacement of the lesser trochanter and diaphyseal external rotation. The larger lesser trochanteric/calcar fragment and comminution of the intertrochanteric region can make assessment of rotational reduction difficult and requires a keen fluoroscopic awareness in multiplanar views to prevent malreduction.

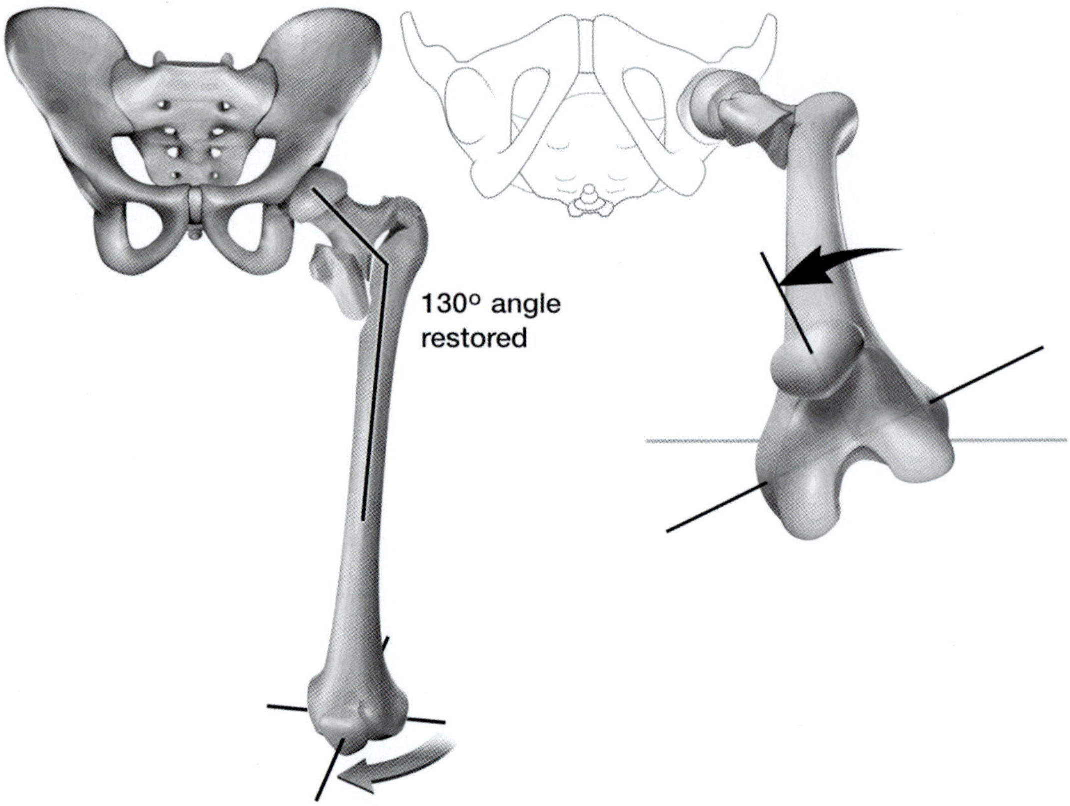

Figure 18-17 | Intraoperative axial traction with internal rotation is often successful in achieving a closed reduction. On occasion, the head-neck fragment can remain within the acetabulum with natural anteversion and persistent displacement from the diaphyseal–greater trochanter fragment (often due to posterior sag). Here axial traction successfully removes the varus neck–shaft angle making the peritrochanteric region appear reduced. However, the classic internal rotation reduction maneuver creates an internally rotated malreduction with anterior cortical compression and posterior cortical gapping. The displaced lesser trochanteric/calcar fragment is often large enough to prevent its use as a reliable marker of rotation.

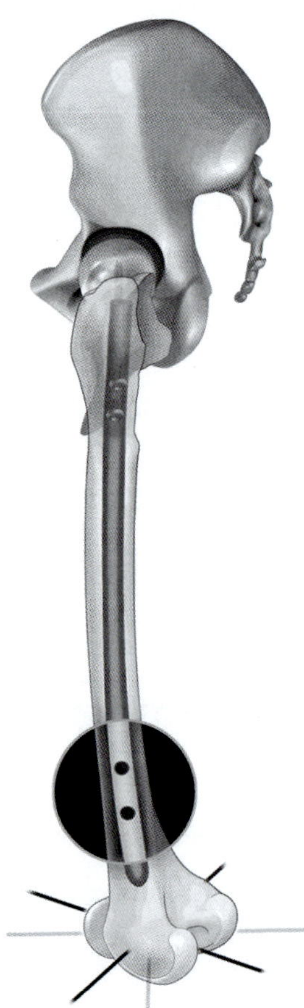

Figure 18-18 | Failure to recognize this malrotation and peritrochanteric compression with a long cephalomedullary nail will often lead to difficulty with distal interlocking due to implant rotational mismatch. A true lateral fluoroscopic view of the distal femur should demonstrate overlap of the medial and lateral condyles with presentation of the distal interlocking holes. This lateral illustration demonstrates proximal fixation of the poorly reduced intertrochanteric fragments and the resulting internal rotation of the distal femoral condyles away from the "perfect circle" interlocking holes. Commitment to this fixation construct leads to an undesirable internal rotation malreduction, greater proximal implant mechanical stress, risk of nonunion, and functional consequences. This can be prevented with numerous roll over and back AP and lateral fluoro views and assessment of the patellar position (as a surrogate for rotation) before, during, and after fixation. Also, a clinical exam of rotation is recommended in complex fracture patterns before the patient leaves the operating room.

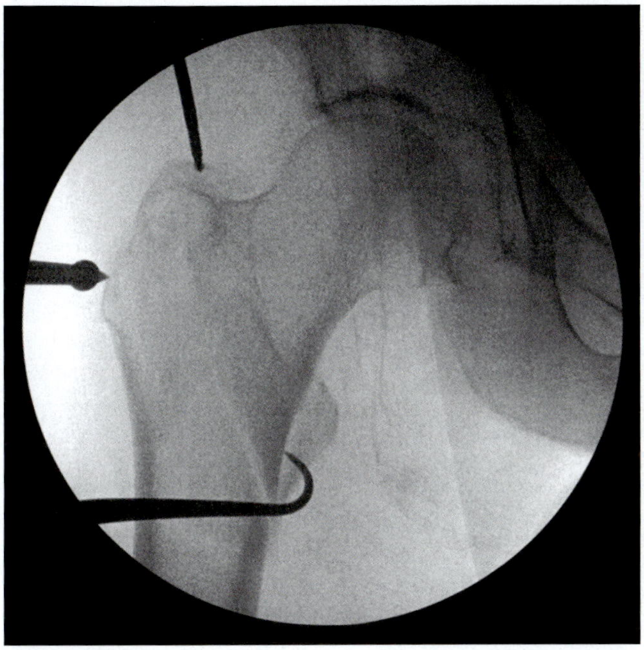

Figure 18-19 | Percutaneous fracture reduction prior to intramedullary fixation.

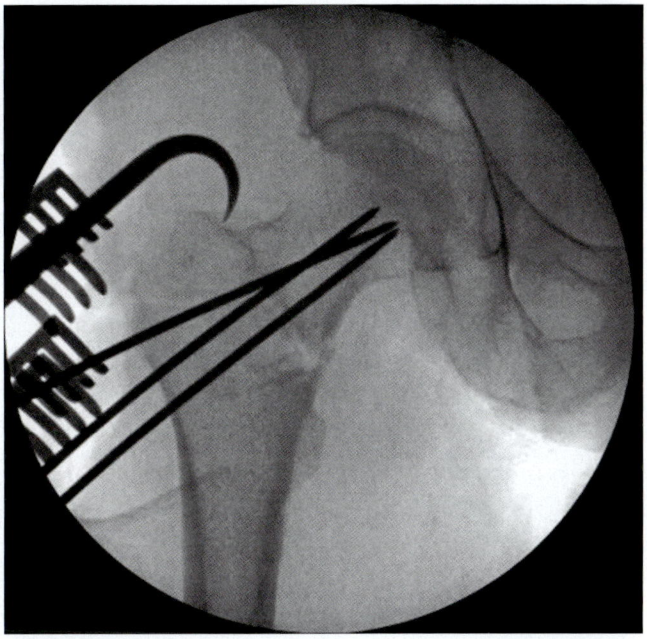

Figure 18-20 | Provisional pin fixation of a reduced fracture.

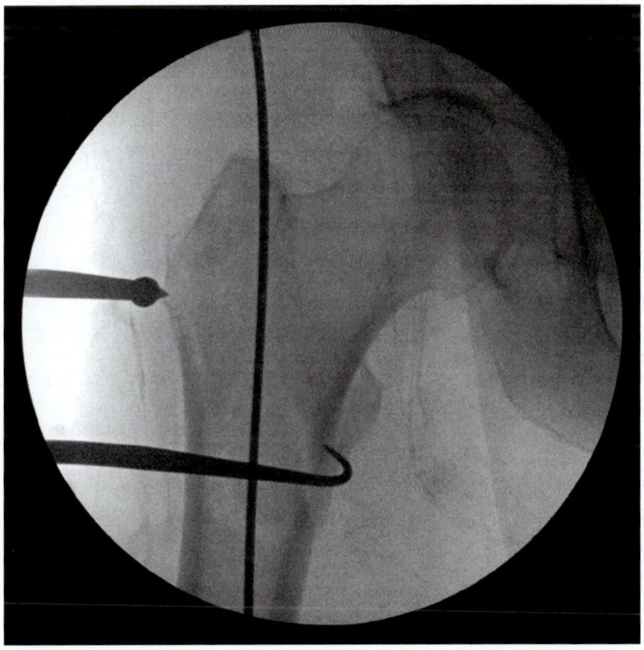

Figure 18-21 | The proper starting point for a cephalomedullary nail is slightly medial to the tip of the greater trochanter.

Tip-to-Apex Distance

- Accurate placement of implants is imperative. A cephalic lag screw should be placed deep and central within the head. The tip-to-apex distance is the sum of the measured distances from the tip of the screw to the apex of the femoral head on both the AP and lateral projections. A tip-to-apex distance of <25 mm decreases the risk of implant failure (Fig. 18-22).[4]
- Making accurate measurements with fluoroscopic images is difficult because of magnification error. Using the known diameter of the lag screw, the tip-to-apex distance can be estimated intraoperatively. Depending on the specific implant, cephalic lag screws have a shaft diameter of 8 to 12 mm. Therefore, ideal placement of the tip of the lag screw is within one screw diameter from the apex of the femoral head.

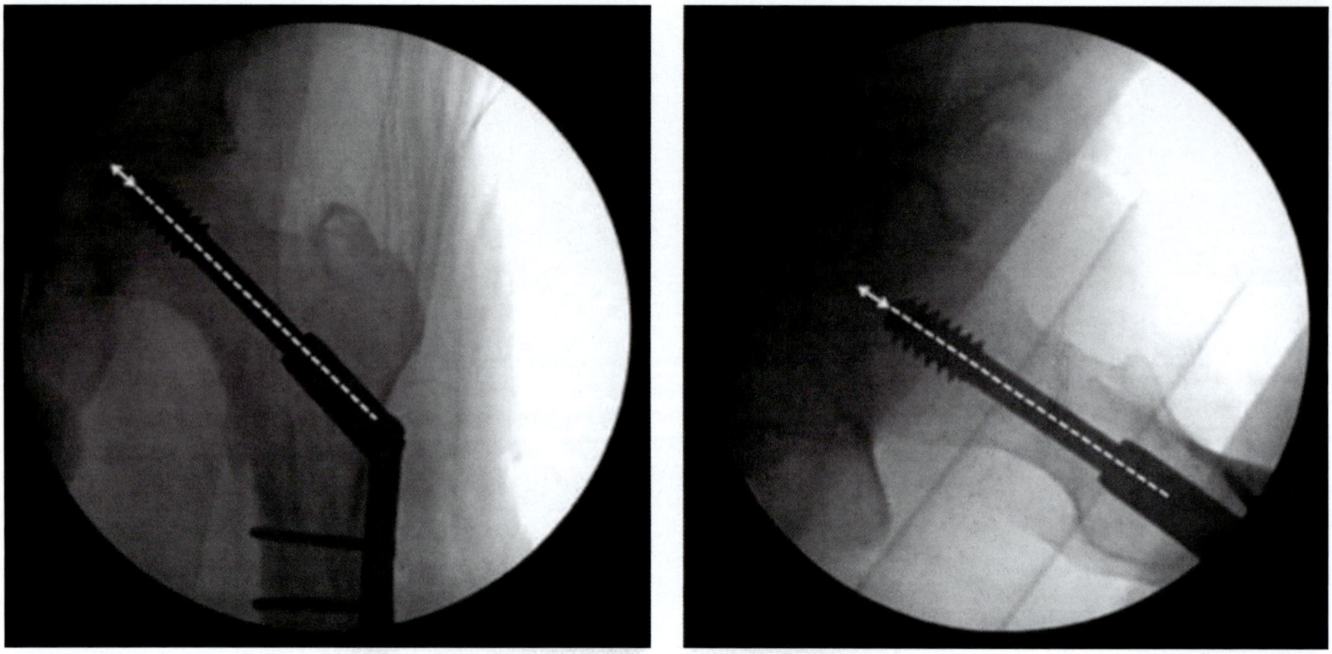

Figure 18-22 | A tip-to-apex distance <25 mm decreases the risk of implant failure.

Conclusion

Patient-specific factors such as medical comorbidities and osteoporosis make the management of intertrochanteric fractures challenging. Surgeon-controlled factors can be optimized with quality imaging and a thorough understanding of the radiographic anatomy of the proximal femur. Appropriate implant selection, adequate fracture reduction, and proper implant placement decrease complications and improve outcomes.

References

1. Haidukewych G. Intertrochanteric fractures: ten tips to improve results. *J Bone Joint Surg Am.* 2009;91(3):712–719.
2. Lubovsky O, Liebergall M, Mattan Y, et al. Early diagnosis of occult hip fractures: MRI versus CT scan. *Injury.* 2005;36:788–792.
3. Carr JB. The anterior and medial reduction of intertrochanteric fractures: a simple method to obtain a stable reduction. *J Orthop Trauma.* 2007;21:485–489.
4. Baumgaertner MR, Curtin SL, Lindskog DM, et al. The value of the tip-apex distance in predicting failure of fixation of peritrochanteric fractures of the hip. *J Bone Joint Surg Am.* 1995;77:1058–1064.

Chapter 19
Subtrochanteric Femur Fractures

TIMOTHY S. ACHOR

Bony Anatomy

- The subtrochanteric region of the femur includes the area from the lesser trochanter to a point 8 cm distally. However, any fracture occurring in the diaphysis of the proximal one-third of the femur can generally be referred to as subtrochanteric (Fig. 19-1).
- The anatomy of the proximal femur is complex from both bone and soft tissue standpoints.
- There are multiple deforming forces acting on the subtrochanteric region that result in a classic pattern of proximal fragment flexion with abduction and external rotation and distal fragment adduction and shortening. Failure to correct varus and flexion moments at the fracture often lead to malunion, nonunion, or implant failure.
- The cortical bone in this region is particularly dense, as the proximal femur sees tremendous forces. Comminution, especially medially, is not uncommon and can pose a challenge to restoring coronal alignment.

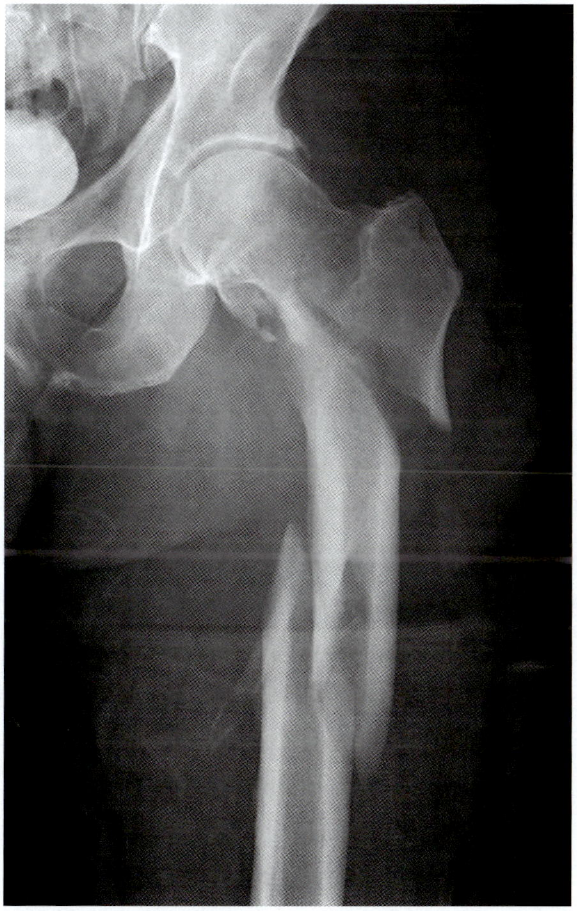

Figure 19-1 | A classic "reverse oblique" intertrochanteric femur fracture with segmental subtrochanteric extension.

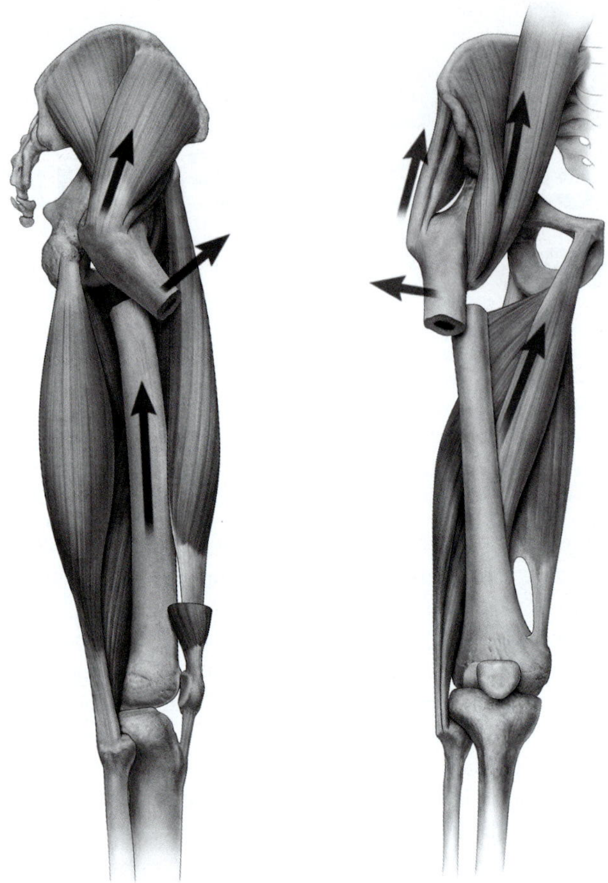

Figure 19-2 | Typical displacement pattern of subtrochanteric femur fractures. The proximal segment is flexed, abducted, and externally rotated; the distal segment is shortened and externally rotated.

- There is no true spongy "metaphyseal bone" in the proximal femur.
- The isthmus of the femur is typically located at the junction of the proximal and middle thirds.

Radiographic Anatomy

- The piriformis fossa is in line with the medullary canal (anatomic axis) of the femur on the AP projection. In cases of medial subtrochanteric comminution, a piriformis nail offers a favorable mechanical advantage to preventing varus malalignment but requires adequate intraoperative reduction techniques during reaming and nail insertion.
- AP and lateral radiographs of the proximal femur will reveal the injury with predictable displacement patterns.
- Lateral projection images are usually obtained in a cross-table manner with contralateral hip and knee flexion.
- Typical displacement pattern of the proximal segment includes flexion, abduction, and external rotation due to the muscle pull of the iliopsoas, gluteus medius/minimus, and external rotators, respectively (Fig. 19-2).
- Distally, there can be an adduction deformity (Fig. 19-3).
- Low-energy subtrochanteric fractures with a history of bisphosphonate use must raise suspicion of a pathologic fracture.
- Radiographic findings associated with bisphosphonate fractures include cortical thickening, lateral cortical beaking, and a relatively transverse pattern (Fig. 19-4).

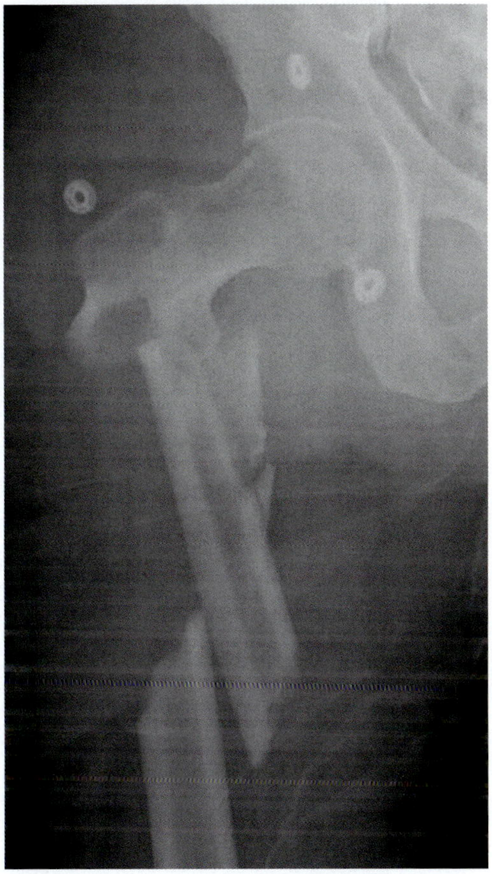

Figure 19-3 | Radiographic appearance of typical displacement patterns about the proximal femur.

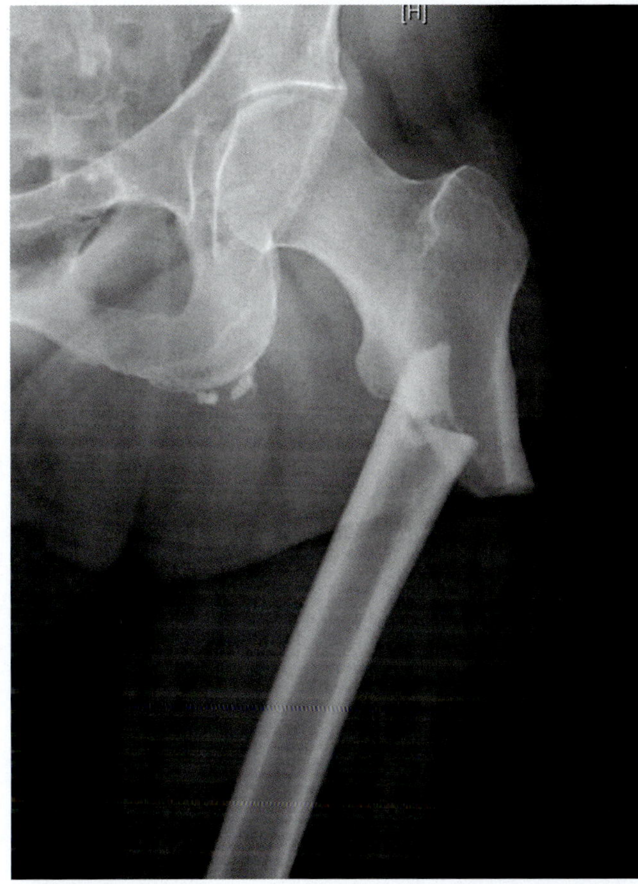

Figure 19-4 | Bisphosphonate-associated fracture with pathognomonic radiographic findings: cortical thickening, lateral beaking, and a relatively transverse pattern, with or without a medial spike.

Preoperative Imaging

- As proximal femur fractures are typically high-energy injuries, a screening AP pelvis radiograph is indicated to rule out any associated injuries (Fig. 19-5).
- Plain films radiographs are typically sufficient for diagnosis and preoperative planning; however, CT scan can be helpful in identifying occult fracture lines, and 3-D reconstructions can be utilized as well.
- Full-length orthogonal images of the femur are critical to rule out associated segmental injuries (Figs. 19-6 and 19-7).

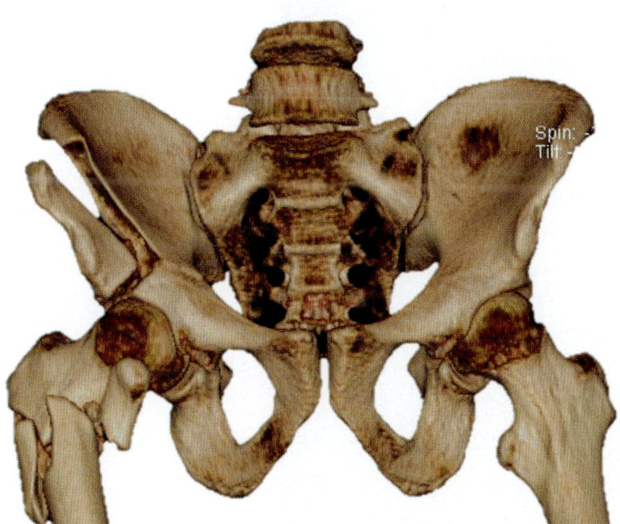

Figure 19-5 | 3-D surface rendered CT reconstruction of a 38 year-old male after a fall off roof. Notice the comminuted subtrochanteric fracture with associated ipsilateral ilium fracture.

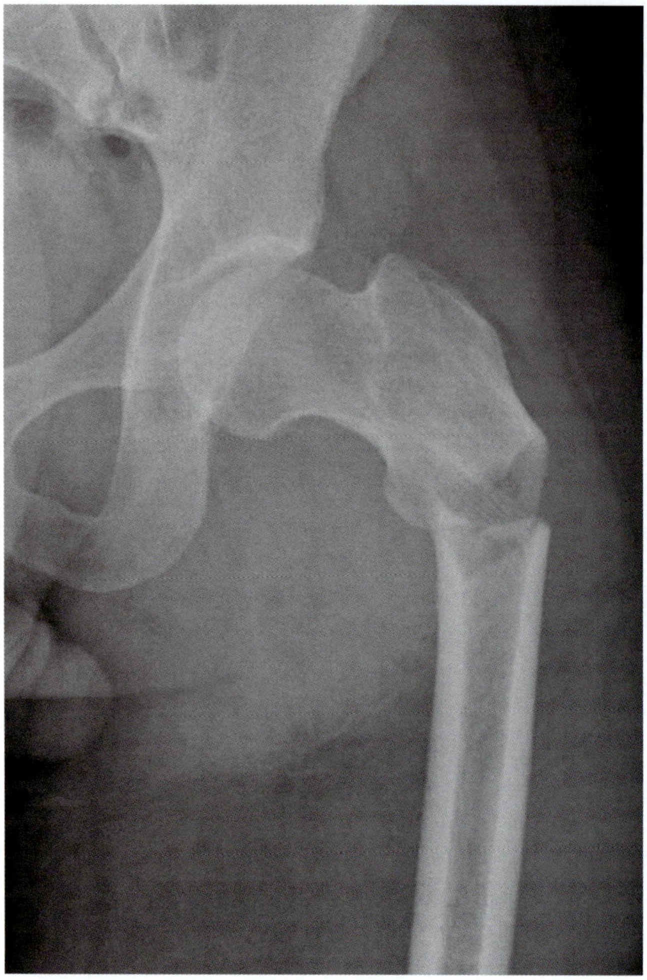

Figure 19-6 | 27 year-old male s/p motorcycle crash with high energy subtrochanteric fracture. Limited views of the hip would have missed the segmental injury noted in Figure 19-7.

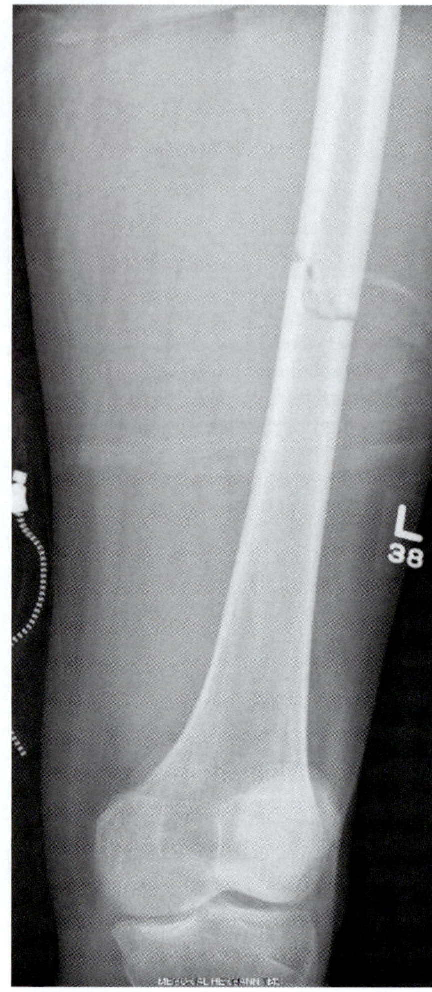

Figure 19-7 | Full-length radiographic studies are mandatory and should be obtained in all instances.

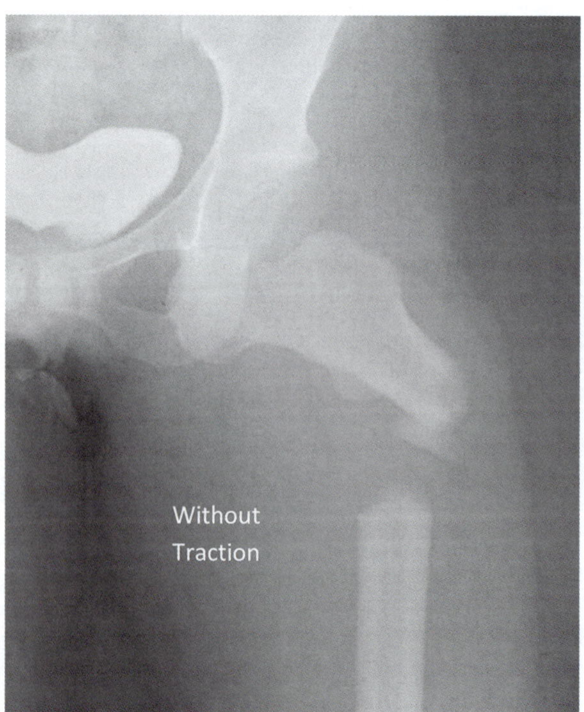

Figure 19-8 | Injury film reveals a hip dislocation and a relatively short proximal segment. The length of the proximal segment can have implant choice implications.

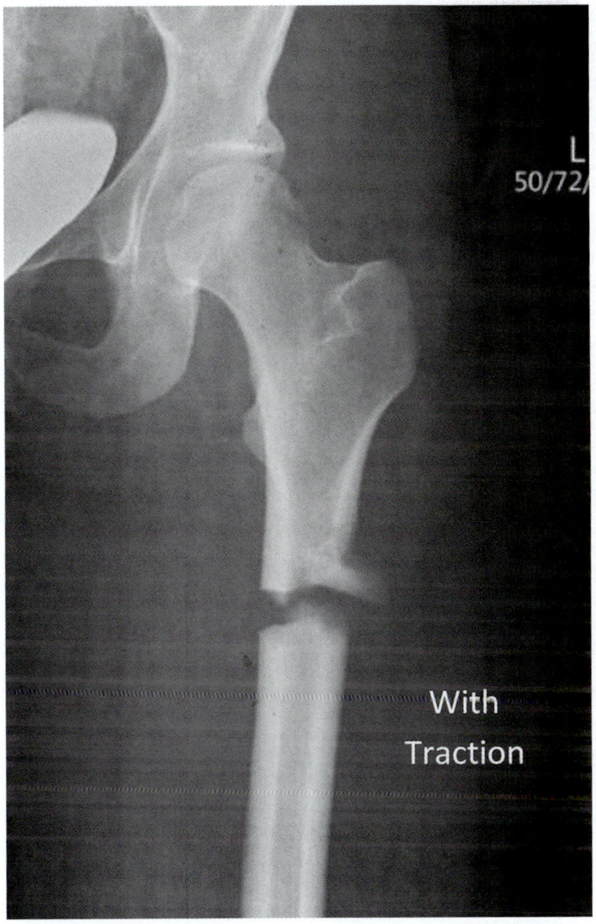

Figure 19-9 | Same patient from Figure 19-8, now after hip reduction and traction view. The true length of the proximal segment is revealed.

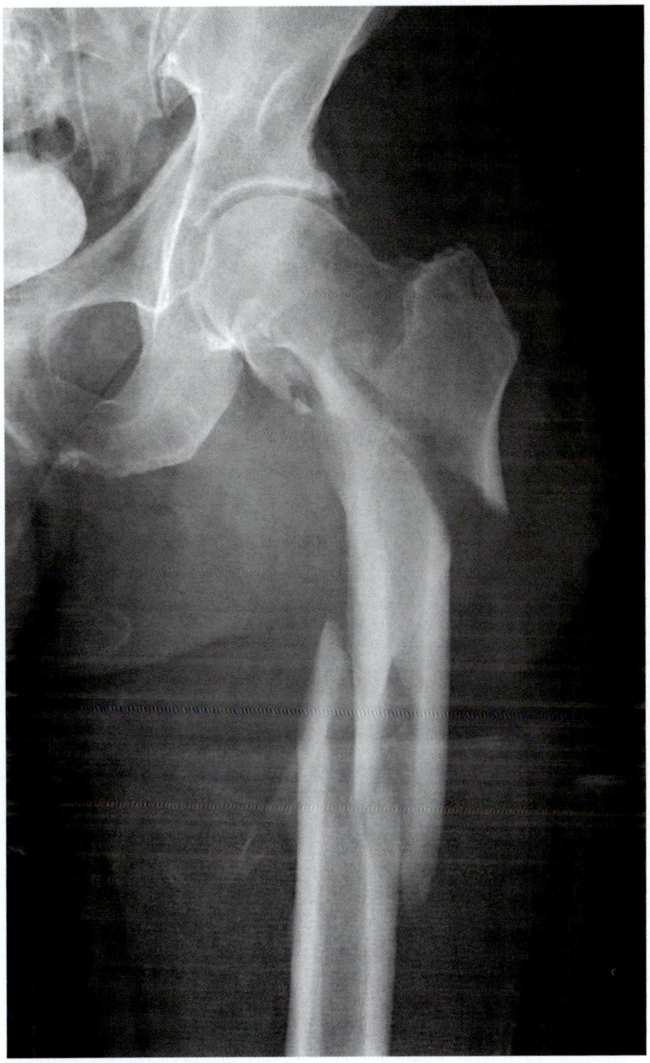

Figure 19-10 | AP radiograph of the proximal femur reveals an obvious reverse oblique intertrochanteric fracture proximally, but involvement of the femoral neck is unclear.

- Traction views can be helpful to determine the exact level of the fracture. This is important in determining the appropriate implant (nail vs. plate) and proximal interlocking bolt options (standard vs. reconstruction/cephalomedullary) (Figs. 19-8 and 19-9).
- Any suggestion on plain films or clinical suspicion of an ipsilateral femoral neck fracture warrants additional advanced imaging studies (i.e., CT scan) (Figs. 19-10 and 19-11).
- Again, medial comminution associated with subtrochanteric fractures is common and must be noted; these fractures are at risk for varus malreduction/displacement due to loss of medial support.

Intraoperative Positioning

- Positioning of patients with subtrochanteric femur fractures is based on patient and fracture characteristics, as well as surgeon preference. Options for positioning include supine or lateral on a radiolucent table or on a fracture table (Fig. 19-12).
- The use of a piriformis entry nail is exceedingly difficult on a fracture table as compared to the free-leg radiolucent table technique where the extremity can be manipulated to achieve a proper nail starting point and fracture reduction.
- The author prefers to perform the procedure supine on a radiolucent flat-top table. The entire leg is draped free from the flank to the toes. Care is taken not to drape out the nail insertion site proximally.

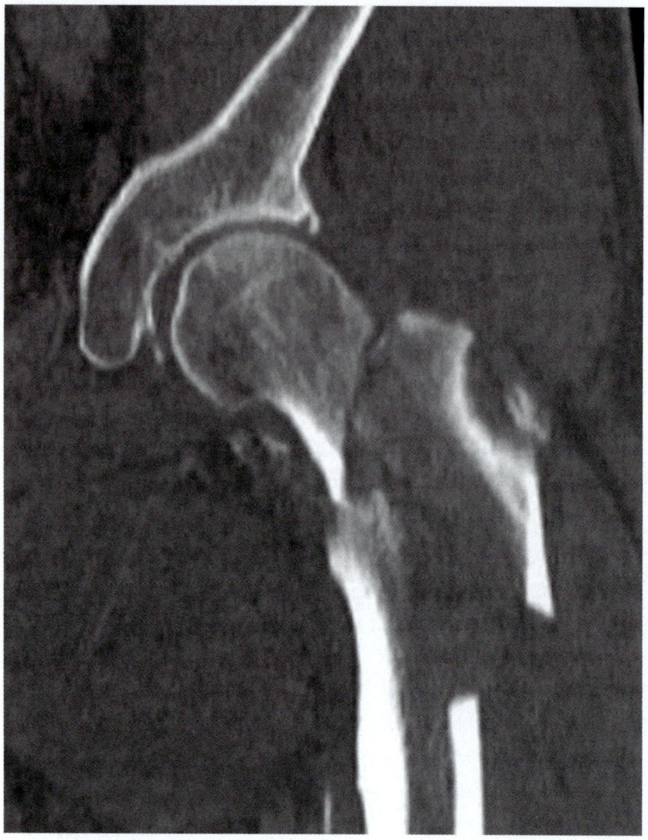

Figure 19-11 | CT scan coronal recontruction of the patient in Fig 19-10. With advanced imaging studies, the femoral neck fracture becomes more apparent.

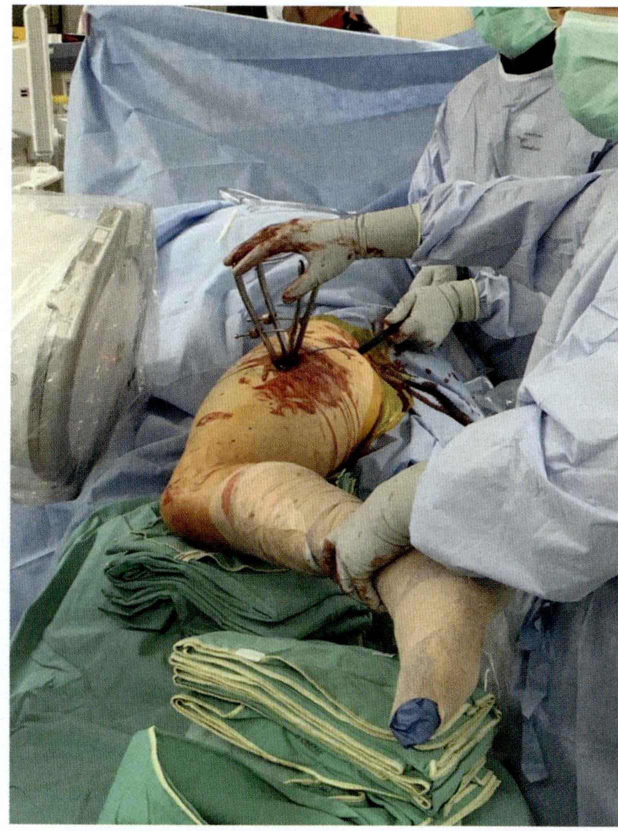

Figure 19-12 | Intraoperative photograph showing a patient in the lateral position undergoing an open reduction and intramedullary nailing of a subtrochanteric fracture.

- Prior to prepping and draping, fluoroscopic images of the contralateral limb are taken for later comparison of length, alignment, and rotation. This is performed in every case regardless of the severity of injury or complexity of proposed procedure. Images can be printed and taped to the image intensifier for intraoperative comparison. This can be particularly useful in comminuted fractures where accurate length assessment is impossible (Fig. 19-13).
- A bump can be placed under the ipsilateral hip; however, this can introduce rotatory deformity if the surgeon is not compulsive about the rotatory position of the distal femoral segment. The author prefers no bump under the hip but just a small bump under the leg to aid in presentation of the limb.
- The author utilizes the same positioning regardless of the implant to be used.
- The C-arm is positioned on the contralateral side of the patient where various AP and lateral views are assessed throughout the case. Note that imaging of the proximal femoral fragment may require a combination of true lateral and roll-up lateral images to assure that screws are appropriately placed within the femoral head and neck (Fig. 19-14).
- Note that imaging of the proximal femoral fragment may require a combination of true lateral and roll-up lateral images to assure that screws are appropriately placed safely within the femoral head and neck (Fig. 19-15).
- There can be wide fracture displacement, and accordingly, closed reduction techniques are often unsuccessful (Fig. 19-16).
- Often percutaneous or even open reduction techniques are utilized:

An anterior to posterior Schanz pin carefully placed along the inferior femoral neck calcar and out of the way of subsequent nail screws can be percutaneously placed under true AP fluoro view (roll over to match flexion-abduction and external rotation of proximal fragment). This pin allows a powerful vector

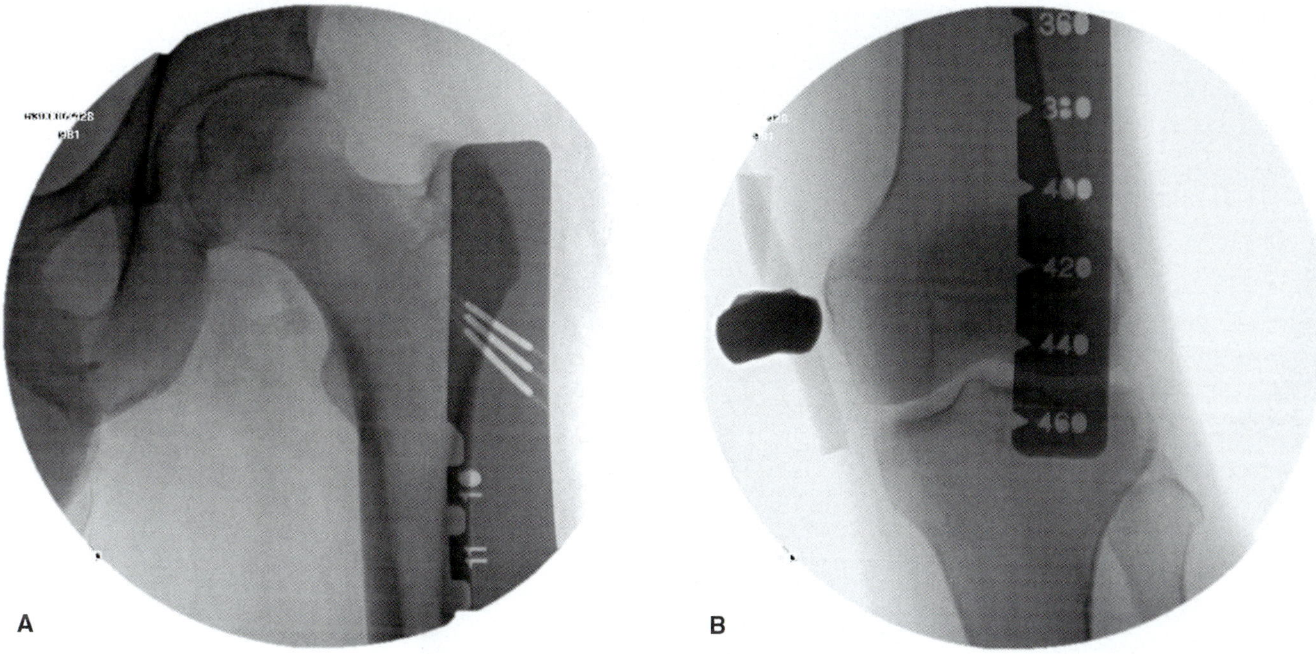

Figure 19-13 I Intraoperative utilization of a radio-opaque ruler to measure the length of the uninjured femur. This allows for later comparison to the fractured femur to improve accuracy of length restoration.

to control sagittal plane reduction along with other coronal plane reduction aids (Schanz pin or bone hook). Note that an AP starting point just medial to the tip of the greater trochanter is mechanically advantageous to prevent varus malalignment when using a trochanteric entry nail for subtrochanteric fractures (Fig. 19-17).

Failure of closed or percutaneous reduction techniques to prevent varus and flexion malalignment should prompt an open reduction with clamps (Fig. 19-18).

If an anatomic reduction can be maintained, cerclage cables placed in a soft tissue–friendly manner are another option to maintain a reduction (Fig. 19-19).

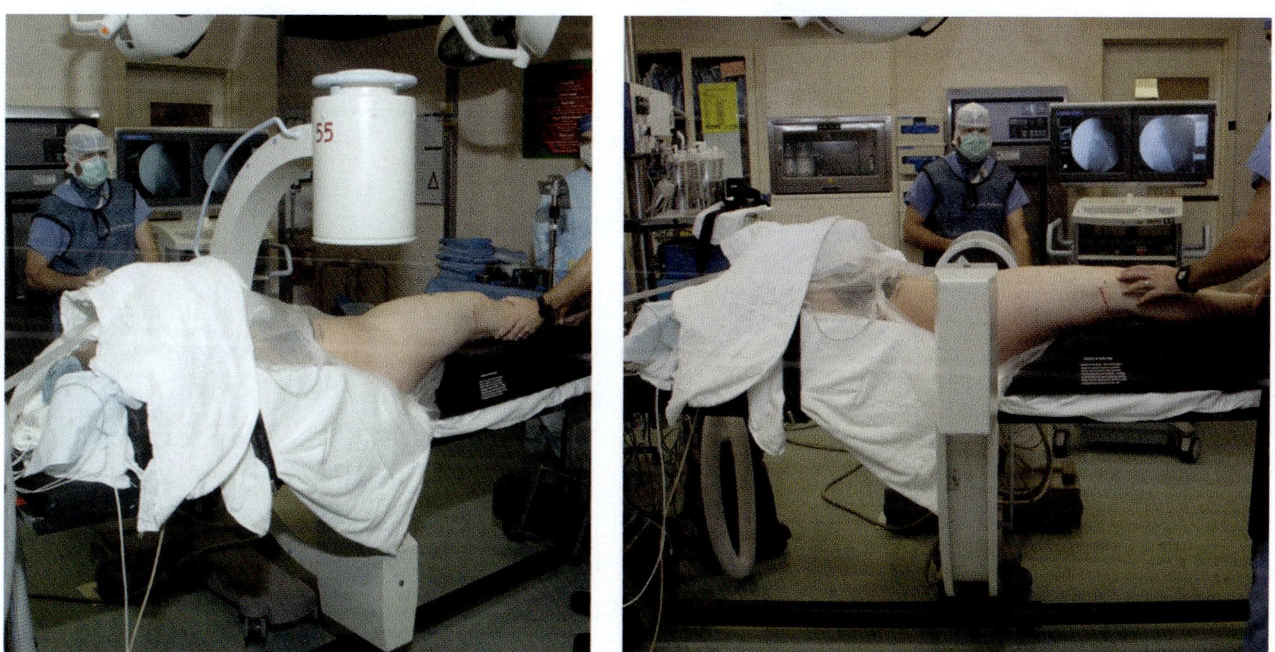

Figure 19-14 I Intraoperative photographs showing the typical patient position, bump, and position of the C-arm in preparation for nailing of a subtrochanteric fracture.

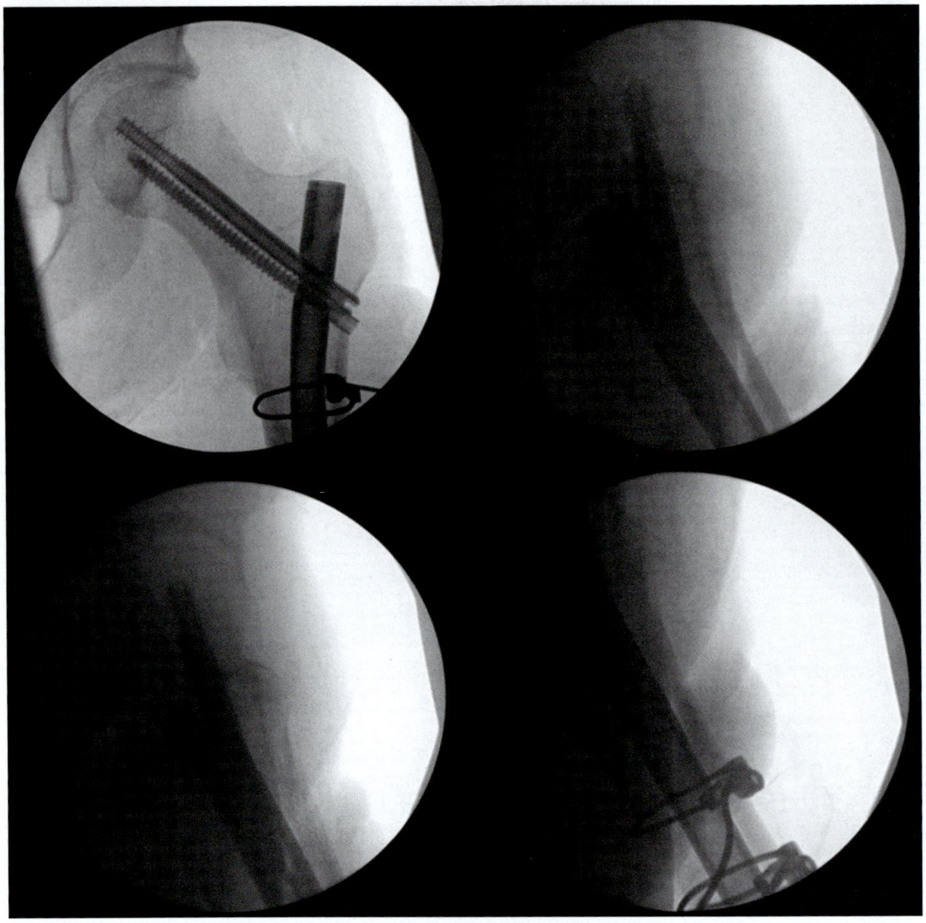

Figure 19-15 | Multiple lateral projections can be taken to ensure safe placement of screws contained within the femoral head.

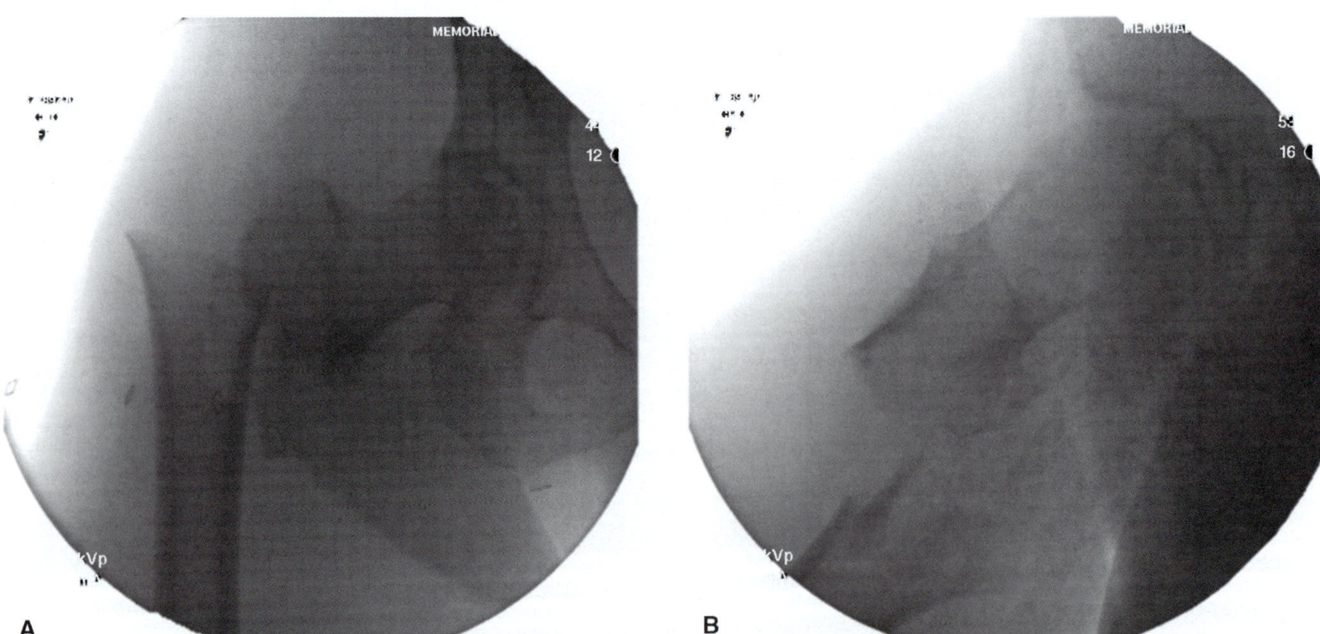

Figure 19-16 | This 29 year-old male sustained a high energy subtrochanteric fracture. Even with appropriate anesthesia, the fracture does not reduce well with attempted closed means. Often, high energy proximal femur fractures benefit from a percutaneous or open reduction.

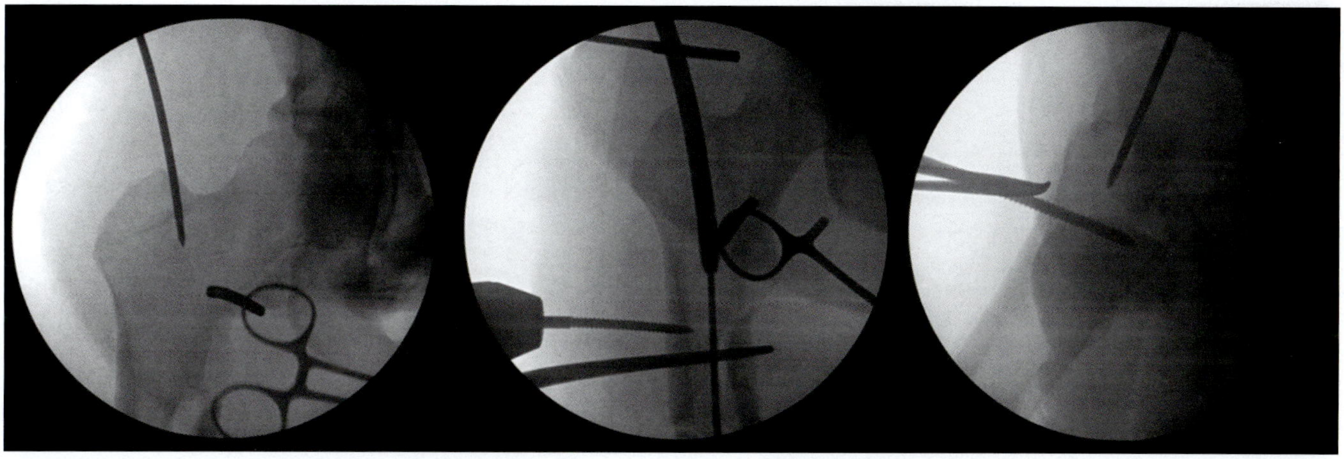

Figure 19-17 | Multiple reduction aides are often necessary. Here, an anterior-to-posterior Schanz pin has been placed to control the flexion deformity, and a lateral-to-medial pin has been placed to control the abduction deformity. When a trochanteric implant is utilized, a medial start site can decrease likelihood of a varus reduction.

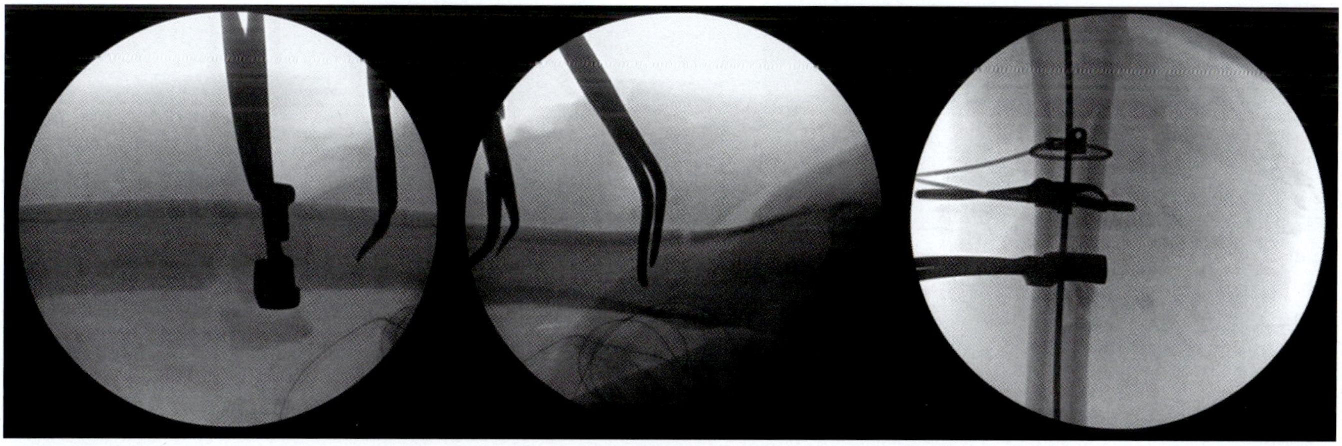

Figure 19-18 | Open reduction with clamps placed in strategic locations are necessary when closed or percutaneous techniques have failed.

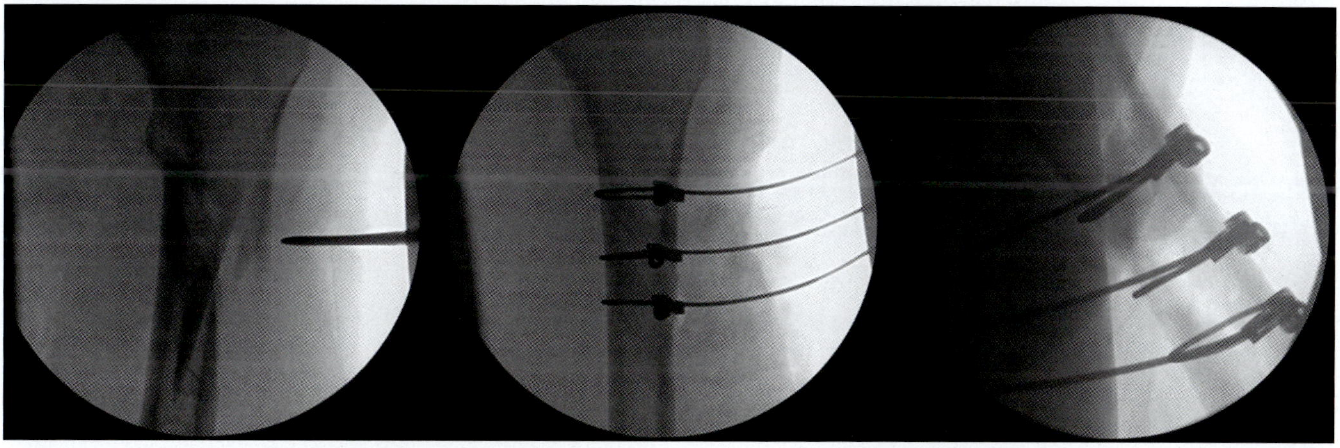

Figure 19-19 | In addition to clamps, well-placed and positioned cables can help maintain reduction as well.

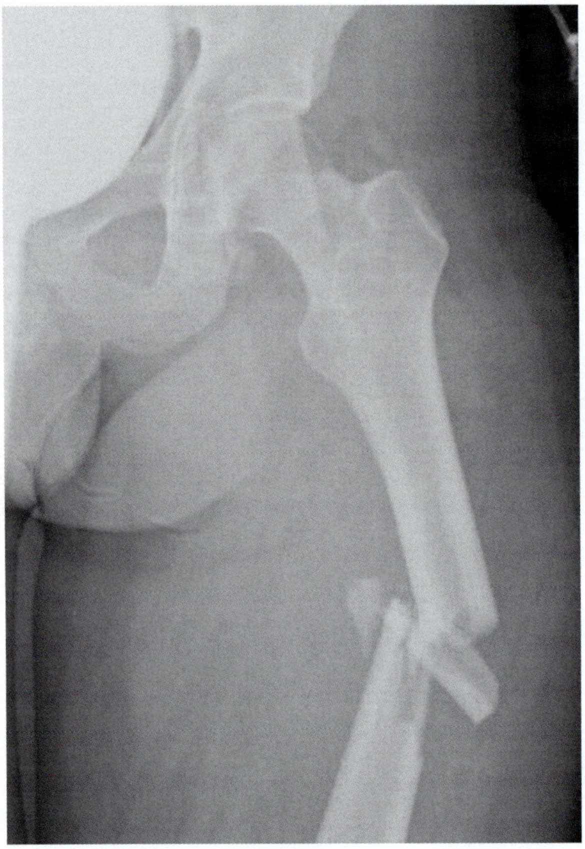

Figure 19-20 |

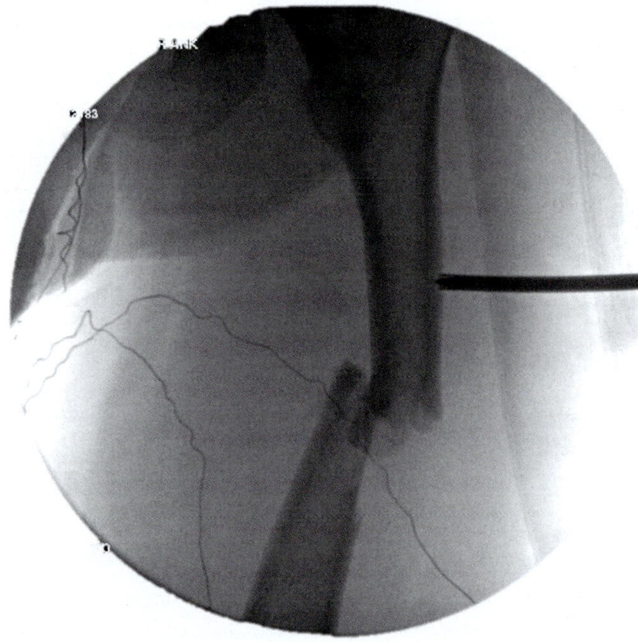

Figure 19-21 |

Case 1: This 28-year-old male was involved in a high-speed motor vehicle collision (Fig. 19-20).

It can be difficult to adduct the proximal segment enough to allow for appropriate starting guidewire placement for a piriformis nail. As such, a 5.0-mm Schanz pin can be utilized as a "joystick" to adduct this segment. Note in this image, the Schanz pin is not on the *exact* lateral cortex, but rather is slightly anterior or posterior (Fig. 19-21).

Here, the starting position of the Schanz pin has been corrected, and it is now seated squarely on the lateral cortex (Fig. 19-22).

The Schanz pin is inserted in a bicortical manner (Fig. 19-23).

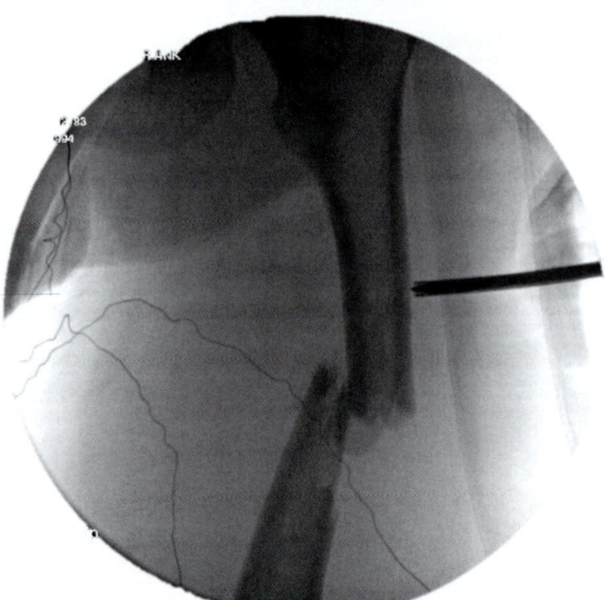

Figure 19-22 |

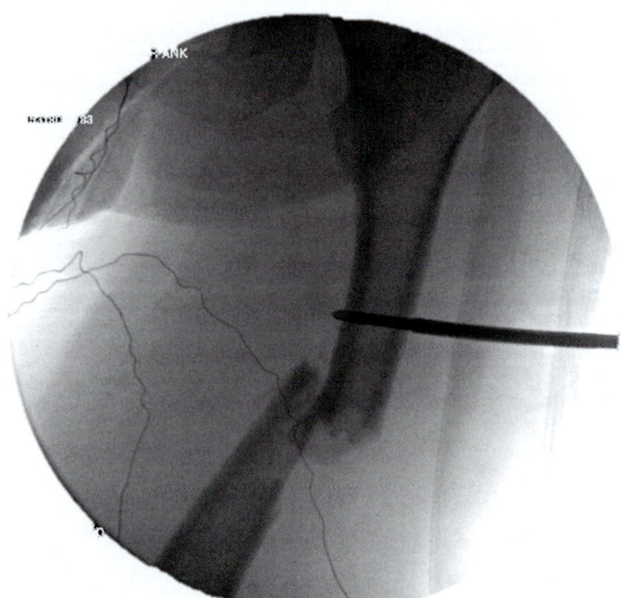

Figure 19-23 |

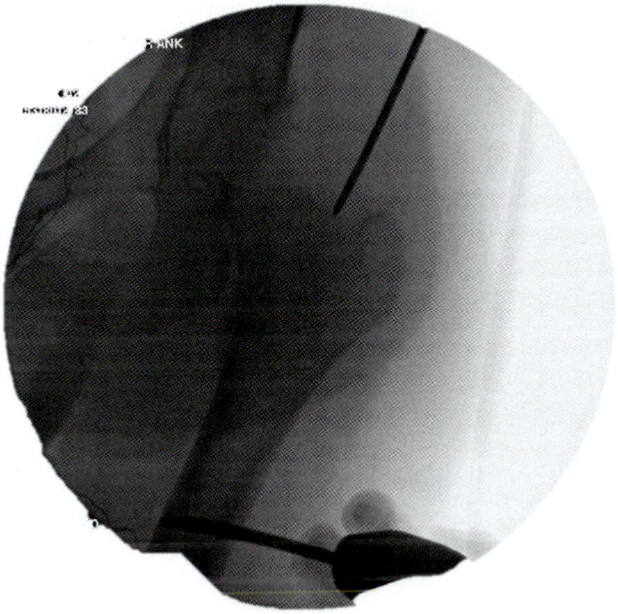

Figure 19-24 |

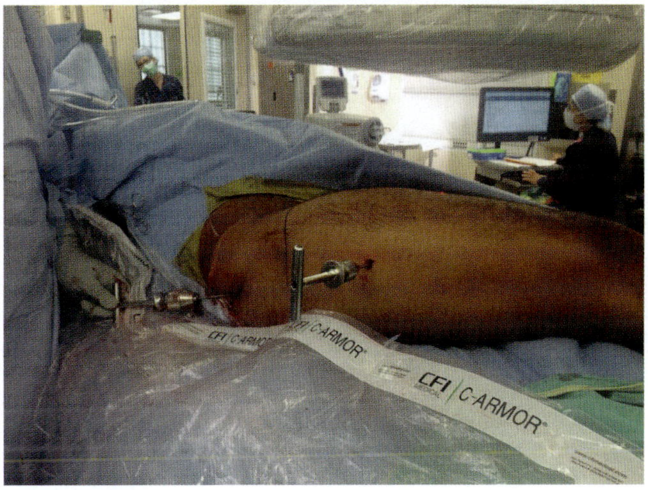

Figure 19-25 |

A T-handle chuck is then used to manipulate the proximal segment. Note in this image, the starting guidewire is positioned too anterior. The wire must be walked posterior until it falls into the piriformis fossa (Figs. 19-24 and 19-25).

This image shows a more appropriate starting point within the piriformis fossa (Fig. 19-26).

Now the cannulated canal opening reamer can be utilized to open the proximal femoral canal. Note that the fluoroscopic image allows the surgeon to visualize that the soft tissue protection sleeve is in good position (Fig. 19-27).

It is critical that the opening reamer be in line with the medullary canal; for subtrochanteric fractures, any deviation of the wire in a medial direction will lead to a varus deformity (Fig. 19-28).

- Although the bicortical Schanz pin can be used for manipulation of the fracture fragments and passage of the ball-tipped guidewire across the fracture, it must be removed prior to reaming.
- Alternatives to maintain reduction during reaming include a unicortical Schanz pin or the ball-spiked pusher (Picador) (Fig. 19-29).

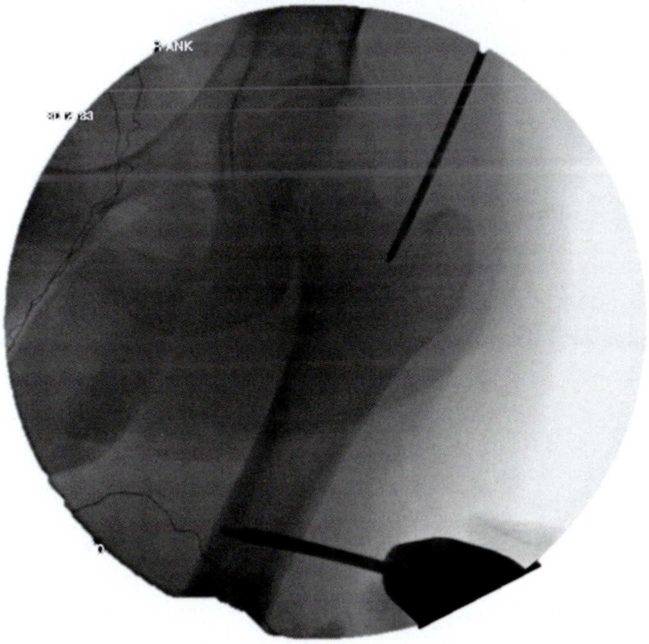

Figure 19-26 |

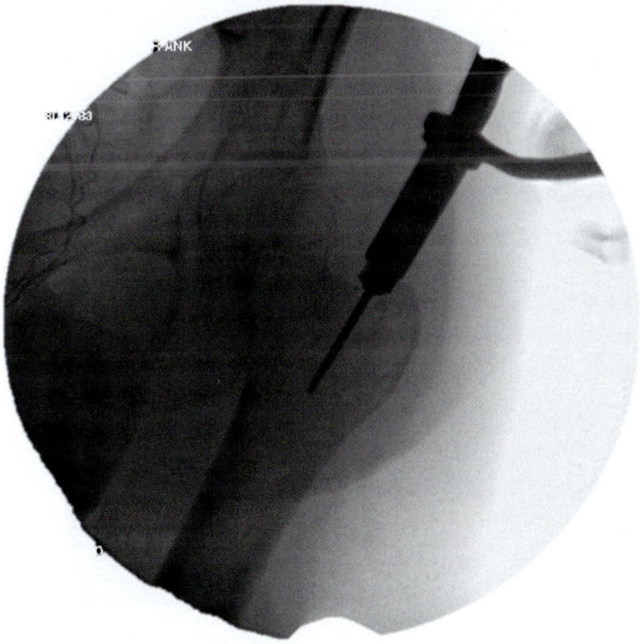

Figure 19-27 |

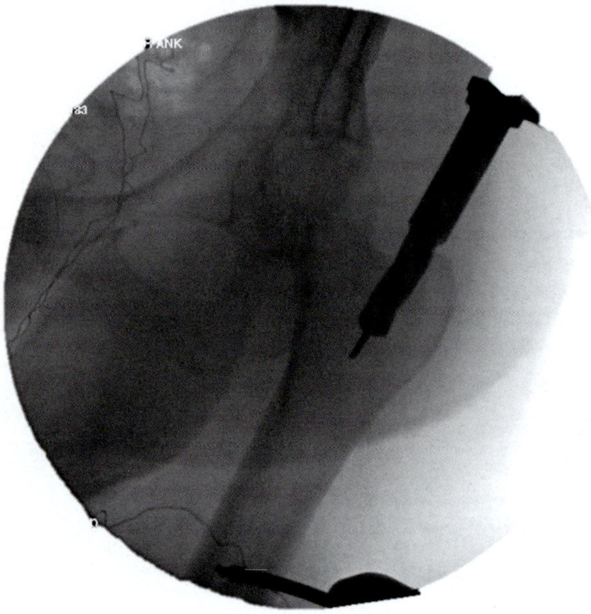

Figure 19-28 |

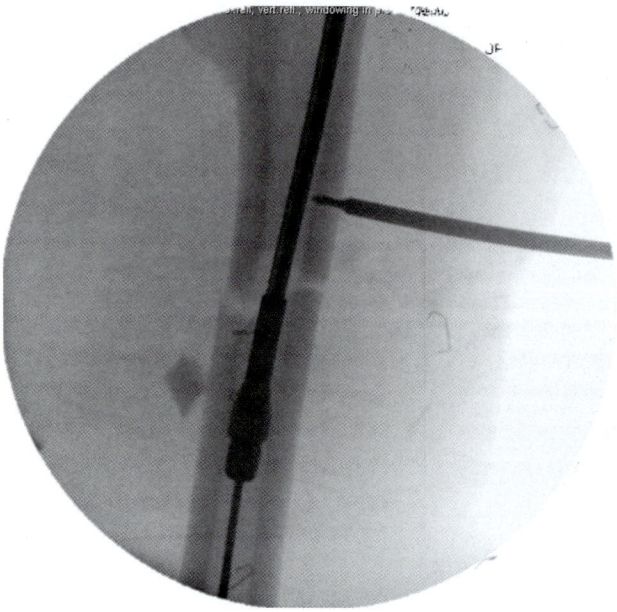

Figure 19-29 |

Case 2: This 22-year-old male was involved in a high-speed motorcycle crash. He sustained multiple injuries, including this severely comminuted subtrochanteric femur fracture (Fig. 19-30).

Here, a ball-spiked pusher is used to maintain alignment during reaming. This can be done in a percutaneous manner (Figs. 19-31 and 19-32).

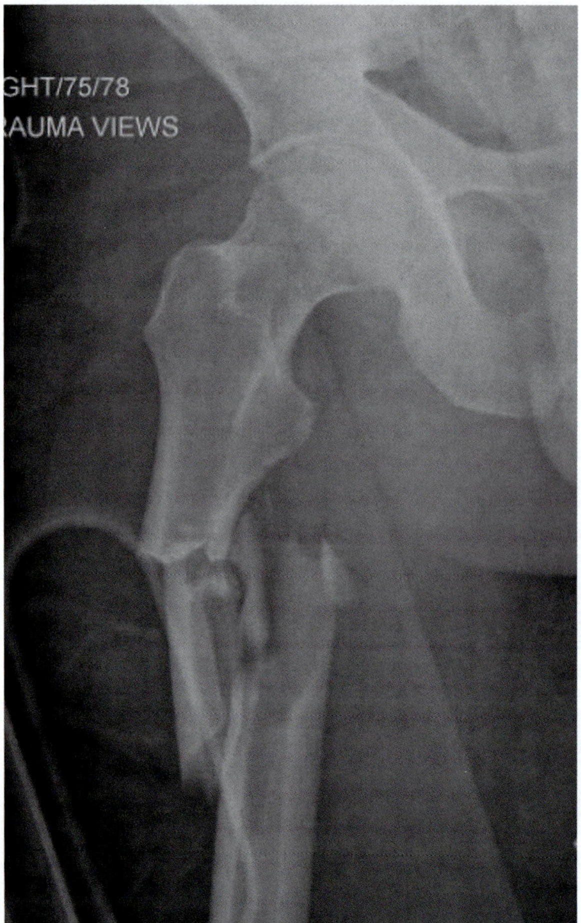

Figure 19-30 |

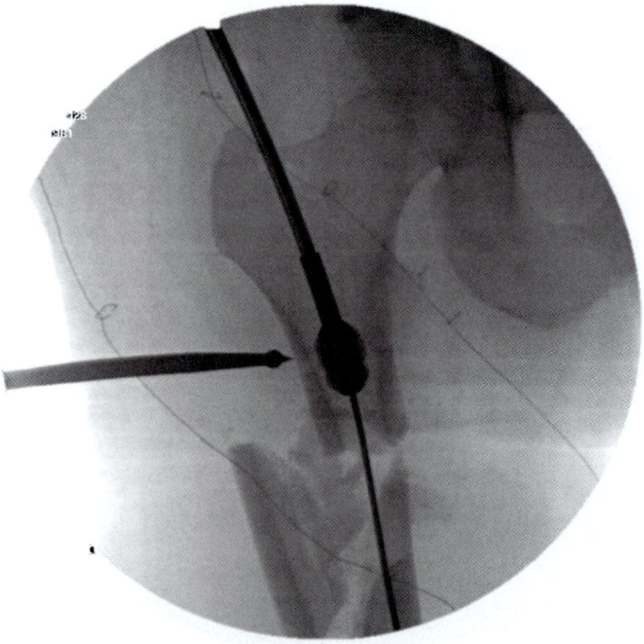

Figure 19-31 |

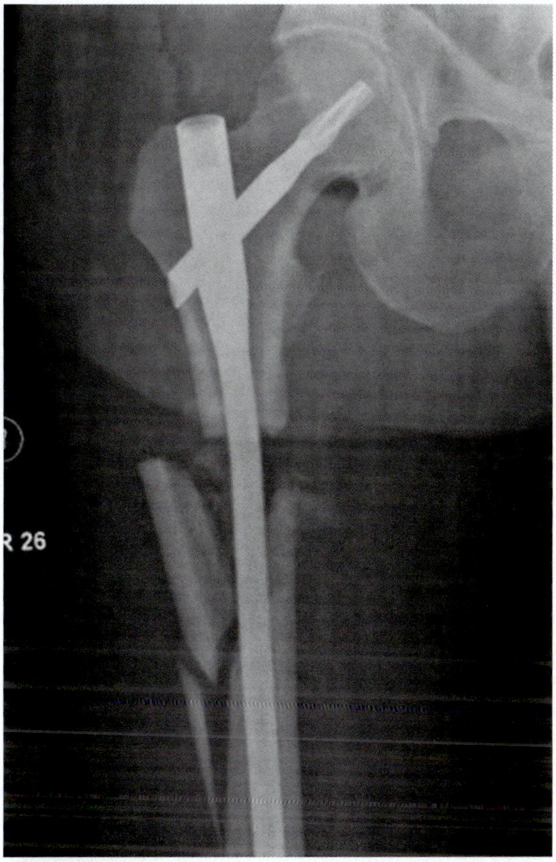

Figure 19-32 |

Fracture Table Imaging

If the surgeon's preference is to utilize a fracture table for subtrochanteric stabilization, it should be noted that absolute reduction of the deforming forces may not be feasible. Thus, a combination of percutaneous or open reduction techniques along with repositions of the extremity in traction may be necessary. Reduction should be maintained before and during reaming along with nail insertion.

- One technical trick is to slightly flex the distal fragment in traction with the table to improve the sagittal plane alignment (Fig. 19-33).
- Note that internal malrotation can be common with use of a fracture table and meticulous attention to rotation is necessary throughout the case.

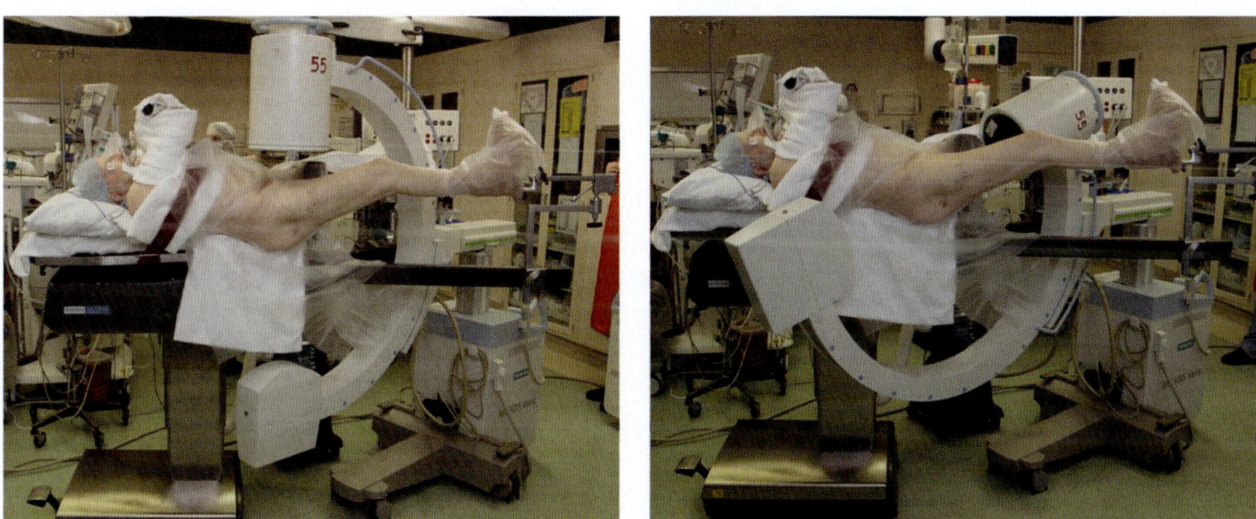

Figure 19-33 | Use of traction table to aid in closed reduction. Here, traction can be applied with elevation of the distal segment to improve the reduction and "deliver" the distal segment to the proximal segment.

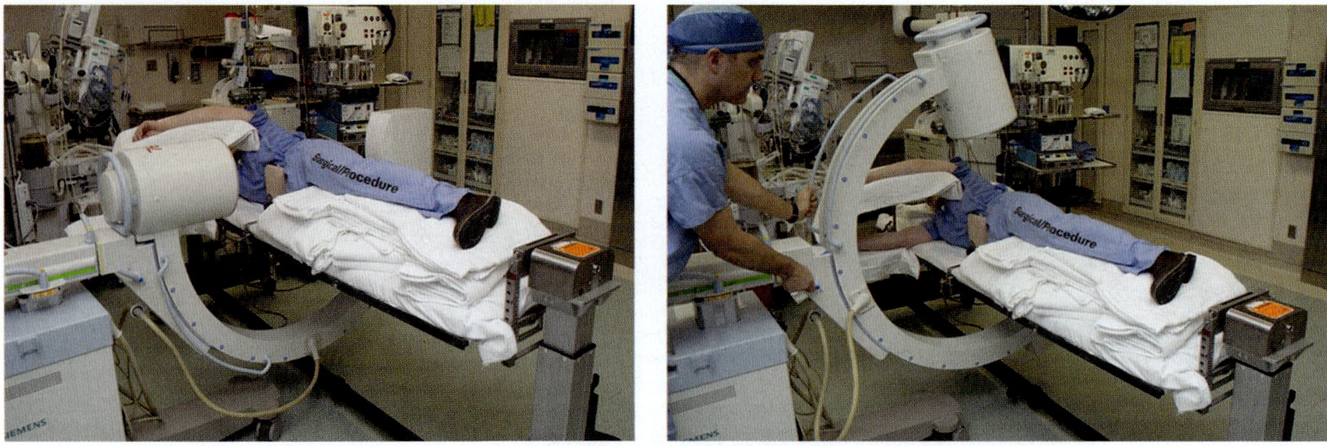

Figure 19-34 | Simulated patient in the lateral position showing ease of fluoroscopic imaging. Deforming forces about the proximal femur can be mitigated using this position.

Free-Leg Lateral Position on Radiolucent Table

One distinct advantage to this positioning technique is the relative ease of free-leg fracture reduction based upon moving the limb within the planes of deformity (*when compared to the supine position*). The distal limb can be forward flexed to meet the proximal fragment (sagittal reduction) with radiolucent pillows/blankets or bolsters to restore the coronal plane and prevent varus malalignment. The lateral-based flexion moment of subtrochanteric fractures also tends to be less accentuated in this position (Fig. 19-34).

- This position often allows improved access for either a piriformis or trochanteric start point, even in an obese patient.
- Lateral fluoroscopic imaging of the proximal segment (head/neck) can be more challenging with overlap of the contralateral limb within the field. Again, flexion of the limb can help direct the injured leg away from the down leg and prevent superimposed bony anatomy.

Chapter 20
Femoral Shaft Imaging

JEAN-CLAUDE G. D'ALLEYRAND
THEODORE T. MANSON

Bony Anatomy

- The femoral diaphysis is straight in the AP plane, with an apex anterior bow in the sagittal plane and its epiphyses rotated with respect to one another in the transverse plane.
  - This rotation, or version, can vary quite a bit between patients, and some modest side-to-side variability may exist between the femora of individuals.[1]
  - There is also variability in the morphology of the greater trochanter between individuals, which can have implications on intramedullary rod placement from a trochanteric starting point.
- The gold standard for treating femoral shaft fractures is by means of intramedullary rodding.
  - This can be done in antegrade fashion, from either the piriformis or trochanteric starting points, or in retrograde fashion from a starting point at the junction between the trochlea and intercondylar notch.

Radiographic Anatomy

Preoperative Imaging

- Imaging of a femoral shaft fracture is straightforward, requiring only standard radiographic technique. Specifically, one should use orthogonal, true AP, and lateral views, using the patella as the rotational reference, taking care to move the x-ray emitter and cassette, not the limb, when changing between views. Due to the length of the adult femur, it is important that the radiographer orient the cassette obliquely, such that the thigh forms a hypotenuse running diagonally across the cassette, so that a maximum amount of femur is captured on each image. This limits the chances of missing or underevaluating a mid-diaphyseal fracture.
- Adequate radiographic imaging includes an AP pelvis and orthogonal views of the entire femur. An incompletely sedated patient may not tolerate the positioning needed for quality radiographs, and there is evidence that radiography alone is insufficient to evaluate for an associated femoral neck fracture.[2] With few exceptions, evaluation of a femoral shaft fracture should include a fine-cut CT through the femoral neck. Fractures that involve the distal one-third of the diaphysis may extend into the knee joint or have an unidentified, noncontiguous intra-articular fracture; thus, a CT scan of the knee should be considered for these injuries.

Radiographic Evaluation of Intramedullary Fixation Start Points

Piriformis Starting Point

- On an AP view, the piriformis start point appears as an L-shaped radiodensity, in line with the medullary canal and approximately 2 to 3 cm distal to the proximal border of the femoral neck (Fig. 20-1A). On the lateral view, the piriformis fossa is visualized by following the slope of the posterior femoral neck. As the contour of the neck slopes obliquely posteriorly and distally, the cortical surface flattens out for a few millimeters before continuing its oblique course toward the lesser trochanter. The apex between this flattened section and the posterior cortex of the neck is the piriformis fossa (Fig. 20-1B). The trajectory of a piriformis nail is in line with the medullary canal of the femur; thus, the guidewire should be aligned with the center of the canal on both views prior to insertion into the femur (Fig. 20-2A and B).

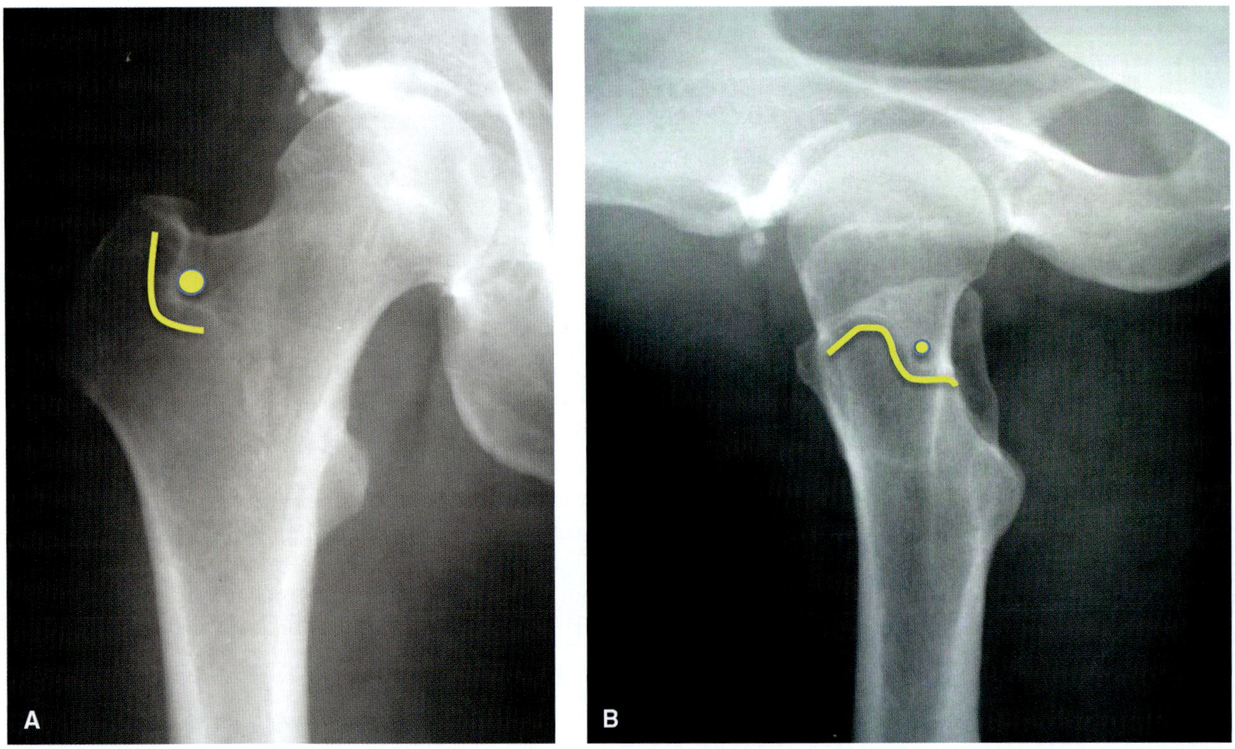

Figure 20-1 | A and B: Piriformis starting point. *Curved line*: Contours of piriformis fossa. *Solid circle*: Starting points.

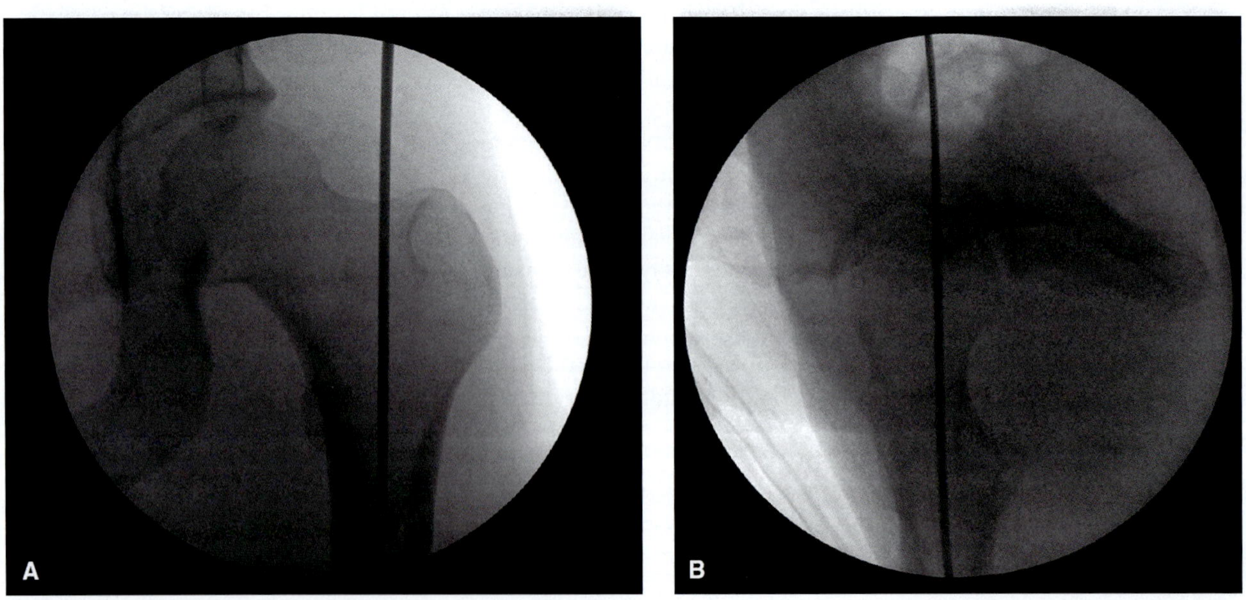

Figure 20-2 | A and B: Piriformis guidewire. Starting point and trajectory keep the wire in line with the medullary canal on AP and lateral views.

Trochanteric Starting Point

- The morphology of the greater trochanter varies between individuals. In order to obtain an optimal AP view for a trochanteric starting point, the C-arm should be rotated such that the anteromedial and posteromedial edges of the greater trochanter are superimposed. The guidewire is then placed on the superior tip of the trochanter, aiming for the center of the canal at the level of the lesser trochanter (Fig. 20-3A). Many surgeons will actually start this guidewire slightly medial to the tip of the trochanter, especially with more proximal fractures to resist varus deformity caused by too lateral of a starting point.
- The lateral view of the trochanteric starting point is obtained by rotating the C-arm until the femoral head, neck, greater trochanter, and shaft are all collinear, or at least as collinear as allowed by the patient's morphology. Delineation of the femoral neck is enhanced by adding cephalic tilt to the C-arm (Figs. 20-3B and 20-9B). Rather than focusing on a "one-third, two-thirds" starting point as is recommended in most technique guides, it is more important to consider the position of the implant with respect to the femoral head and neck. By obtaining a perfect lateral image,

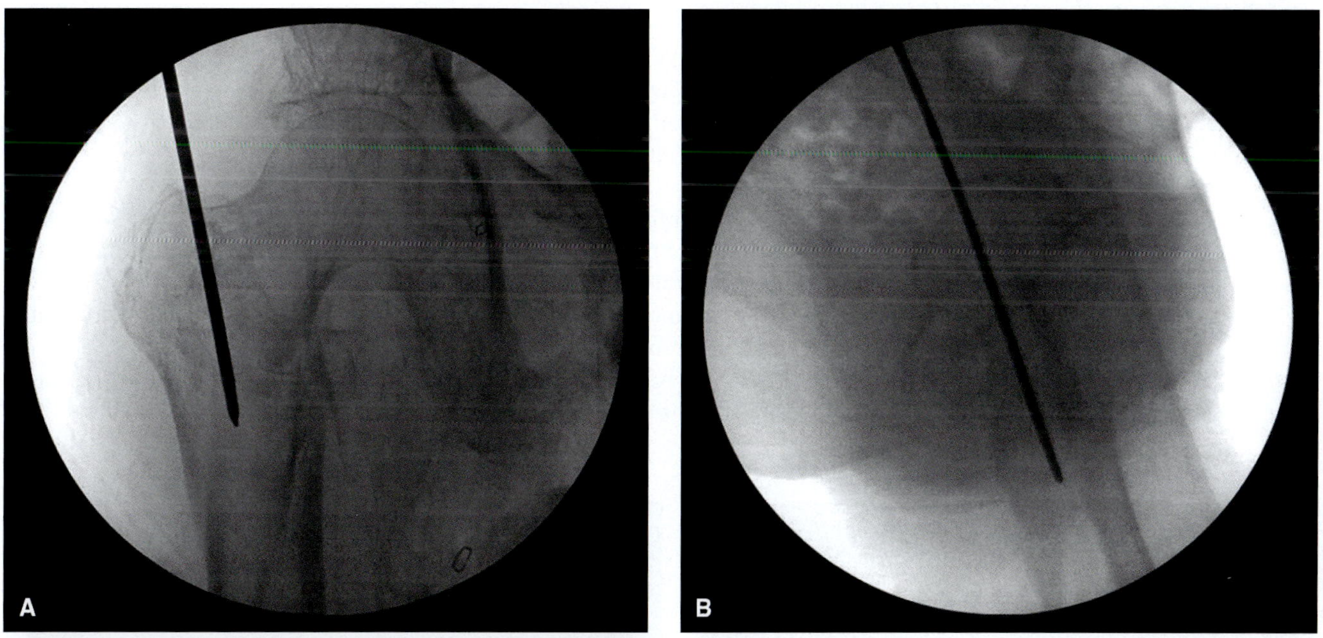

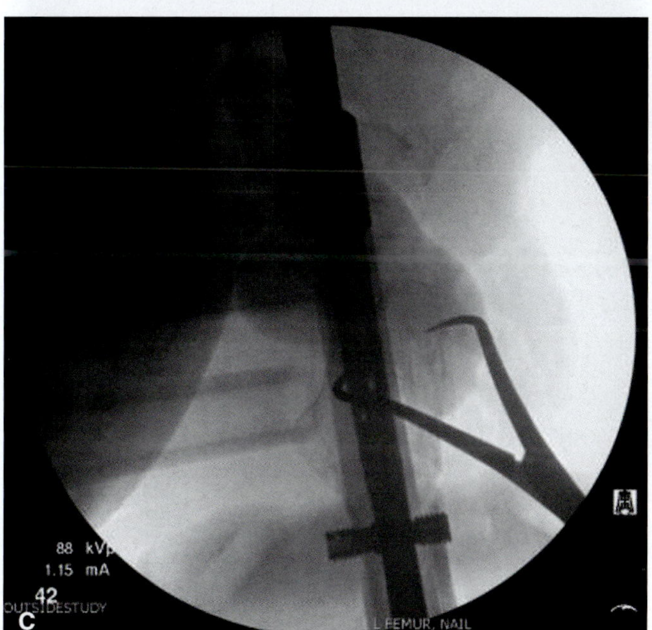

Figure 20-3 | Trochanteric guidewire placement and proper jig orientation. **A:** In the AP projection, the wire is placed just medial to the tip of the greater trochanter, in line with the medullary axis. **B:** On a perfect lateral view, the wire bisects the head, neck, and shaft. Note the excellent visualization of the neck afforded by canting the C-arm toward the patient's head. **C:** Perfectly placed cephalomedullary fixation is achieved by making the head, neck, nail, and jig perfectly collinear on a true lateral of the hip. Again, note the visualization of the neck achieved by proper cephalic tilt of the C-arm receiver.

and bisecting the head and neck with the path of the guidewire (Fig. 20-3B), the surgeon ensures that the nail will be in a position to allow the safest possible placement of fixation into the femoral head, if needed. Where that trajectory traverses the greater trochanter is irrelevant, and it often bisects the trochanter, rather than being at the junction of the anterior one-third and posterior two-thirds. The trajectory of the guidewire should be aiming down the center of the proximal diaphysis. At times, the proximal femoral morphology is such that the starting point must be slightly off of the head-neck axis in order to allow the nail to easily pass through the diaphyseal canal.

- Prior to locking the proximal aspect of a trochanteric nail, it is vital that the surgeon obtain a perfect lateral of the head and neck, ensuring that they are collinear with each other, and that the head-neck axis is perfectly superimposed with both the nail and the radiolucent jig (Fig. 20-3C). Even a small amount of rotation of the nail, such that the jig is noticeably anterior or posterior to the nail on this view, will cause the head fixation to deviate from the head-neck axis, thus increasing the chance of penetration into the joint.

Retrograde Starting Point

- Like a nail properly placed through the piriformis fossa, a retrograde nail follows the axis of the femoral canal on both AP and lateral views. Thus, the surgeon's goal is to bisect the canal on both views with the trajectory of the guidewire and, eventually, the nail itself. While the true medullary axis exits the distal femur a millimeter or two medial to the nadir of the intercondylar notch, this deviation is so small that the apex of the trochlea is used as the starting point, since this is a very easy point to identify on fluoroscopy.
- On a perfect AP view of the knee, with the fibular head bisected by the lateral aspect of the tibial plateau, the guidewire is placed at the nadir of the intercondylar notch, in line with the diaphyseal canal (Fig. 20-4A). On a perfect lateral of the knee, with the femoral condyles superimposed on each other, the start point is at the junction of the floor of the trochlea and Blumensaat's line, with the wire in line with the diaphyseal canal (Fig. 20-4B).
- When locking a retrograde nail, it is important to ensure that the nail is fully inserted within the bone, with no portion of it protruding into the patellofemoral joint (Fig. 20-4B).

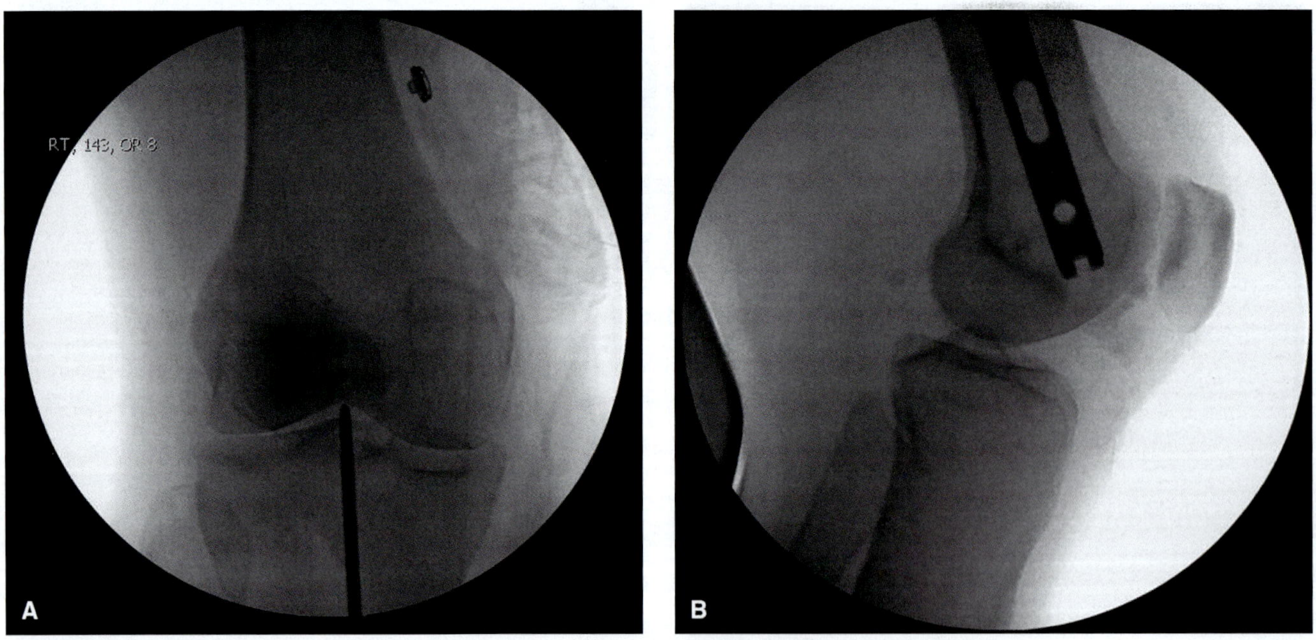

Figure 20-4 I Retrograde nail placement. **A:** AP view shows placement of wire at apex of trochlea, in line with femoral shaft. **B:** On lateral view, the guidewire and nail enter at the junction between Blumensaat's line and the posterior limit of the trochlea. Note that the nail can be visualized deep to the subchondral bone of the trochlea on this true lateral, although confirmation should be made via direct palpation.

Radiographic Assessment of Reduction

- Judging the fracture's reduction is sometimes easily done via "cortical keys," whereby the fracture is manipulated until the fragments appear to be reduced on orthogonal views, with no step-off seen between the cortices on either side of the fracture[3] (Fig. 20-5A). This is most easily done with minimally to mildly comminuted fractures, although the reduction of purely transverse fractures can be difficult to judge with this method (Fig. 20-5B). Less direct methods must be used to judge the reduction of substantially comminuted fractures and for some simple fracture patterns that lack enough irregular edges to use the above method. The goal of diaphyseal fracture treatment is to restore the length, alignment, and rotation of the diaphysis; thus, the surgeon needs a means to assess these without the aid of cortical keys.
- Restoration of length can usually be confirmed by ensuring that there is no overlapping of, nor diastasis between, fragments. A radiographic ruler can also be used to compare the length of the injured femur with that of the uninjured side (Fig. 20-6A–D). If the restoration of length is in doubt, a postoperative scanogram with a radiographic ruler should provide an accurate assessment of length and allow precise planning of revision, if needed.
- When assessing fracture alignment, one should obtain the widest possible view of the diaphysis. The amount of angulation will be increasingly underestimated as the width of view of the bone decreases. In order to get the widest field of view, the fluoroscope receiver should be placed as close to the skin as possible. Also, fluoroscopes have differently sized receivers, and a larger receiver allows a greater width of view. With fractures that involve much of the diaphysis, judgment of alignment can be very challenging. There are some aids to achieving proper alignment, such as ensuring the intramedullary rod is perfectly aligned in both the proximal and distal fragments, but confirmation will require portable radiographs with large cassettes. This can be done intraoperatively at the end of the case, maintaining sterility of the room and back table. Thus, a revision could be done during the same surgery if necessary.
- Fracture malrotation is usually the deformity that is most difficult to evaluate. Due to the variability of femoral version between individuals, there is no standardized version with which to judge a reduction.[1] If any doubt exists about the fracture's rotation, comparison should be made with the uninjured side. This can be done both **qualitatively** and **quantitatively**. A qualitative comparison can be done by obtaining a perfect AP of the knee and translating the fluoroscope proximally and obtaining an AP image of the hip. The leg should be held immobile and the fluoroscope boom locked in place between obtaining these two images. The overall morphology

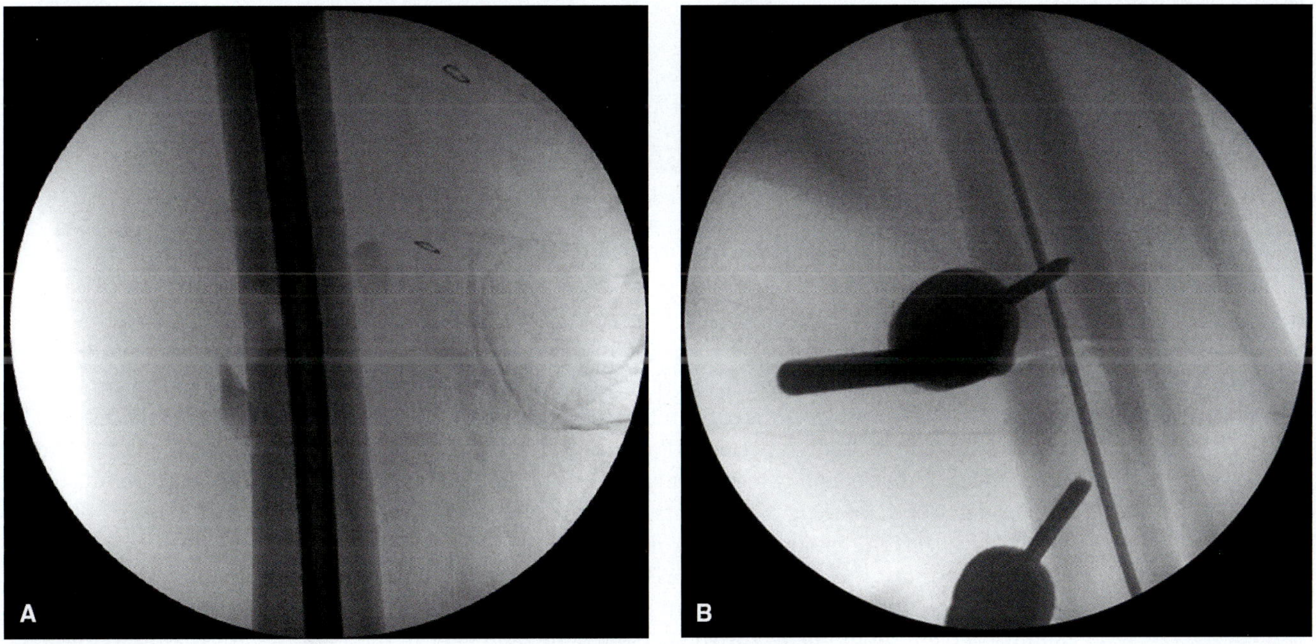

Figure 20-5 | **A:** Absence of a cortical step sign on AP view. The donor site for the lateral butterfly fragment lines up perfectly, confirming a proper rotational reduction. **B:** A purely transverse fracture without comminution. Assessing rotation is much harder and usually requires more than one method of confirming restoration of rotation.

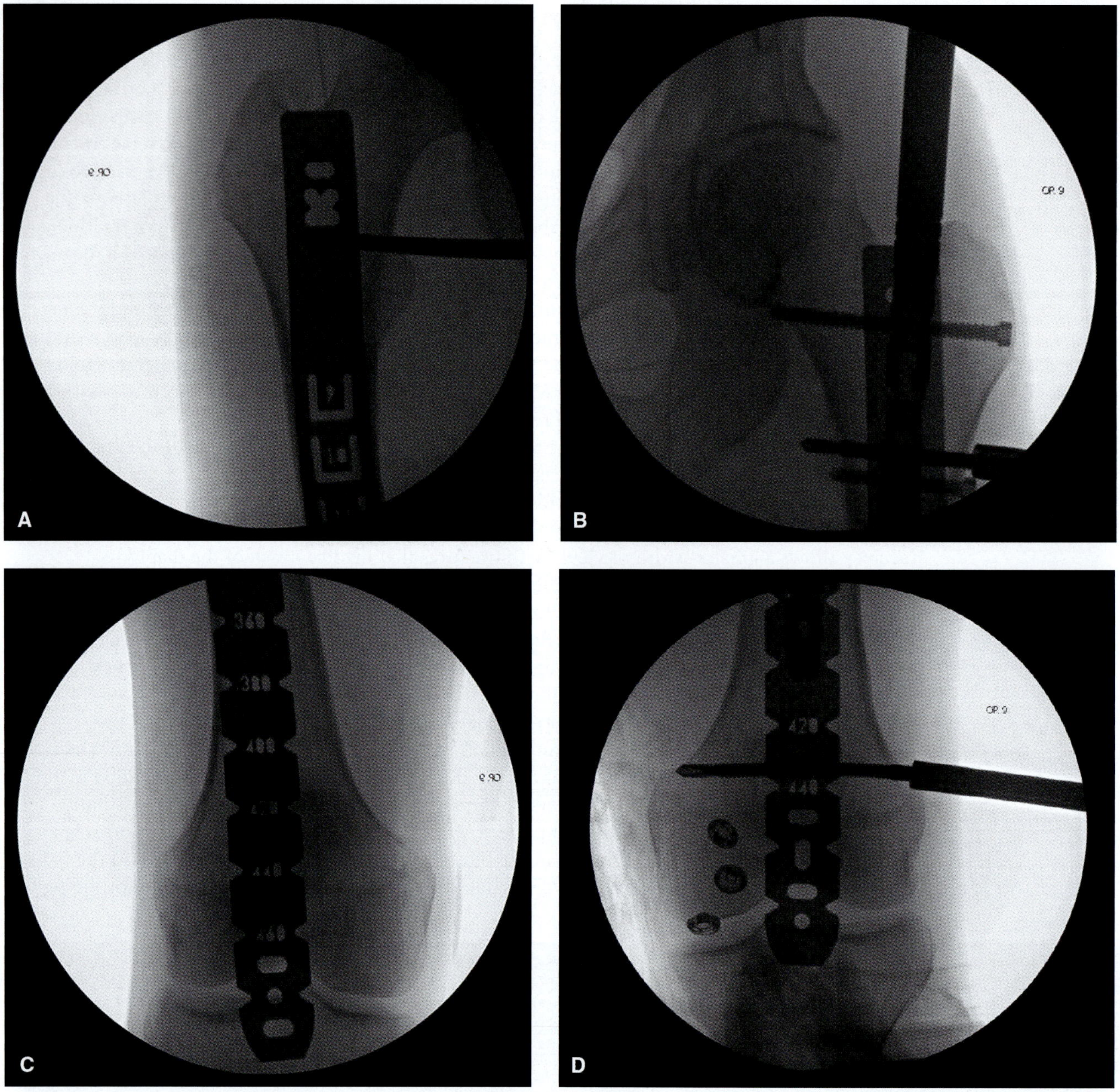

Figure 20-6 | Use of radiographic to assess length. **A and B:** Proximal edge of ruler placed on same location of bilateral proximal femora. **C and D:** The same radiographic feature should be used distally. In this patient, using two rulers, the physeal scar of each femur measures 445 mm from the superior aspect of the neck, confirming the anatomic restoration of length.

of the proximal femora should appear identical after performing this method on both femora (Fig. 20-7A and B). A quantitative comparison of femoral version can be made by measuring the amount of C-arm "roll" needed to transition between a perfect image of the hip and one of the knee. Judging what is a perfect AP image of the hip can be very difficult; thus, a quantitative assessment of the version is more easily achieved using lateral images of the hip and knee.[4] Obtaining proper imaging of the contralateral femur can sometimes be difficult intraoperatively; thus, any suspicion that judging the rotation will be difficult should prompt the imaging of it (if uninjured) prior to draping. The AP image of the contralateral hip, while holding the knee in a true AP position, should be saved in the C-arm image directory, and the measurement of that femur's version should be recorded. These will be used later in the case for comparison to the injured side prior to locking in its rotation.

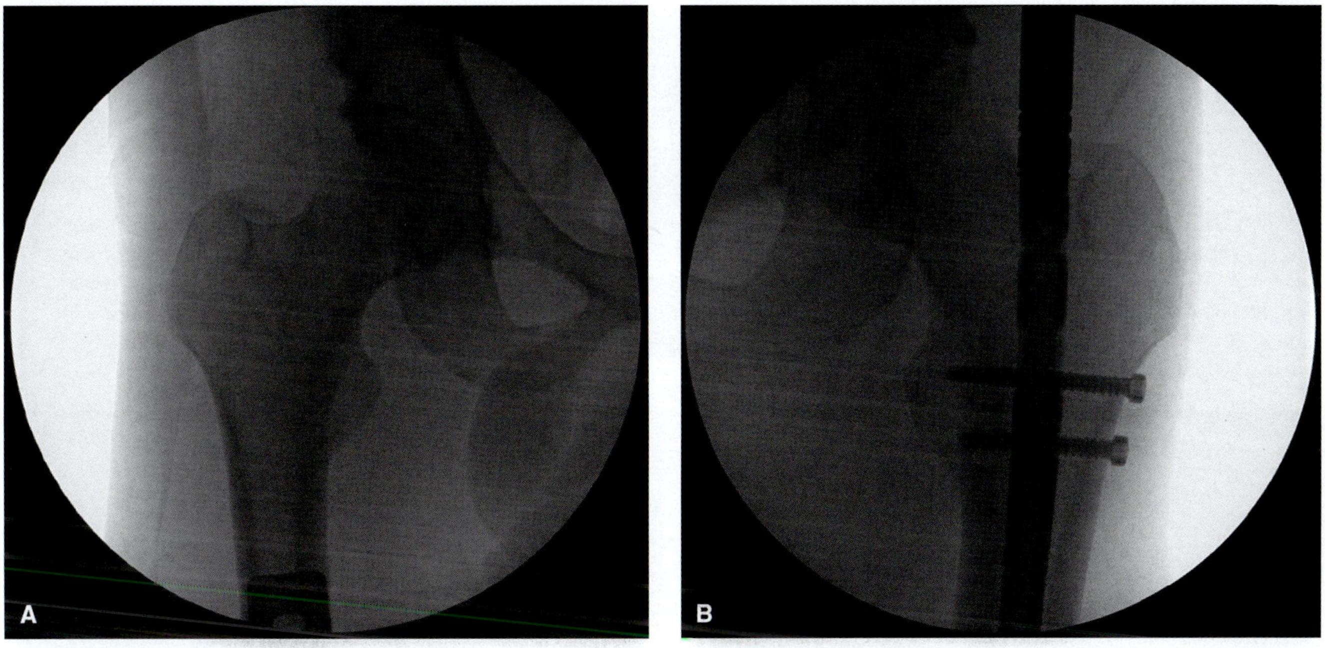

Figure 20-7 | A and B: Qualitative comparison of rotational profile after obtaining a true AP of the knee. The proximal femora look identical in terms of shape of lesser trochanter and where the posterior border of the greater trochanter intersects the femoral neck. This strongly suggests that anatomic or near-anatomic rotation has been restored.

Intraoperative Positioning

- Femoral nailing can be performed in both the supine and lateral position, either using freehand technique on a radiolucent table or using a traction table. There are advantages and disadvantages to each method; thus, it is advantageous for the surgeon to be comfortable with more than one of them. Irrespective of the method used, the fluoroscope is placed on the contralateral side of the table, with the receiver placed above the patient.

Supine Positioning

Antegrade Nailing

- Regardless of the table used, it is imperative to move the hip to the edge of the table, ideally creating a lateral bend through the pelvic region so that the flank is not impeding the passage of instruments and so that the proximal femur is easily accessible to the starting guidewire. To facilitate the passage of reamers while preparing the canal, the ipsilateral upper extremity can be positioned across the torso prior to draping. A pillow is placed between the forearm and the chest, with foam padding placed over the elbow prior to circumferentially taping the limb into position. A bump of two to three sheets should be placed under the ipsilateral hemipelvis when using a radiolucent table, in order to facilitate access to the guidewire starting point. Due to the uneven pressure that would be caused by the perineal post, a bump is not usually placed under the pelvis when using a fracture table.

Retrograde Nailing

- A bump is generally not placed under the pelvis when nailing retrograde. Since the distal femur is generally oriented orthogonally to the table, bumping the pelvis might introduce an external rotation deformity through the fracture. If significant concerns exist regarding the restoration of anatomic rotation, the uninjured leg can be prepped into the field for comparison. The thigh can be supported on a stack of gowns or towels, but a radiolucent triangle is more stable and less likely to move during the case. Use of a large triangle also allows the application of traction when levering the proximal tibia over the corner of the triangle. A stack of sterile towels is placed between the thigh and the triangle in order to negate the posterior sag through the fracture. Occasionally, the edge of the triangle blocks the view of the starting point on a perfect AP projection (Fig. 20-8). Removing a few degrees of cephalic tilt will prevent this superimposition, without affecting the ability to assess the starting point or trajectory on this view.

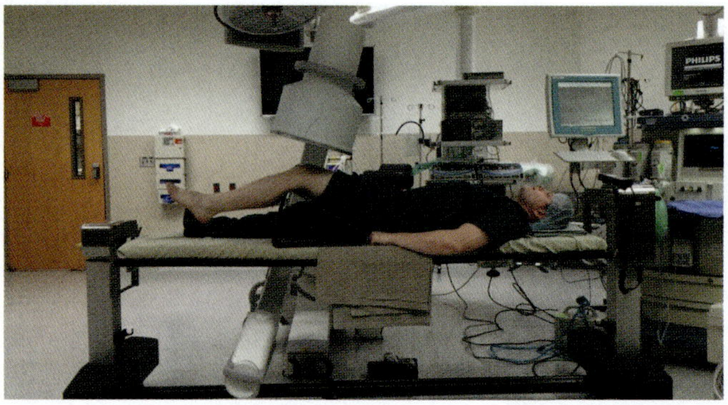

Figure 20-8 | Positioning for a retrograde nail. The C-arm is currently canted to match the hip's flexion and obtain a true AP of the knee. By flexing the knee over the fulcrum of the triangle's corner, added length will be restored. However, this will bring the apex of the trochlea in line with the distal surface of the triangle, which will then obscure the starting point. This can be avoided by canting the C-arm a few degrees more vertically, sacrificing a true AP for clear visualization of the starting point.

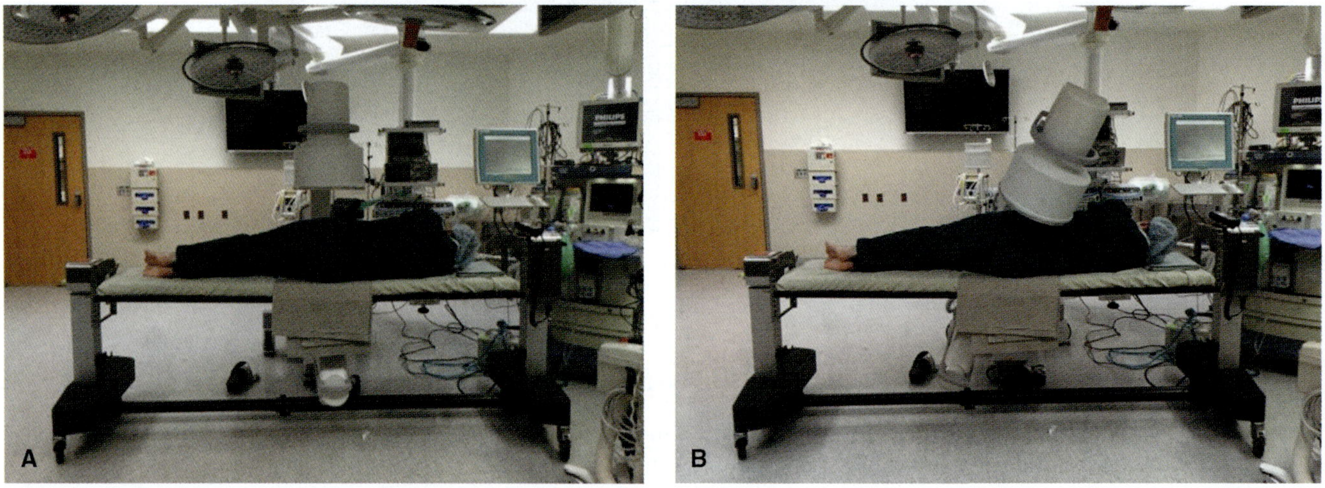

Figure 20-9 | Lateral positioning. **A:** The C-arm is oriented perpendicular to the floor, and is thus not likely to generate true images of the femoral neck. **B:** The C-arm is tilted in the cephalad direction, allowing good delineation of the femoral neck, and is "overrolled" to match the current rotation of the proximal fragment. A perfect lateral of the neck is now achievable, allowing precise nailing and accurate, safe placement of fixation in the femoral head.

Lateral Positioning

- This position is almost exclusively used for antegrade nailing, although retrograde nailing is possible in the lateral position, if the surgery is not being performed on a traction table. Lateral positioning is very straightforward and allows easy access to the proximal femoral starting point, even in obese patients. Care must be taken to adequately pad the fibular neck and all bony prominences. For mid-diaphyseal fractures, placing the patient's feet and knees together will usually bring the fracture rotation close to normal (Fig. 20-9A and B). Care should be taken when allowing the operative limb to fall posterior to the contralateral one, as this will externally rotate the fracture, which may not be desirable.

References

1. Eckhoff DG, Jacofsky D, Springer B, et al. Bilateral symmetrical comparison of femoral and tibial anatomic features. *J Arthroplasty.* 2016;31(5):1083–1090. Available at: http://www.arthroplastyjournal.org/article/S0883540315010311/fulltext
2. Tornetta P, Kain MSH, Creevy WR. Diagnosis of femoral neck fractures in patients with a femoral shaft fracture. Improvement with a standard protocol. *J Bone Joint Surg Am.* 2011;89(1):39–43.
3. Langer JS, Gardner MJ, Ricci WM. The cortical step sign as a tool for assessing and correcting rotational deformity in femoral shaft fractures. *J Orthop Trauma.* 2010;24(2):82–88.
4. Tornetta P, Ritz G, Kantor A. Femoral torsion after interlocked nailing of unstable femoral fractures. *J Trauma.* 1995;38(2):213–219.

Chapter 21
Distal Femur Fractures

ANDREW J. SHEEAN
MICHAEL J. BELTRAN

Bony Anatomy

- The distal femur has unique geometry in three planes: axial, sagittal, and coronal. A thorough appreciation of this anatomy is critical to obtaining an anatomic reduction of fractures and for appropriate placement of precontoured plates and periarticular screws.
- In the axial plane, the distal femur is trapezoidal, with a lateral slope of 10 degrees and a medial slope of 25 degrees. The lateral condyle projects anteriorly relative to that of the medial condyle at an angle of 10 degrees. In the coronal plane, the medial condyle extends further distally than does the lateral condyle, resulting in an average lateral distal femoral angle of 81 degrees (Fig. 21-1).[1,2]

Radiographic Anatomy and Preoperative Imaging

- AP and lateral plain film radiographs are obtained in order to appreciate the extent of coronal and sagittal plane deformity. Figure 21-2 demonstrates the shortening and recurvatum deformity typical of distal femur fractures, which occurs secondary to the unopposed pull of the extensor mechanism and gastrocnemius.
- In addition to orthogonal radiographs of the knee, the entire femur should be imaged to assess for proximal fractures or extension, retained previous hardware, or associated bony deformity. The presence of any of these situations may alter the anticipated surgical treatment plan.
- The presence of an intercondylar fracture line indicates that a preoperative CT scan is necessary to properly assess for associated coronal split condylar fractures ("Hoffa fragments," Figs. 21-3 and 21-4). The incidence of these injuries in the setting of an intercondylar fracture on plain films is 38%, and they are easily missed in the absence of a CT scan.[3]

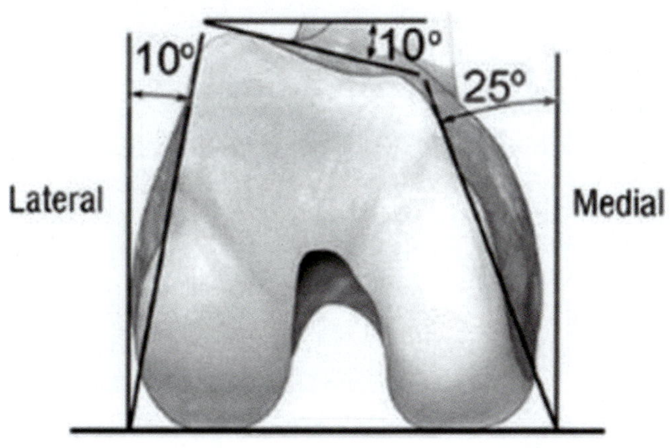

Figure 21-1 Axial geometry of the distal femur. (From Beltran MJ, Gary JL, Collinge CA. Management of distal femur fractures with modern plates and nails: state of the art. *J Orthop Trauma.* 2015;29:165–172.)

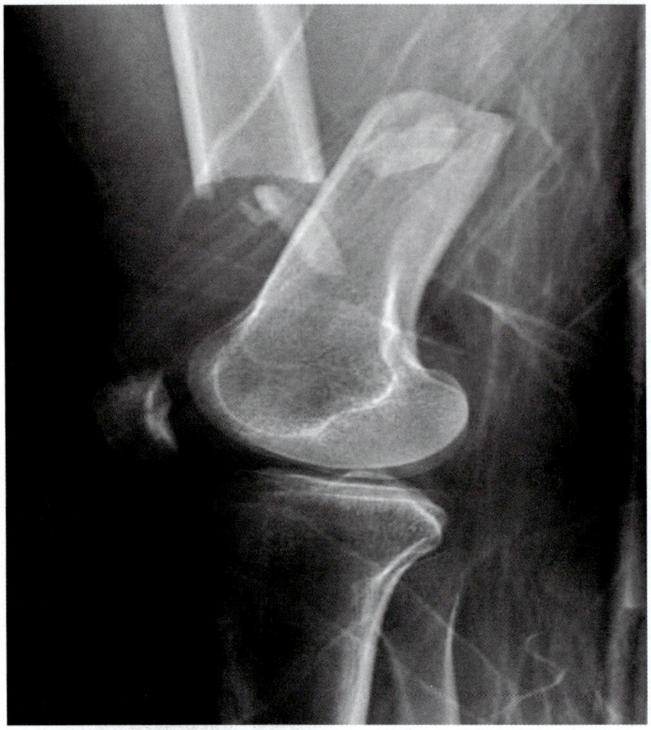

Figure 21-2 | Lateral radiograph of an extra-articular distal femur fracture. The shortened, recurvatum deformity typical of these fractures is demonstrated.

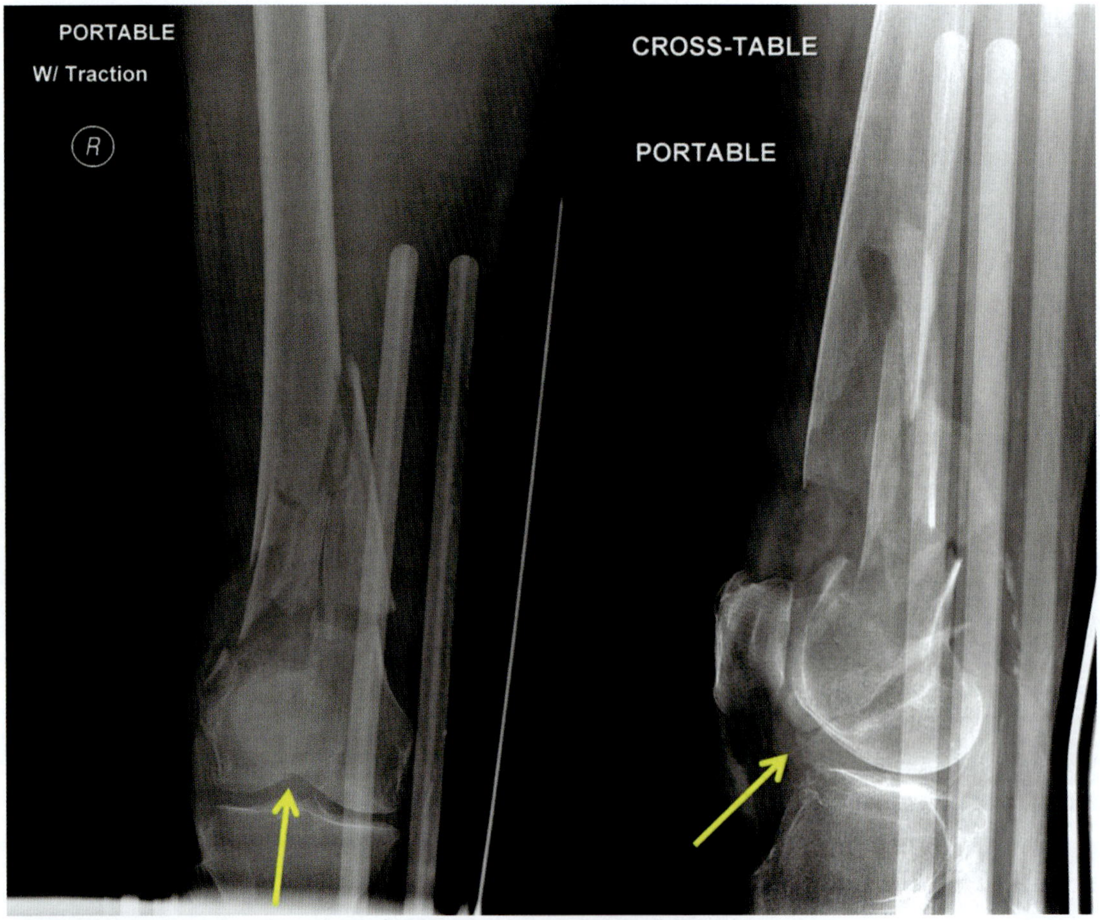

Figure 21-3 | Careful assessment of injury traction images affords the opportunity to recognize subtle intra-articular splits and Hoffa fractures (*yellow arrows*).

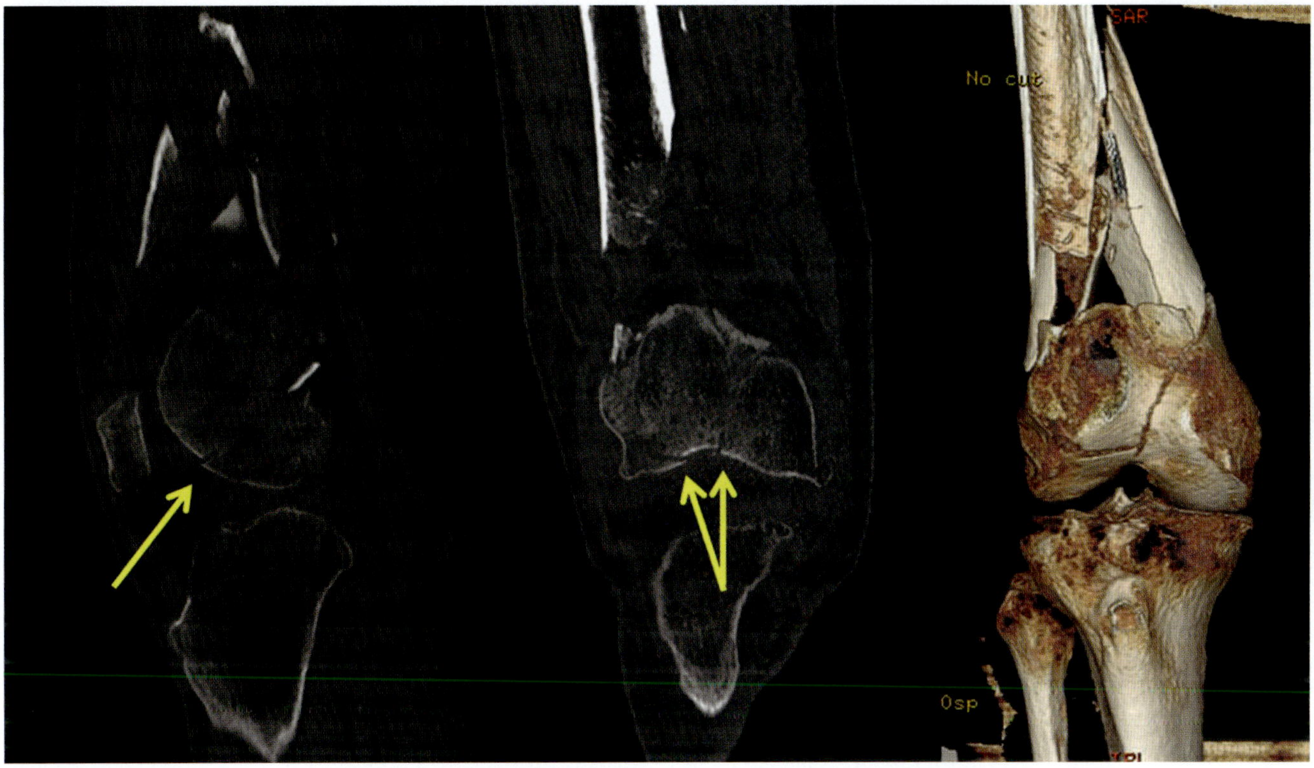

Figure 21-4 | These fracture lines (represented with *yellow arrows*) can be better appreciated with preoperative CT scans to plan for intraoperative reduction techniques and fixation methods. Failure to recognize them can lead to inefficient articular reduction and increased posttraumatic degenerative changes.

Intraoperative Positioning and Imaging—Plating and Retrograde Nailing

- The patient is positioned supine on a radiolucent table with the C-arm positioned opposite the injured extremity. A bump should be placed under the hip and buttock to aid with imaging and rotational alignment during the procedure (Fig. 21-5).
- Prior to draping, fluoroscopic images of the contralateral femur should be obtained to aid with intraoperative assessment of rotation. A perfect AP of the knee is first obtained, and then the C-arm is directed proximally to obtain a corresponding true AP of the hip, allowing the contour of the lesser trochanter to be used as a guide for comparison (specifically, rotation) (Fig. 21-6). Positioning the C-arm for obtaining an AP intraoperative fluoroscopic image.

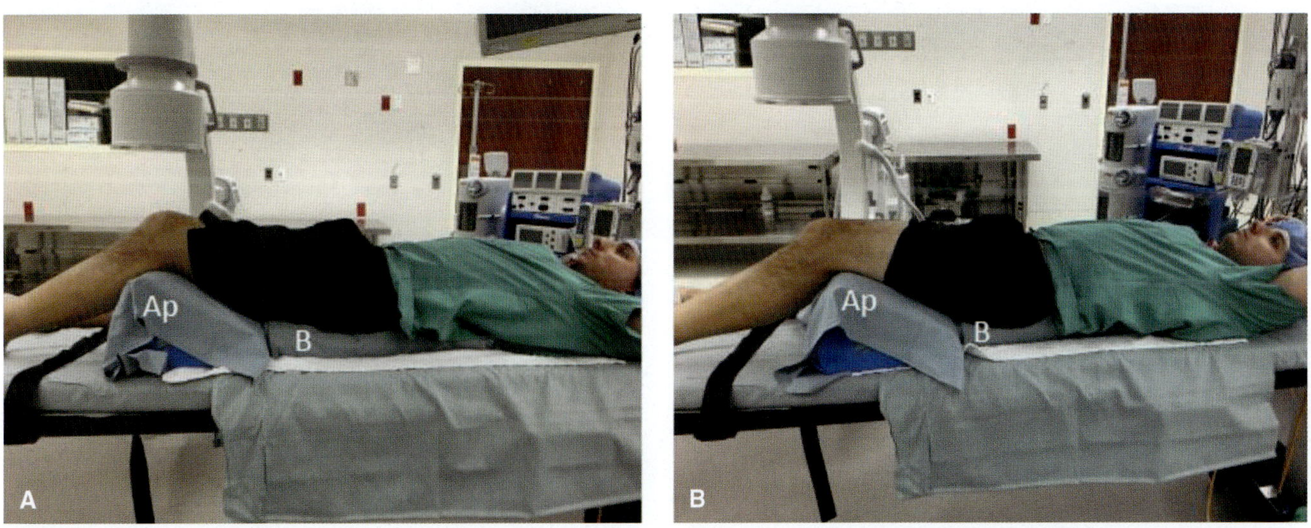

Figure 21-5 | A bump (*B*) is placed under the operative hip. Note the effect of positioning the bump too distal as the apex of the triangle (*Ap*) is situated distal to the popliteal fossa **(A)**. With the bump positioned more proximally, the triangle can be positioned such that the apex of the triangle is situated directly posterior to the popliteal fossa, thereby aiding with reduction of the distal fracture fragment **(B)**.

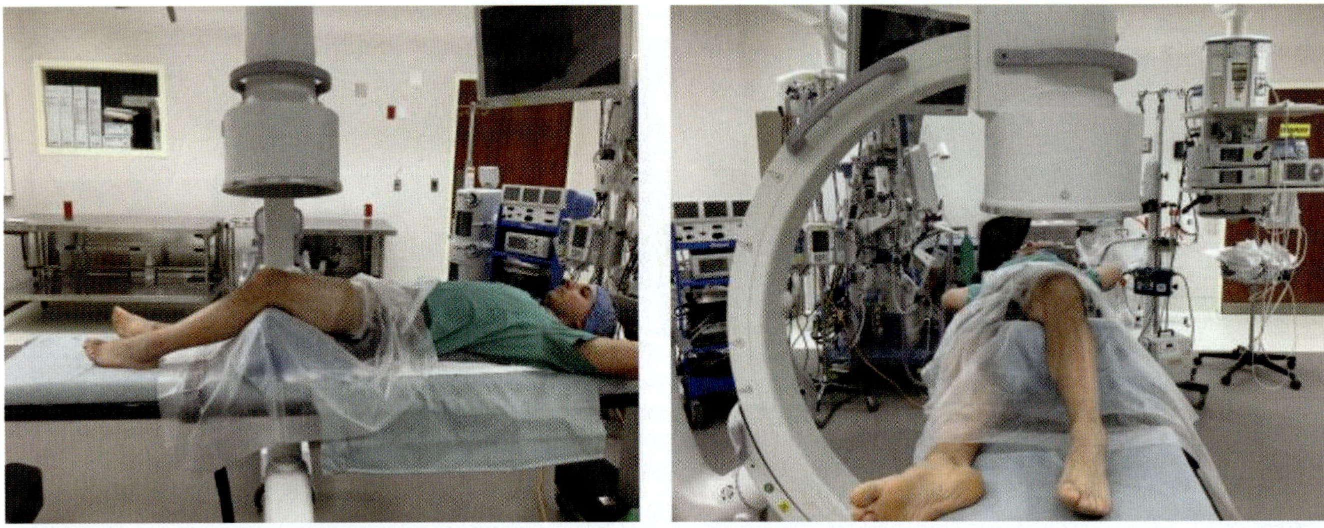

Figure 21-6 | Positioning the C-arm for obtaining an AP intraoperative fluoroscopic image.

The surgeon must ensure that quality AP (Fig. 21-6) and lateral (Fig. 21-7) intraoperative fluoroscopic images can be obtained prior to beginning the case. Additionally, several additional fluoroscopic images may be employed intraoperatively to verify the accuracy of fracture reduction and positioning of hardware, especially screws. Ensuring that correct AP and lateral views can be obtained becomes critically important when assessing fracture reduction and placement of implants. For retrograde nailing of metaphyseal and metadiaphyseal fractures where isthmal fit of the nail will not occur, nail starting point and trajectory must be correct; otherwise, a translational or angular deformity may occur during nail placement.

- *AP of the knee*: Obtained by ensuring that the lateral aspect of the tibia bisects the proximal fibula and that the patella is centered over the femoral condyles (Fig. 21-8). Alternatively, the surgeon can obtain a perfect lateral image and then rotate the C-arm 90 degrees for the corresponding AP image.
- *Lateral of the knee*: obtained by superimposing the posterior aspects of the medial and lateral femoral condyles. The lateral femoral condyle extends further anterior compared to the medial femoral condyle; these landmarks should be used when determining appropriate placement of plates (Fig. 21-9). Blumensaat's line represents the anterior and proximal extent of the intercondylar notch and is a critical landmark for nail starting point and plate/screw placement (Figs. 21-10 and 21-11).

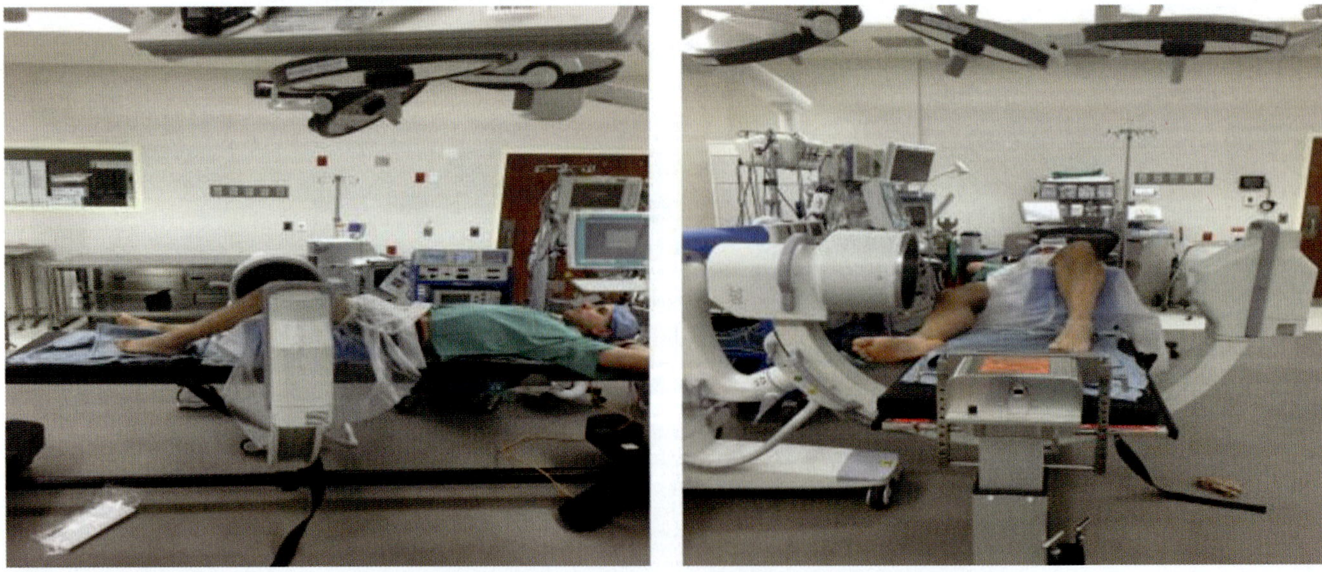

Figure 21-7 | Positioning the C-arm for obtaining a lateral intraoperative fluoroscopic image.

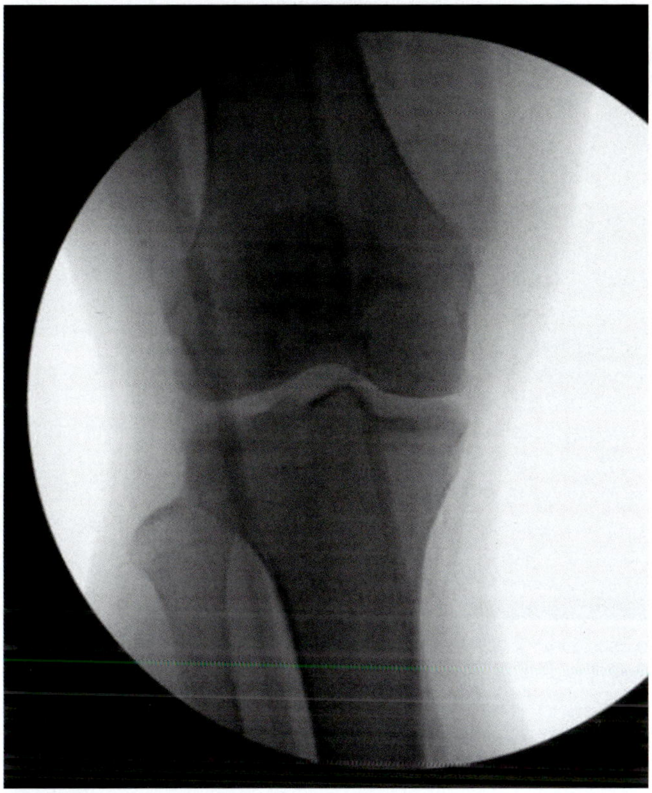

Figure 21-8 | AP view of the femur demonstrating the patella centered between the condyles and the fibula bisected by the lateral tibia.

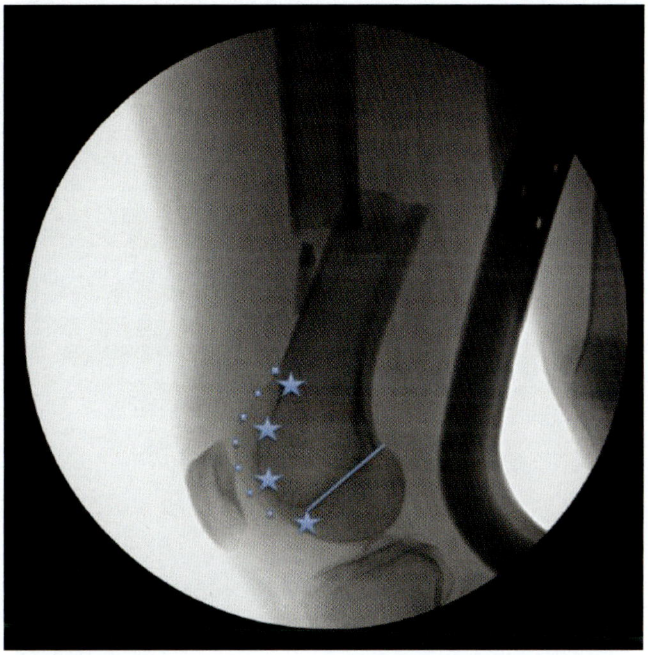

Figure 21-9 | The relationship between the medial and lateral femoral condyles on the lateral view of the distal femur. The lateral femoral condyle (*dotted line*) extends anterior to the medial femoral condyle (*stars*). Blumensaat's line is visualized as the anterior and proximal extent of the intercondylar notch.

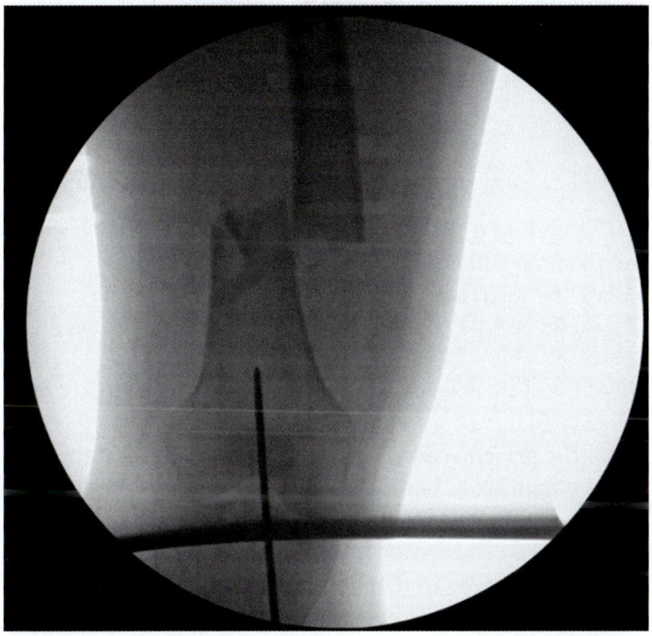

Figure 21-10 | AP fluoroscopic image of the knee demonstrating the appropriate starting point and trajectory for a retrograde nail, beginning just medial to the posterior cruciate ligament (PCL) insertion and in line with the canal.

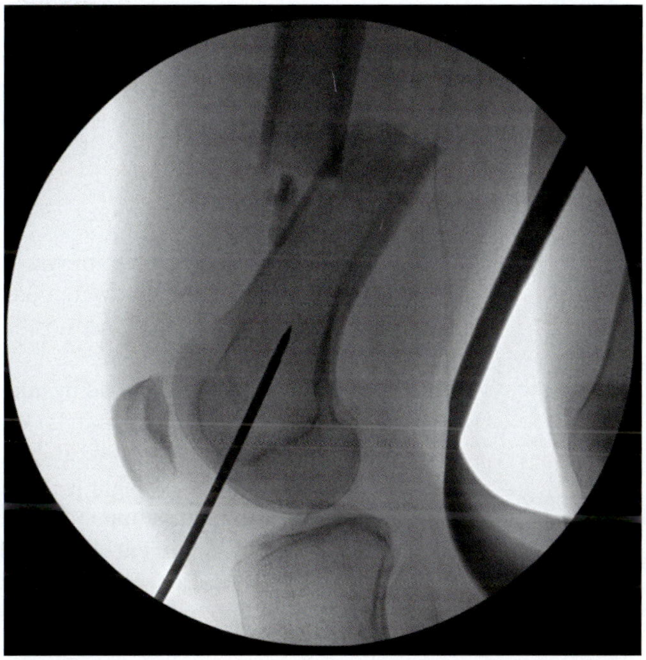

Figure 21-11 | The corresponding perfect lateral image demonstrating the correct starting point just anterior to Blumensaat's line with wire trajectory in line with the canal.

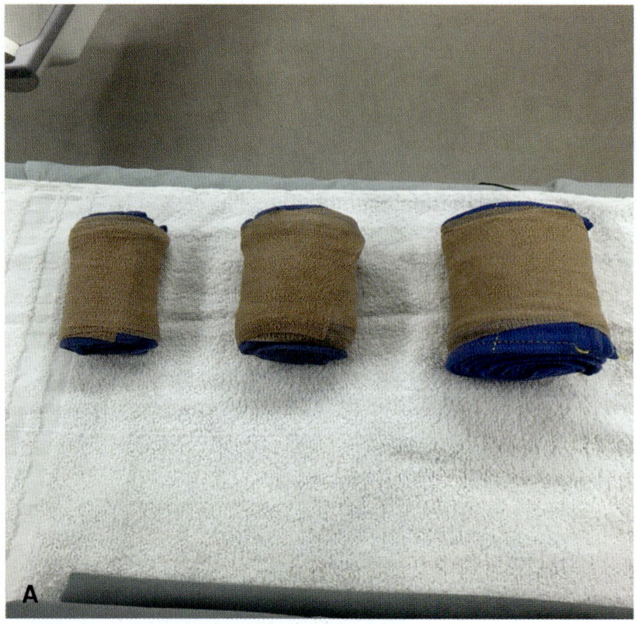

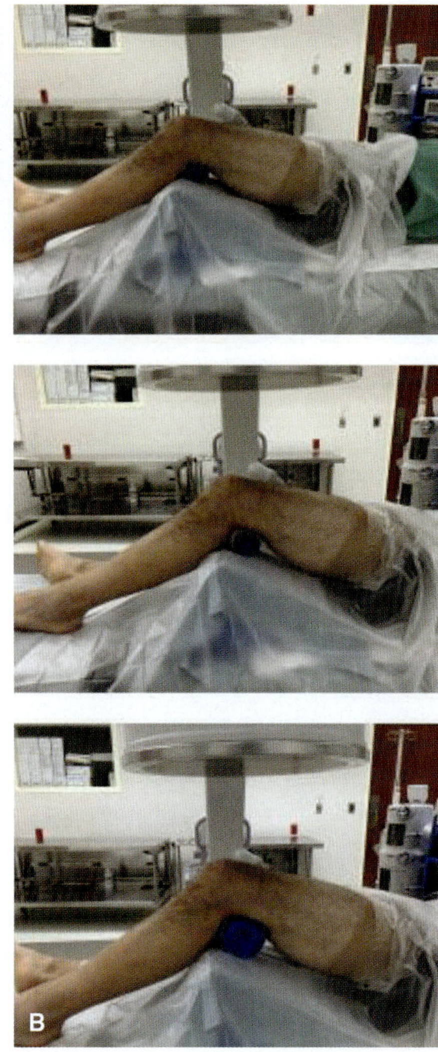

Figure 21-12 | Bumps of varying thickness **(A)** are used to counteract the recurvatum deformity encountered with the distal segment. **B:** The size of the bump used is predicated on the patient's anatomy and the extent of the deformity present.

Bumps of varying thickness can be employed to combat the commonly encountered recurvatum deformity of the distal segment (Fig. 21-12).

- When a fracture is more amenable to plate fixation, additional fluoroscopic views become necessary to ensure hardware does not violate the intercondylar notch or medial soft tissue structures of the knee. The most important views are the "notch view" and "25-degree rollover view."
- The notch view is obtained by adding caudal tilt of the C-arm and is used to confirm that screws do not violate the intercondylar notch (Fig. 21-13).
- The surgeon should also be able to recognize the presence of a "paradoxical notch view." If the intercondylar notch height is increased while obtaining a routine AP of the knee, then the distal segment is in recurvatum and sagittal plane reduction is still required. A lateral should be obtained to correct the alignment (Figs. 21-14 and 21-15).
- Because of the axial geometry of the distal femur (Fig. 21-1), medially directed screws have the potential to impinge on soft tissue structures such as the MCL when they are too long. The 25-degree rollover view is useful to assess for appropriate screw length, by imaging directly in the plane of the medial slope of the distal femur (Figs. 21-16, 21-17, and 21-18A and B).

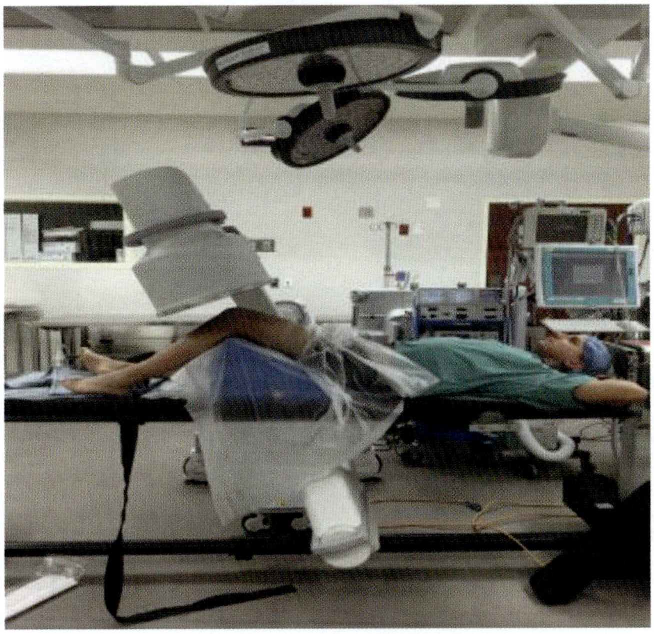

Figure 21-13 | C-arm orientation in order to obtain a "notch view." With the knee flexed to 30 degrees over a generous bump or sterile triangle, the C-arm is tilted 15 degrees caudad in order to orient the beam 45 degrees to the knee.

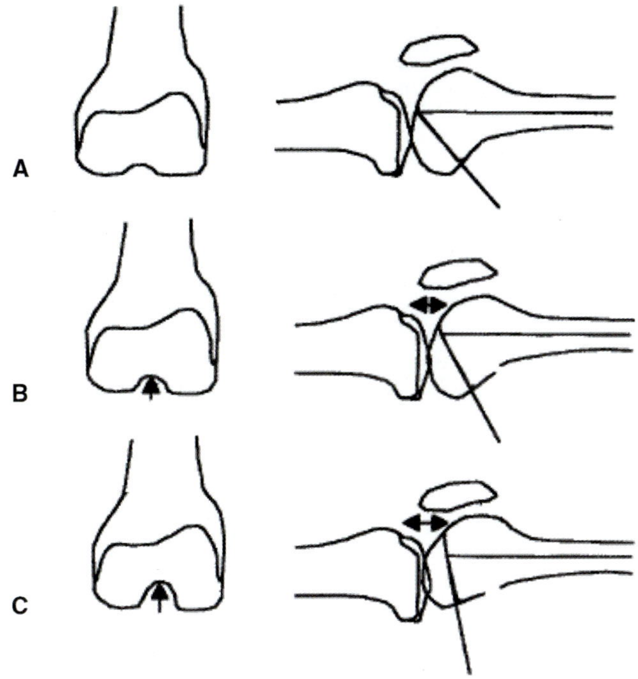

Figure 21-14 | The "paradoxical notch view" is an indicator of recurvatum deformity of the distal femur. **A:** The normal appearance of the intercondylar notch centered in the radiographic beam. **B and C:** The increasing recurvatum deformity of the distal femur on the AP view results in an increase in the height of the intercondylar notch. (From Krettek C, Schandelmaier P, Miclau T, et al. Intraoperative control of axes, rotation and length in femoral and tibial fractures—a technical note. *Injury.* 1998;29(suppl 3):C29–C39. Ref. 4.)

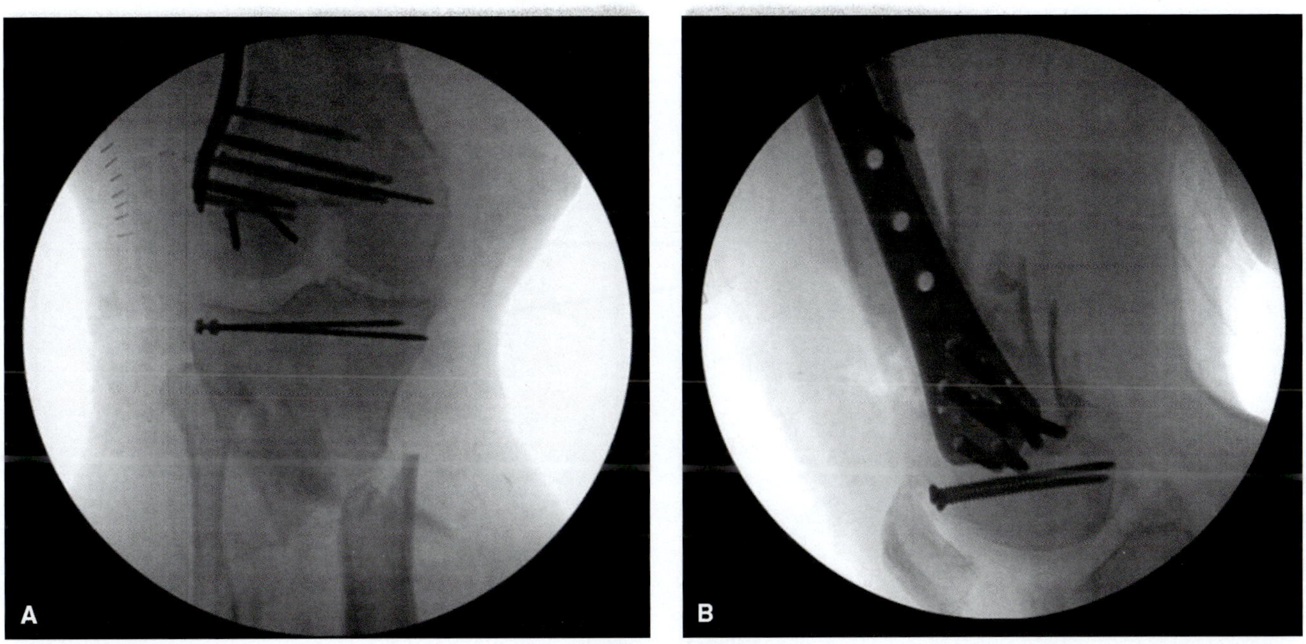

Figure 21-15 | Complex combined distal femur and proximal tibia fracture pattern. Increased notch height is readily apparent on the AP **(A)**, indicating the presence of severe recurvatum deformity. A lateral view **(B)** confirms the finding. Plate removal was required to re-reduce the fracture in the sagittal plane after fixation of the tibia.

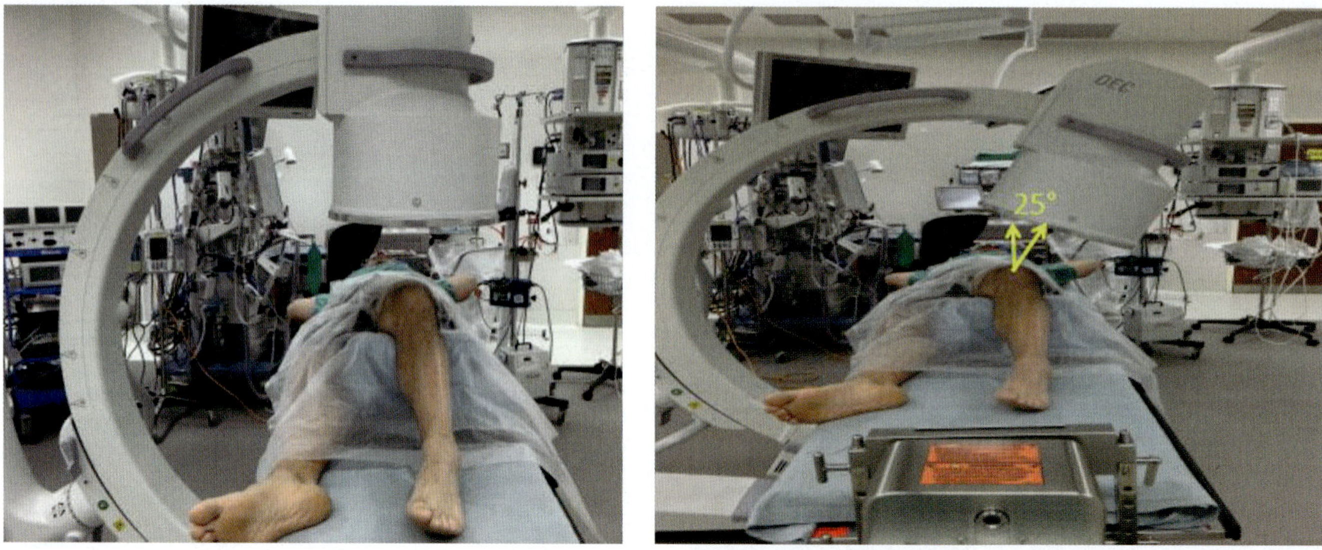

Figure 21-16 | C-arm orientation in order to obtain a "25-degree rollover view" to confirm that screws are not long medially. Irritation of the MCL is common with inappropriately long screws and may affect knee ROM and rehabilitation, in addition to the potential need for removal of implants after fracture healing.

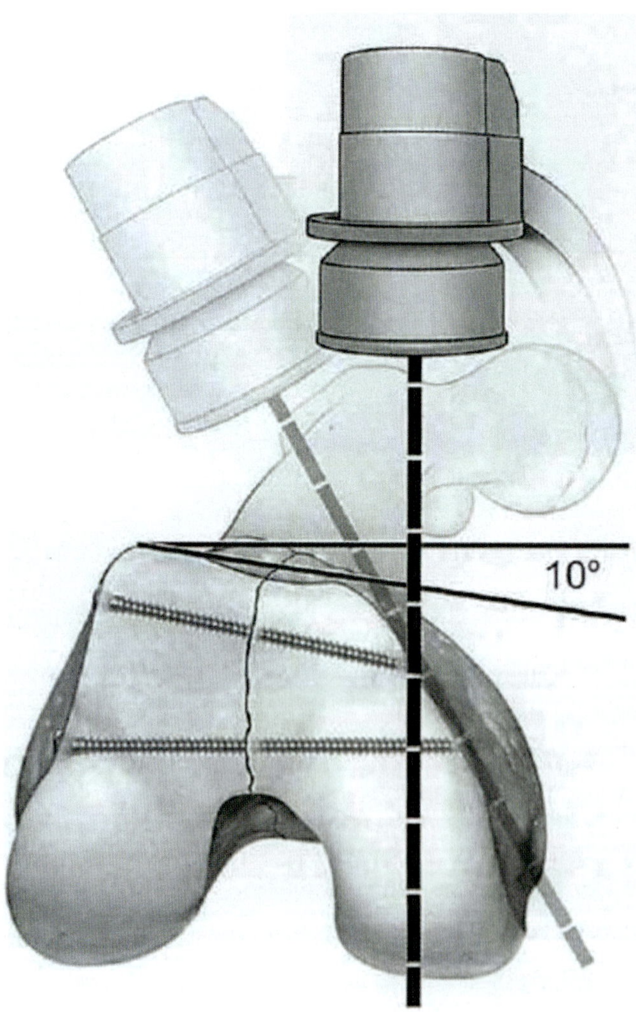

Figure 21-17 | Illustration depicting the orientation of the beam tangent to the medial condyle required to accurately assess the length of medially directed screws. (From Wright Raymond D, Gardner MJ, Bradford Henley M. Distal femur fractures. In: *Harborview Illustrated Tips and Tricks in Fracture Surgery*. 1st ed. Philadelphia, PA: Lippincott Williams & Wilkins, a Wolter Kluwer Business; 2011:232. Ref. 5.)

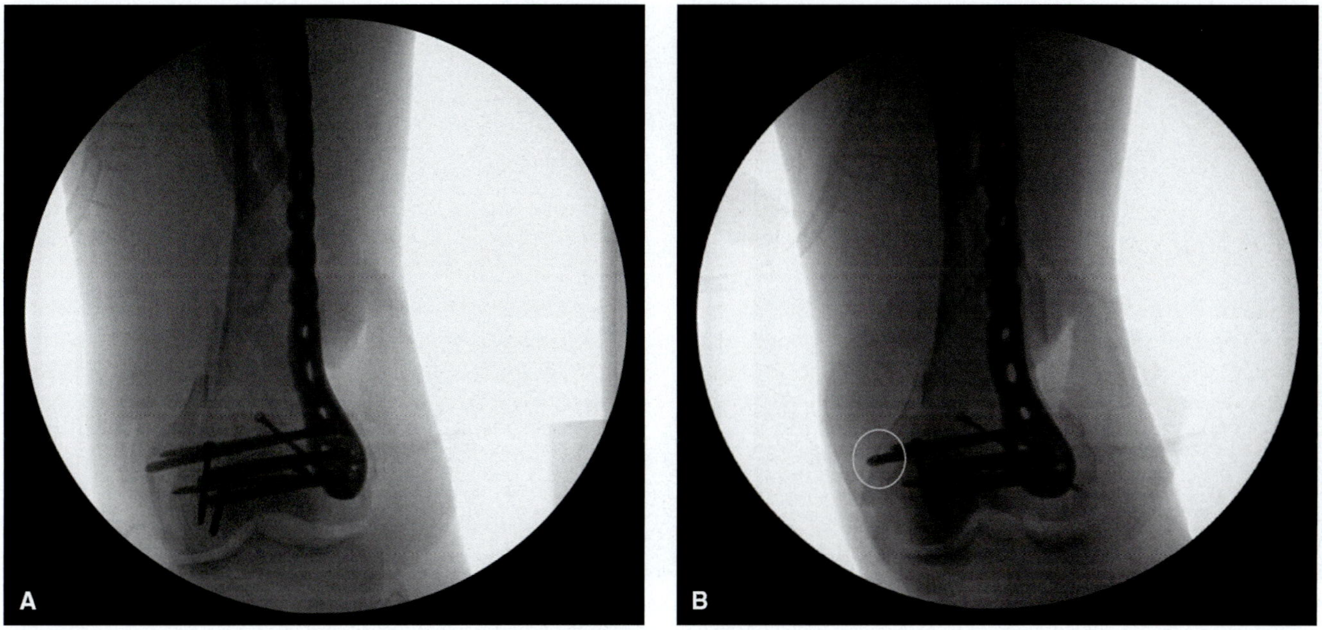

Figure 21-18 | AP of the knee **(A)** in which all screws appear to be of appropriate length as no screw appears to extend past the medial cortex. By obtaining a 25-degree rollover view **(B)**, a prominent screw is visualized and requires exchange for a shorter screw. These are typically anterior screws due to the trapezoidal shape of the distal femur (see Fig. 21-1). For laterally directed hardware (most commonly interlocking screws), a 10-degree rollback view can be obtained if screw length is a concern.

- A number of predictable deformities and complications are associated with errant plate and screw placement, but are easily assessed intraoperatively with fluoroscopic imaging.[1,2] It is important to critically assess plate placement after provisional reduction and fixation has been applied but prior to placement of all remaining fixation. The plate should be slightly anterior of center on the lateral view and matching the flare of the femur on an AP (Fig. 21-19).

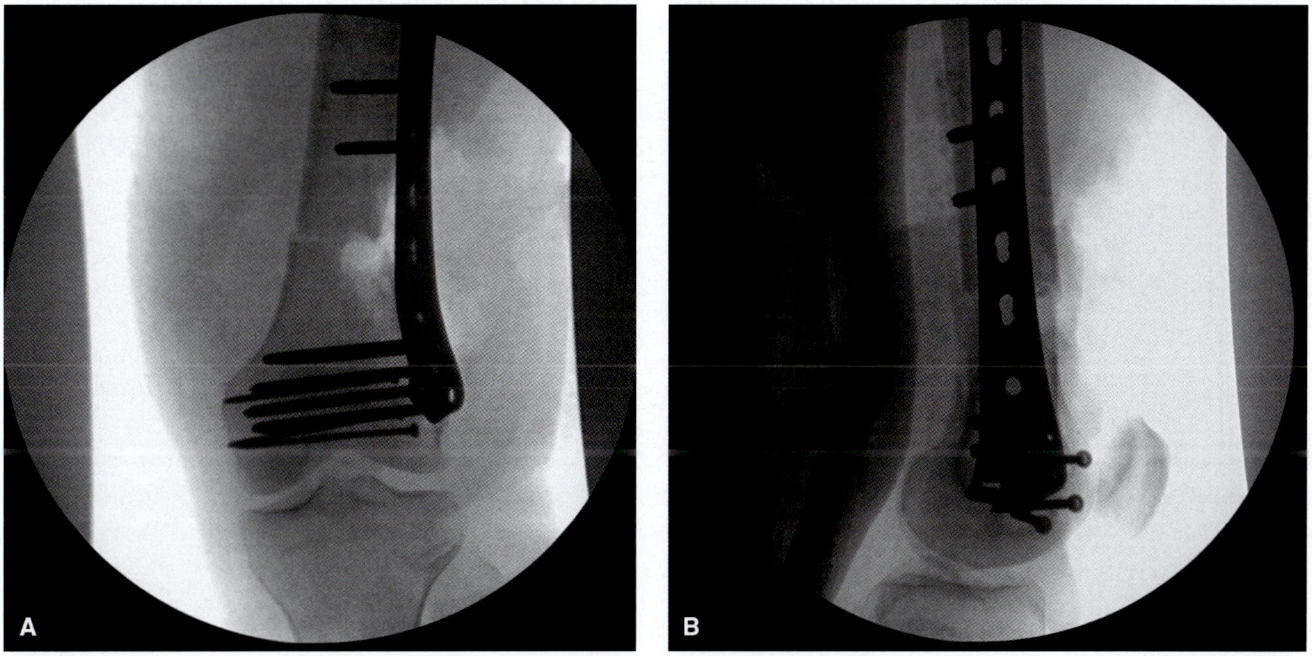

Figure 21-19 | AP **(A)** and lateral **(B)** images demonstrating correct plate placement. On the AP image, screws are oriented parallel to the knee joint indicating that coronal alignment has been restored, and flare of plate matches the lateral condyle. The absence of a paradoxical notch sign alerts the surgeon to an appropriate sagittal axis. On lateral image, plate is centered on articular block with anterior edge of plate just anterior to medial condyle. Note all screw holes are anterior to Blumensaat's line.

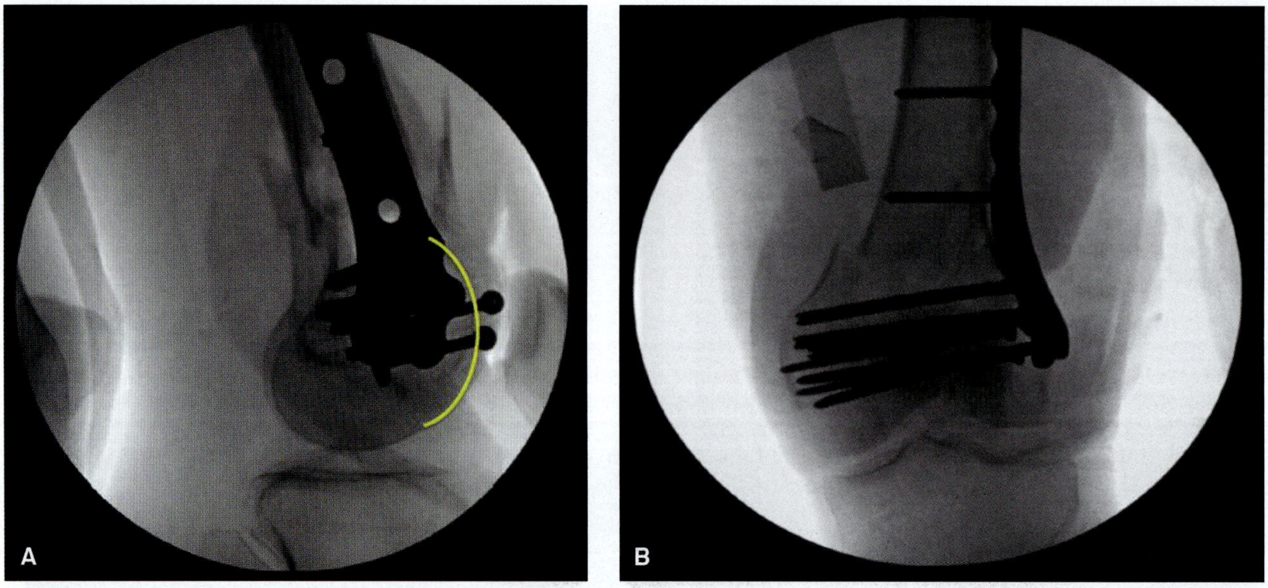

Figure 21-20 | AP **(A)** and lateral **(B)** images demonstrating an induced "golf club" deformity. On lateral view, the plate appears centered. However, the anterior edge of plate is entirely posterior to anterior margin of medial femoral condyle (*yellow line*). When proximal segment is reduced to the precontoured plate, the entire articular block becomes medialized.

Common pitfalls in plate placement include the following:

1. Too anterior: Screws can violate the trochlear groove. This error is avoided with direct visualization of the knee joint.
2. Too posterior: Screws can violate the intercondylar notch, and plate placement can induce a "golf club" deformity due to the trapezoidal nature of the distal femur (Fig. 21-20). Avoid errant screws with the notch view, and on lateral image, ensure that the anterior margin of plate is at or just anterior to margin of medial femoral condyle to avoid golf club deformity.
3. Too valgus-varus: Coronal plane deformities are avoided by understanding that the fixed-angle screws placed through modern precontoured implants are designed to restore correct alignment. Provisional pins and screws placed should be parallel to the knee joint.

References

1. Beltran MJ, Gary JL, Collinge CA. Management of distal femur fractures with modern plates and nails: state of the art. *J Orthop Trauma.* 2015;29(4):165–172. doi:10.1097/bot.0000000000000302.
2. Collinge CA, Gardner MJ, Crist BD. Pitfalls in the application of distal femur plates for fractures. *J Orthop Trauma.* 2011;25(11):695–706. doi:10.1097/BOT.0b013e31821d7a56.
3. Nork SE, Segina DN, Aflatoon K, et al. The association between supracondylar-intercondylar distal femoral fractures and coronal plane fractures. *J Bone Joint Surg Am.* 2005;87(3):564–569. doi:10.2106/jbjs.d.01751.
4. Krettek C, Miclau T, Grun O, et al. Intraoperative control of axes, rotation and length in femoral and tibial fractures. Technical note. *Injury.* 1998;29(suppl 3):C29–C39.
5. Wright R, Gardner MJ, Bradford Henley M. Distal femur fractures. In: Gardner MJ, ed. *Harborview Illustrated Tips and Tricks in Fracture Surgery.* 1st ed. Philadelphia, PA: Lippincott Williams & Wilkins, a Wolters Kluwer Business; 2011:232.

Chapter 22
Patella Fractures

MILTON T.M. LITTLE
MARSCHALL B. BERKES
DEAN G. LORICH

Bony Anatomy

- The patella is a complex three-dimensional bone.
- The anterior, nonarticular surface is shield shaped with distal taper at inferior pole.
- The posterior (articular surface) is elliptical shaped with three facets with thickened cartilage (Fig. 22-1).
  - Lateral facet—largest facet, concave, and plateaus laterally
  - Medial facet—convex, smaller than lateral facet
  - Odd facet—most medial aspect of the patella
    - Central articular ridge separates lateral and medial facet.
- The blood supply is provided by dorsal vessels and also ascending vessels via the fat pad inferomedially into nonarticular portions of patella.[1]
- Critical soft tissue attachments:
  - All soft tissues attach at nonarticular portions of the patella.
  - Soft tissue attachments are critical to extensor mechanism function.
  - Patella tendon inserts at inferior pole of the patella and can be affected by inferior pole comminution, leading to unrecognized displacement and extensor mechanism incompetence if not treated appropriately.
  - Quadriceps tendon inserts at superior pole of the patella.
  - Lateral retinaculum and medial retinaculum (including medial patellofemoral ligament) insert along the respective medial and lateral portions of the patella and frequently disrupted in patella fractures.

Radiographic Anatomy

Radiographic views[2]

- True lateral of the patella: obtained with limb in neutral rotation (Fig. 22-2)
  - Salient features
    - Articular tangent; correlates with articular ridge between medial and lateral facets
    - Secondary articular density; created by confluence of edge of the lateral facet with variable contributions from the edge of the medial facet or intersection of the medial and odd facet
    - Anterior cortical density
- Accessory view of the lateral facet: obtained with patella in approximately 20 degrees (range 12 to 35 degrees) of external rotation (Fig. 22-3)
  - Salient features
    - Tangent to the lateral facet.
    - Best view to visualize displacement at the lateral facet articular surface.
    - Articular surface will appear as a straight line.
    - Proximal beaking visualized.

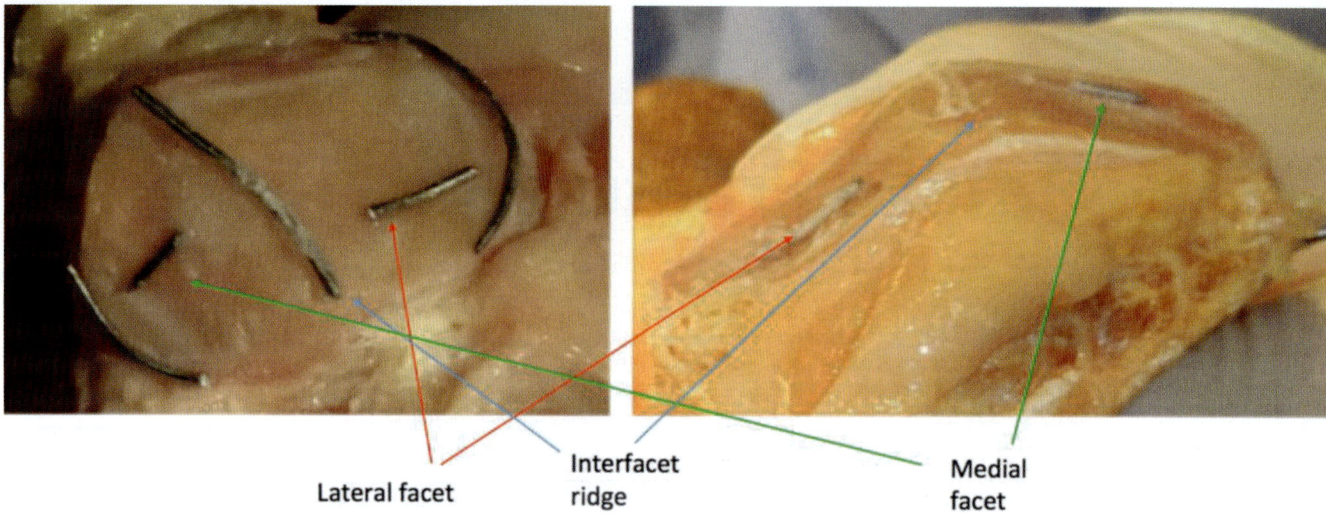

Figure 22-1 I Bony anatomy of patella.

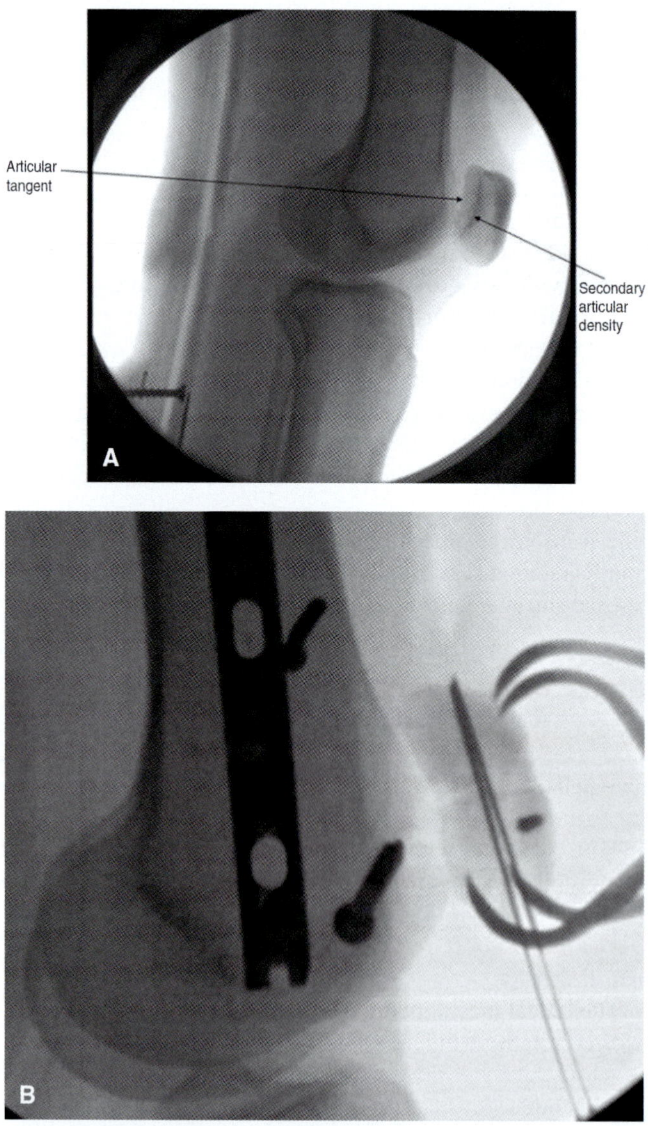

Figure 22-2 I A and B: True lateral view of the patella.

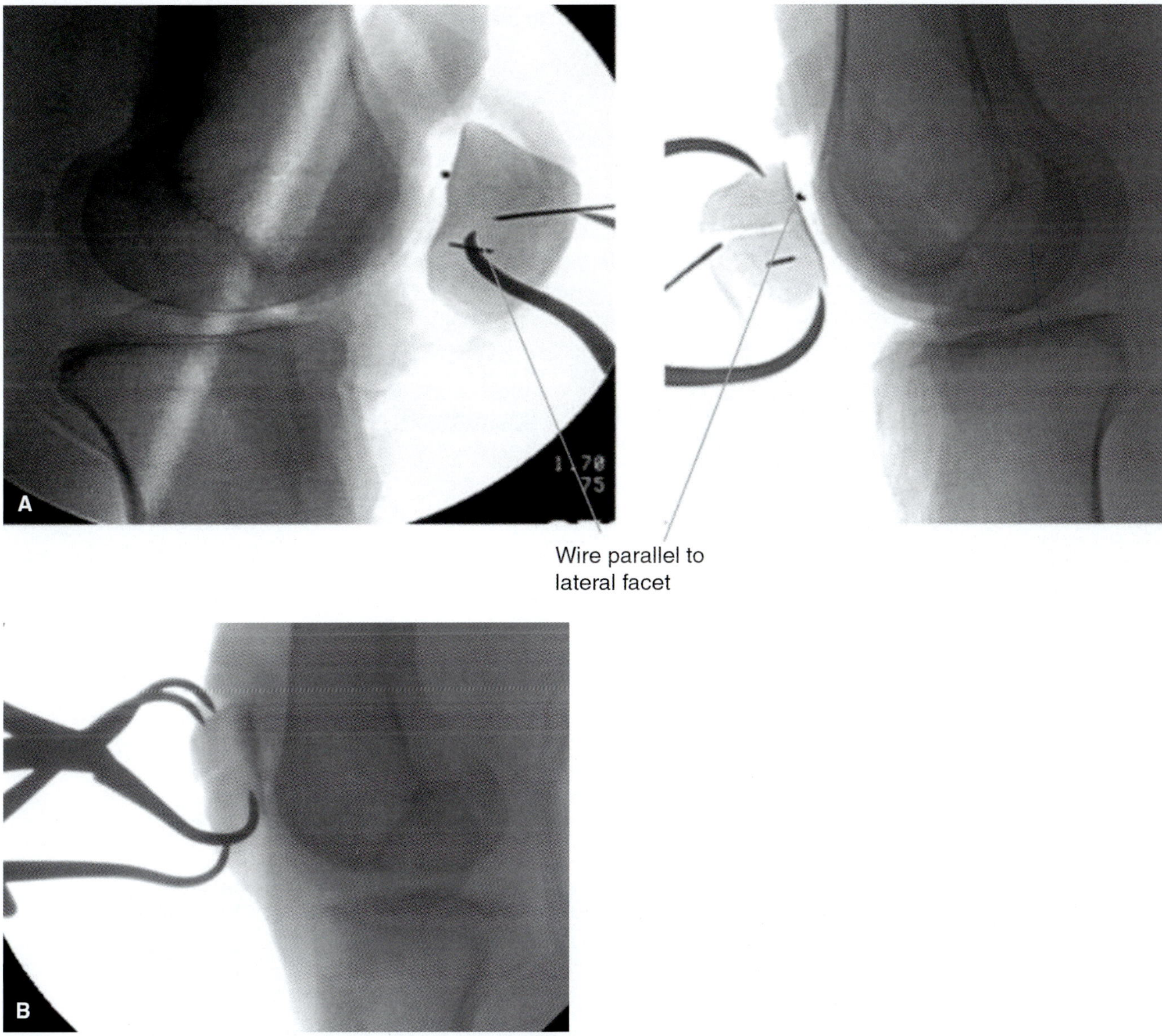

Figure 22-3 | **A and B:** Accessory view of lateral facet.

- Accessory view of the medial facet: obtained with patella in approximately 30 degrees (range 15 to 45 degrees) of internal rotation (Fig. 22-4)
  - Salient features
    - Tangent to the medial facet
    - Best view to visualize displacement at the medial facet articular surface
    - Hexagonal or sail shape

Preoperative Imaging

AP and lateral views of the knee are usually adequate to determine if surgical or nonsurgical treatment is indicated (Fig. 22-5).

- CT scan should be performed for most operative patella fractures (Fig. 22-6).
- Allows true assessment of comminuted fractures.
- Rule out and plan accordingly for inferior pole comminution as this is usually not fully appreciated with plain radiographs.[3]
- Determine major fracture fragments and plan fixation strategy accordingly.

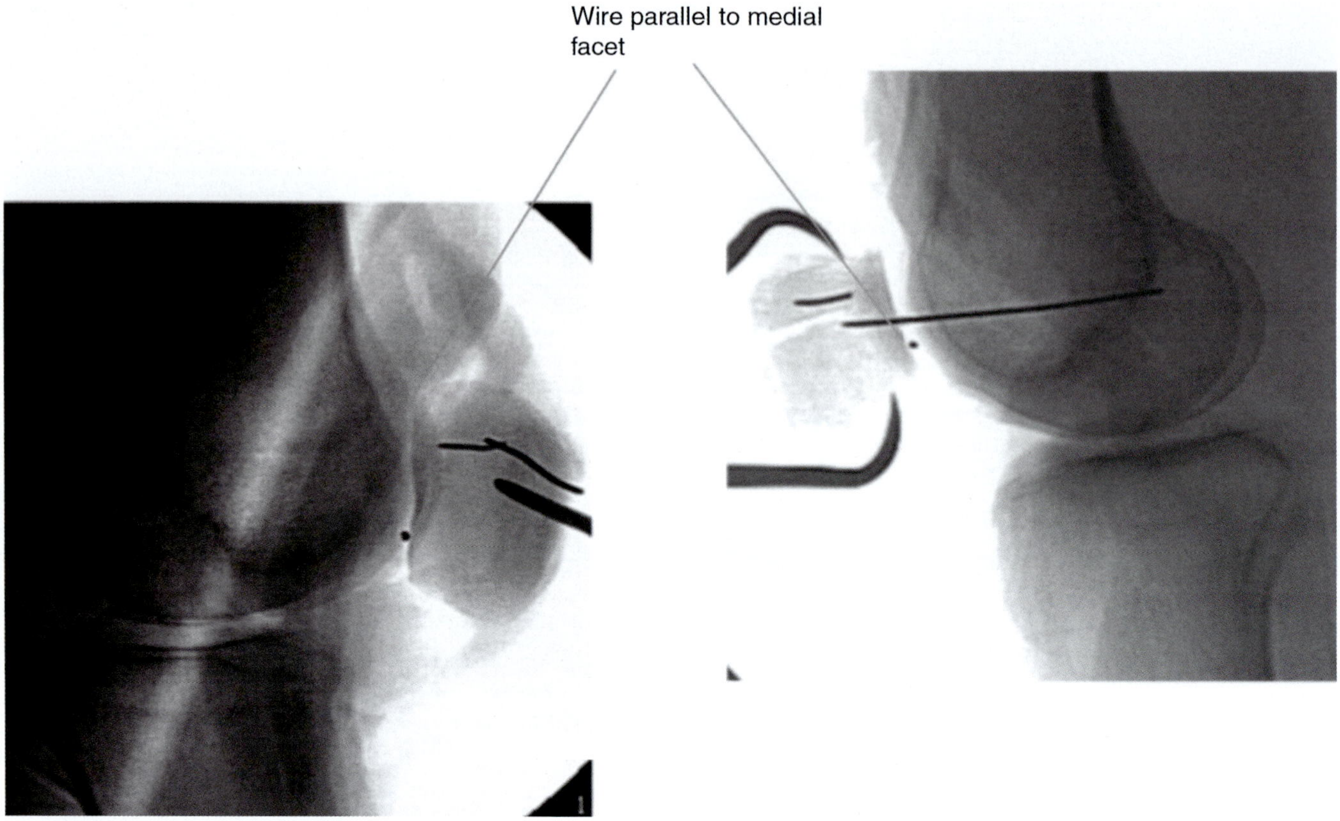

Figure 22-4 | Accessory view of medical facet.

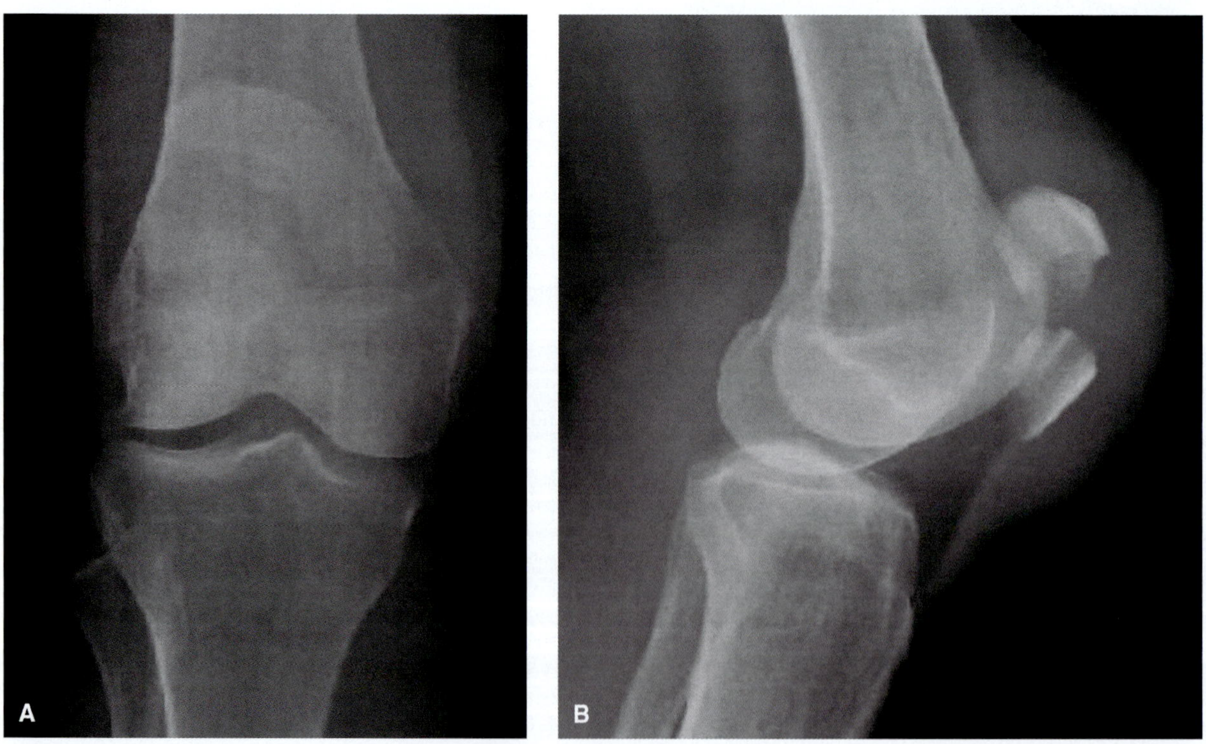

Figure 22-5 | **A and B:** AP and lateral views of the patella.

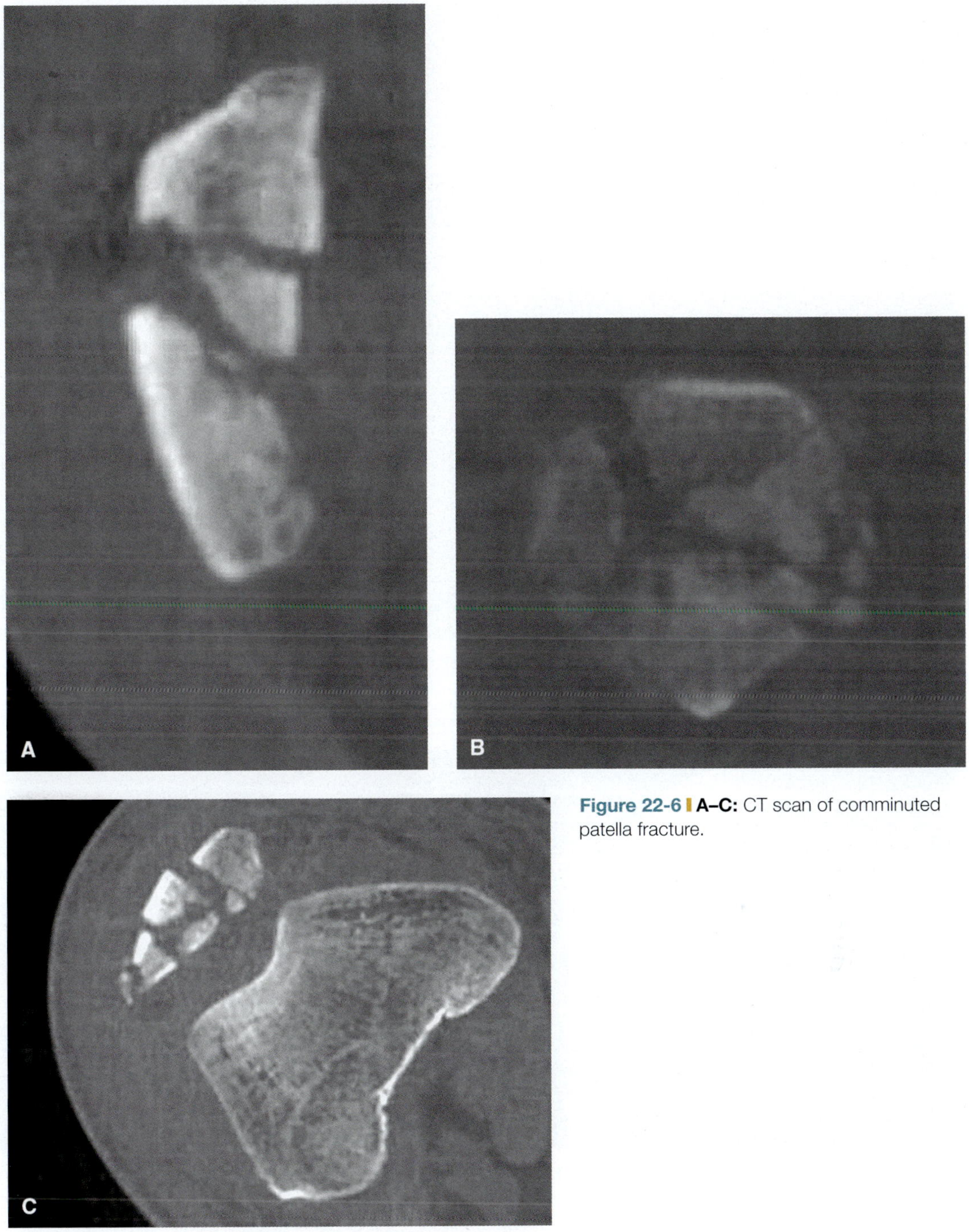

Figure 22-6 | A–C: CT scan of comminuted patella fracture.

Intraoperative Positioning

- Implant and fixation strategies are dictated by fracture (Fig. 22-7).
  - Simple fractures can be treated with tension band and screw construct.
    - Use both AP and lateral views to ensure cannulated screws (for modified tension band construct) are short of superior cortex, so wires contacts bone and not metal as it bends.
  - Complex/comminuted fractures require multiplanar fixation.
    - Consider live fluoroscopy with internal and external rotation to ensure all screws remain extra-articular.
- **Supine Positioning**
  - OSI/Jackson or other radiolucent diving board-type table.
  - Rolled blanket bump under ipsilateral buttock.

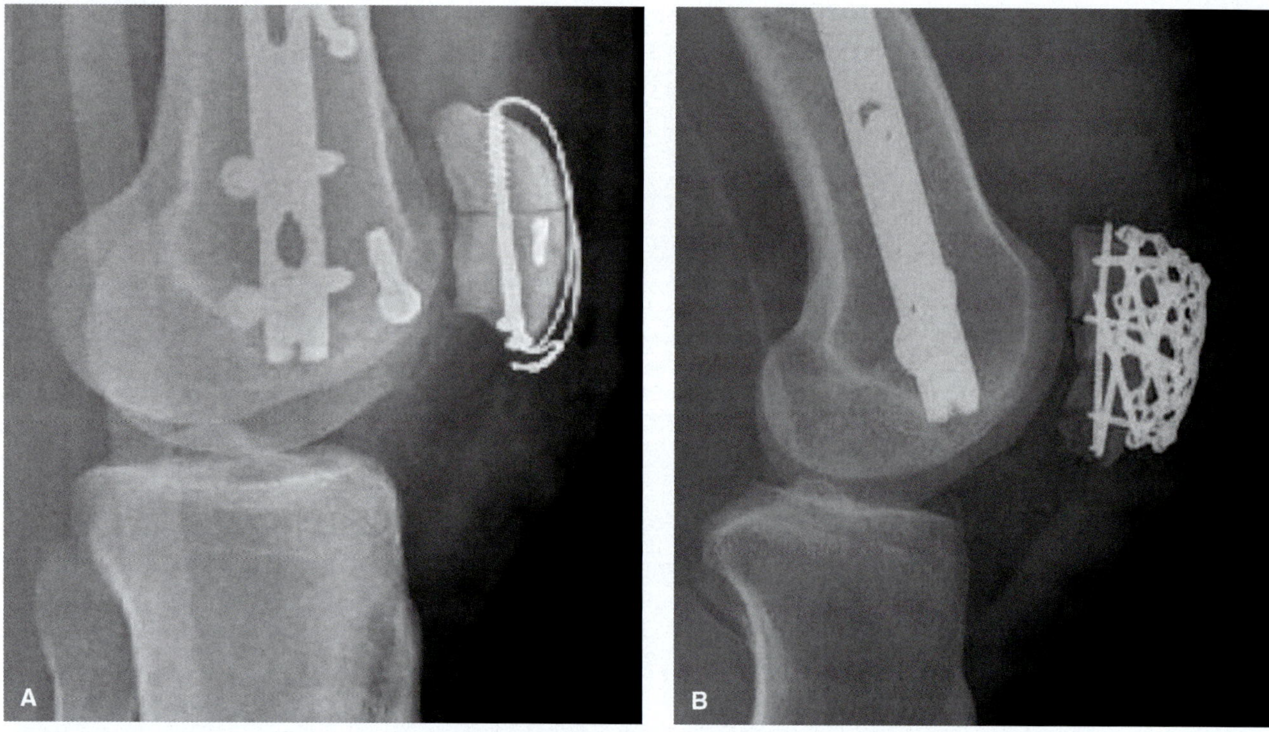

Figure 22-7 | A and B: Cannulated screws with tension band for simple, transverse fracture and multiaxial fixation K-wires and dorsal minifragment mesh plate for highly comminuted fracture pattern.

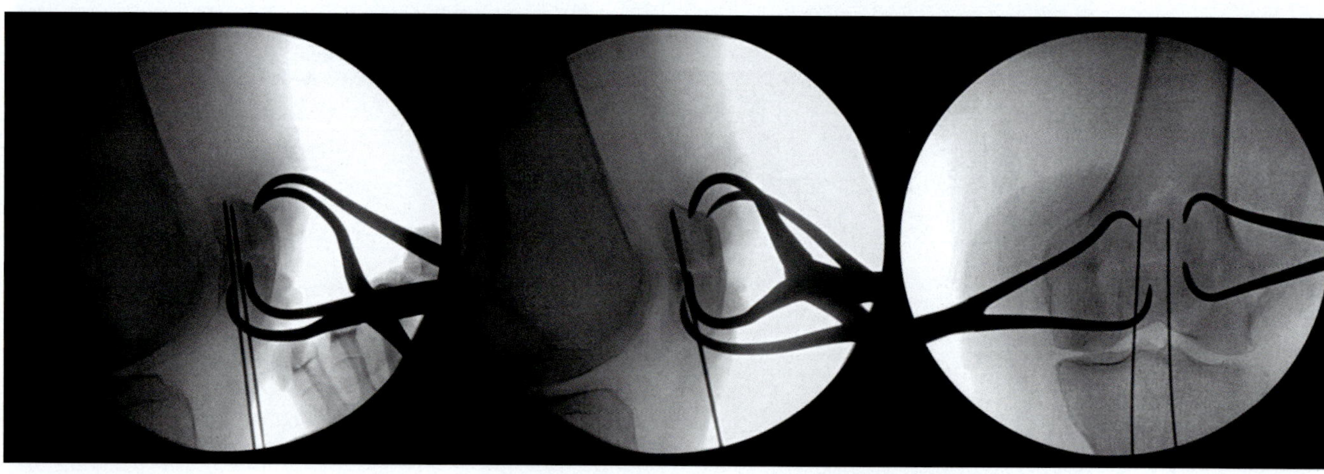

Figure 22-8 | To prevent wire fatigue in cannulated screw and tension band constructs, guidewires should be placed near the articular surface subchondral bone from distal to proximal without penetration of the superior patellar cortex. This can be correlated between AP and lateral images as depicted above. Screw lengths should be calculated less than this distance to allow fracture compression through the figure-of-8 tension band wire that leaves the screw tips within bone and mechanically loads the patella rather than exiting and coursing over the edge of a sharp screw that projects out of the bone.

- Foam leg ramp or stack of blankets for positioning the operative extremity (Fig. 22-8).
- Bump utilized under ankle during clamping and fixation to hyperextend knee and assist with reduction (Fig. 22-9).
- C-arm should come from contralateral side and orthogonal to the limb/table to facilitate AP and lateral views.
- Assess fixation strength and flexion post fixation to determine rehabilitation protocol (Figs. 22-10–22-12).

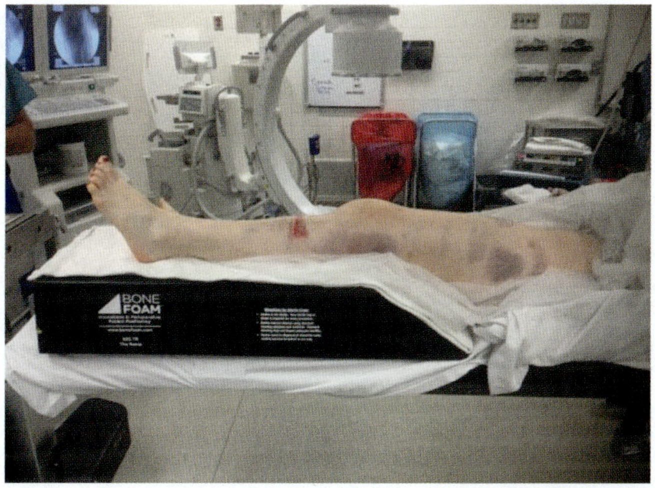

Figure 22-9 | Ramp in place for positioning.

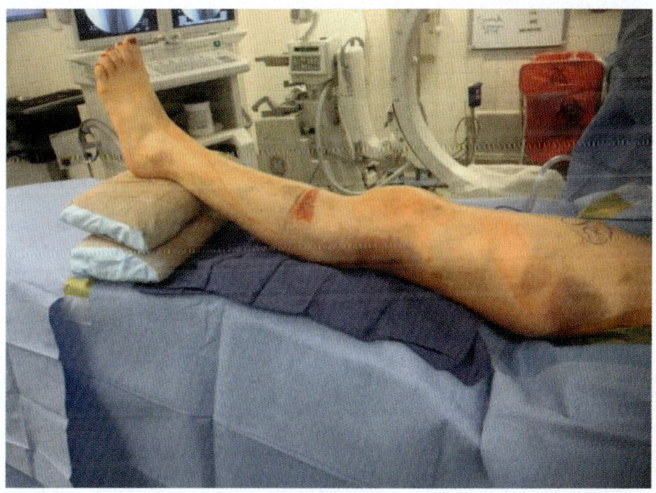

Figure 22-10 | Lower extremity bump in place to extend leg for fixation and repair.

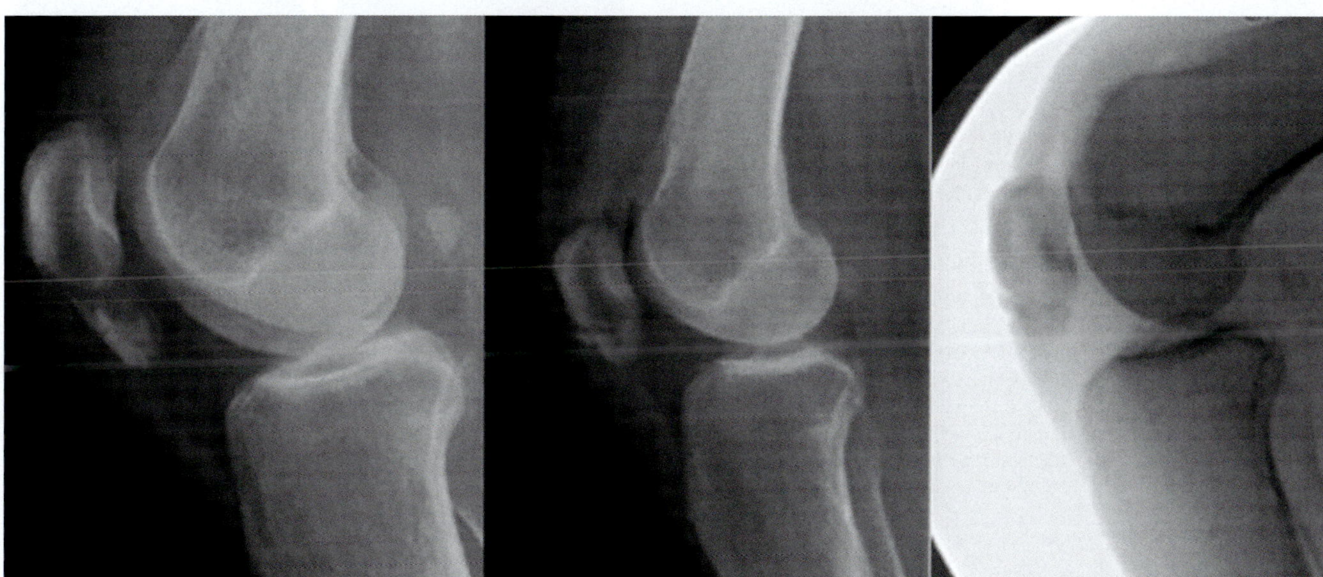

Figure 22-11 | Suture repair inferior pole fracture demonstrating stability with 90 degrees of flexion.

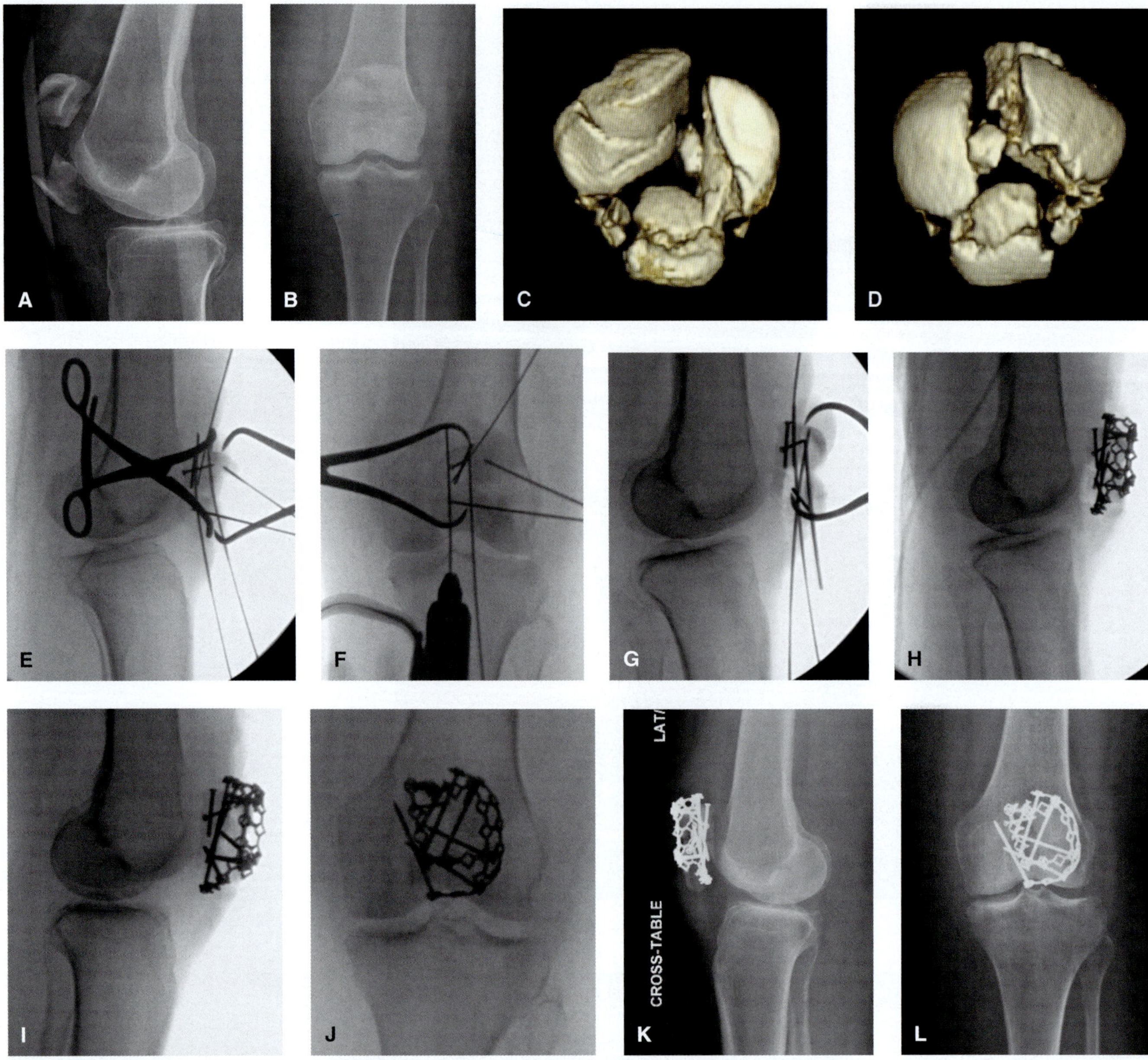

Figure 22-12 | Comminuted patella fracture **(A–D)**, K-wires, subchondral screws, clamps for temporizing fixation **(E–G)**, application of rim plate for polyaxial fixation. Rim plate captures inferior pole and the construct is augmented with patellar tendon Krackow stitch **(H–J)**. Postoperative imaging demonstrating maintenance of reduction in 3 month post-operative imaging **(K,L)**.

References

1. Lazaro LE, Wellman DS, Klinger CE, et al. Quantitative and qualitative assessment of bone perfusion and arterial contributions in a patellar fracture model using gadolinium-enhanced magnetic resonance imaging: a cadaveric study. *J Bone Joint Surg Am.* 2013;95(19):e1401–e1407.
2. Berkes MG, Little MT, Pardee NC, et al. Defining the lateral and accessory views of the patella: an anatomic and radiographic study with implications for fracture treatment. *J Orthop Trauma.* 2013;27(12):663–671.
3. Lazaro LE, Wellman DS, Pardee NC, et al. Effect of computerized tomography on classification and treatment plan for patellar fractures. *J Orthop Trauma.* 2013;27(6):336–344.

Chapter 23
Tibial Plateau Fractures

BHARAT SAMPATHI
JOHN A. SCOLARO

Bony Anatomy

- The tibial plateau is the proximal weight-bearing surface of the tibia and articulates with the medial and lateral distal femoral condyles.
- The intercondylar eminence is positioned between the medial and lateral plateau and does not articulate directly with the femur.
- The lateral plateau is convex in both the coronal and sagittal plane.
- The medial plateau is concave in both the coronal and sagittal plane.
- The articular surface of the lateral plateau is proximal to the medial plateau; an approximate 3-degree varus angle exists between the shaft of the tibia and a line drawn across the articular surface in the nonarthritic knee.
- A posterior slope exists to the proximal tibial plateau that measures approximately 8 degrees.[1]

Radiographic Anatomy

Anterior-Posterior (AP) View

- On the standard AP view of the knee, the patella is centered between the medial and lateral femoral condyles; there is approximately one-third to one-half overlap of the fibular head with the lateral edge of the proximal tibia on this view (Fig. 23-1A and B).
  - Excessive external rotation: the patella overlies the lateral distal femoral condyle, and there is increased overlap of the proximal tibia and fibula.
  - Excessive internal rotation: the patella overlies the medial distal femoral condyle, and there is little to no overlap of the proximal tibia and fibula.

AP with 10-Degree Caudal Tilt

- An AP view of the proximal tibia with 10 degrees of caudal tilt provides an image parallel to the joint surface; this can be particularly useful fluoroscopically in assessment of articular reduction (Fig. 23-2A and B).

Lateral View

- On the standard lateral view of the knee, the posterior aspect of the femoral condyles is perfectly superimposed. The uninjured lateral plateau is seen proximal to the medial plateau (Fig. 23-3).

Modified Lateral Views

- On the lateral view, the leg can be brought into adduction (toward the midline/away from the x-ray source) to elevate the medial plateau into view (Fig. 23-4A and B).
- Similarly, the leg can be brought into abduction (away from the midline/toward the x-ray source) to elevate the lateral plateau into view (Figs. 23-5A and B and 23-6).

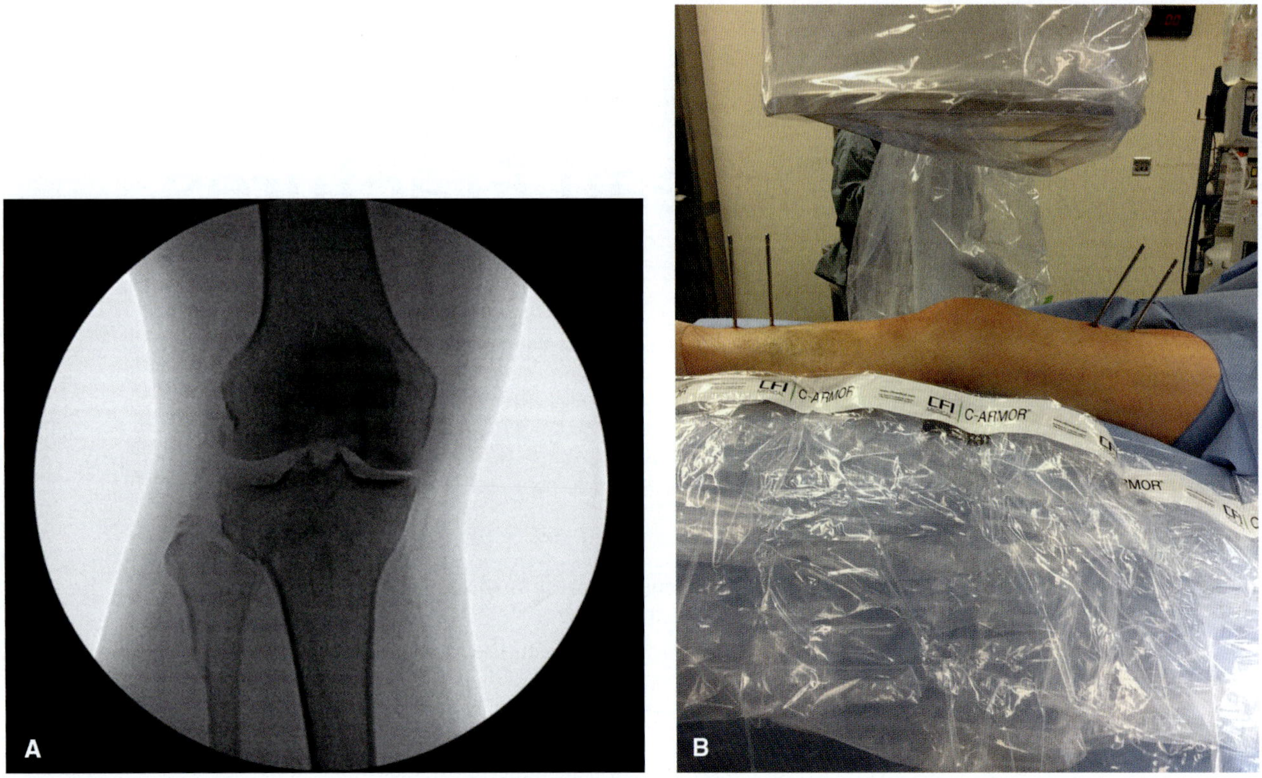

Figure 23-1 | A. Standard AP view of lateral split depression lateral plateau fracture. **B.** Standard C-arm position for true AP of the tibial plateau.

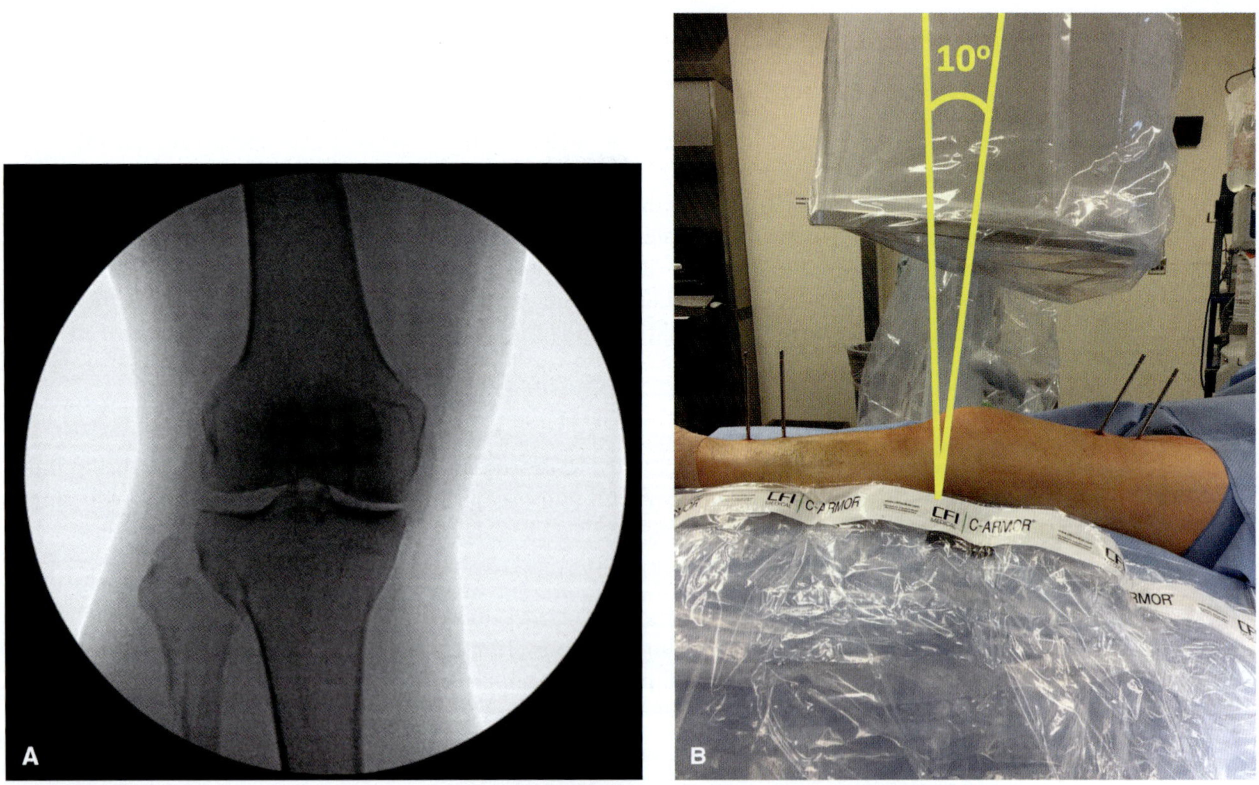

Figure 23-2 | A. AP view with 10 degrees of caudal tilt; beam is nearly parallel to tibial plateaus. **B.** Caudal tilt C-arm position used to efface the true articular joint line view of the tibial plateau.

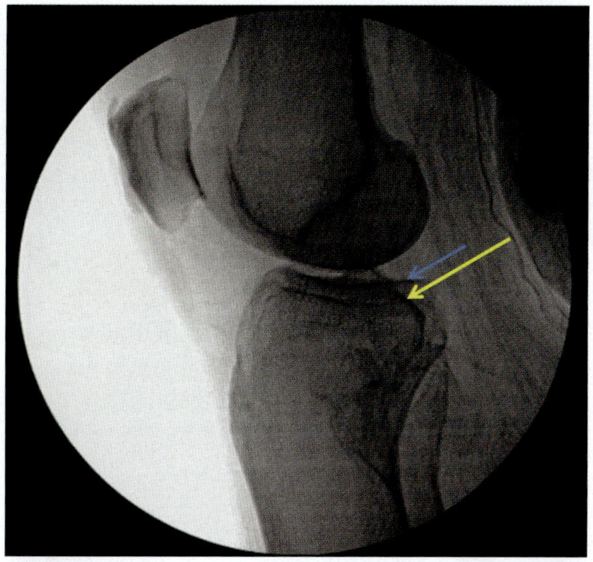

Figure 23-3 | Standard lateral view of lateral split depression lateral plateau fracture. In this image, lateral plateau is depressed (*yellow arrow*) and is lower than the uninjured medial plateau (*blue arrow*).

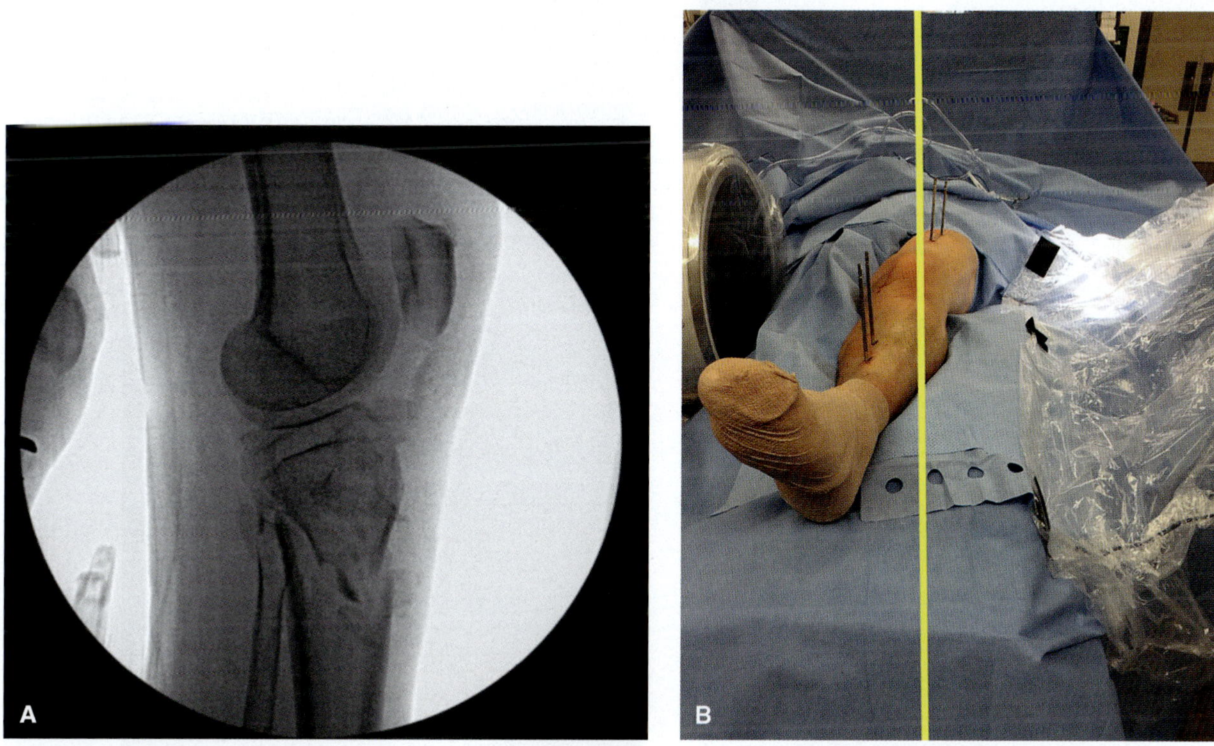

Figure 23-4 | A. Bicondylar plateau fracture; leg is adducted toward image intensifier, elevating medial plateau into view. **B.** Depiction of leg adduction relative to the true C-arm lateral which is used to profile the medial tibial plateau fracture/reduction.

Preoperative Imaging

- Standard AP and lateral radiographs should be obtained prior to any advanced imaging (Figs. 23-7 and 23-8).
- Following evaluation of the plain injury radiographs, a determination should be made as to whether an external fixator will be placed for fracture or soft tissue reasons.
- A computed tomography (CT) scan is commonly obtained following plain radiographs and should be obtained after external fixation, if applicable.
- Axial, coronal, and sagittal CT reconstructions are useful to for fracture classification and preoperative planning[2] (Figs. 23-9–23-11).
- If an external fixator is applied, connecting clamps should be placed so they do not impede AP or lateral fluoroscopy of the knee and proximal tibia. Schanz pins should also be placed away from the joint surface and intended location of fixation hardware (Figs. 23-12 and 23-13).

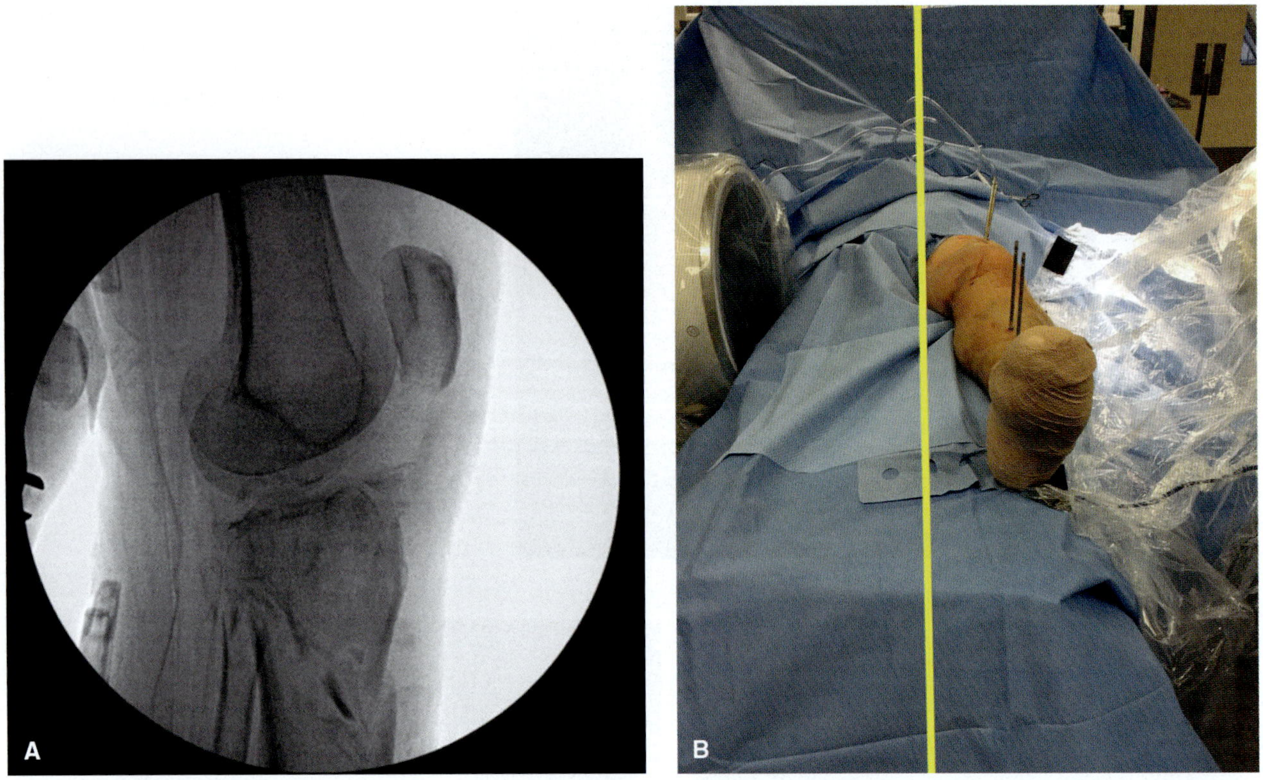

Figure 23-5 | A. Bicondylar plateau fracture; leg is abducted away from image intensifier, elevating lateral plateau into view. **B.** Depiction of leg abduction relative to the true C-arm lateral which is used to profile the lateral tibial plateau fracture/reduction.

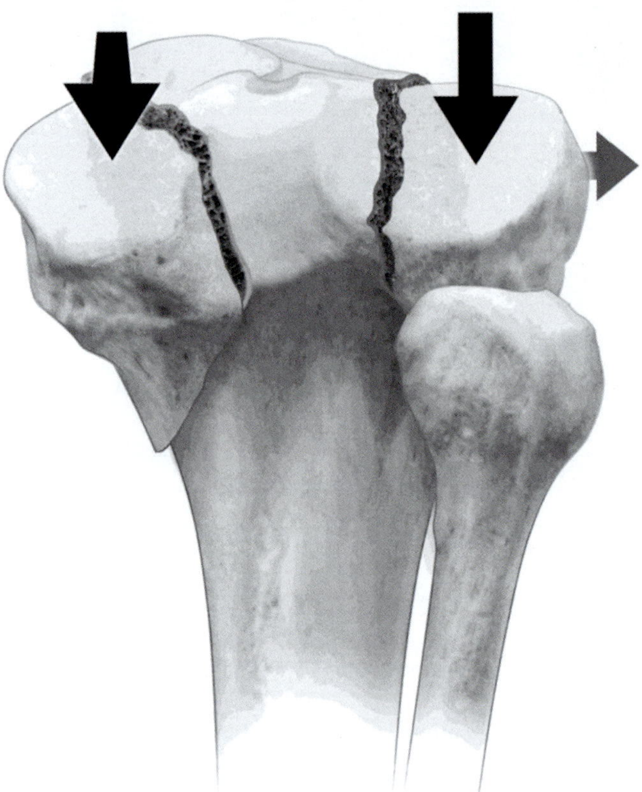

Figure 23-6 | Posterior view of a typical bicondylar tibial plateau fracture pattern. The lateral split depression results in widening of the lateral tibial joint line and an increased posterior slope. The normal gentle convex shape of the lateral tibial articular surface is lost due to the joint depression. The posteromedial coronal shear fragment demonstrates an unstable fragment prone to articular step-off and may be of varying size with tibial eminence or posterior lateral joint extension.

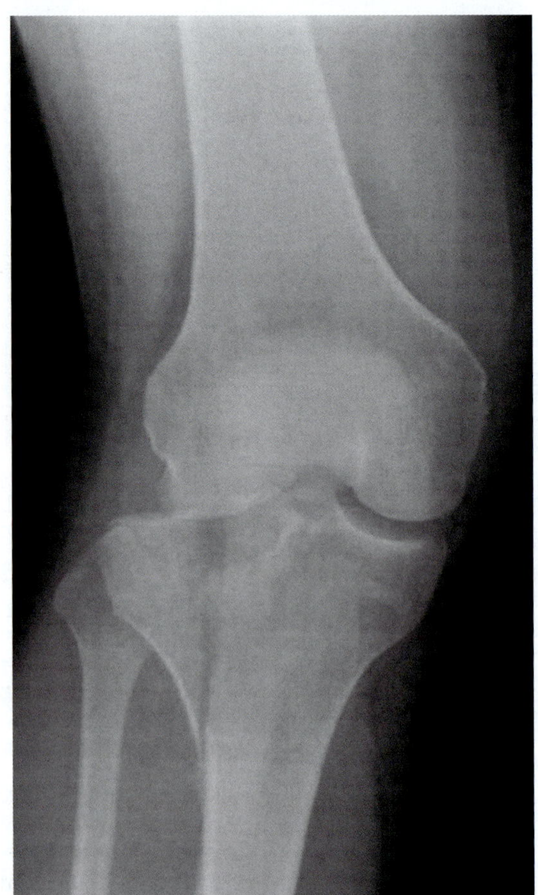

Figure 23-7 | Standard AP (7) and lateral (8) plain radiographs of a split depression lateral plateau fracture.

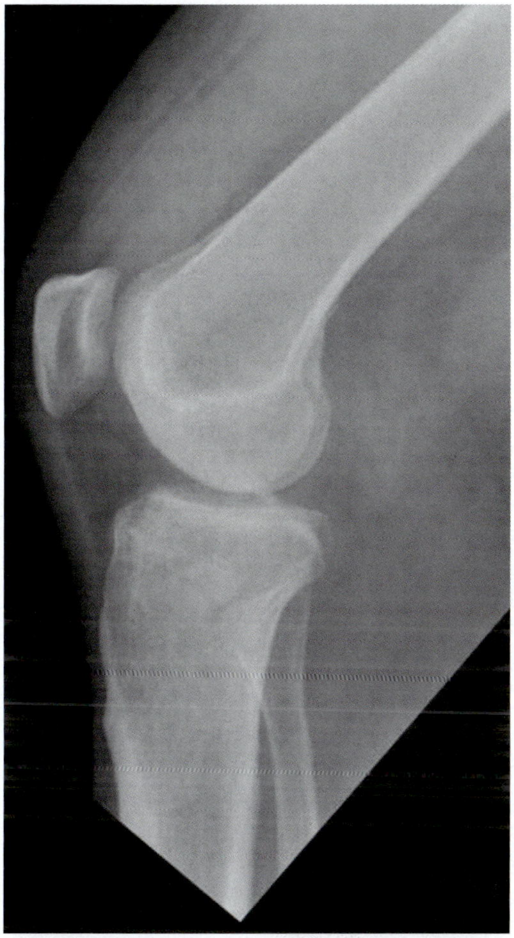

Figure 23-8 | Standard AP (7) and lateral (8) plain radiographs of a split depression lateral plateau fracture.

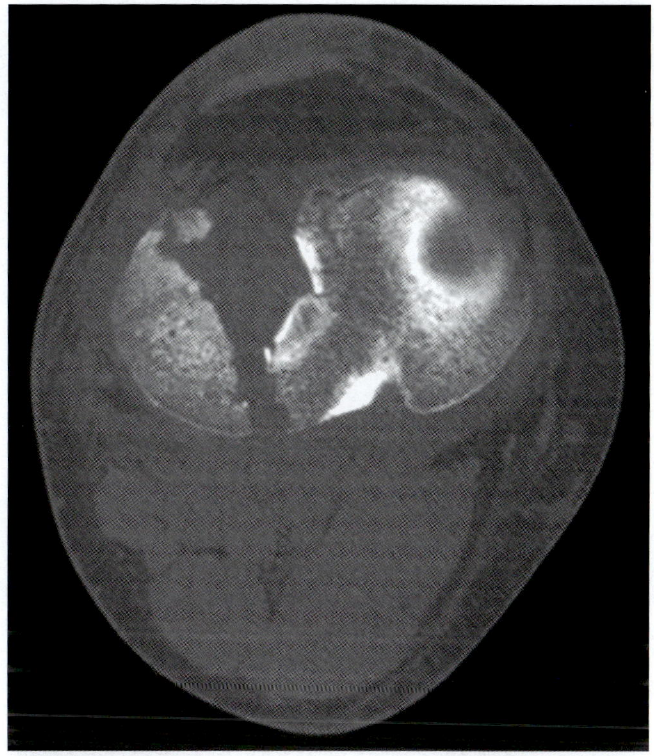

Figure 23-9 | Axial (9), coronal (10), sagittal (11) CT scan images of patient with split depression lateral plateau fracture.

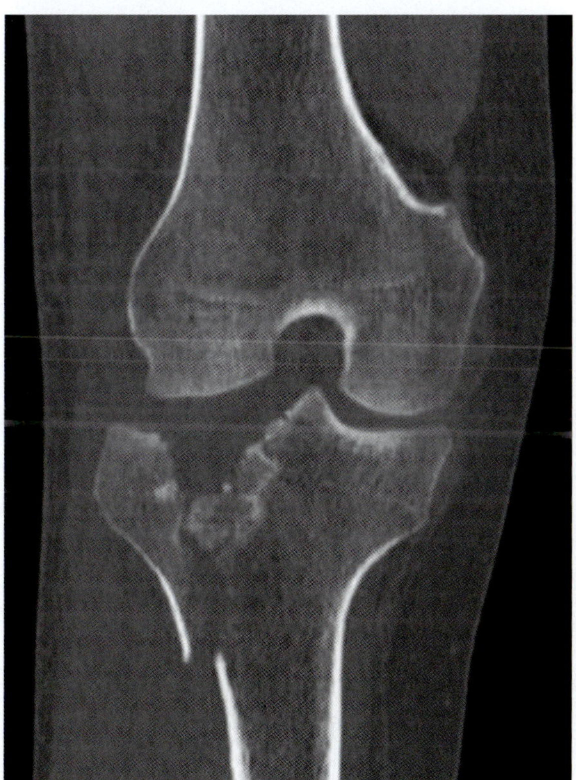

Figure 23-10 | Axial (9), coronal (10), sagittal (11) CT scan images of patient with split depression lateral plateau fracture.

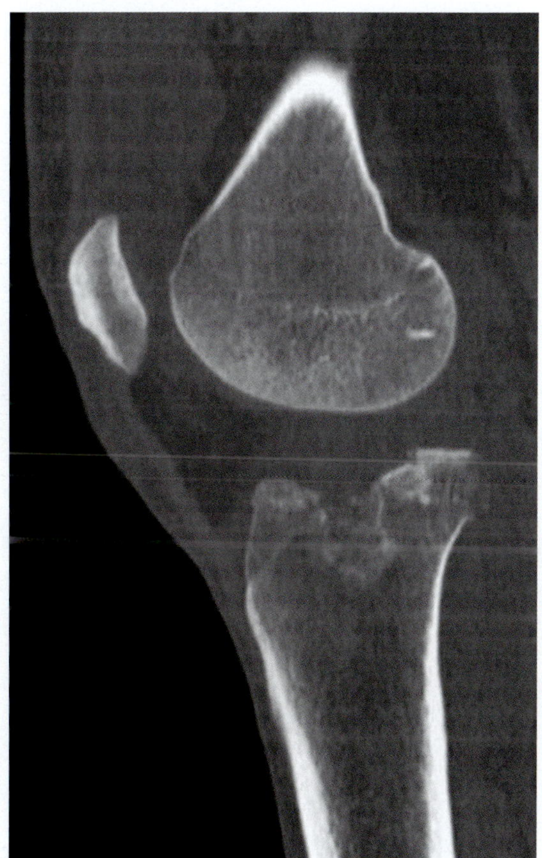

Figure 23-11 | Axial (9), coronal (10), sagittal (11) CT scan images of patient with split depression lateral plateau fracture.

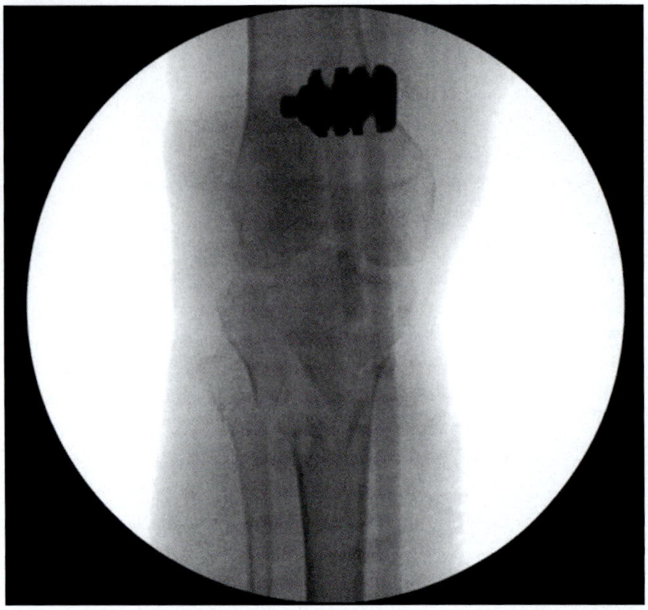

Figure 23-12 | AP (12) view of knee showing bar-to-bar clamp away from visualization of joint line. AP (13) view of the tibia demonstrating Schanz pin placement away from fracture and future implants.

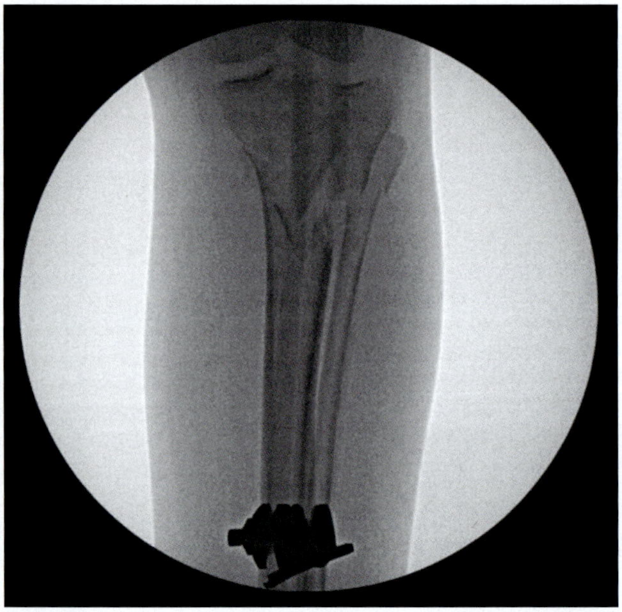

Figure 23-13 | AP (12) view of knee showing bar-to-bar clamp away from visualization of joint line. AP (13) view of the tibia demonstrating Schanz pin placement away from fracture and future implants.

Intraoperative Positioning

- Commonly the patient is positioned supine on a standard operating room table with a small bump placed under the ipsilateral ischium. The size of the bump depends on the size of the patient; the patella of the operative limb should point to the ceiling (Figs. 23-14 and 23-15).
- The ipsilateral arm is placed over the chest, padded with a pillow or egg crate foam and secured to avoid placing stretch on the brachial plexus.
- When a medial approach to the proximal tibia is needed, removal of the ischial bump allows for external rotation of the affected limb and improved working space.

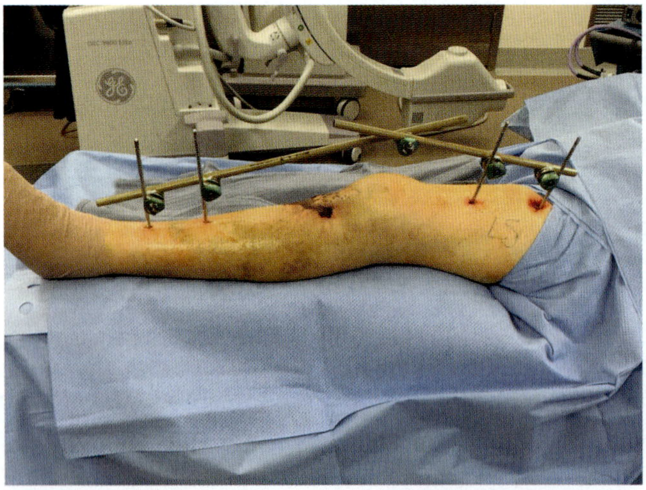

Figure 23-14 | Clinical view from lateral side of leg (14) and foot of bed (15) showing standard supine setup for tibial plateau surgery.

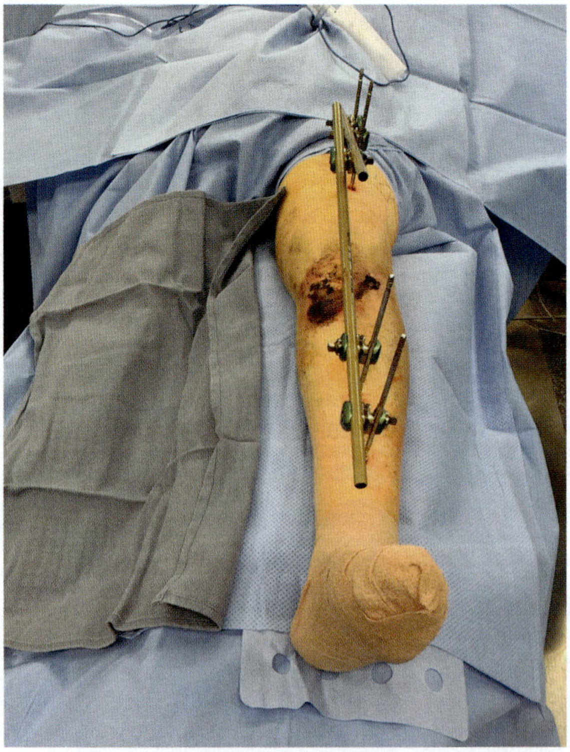

Figure 23-15 | Clinical view from lateral side of leg (14) and foot of bed (15) showing standard supine setup for tibial plateau surgery.

- Some surgeons favor prone positioning for access to the posterior or posterior medial proximal tibia; standard prone positioning considerations are therefore implemented to protect bony prominences and structures at risk.
- An unsterile tourniquet can be placed around the proximal thigh prior to sterile preparation and draping of the operative leg at the surgeons discretion.
- The operative extremity is elevated on a radiolucent foam ramp to allow uninhibited AP and lateral fluoroscopic images to be taken with minimal manipulation of the limb. Other radiolucent positioning options are a stack of blankets or radiolucent triangle.
- The C-arm fluoroscopy machine is positioned opposite the side that the surgeon is working. If medial and lateral approaches are required, the surgeon should plan to work on the same side of the C-arm or request that the machine and technologist switch sides of the room intra-operatively.

Lateral Plateau Fractures

- Femoral distractor
  - The proximal threaded Schanz pin is placed through the lateral incision across the widest portion of the femoral condyles; the distal pin is placed bicortically through a lateral percutaneous incision in the tibial shaft.
  - Distraction results in knee varus and increased space between the lateral distal femur and lateral tibial plateau. In order to maximize lateral joint distraction and minimize abutment of the medial joint or loss of provisional medial fixation, it can be valuable to preload the femoral distractor and coronal alignment into valgus. The lateral based femoral distractor vector will result in favorable distraction of the joint with medial compromise (Fig. 23-16).
- Joint elevation
  - Elevation of depressed joint fragments with a bone tamp can be followed on AP and lateral fluoroscopy (Fig. 23-17).

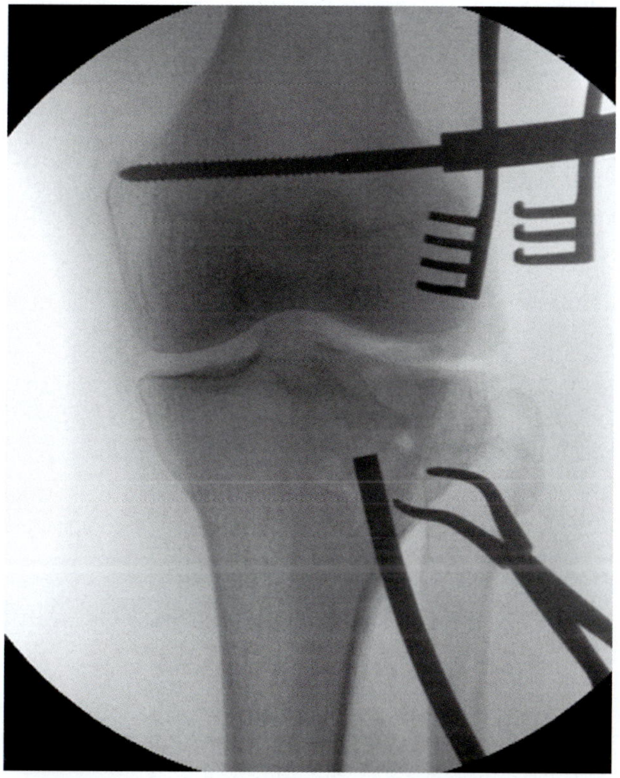

Figure 23-16 | AP view showing proximal distractor Schanz pin placed across femoral condyles. Note that a distal, lateral Schanz pin is placed within the tibial diaphysis below the planned, terminal level of plating allowing the femoral distractor to open up the joint and provide visualization of the reduction through a lateral submeniscal arthrotomy. A lateral clamp is holding the lateral joint split and the curved impactor is seen just below a depressed joint fragment.

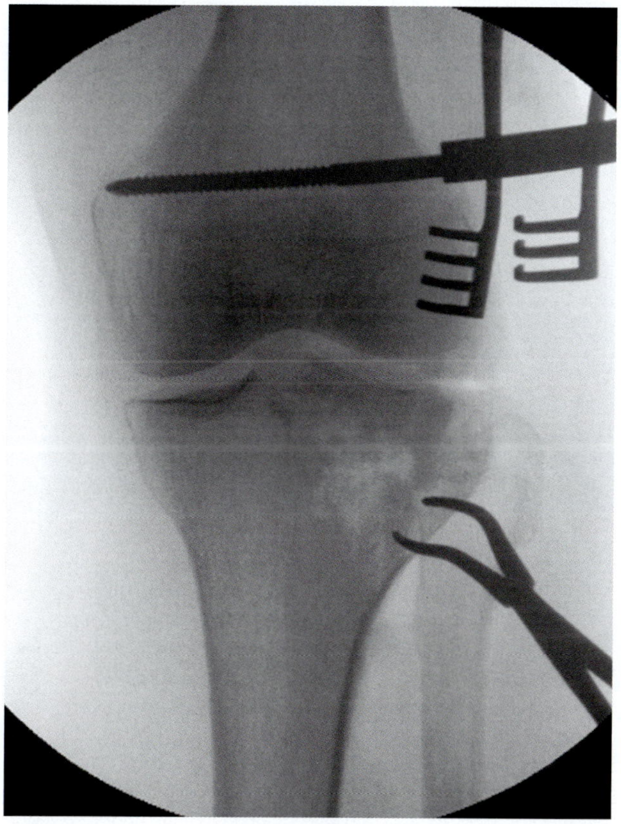

Figure 23-17 | AP view showing elevation of previously depressed joint fragment.

- Small diameter Kirschner wires can be used as provisional or permanent support for elevated chondral fragments.
- Fluoroscopic reduction can be confirmed through a submeniscal arthrotomy and direct visualization of the joint surface; both direct joint visualization and fluoroscopic information best predicts accurate reduction[3] (Fig. 23-18).
- Plate position as well as fill of implanted graft can be confirmed with fluoroscopy prior to definitive placement of fixation hardware (Figs. 23-19 and 23-20).

Medial Plateau Fractures

- Fracture identification and planning
  - AP and lateral plain radiographs as well as CT scan should be used to identify and plan surgical approach (Figs. 23-21–23-23).
  - Medial plateau fractures can occur in isolation or exist as a component of a bicondylar injury.
  - Isolated medial plateau fractures may require a medial approach alone. In bicondylar tibial plateau fractures, the fracture pattern determines whether medial and lateral surgical approaches are needed.
  - Posterior medial fracture fragments require reduction and fixation in most cases as they are not well stabilized by lateral proximal tibial implants (Fig. 23-24).[4]
- Intraoperative positioning
  - The patient can be placed supine with the operative leg allowed to externally rotate.
  - Soft bumps placed proximal to the knee joint and distal, near the ankle, allow the deep and posterior compartment musculature to fall away from the bone.
  - The knee can be bent and placed into a "figure four" type position to also allow access to the posterior medial tibia.
- Isolated medial plateau fractures
  - Joint reduction is performed primarily with fluoroscopy as the medial collateral ligament prohibits a submeniscal arthrotomy (Fig. 23-25).

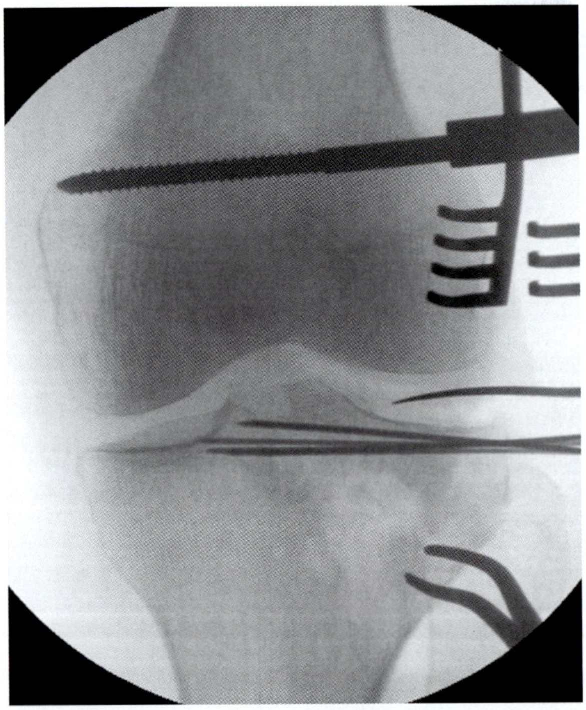

Figure 23-18 | AP view showing provisional Kirschner wires in a subchondral position across the lateral plateau maintaining reduction of the joint. A Freer elevator is visualized coming through the submeniscal arthrotomy, confirming reduction. The subchondral osseous void can also be seen in this image.

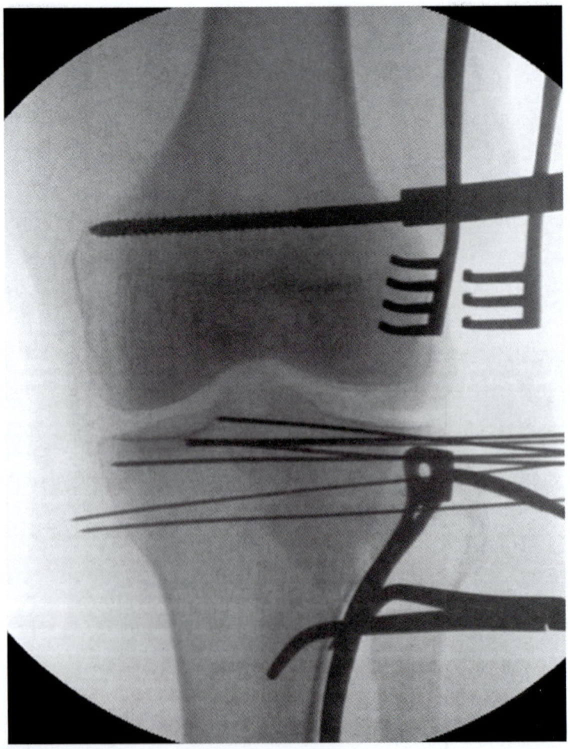

Figure 23-19 | AP view with plate in place, Kirschner wires maintaining reduction and evidence of bone graft within the previous subchondral void.

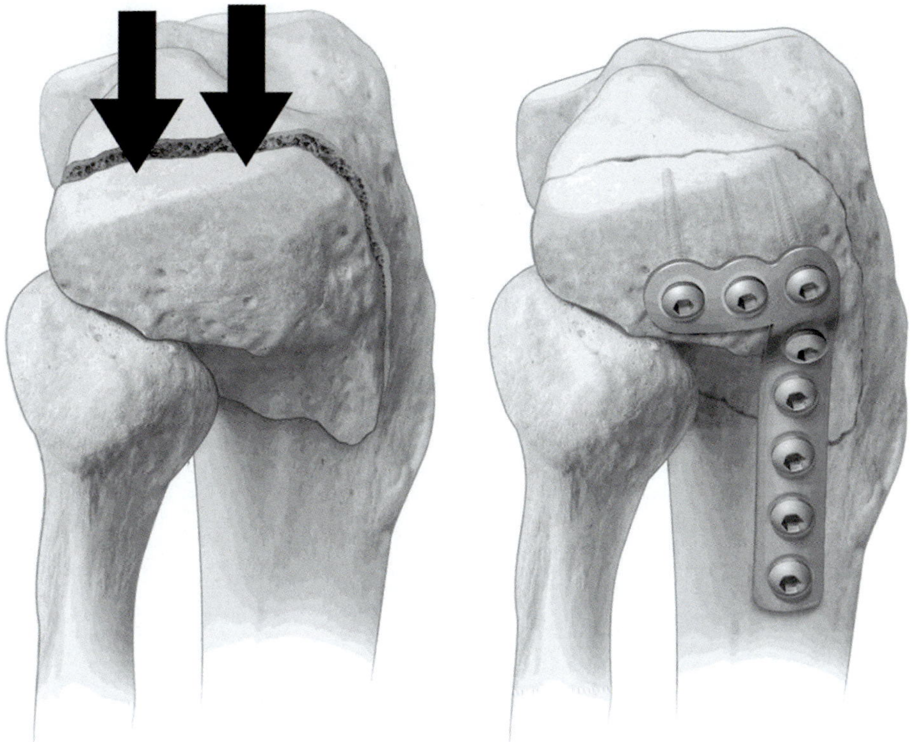

Figure 23-20 | The lateral tibial plateau is approached through an anterolateral window which longitudinally splits the iliotibial band and extends into the origin of the tibialis anterior muscle. A lateral submeniscal arthrotomy allows for assessment of the meniscus and visualization of the joint depression. The articular reduction is achieved either through booking open the lateral tibial condylar split or through a unicortical window with bone tamps. Temporizing K-wires hold the reduction, and restoration of the articular congruity, slope and width on AP, and lateral fluoro images are confirmed before plating. Coronal plane compression of the articular surface is performed through a lateral plate which buttresses the metaphysis. Independent bicondylar lag screws can be positioned above the plate, with fluoroscopy used to confirm the implants remain extra-articular.

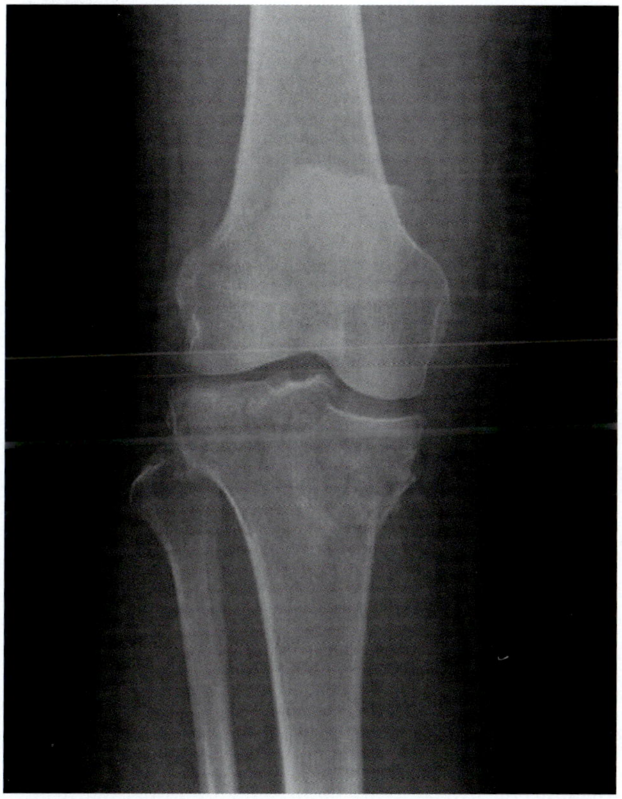

Figure 23-21 | AP (21) and lateral (22) plain radiographs as well as sagittal CT image (23) of isolated medial plateau fracture. Anterior comminution, depression, and a posteromedial fracture fragment can be identified.

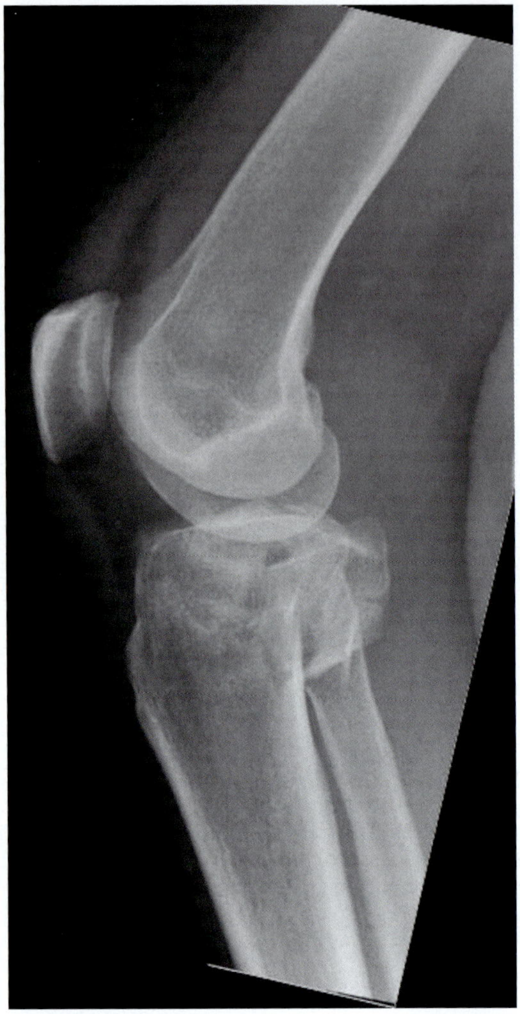

Figure 23-22 | AP (21) and lateral (22) plain radiographs as well as sagittal CT image (23) of isolated medial plateau fracture. Anterior comminution, depression, and a posteromedial fracture fragment can be identified.

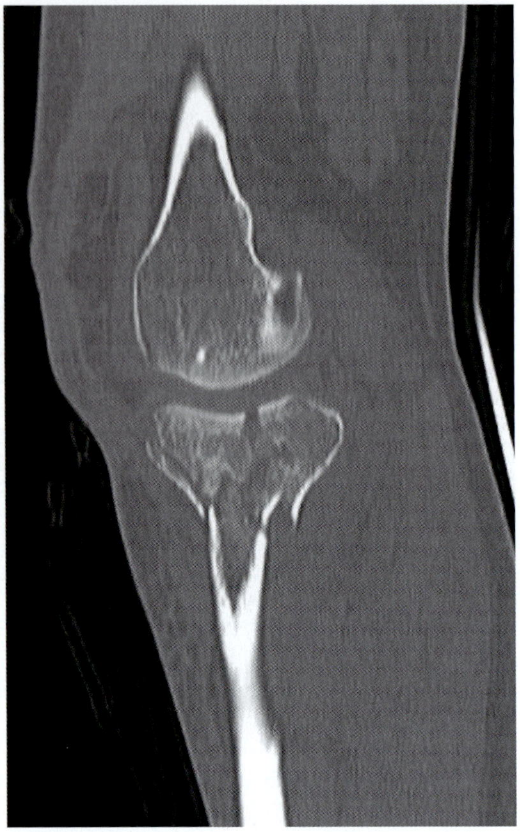

Figure 23-23 | AP (21) and lateral (22) plain radiographs as well as sagittal CT image (23) of isolated medial plateau fracture. Anterior comminution, depression, and a posteromedial fracture fragment can be identified.

  - AP view with caudal tilt is especially useful when performing fluoroscopic medial joint line reduction (Fig. 23-26).
  - AP and lateral fluoroscopy also confirm graft placement as well as hardware position, especially if more than one plate is needed (Fig. 23-27).

- Posterior medial fracture component
  - Lateral fluoroscopy is especially useful to identify the posterior medial fracture fragment (Fig. 23-28).
  - Clamp application for fracture reduction should confirm fracture reduction on both the AP and lateral fluoroscopic view (Figs. 23-29 and 23-30).
  - The AP fluoroscopic image can be used to confirm both joint reduction as well as proper placement of the plate (Fig. 23-31).
  - The lateral fluoroscopic image is used to confirm reduction and proper placement of the plate (Fig. 23-32).

Independent Tibial Tubercle Fragments

- In some bicondylar tibial plateau fractures, a separate tibial tubercle fracture fragment is present and must be stabilized. The axial and sagittal CT reconstructions best show these fractures[5] (Figs. 23-33 and 23-34).
- Lateral fluoroscopic imaging confirms fracture reduction and proper hardware placement (Fig. 23-35).

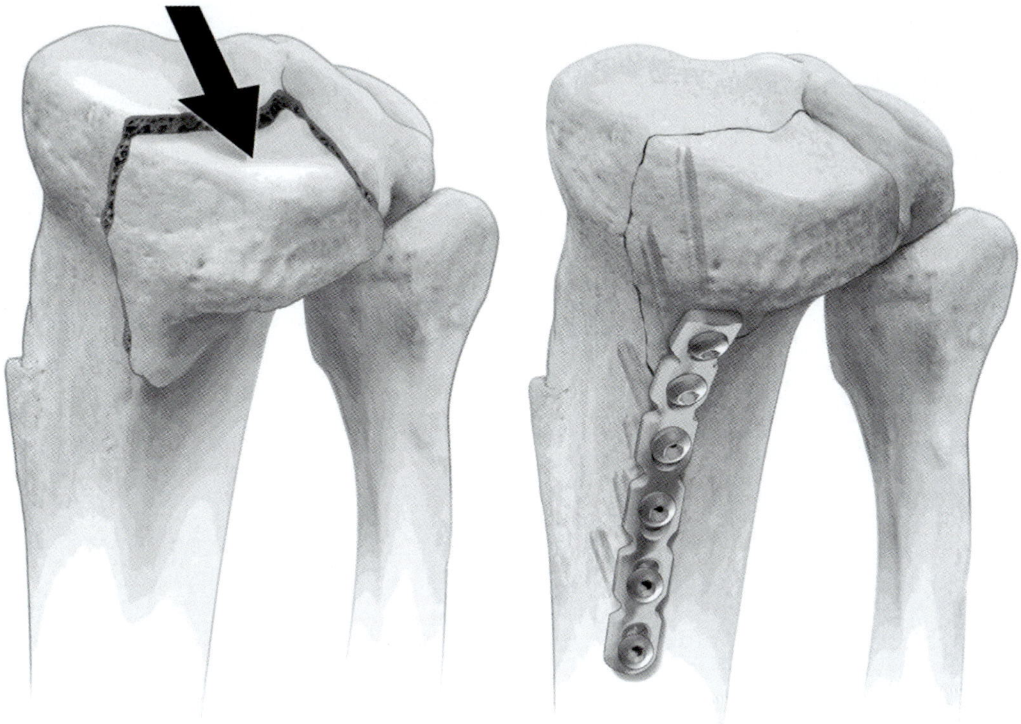

Figure 23-24 I The medial plateau coronal shear fragment is not amenable to reliable fixation from standard lateral plating constructs and often requires its own direct approach, reduction, and buttress plate fixation. Plate placement is based on the fracture orientation. An undercontoured plate positioned proximal to the apex of the fracture is often helpful for reduction with the first screw placed just below the fracture line. The posteromedial pes anserine tendons and origins of the popliteus and flexor digitorum longus muscles may require mobilization for access to the fracture and for plating. Fluoro images should demonstrate restoration of the concave medial joint line.

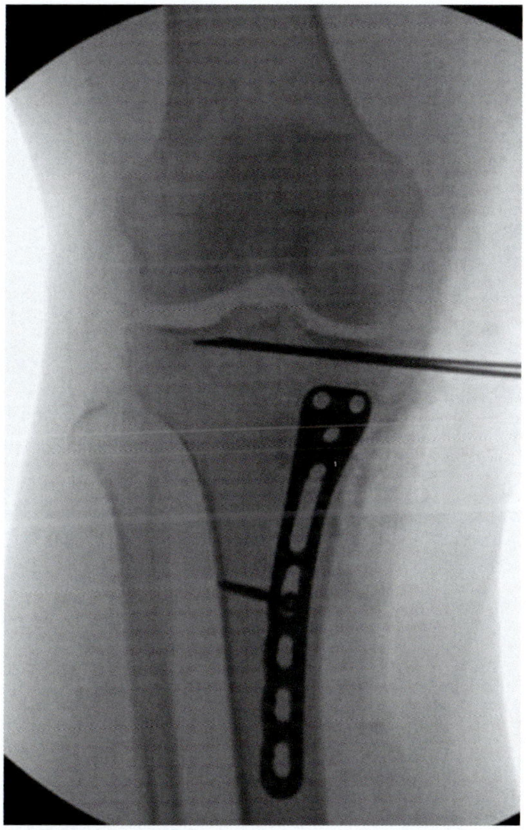

Figure 23-25 I AP view showing provisional Kirschner wire reduction of the medial joint line along with posteromedial plate.

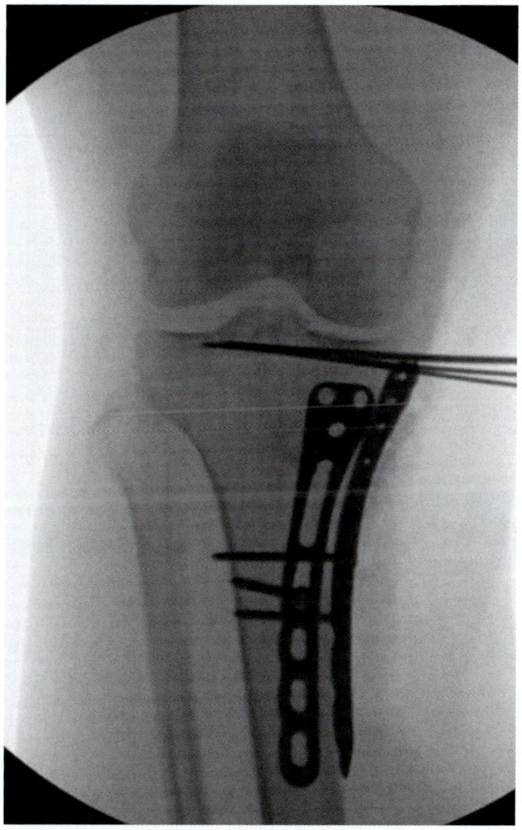

Figure 23-26 I AP view confirming joint reduction, Kirschner wire placement, and placement of supporting direct medial plate.

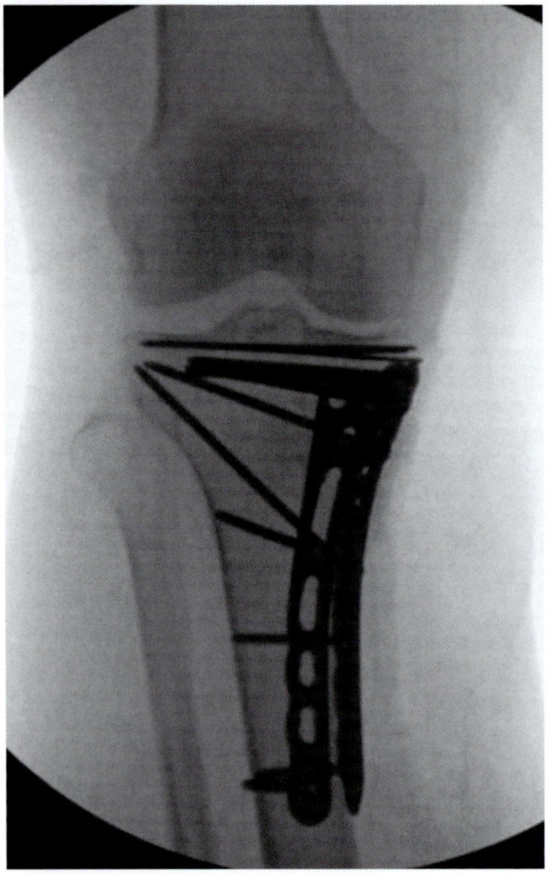

Figure 23-27 | AP view showing dual plate fixation of medial plateau fracture. Kirschner wires have been cut and purposely left in a subchondral position to support the medial joint line.

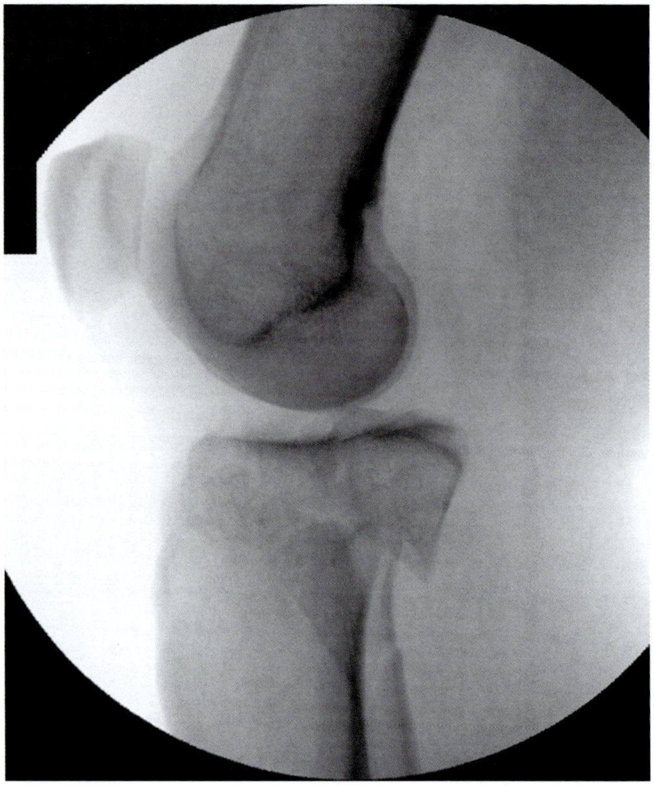

Figure 23-28 | Lateral view of bicondylar tibial plateau fracture showing displaced posteromedial fracture fragment.

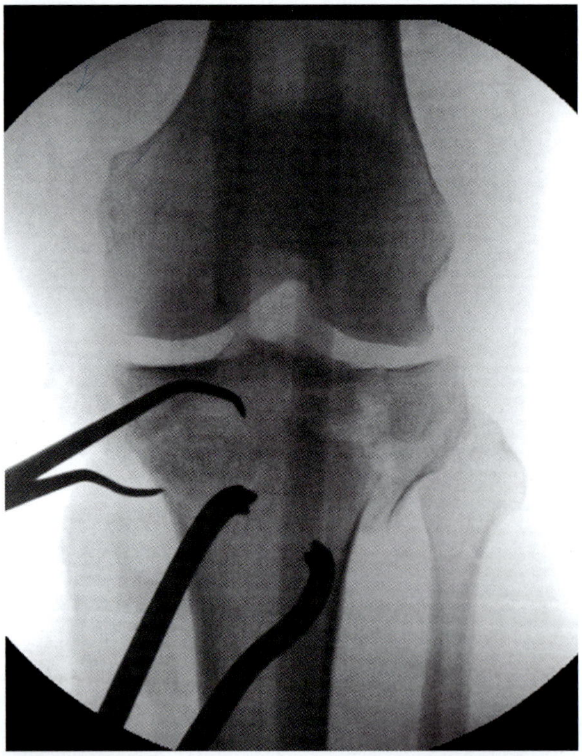

Figure 23-29 | AP (29) and lateral (30) view showing dual clamp reduction of medial plateau component of bicondylar tibial plateau fracture.

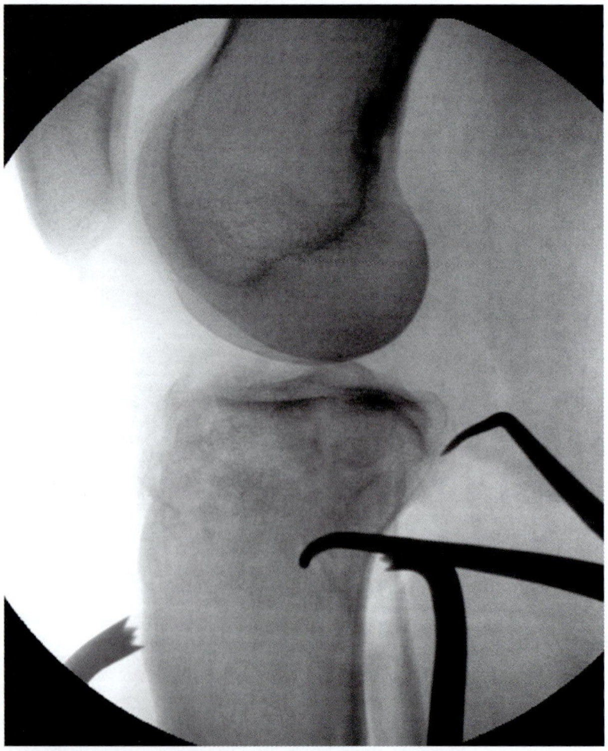

Figure 23-30 | AP (29) and lateral (30) view showing dual clamp reduction of medial plateau component of bicondylar tibial plateau fracture.

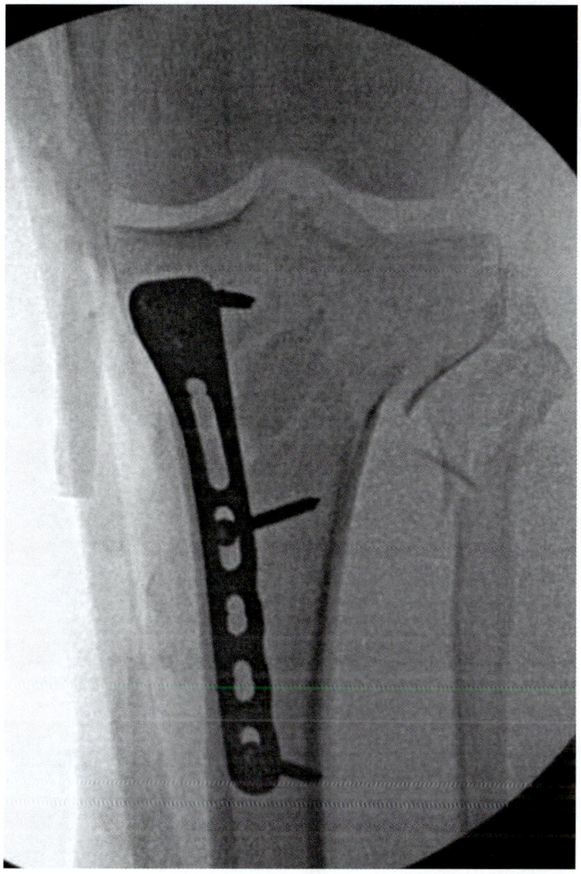

Figure 23-31 | AP (31) and lateral (32) views showing reduction and fixation of posteromedial tibial plateau prior to fixation of lateral plateau.

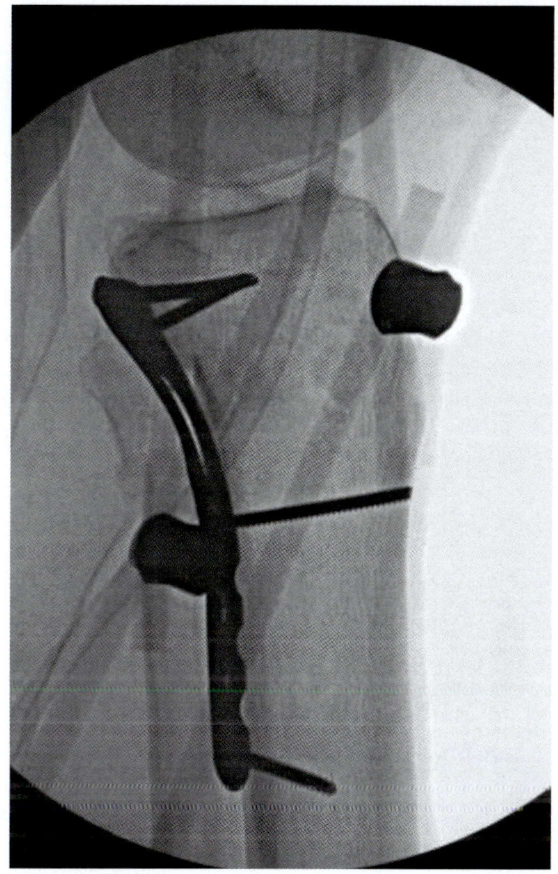

Figure 23-32 | AP (31) and lateral (32) views showing reduction and fixation of posteromedial tibial plateau prior to fixation of lateral plateau.

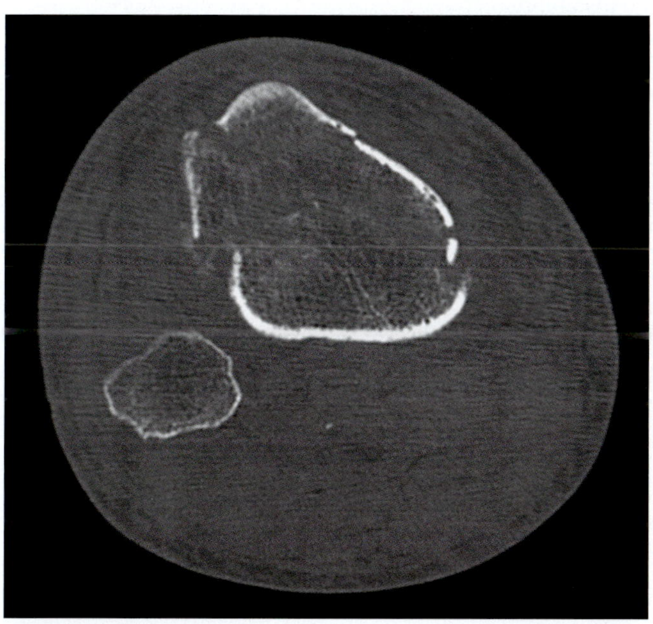

Figure 23-33 | Axial (33) and sagittal (34) CT images showing the independent tibial tubercle fracture fragment component of a bicondylar tibial plateau fracture.

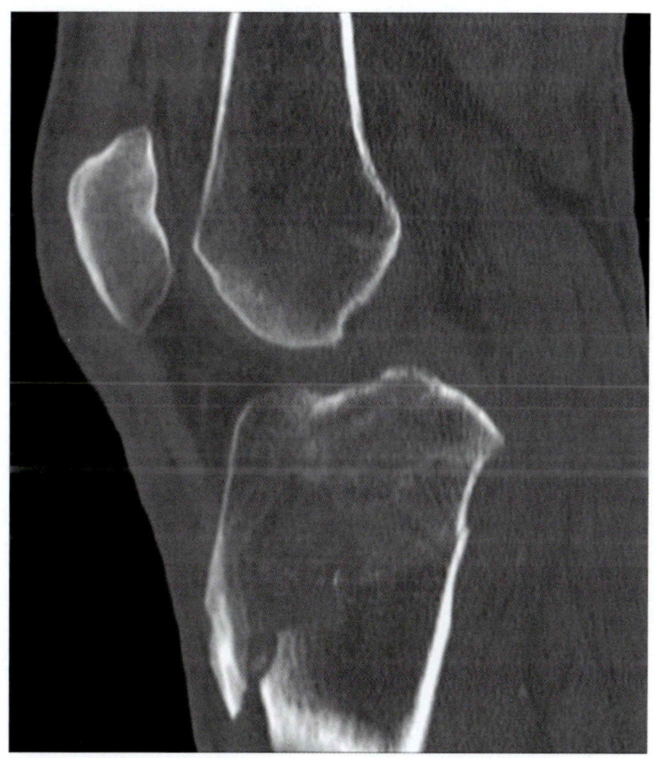

Figure 23-34 | Axial (33) and sagittal (34) CT images showing the independent tibial tubercle fracture fragment component of a bicondylar tibial plateau fracture.

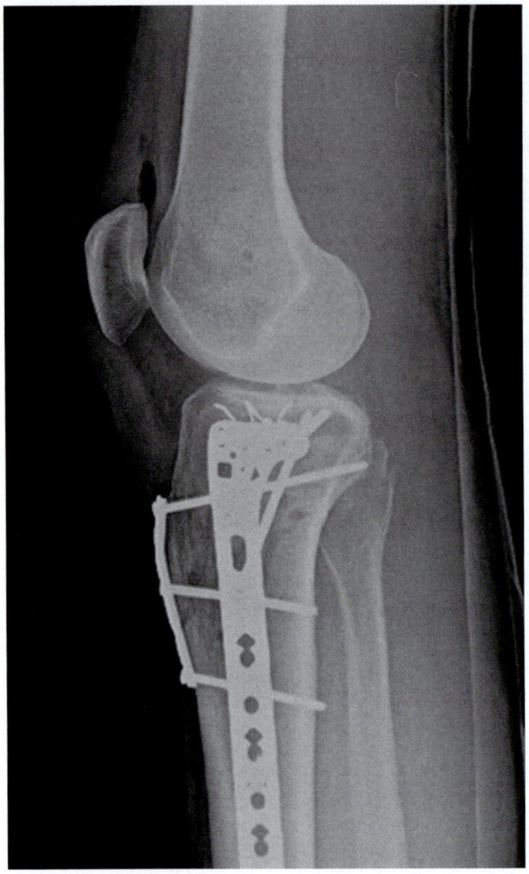

Figure 23-35 | Lateral plain radiograph of anterior plate fixation of the tibial tubercle fracture fragment (typically a 2.7 mm minifragment or 3rd tubular plate.

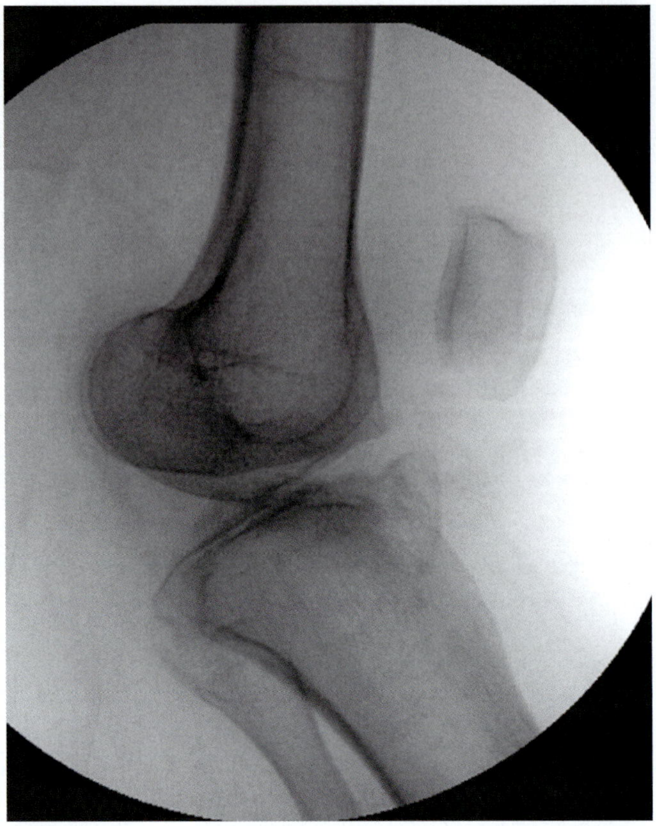

Figure 23-36 | Lateral view of small anterior tibial plateau fracture with hyperextension/recurvatum instability.

Injury Instability

- Intraoperative fluoroscopy can be used to evaluate knee stability. Gentle application of varus or valgus stress can determine coronal plane instability.
- Subtle anterior plateau fractures often represent severe hyperextension injuries; this instability is represented by excessive recurvatum and can be easily seen with examination under fluoroscopy (Fig. 23-36).

References

1. Cinotti G, Sessa P, Ragusa G, et al. Influence of cartilage and menisci on the sagittal slope of the tibial plateaus. *Clin Anat.* 2013;26(7):883–892.
2. Chan PS, Klimkiewicz JJ, Luchetti WT, et al. Impact of CT scan on treatment plan and fracture classification of tibial plateau fractures. *J Orthop Trauma.* 1997;11(7):484–489.
3. Haller JM, O'Toole R, Graves M, et al. How much articular displacement can be detected using fluoroscopy for tibial plateau fractures? *Injury.* 2015;46(11):2243–2247.
4. Barei DP, O'Mara TJ, Taitsman LA, et al. Frequency and fracture morphology of the posteromedial fragment in bicondylar tibial plateau fracture patterns. *J Orthop Trauma.* 2008;22(3):176–182.
5. Maroto MD, Scolaro JA, Henley MB, et al. Management and incidence of tibial tubercle fractures in bicondylar fractures of the tibial plateau. *Bone Joint J.* 2013;95-B(12):1697–1702.

Chapter 24
Tibial Shaft Fractures

ADAM JOHANNSEN
ADAM ADLER
MICHAEL J. GARDNER

Bony Anatomy

- The tibia is a long bone with a neutral coronal and sagittal axis but occasionally prone to variations in the tibial bow (where extreme variants of bow may prevent the use of an intramedullary nail).
- Triangular in shape, the anterior tibial crest is useful in determining alignment/rotation.
- There are wide proximal and distal metaphyseal regions where associated fractures require diligent reduction sequences to prevent malunion (especially with intramedullary nailing). In contrast, the tibial diaphysis is more consistently tubular with thick cortices and an isthmus (located within the distal third) that limits nail diameter.
- Adequate AP and lateral views of the tibial plateau must be obtained to achieve proper nailing start points (medial to the lateral tibial spine on AP view and just at the anterior edge of the articular surface on the lateral view).

Radiographic Anatomy

AP View of the Proximal Tibia

- Proper rotation must be obtained by demonstrating the patella centered over the femoral condyles, one-third fibula overlap at the proximal tibiofibular joint, and well-visualized tibial spines and plateau.[1]
- Correction of apex anterior and valgus deformity in proximal tibia fractures may be necessary with closed or percutaneous methods to assist in adequate imaging and fracture reduction (Fig. 24-1).

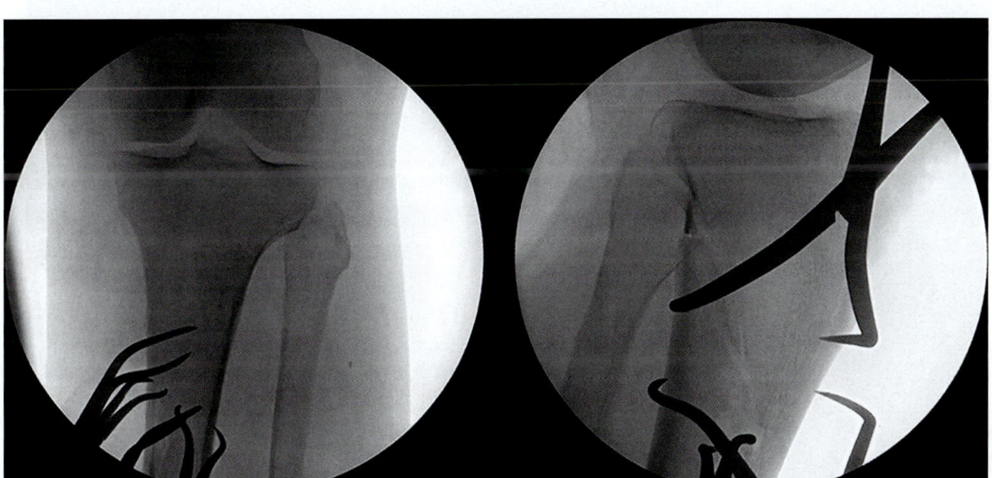

Figure 24-1 | Post-reduction AP and lateral imaging of a proximal third tibial shaft fracture.

Lateral View of the Proximal Tibia

- Proper rotation is confirmed by overlap of the femoral condyles and tibial plateau cortices (Fig. 24-2).
- It is important to ensure that the tibial tubercle and anterior articular margin are well visualized when intramedullary fixation is chosen as the optimal start point is just at the anterior articular edge.

AP View of the Distal Tibia/Fibula

- This image is utilized for proper guidewire placement (centered in the tibia at physeal scar), assessment of rotation, implant placement, and assessment of interlock screw length and ankle alignment (Fig. 24-3).
- The mortise view of the ankle has 15-degree internal rotation from an AP image of the knee. This can be useful to assist in rotational assessment. If syndesmosis is intact, tibiofibular overlap, the incisura, and fibular length (using dime sign) can all be used as markers to aide in fracture reduction. Syndesmotic stress exams should be performed in distal third tibial fractures (Fig. 24-4).

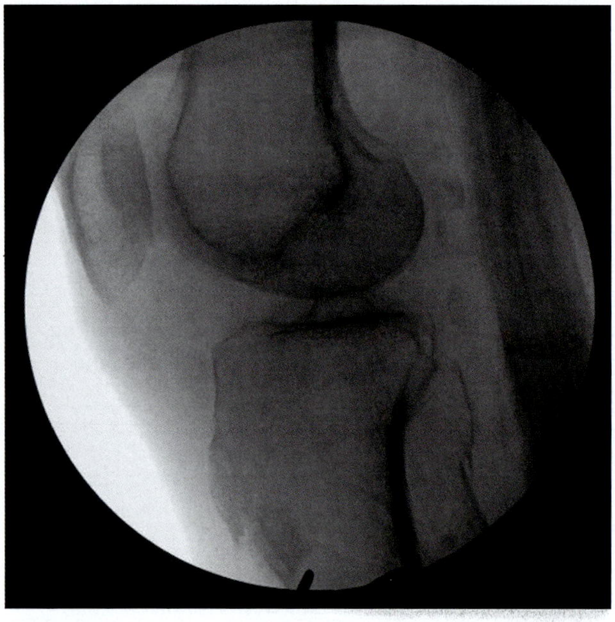

Figure 24-2 | Overlap of tibial articular surfaces and femoral condyles is key to a proper lateral knee image.

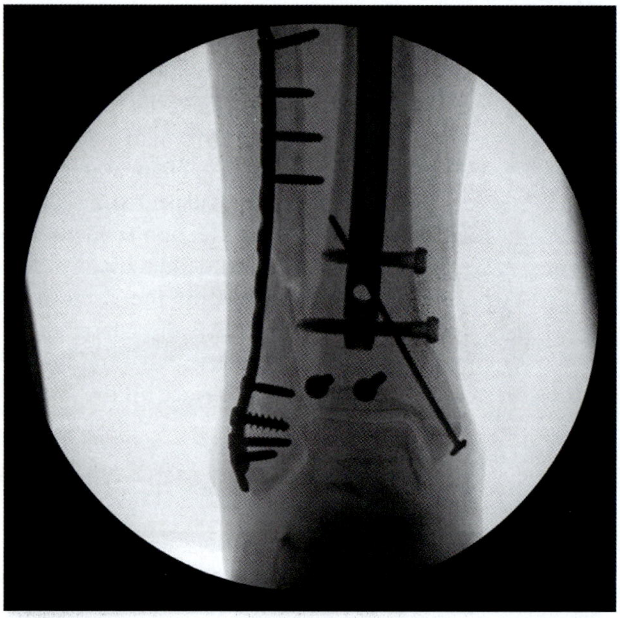

Figure 24-3 |

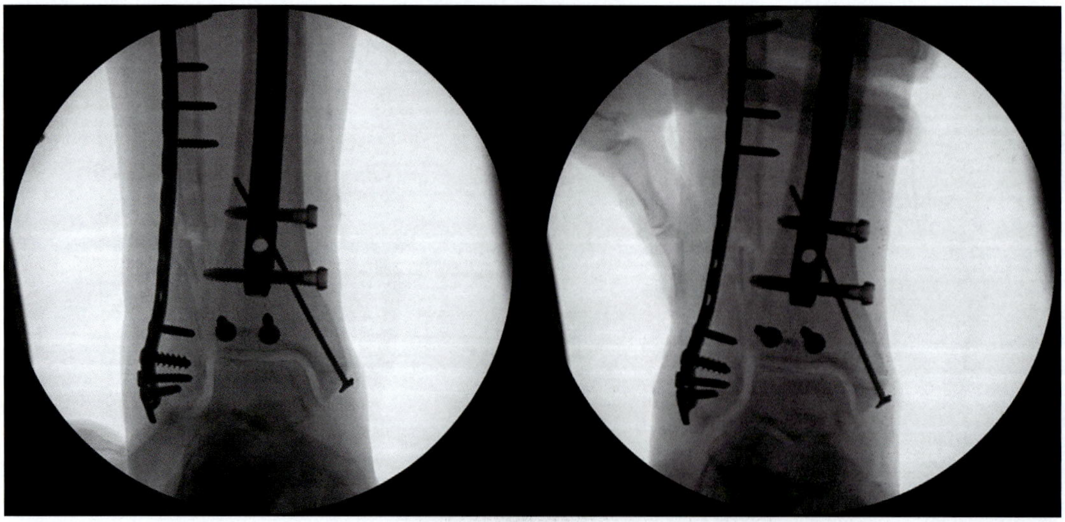

Figure 24-4 | Baseline (*left*) and stress (*right*) mortise ankle films after fixation of tibia and fibula fractures.

Lateral View of the Distal Tibia

- A proper lateral of the ankle should demonstrate a perfect "dome" lateral projection of the talus, which depicts a lateral of the tibial physeal scar and about 50% tib/fib overlap. This is important for the perfect circle distal interlock technique and to ensure adequate reduction, rotation, and ankle alignment (Fig. 24-5).

Preoperative Imaging

- AP and lateral imaging of the entire tibia and fibula is critical for assessing the overall deformity, comminution, and fracture pattern. These images are the mainstay for preoperative planning (Figs. 24-6 and 24-7).
- Dedicated XR imaging of the knee and ankle is important to determine intra-articular extension, isolated posterior malleolus fractures (oblique or spiral distal tibia fractures),[2] or other associated pathology (Figs. 24-8 and 24-9).

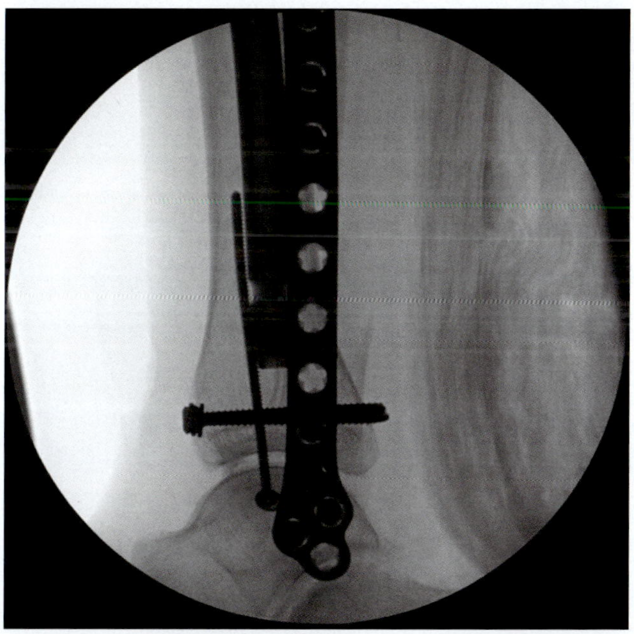

Figure 24-5 | Note that post-fixation hardware can occasionally obscure visualization. In these instances, obliques may be utilized for confirmation of screw length and anatomic reduction.

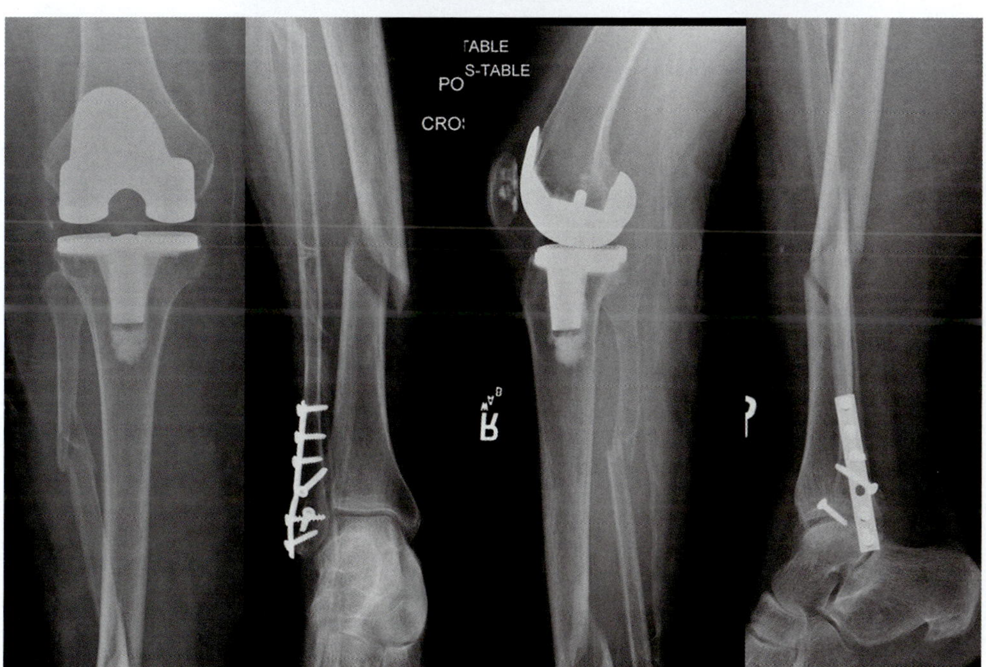

Figure 24-6 | Note that implants above or below may influence surgical planning and implant selection. In this case, the tibial arthroplasty component prevented optimal access for tibial nail insertion in this osteoporotic fracture, thereby necessitating open reduction internal fixation and a neutralization plate protecting the remainder of the tibia.

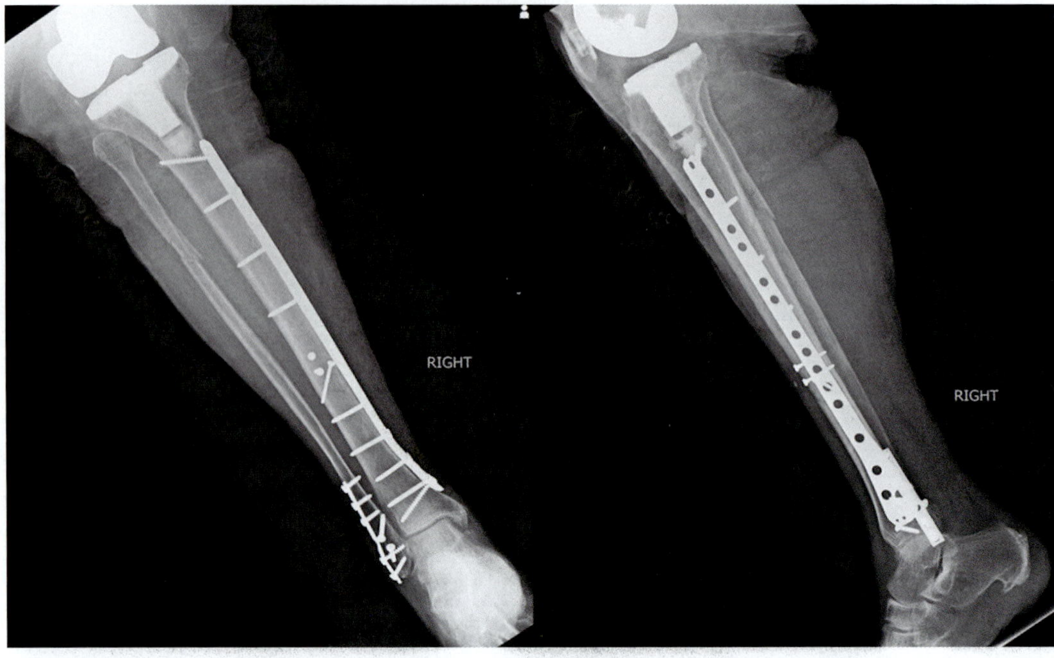

Figure 24-7 | Full length tibia XR's demonstrating total knee arthroplasty hardware limiting the approach for a intramedullary nail. In these instances, minimally invasive reduction and plate fixation may be more easily applied.

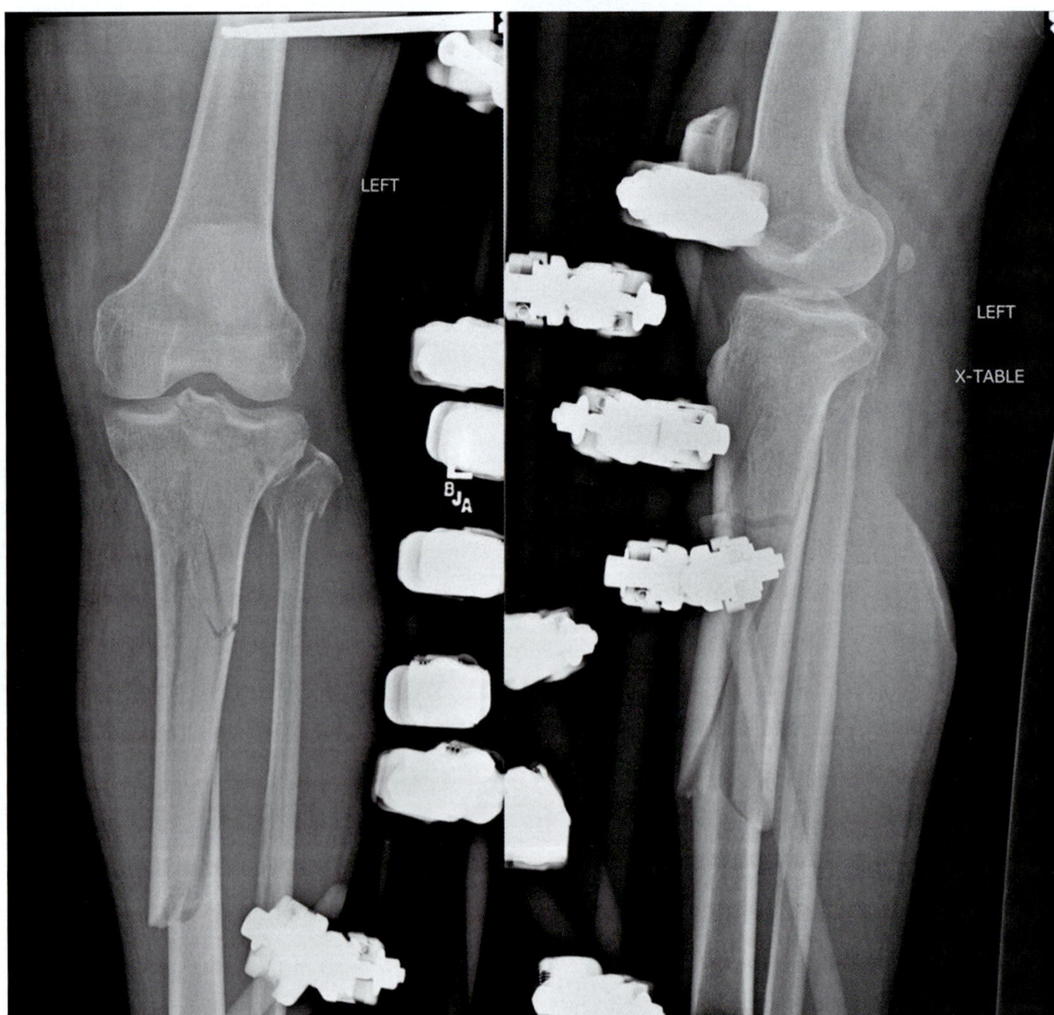

Figure 24-8 | Note the comminution to this proximal tibia fracture having both a plateau and shaft component. This was amenable to compression and plate fixation of the plateau with nail stabilization of the diaphysis.

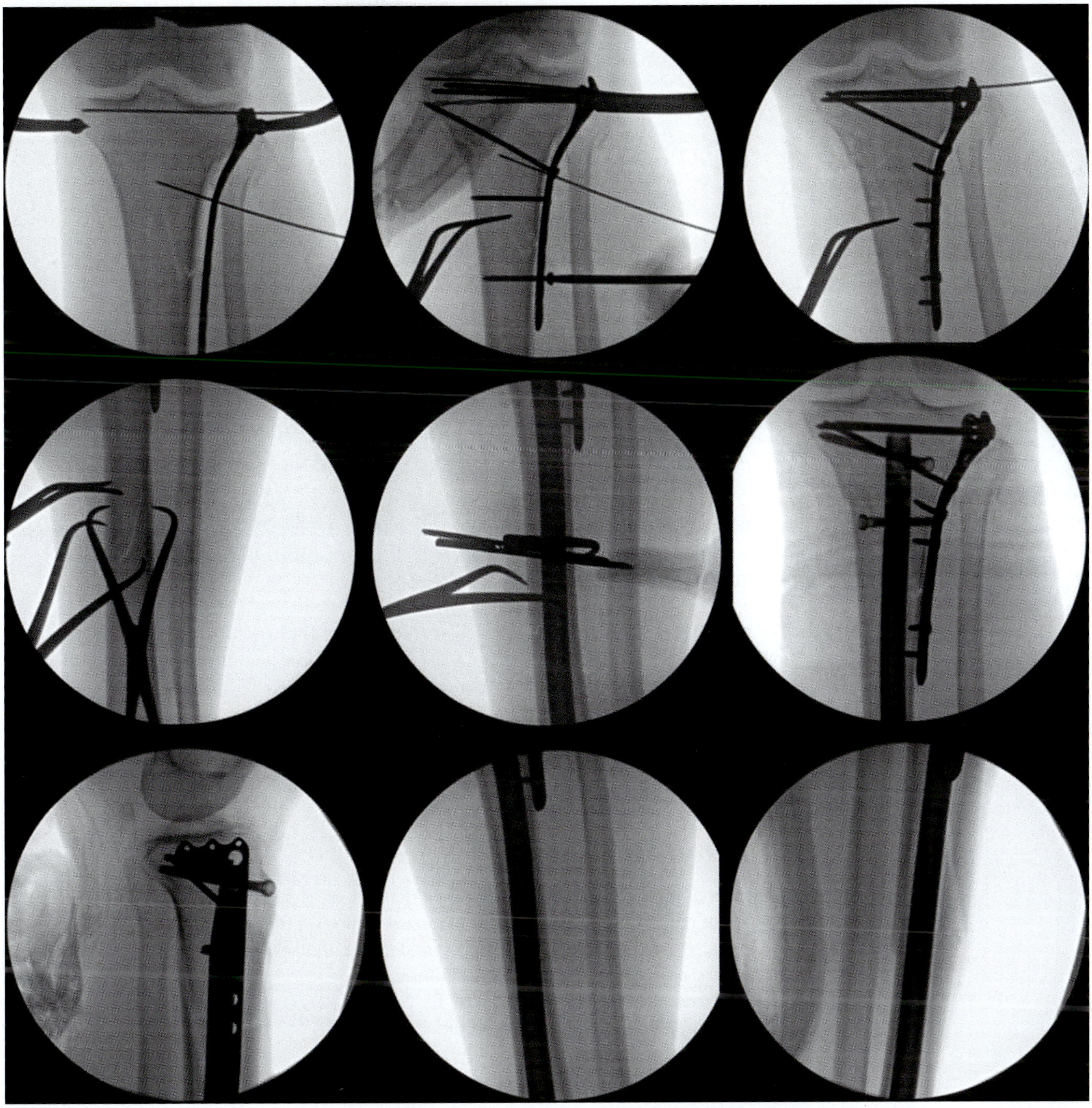

Figure 24-9 | Note the sequence of fixation of the articular surface, followed by independent treatment of the tibial shaft fracture with an intramedullary implant.

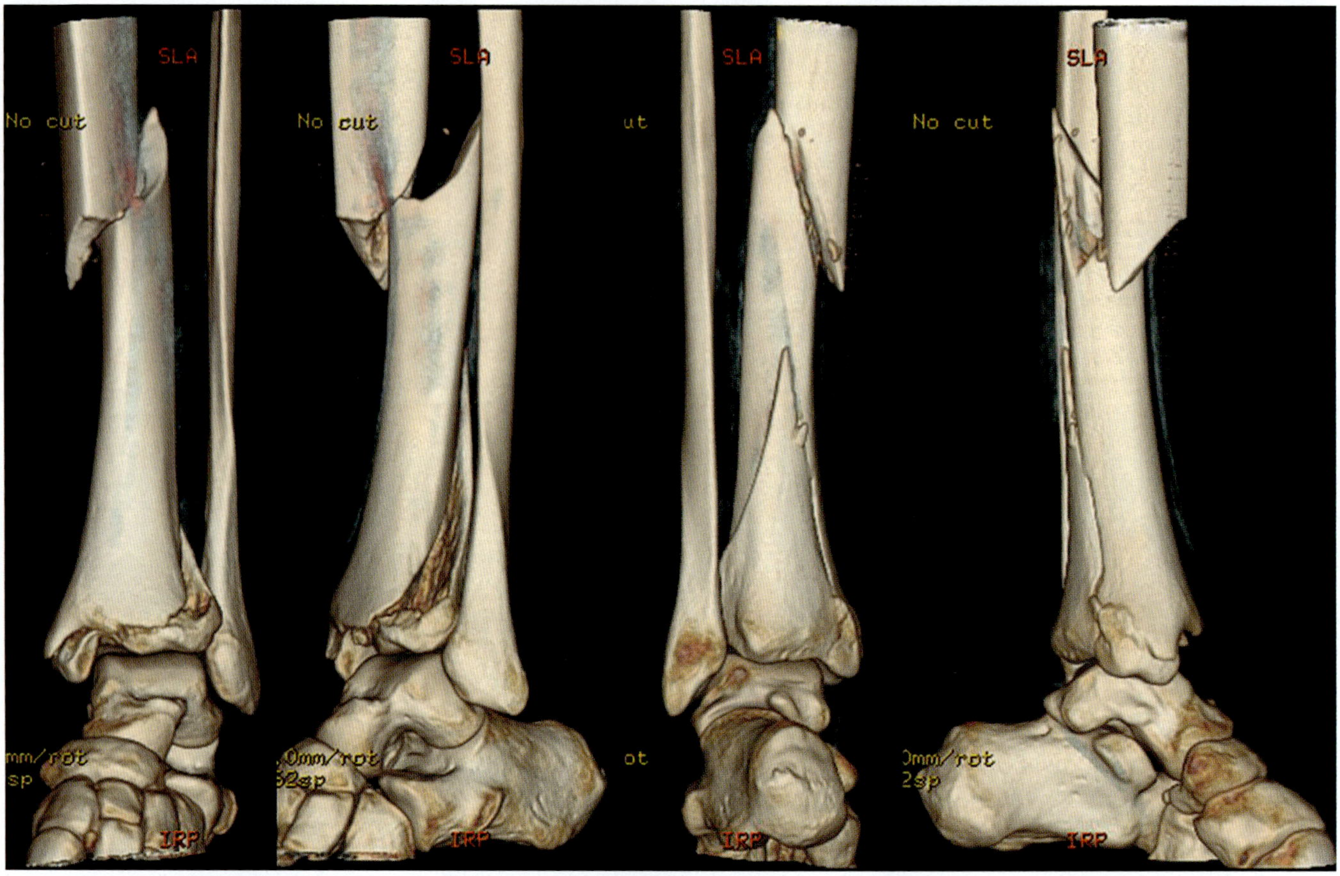

Figure 24-10 | Despite a distal tibial fracture component, careful assessment of this CT scan demonstrated insight for the proper clamp vectors for reduction and fixation with distal lag screws and intramedullary nail stabilization.

- Consider CT imaging to assess for occult articular fractures, or limited cuts to determine alignment and rotation. CT imaging may also assist in preoperative planning (reduction and fixation techniques) (Figs. 24-10 and 24-11A and B).
- Consider AP and lateral imaging of contralateral leg with measurement device to assess length, alignment, and rotation for comminuted or length unstable injuries.
- Calibrated diameter measurements of orthogonal views of the isthmus can aid preoperative planning nail diameter.

Intraoperative Positioning Tips

- Supine patient with a bump under ipsilateral hip so that patella is positioned directly anterior
- Cantilever-type OR table with radiolucent diving board extension for C-arm access
- Note that there are several positioning methods that depend upon the following:
  - The fracture pattern (articular, diaphyseal, or combined)
  - Selected fixation method (IMN vs. plate vs. ex-fix vs. ring fixator)
  - Infrapatellar versus suprapatellar or semiextended nailing
  - Associated injuries or fractures
  - Patient body habitus

Infrapatellar (Transpatellar or Medial/Lateral Parapatellar) IMN Approach in Flexed Position

- Supine, bump under ipsilateral hip.
- Radiolucent triangle.
- Fluoroscopic imaging is more tedious, and tech dependent as axial tilt must be changed between AP and lateral images.

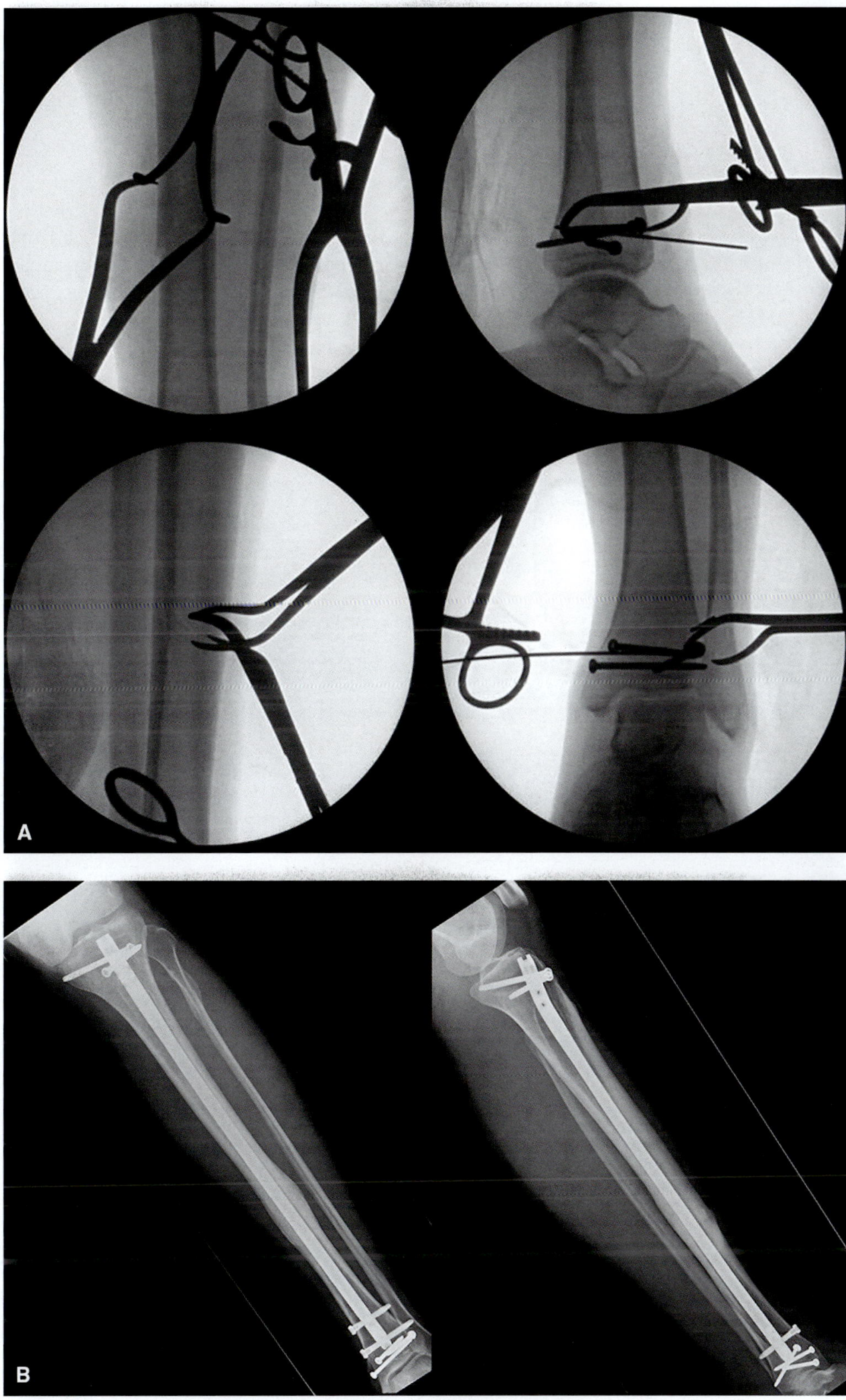

Figure 24-11 | Intraoperative imaging **(A)** and postoperative imaging **(B)** of a distal tibia fracture with intra-articular extension treated with independent leg screws and an intramedullary implant.

- AP imaging in flexed position
  - Proximal tibia
    - Axial C-arm tilt is necessary to match the tibial plateau, but this is often limited by overlap with the distal femur and tilt of the C-arm with respect to table height (requiring some extension to achieve image) (Fig. 24-12).
  - AP of fracture site
    - Used when determining adequacy of reduction, passing of guidewire, reaming, and final implant placement.
    - After optimal rotation of the fracture is assessed with clinical exam and imaging of the proximal and distal tibia, the fluoroscope rotation should not change in order to minimize the risk of malrotation. The only exception is the 15-degree external rotation view for a proper mortise image at the ankle.
  - Distal tibia
    - Axial tilt to match tibial plafond. Again, tilt may be limited by the degree of knee flexion and C-arm tilt/table height (Fig. 24-13).
    - Rotation to show AP and mortise views of the ankle (incisura, medial malleolus, lateral malleolus, dime sign).

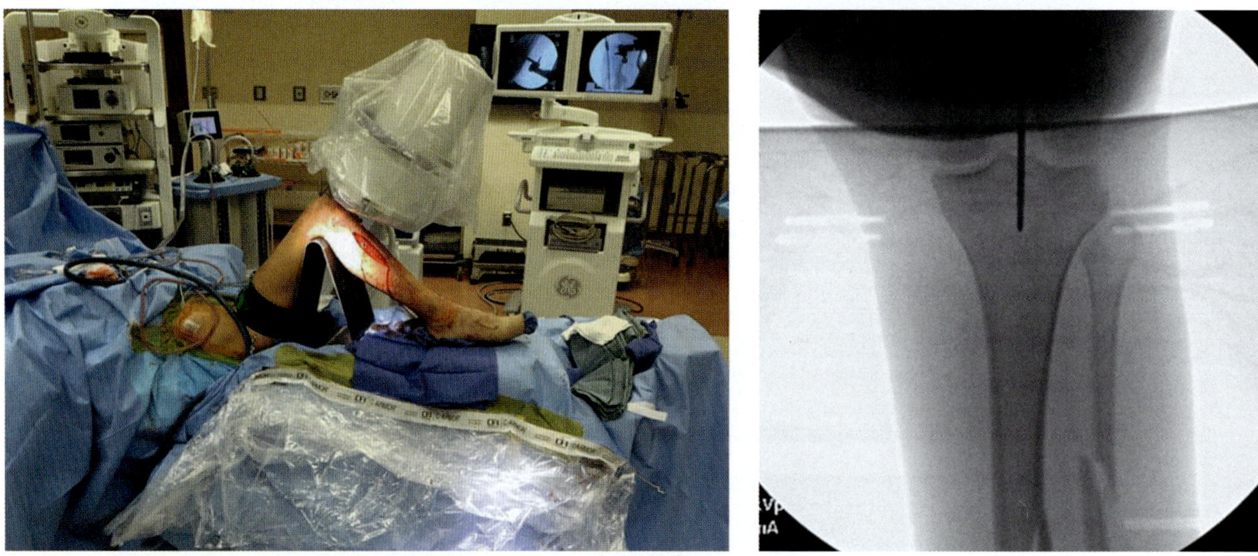

Figure 24-12 | Proper rotation must be obtained by demonstrating the patella centered over the femoral condyles, one-third fibula overlap at the proximal tibiofibular joint, and well-visualized tibial spines and plateau.

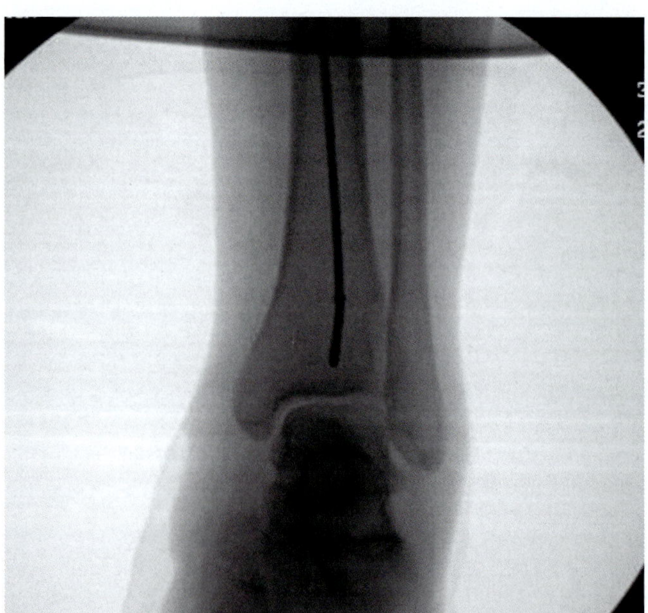

Figure 24-13 | AP image of the ankle confirming proper guidewire placement in the center of the distal tibia.

- Lateral imaging in the flexed position
  - Often, it is best to lock C-arm in direct lateral position and adjust leg (abduction-adduction and rotation) to fit proper orientation in order to minimize risk of malrotation.
  - Proximal tibia
    - Must correct axial rotation on C-arm to rotate to lateral image (mark on floor and machine proper positioning for each image).
    - Assess image quality with femoral condyle overlap, lateral of patella, articular overlap of tibial plateau (Fig. 24-14).
    - In proximal fractures, apex anterior and valgus deformities can make adequate imaging difficult, but this must be obtained via closed or percutaneous methods prior to identifying the appropriate start point.
  - Fracture site
    - Use cortical thickness and fibular length to assess rotation and length.
    - This image may utilize provisional plating or other reduction techniques.
  - Distal tibia
    - Proper lateral of the ankle should demonstrate 50% tib/fib overlap, lateral of physeal scar, perfect lateral of talar dome, and posterior cortex of the fibula aligning with posterior curve of posterior malleolus (Fig. 24-15A and B).

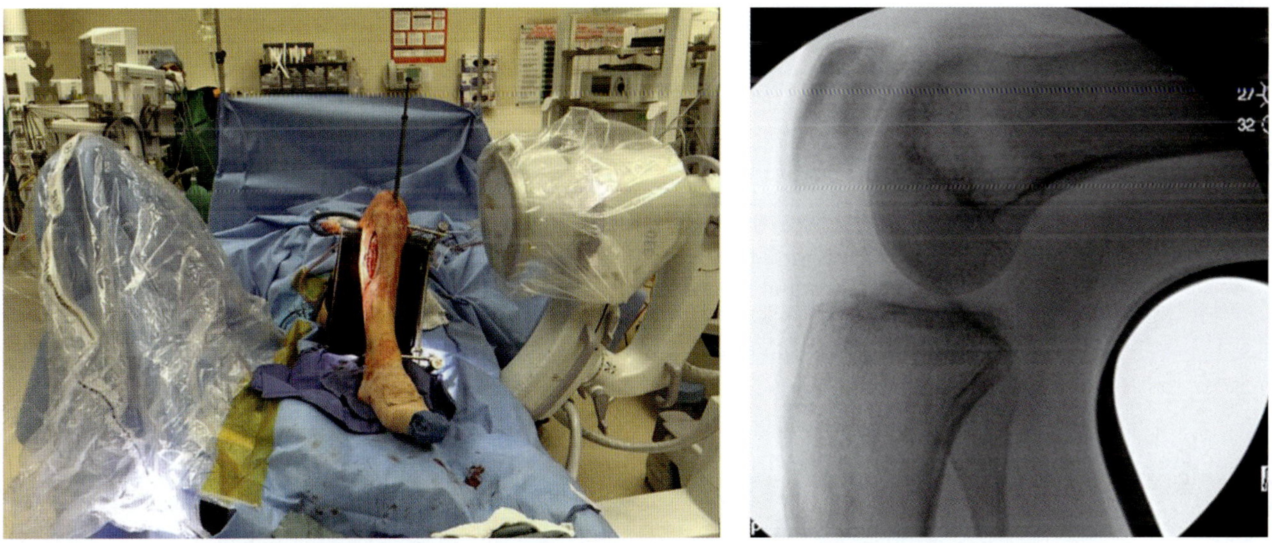

Figure 24-14 | Lateral image of the knee in the hyperflexed position. Note the overlap of the femoral condyles, and parallel appearance of the tibial articular surfaces.

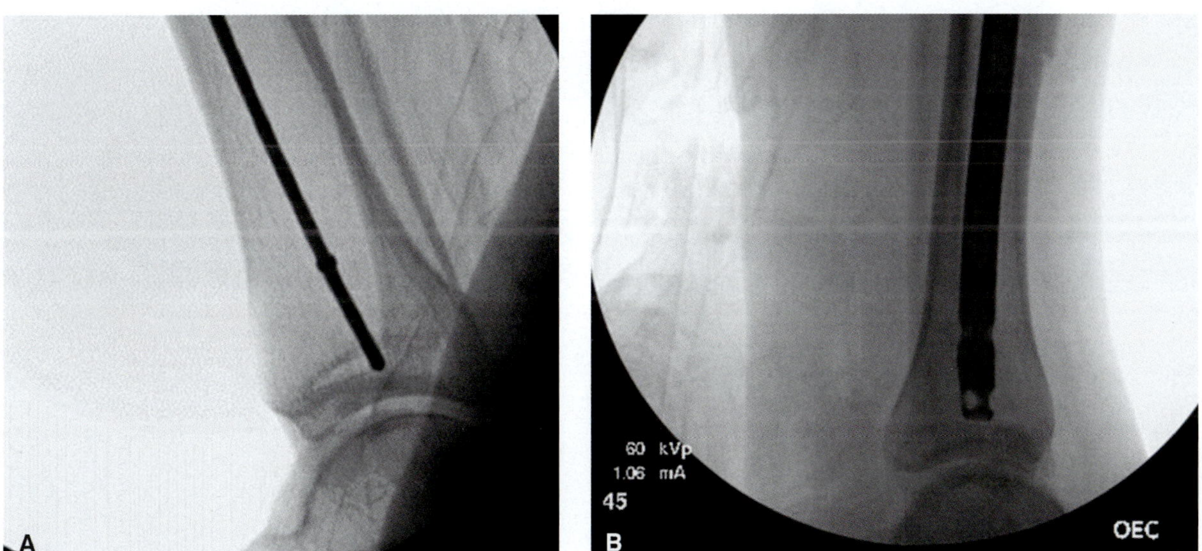

Figure 24-15 | Lateral imaging of the distal tibia demonstrating placement of the intramedullary implant along the course of the guidewire. Burying the guidewire in the subchondral bone will prevent migration or backout during reaming.

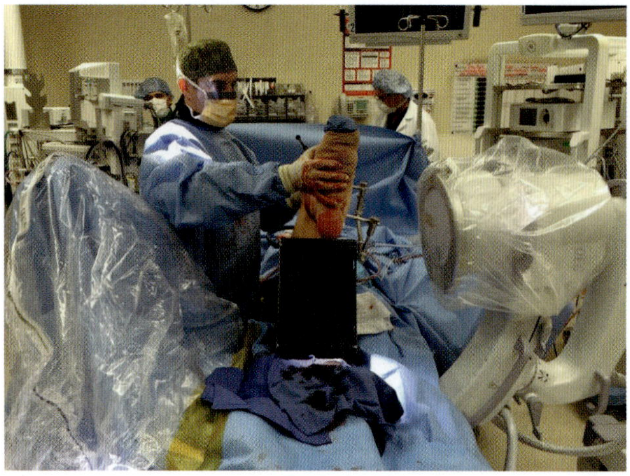

Figure 24-16 | Lateral imaging of the distal tibia in the hyperflexion position of the hip and knee. This is only possible after stability has been achieved at the fracture site.

- Used for perfect circles and to ensure adequate rotation.
- With the C-arm in the lateral position, the surgeon may either flex the hip and knee to obtain a lateral of the distal tibia (assuming stable provisional fixation) (Fig. 24-16), or maintain alignment and move the C-arm distal.

Semiextended (Suprapatellar, Lateral Parapatellar IMN, or Direct Tibial Shaft ORIF) Approach

- Supine patient with a bump under the ipsilateral hip so that patella is directly anterior.
- Bone foam or padded ramp to support proximal and distal to fracture site. Also positions away from contralateral limb for lateral imaging.
- Benefit is that AP and lateral imaging are performed in the same axial tilt to minimize C-arm changes intraoperatively (Figs. 24-17 and 24-18).
- Less fluoro correction is required, often leading to fewer struggles in maintaining reduced alignment.

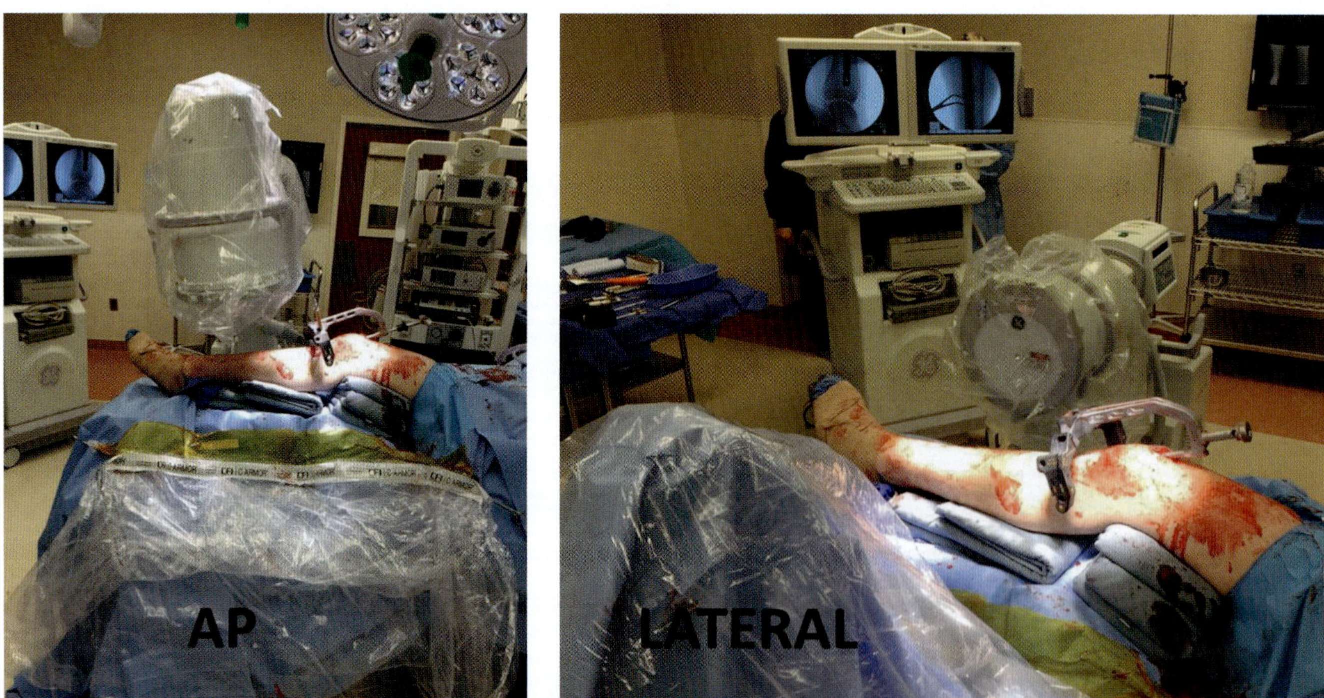

Figure 24-17 | Suprapatellar nailing C-arm positioning.

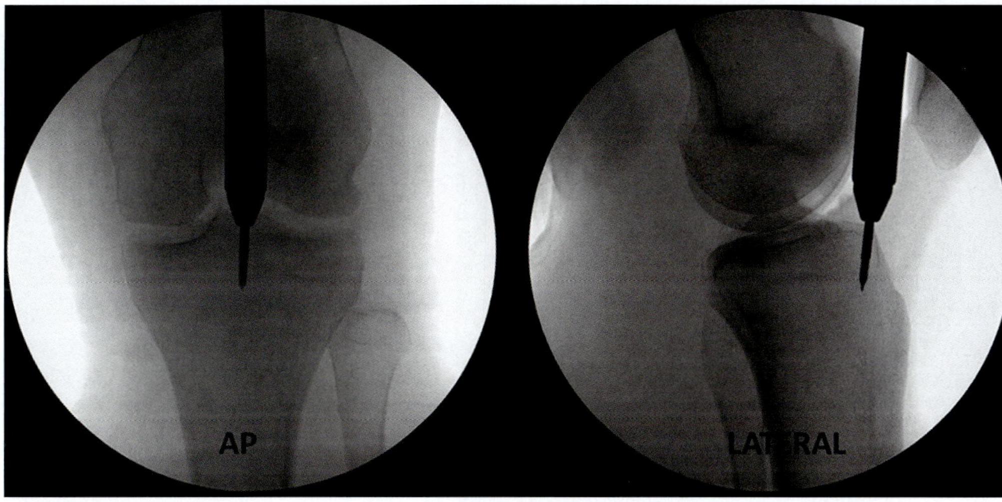

Figure 24-18 | Suprapatellar nailing C-arm fluoro images of ideal start point. Note the semiextended position.

- The semiextended position also creates less deformity in proximal tibia fractures due to decreased tension through patellar tendon and has been found to be an advantageous position for reducing and nailing fractures of the proximal and distal third.
  - AP imaging in semiextended position
    - AP image of proximal tibia
      - Assess image quality with femoral condyle overlap, lateral of patella, articular overlap of tibial plateau (Fig. 24-19).
    - AP image of fracture site
      - This image best assesses for varus/valgus deformity and may be used for percutaneous or open reduction techniques.
    - AP image of the distal tibia
      - Use long clamp or mallet to hold position.
      - If rotating to mortise, rotate C-arm, not leg, to minimize risk of malrotation during imaging.
      - Use this image to assess implant length and distal interlock screw length (Fig. 24-20).
  - Lateral imaging in semiextended position

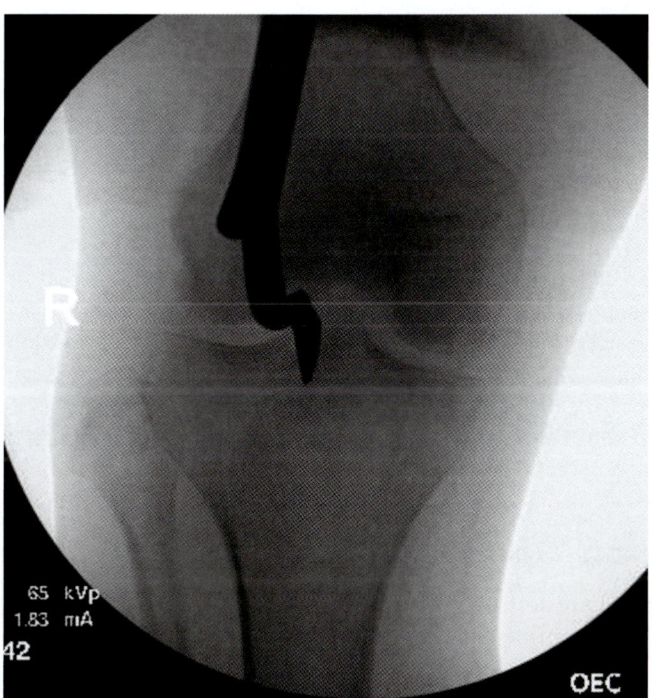

Figure 24-19 | Proper startpoint with the awl in the lateral semi-extended position.

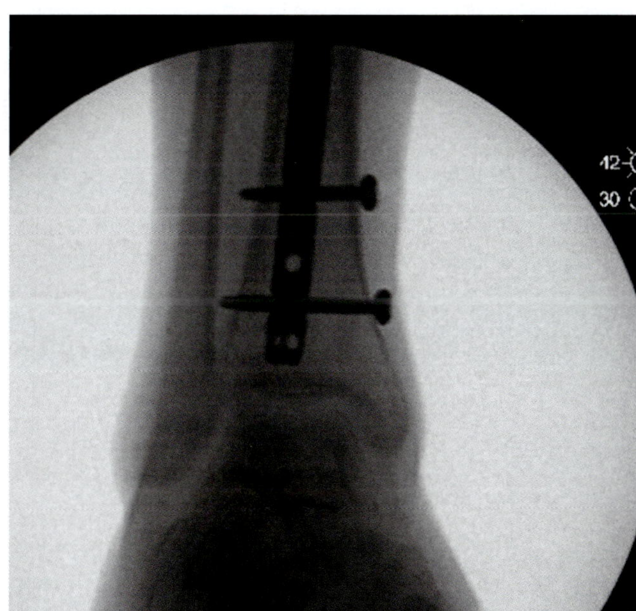

Figure 24-20 | AP imaging of the distal tibia after placement of interlocking screws.

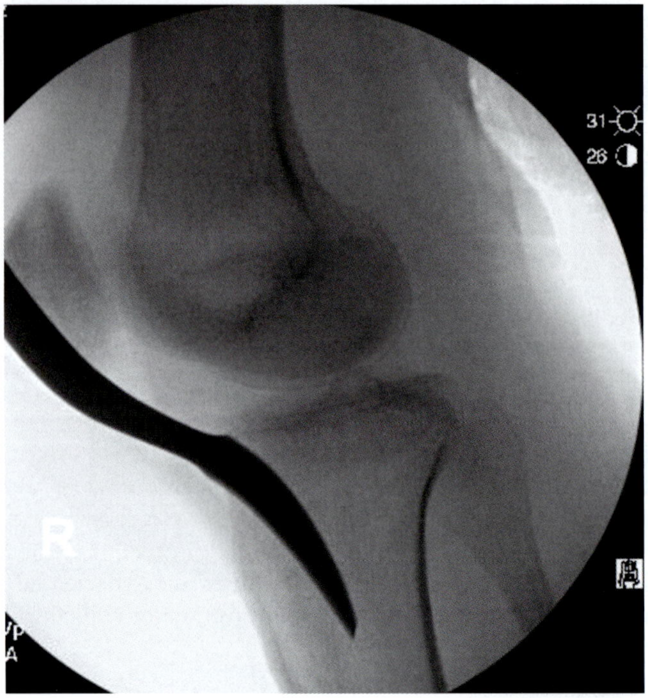

Figure 24-21 | Lateral imaging of the knee confirming proper start point in the lateral semi-extended position.

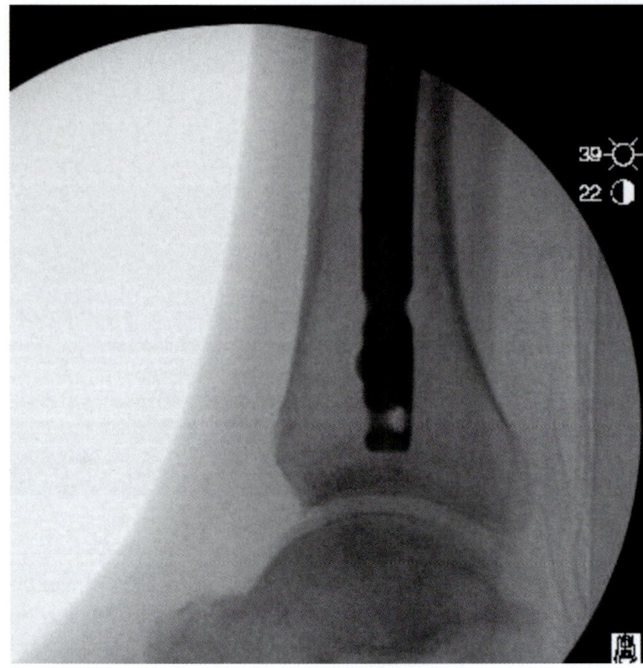

Figure 24-22 | Lateral imaging of the distal tibia confirming proper placement of interlocking screws.

- Lateral image of proximal tibia
  - Do not need to change axial tilt between AP and lateral views.
  - Assess image quality with femoral condyle overlap, lateral of patella, articular overlap of tibial plateau (Fig. 24-21).
  - Must obtain adequate lateral prior to opening reaming of start site.
- Lateral image of fracture site
  - Semiextended position allows gravity to counteract apex anterior forces at fracture site but often requires more traction for adequate length.
- Lateral image of distal tibia
  - Use long clamp or mallet to dorsiflex ankle to neutral. This will ensure perfect lateral of the talus.
  - Image used for perfect circles during fixation of implant or prior to backslapping (Fig. 24-22).

Perfect Circles for Intramedullary Fixation

- Critical for accurate, efficient placement of interlocking screws.
- Small amounts of malrotation or wag can cause oblique or missing drill trajectories.
- Perfect circles should show symmetric shape with no overlapping edges (Fig. 24-23).
- A reliable fluoro sequence for freehand perfect circle distal interlocks is as follows: (1) localize skin incision with perfect circle fluoro technique, (2) localize drill bit orthogonal to IMN with tip 50% across interlock hole, (3) raise drill in opposite orthogonal direction to confirm tip is 50% across hole, (4) advance drill through IMN and confirm before measuring, (5–6) confirm lateral and AP screw location (Fig. 24-24).

Percutaneous Reduction Tips

- Provisional percutaneous clamping can help restore alignment of the tibia with occasional fibular malreduction (red arrow). IMN insertion helps fine-tune restoration of tibial alignment with indirect fibular alignment through an intact interosseous membrane (green arrow) (Fig. 24-25).
- Distal third tibial fractures are usually of a spiral nature requiring reduction sequences to restore alignment. This can be challenging to maintain throughout the reaming and nailing process, especially in the infrapatellar/knee-flexed position (Fig. 24-26).

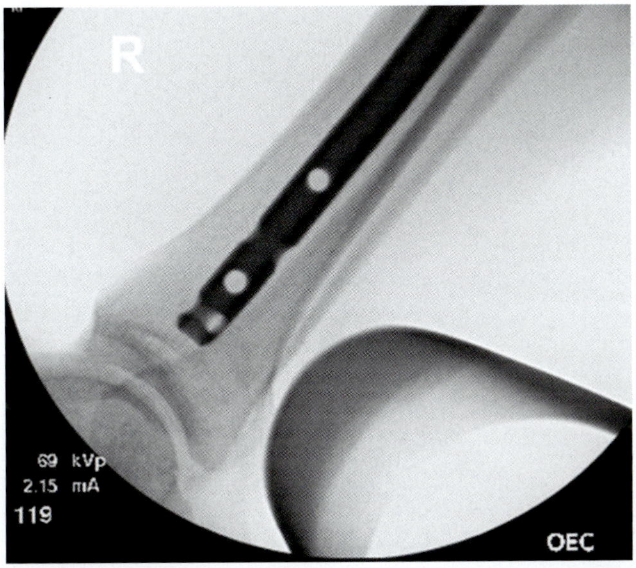

Figure 24-23 | Note the symmetric appearance of perfect circles prior to placement of interlocking screws. This is critical to avoiding improper placement of screws.

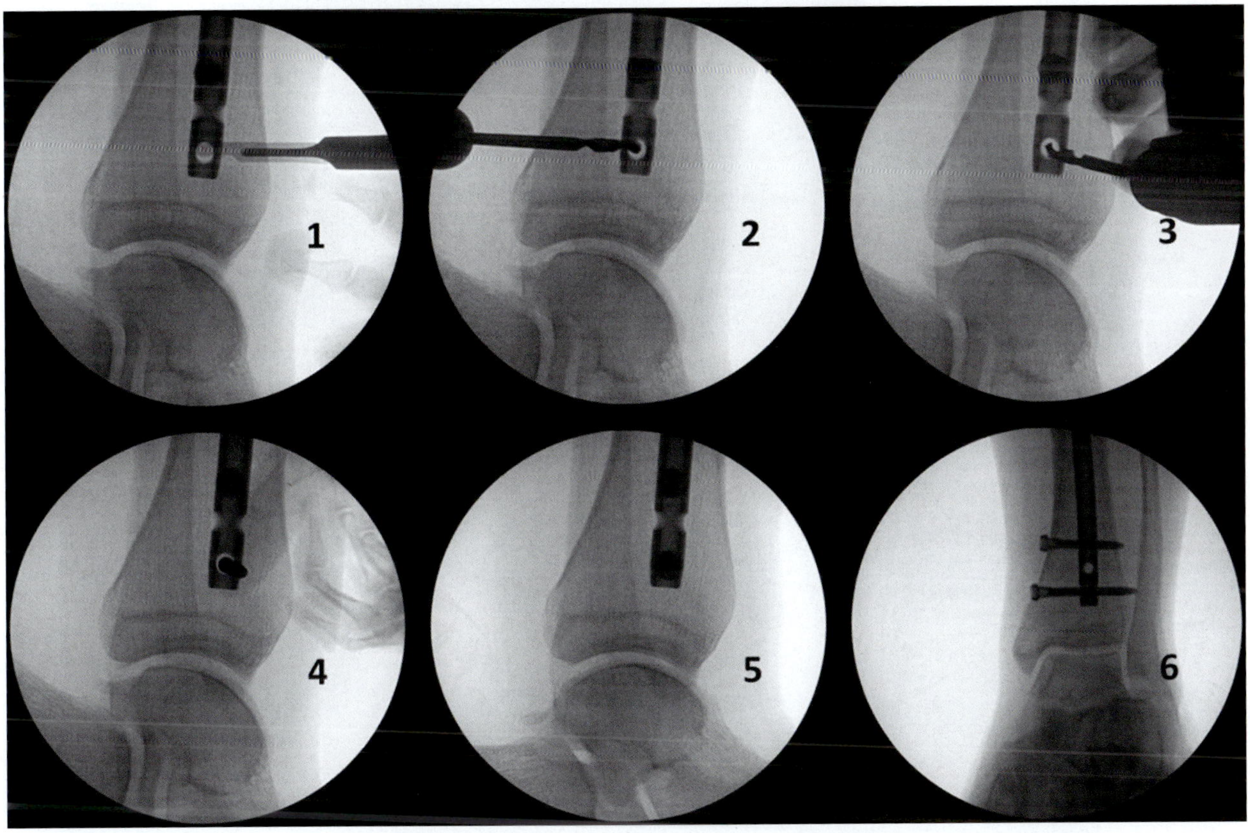

Figure 24-24 | Note the sequence of imaging for placement of interlocking screws using the perfect circle technique.

- The use of a semiextended position and percutaneous clamps at ideal vectors can achieve temporizing reduction to maintain alignment during the nailing process. Notice the sequence of malreduction (red arrows) to reduced (green arrows) that occurs with slight alterations of clamp vector. Supplemental K-wire outside of IMN path allows for additional provisional reduction for reaming and nail insertion. In this case, the lateral malleolar fracture also required plating to restore ankle stability but a stress exam of the syndesmosis did not identify instability (Fig. 24-27).

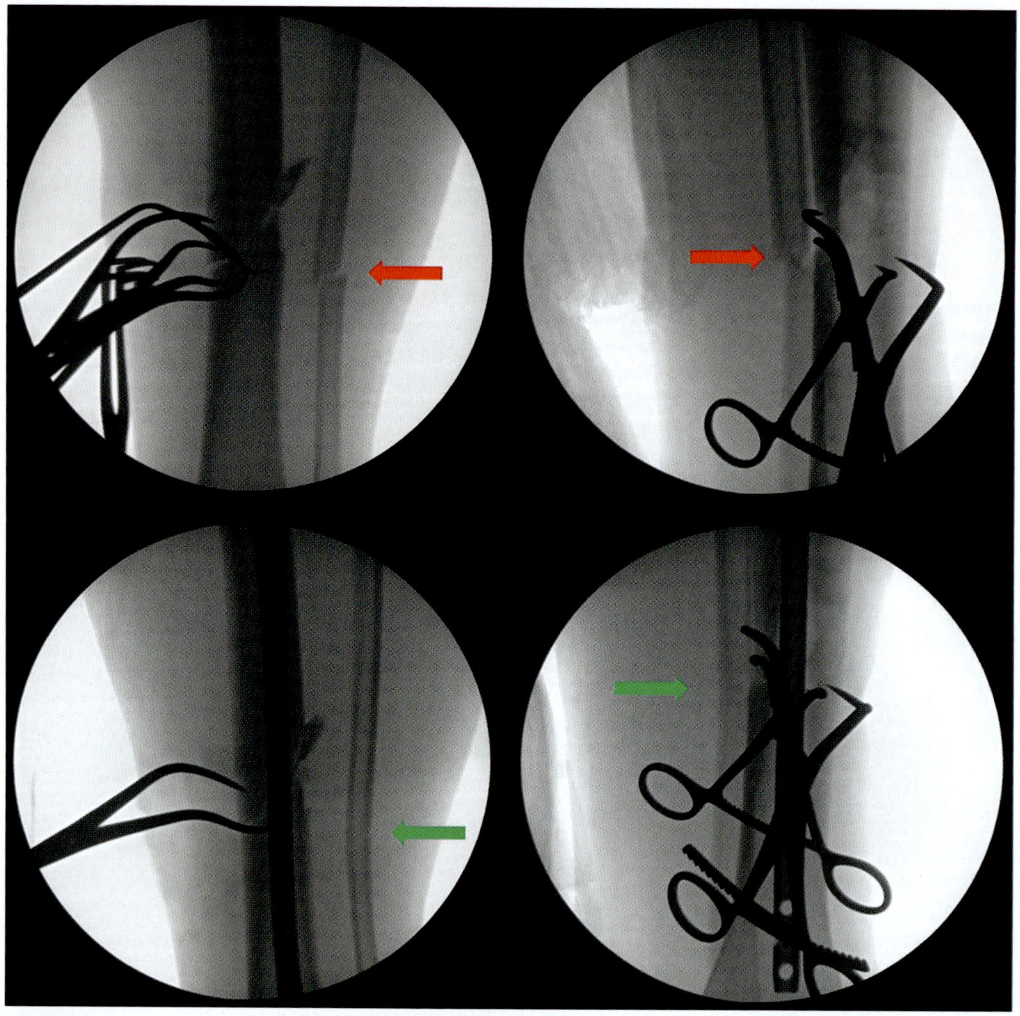

Figure 24-25 | Note the indirect reduction of the fibula once the tibial reduction has been performed.

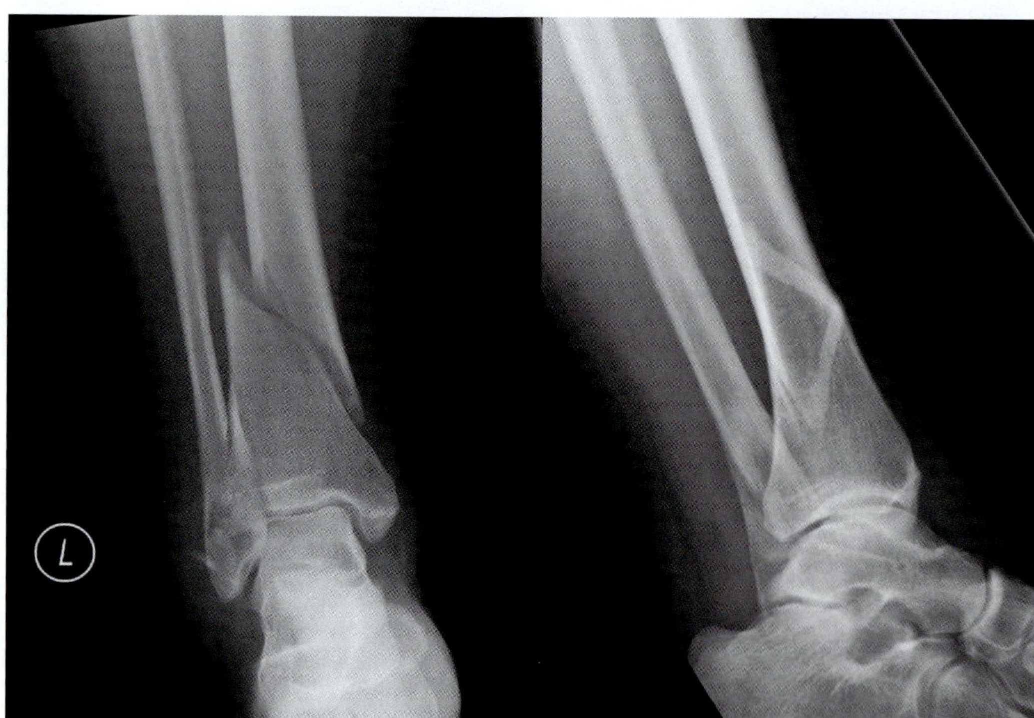

Figure 24-26 | Always carefully assess for an isolated posterior malleolar fracture in distal third spiral tibial fractures.

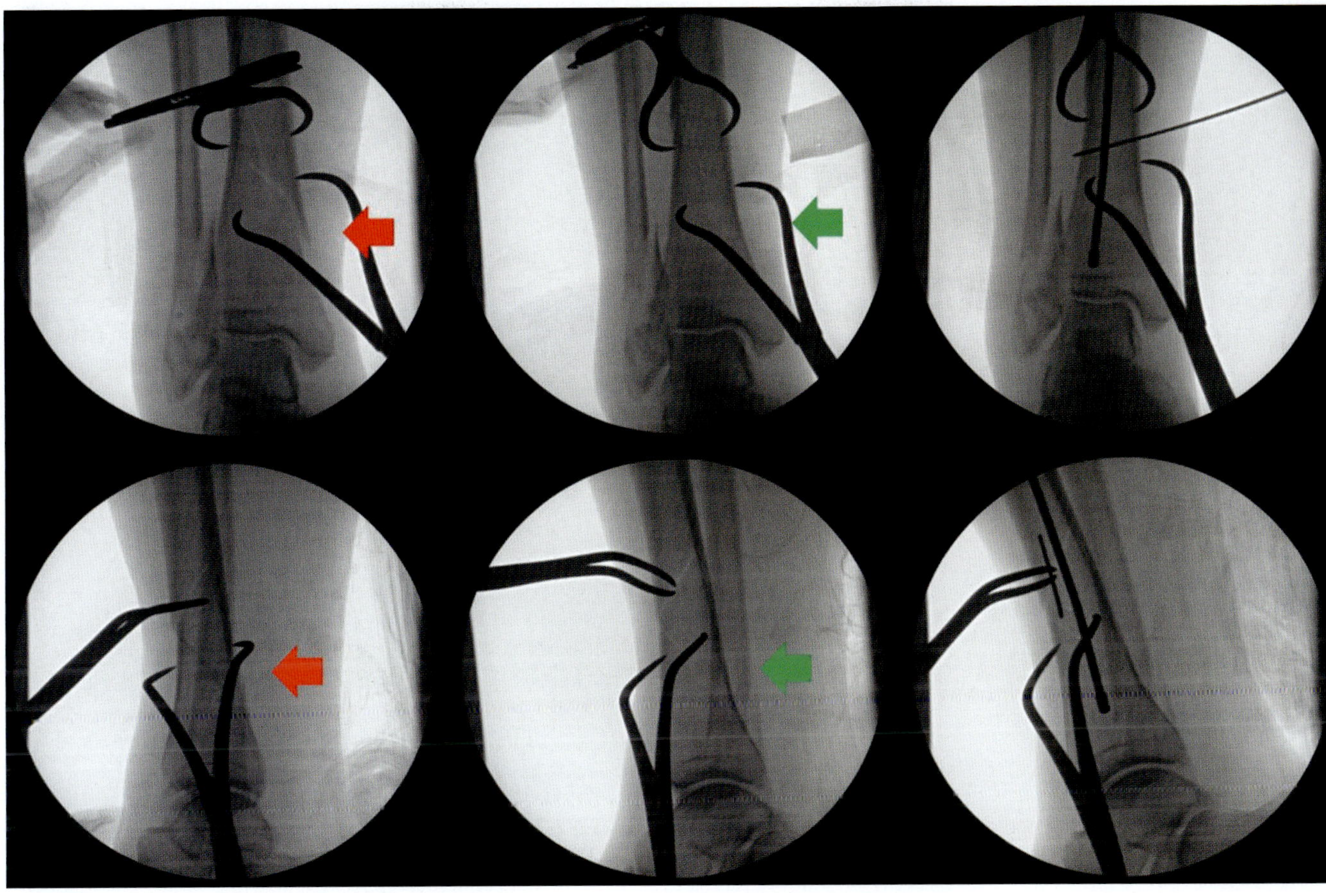

Figure 24-27 | Note the sequence of reduction maneuvers in restoring the length, alignment, and rotation in distal tibial shaft fractures.

Additional Positioning Tips

- Resting AP of knee and view unencumbered from contralateral extremity prior to draping are critical.
- Bed must be clear underneath of all nonnecessary equipment, tubes, and lines secured on bed, for smooth C-arm positioning.
- Ensure that anesthesia equipment, overhead lights, etc., are out of the path of the guidewire and implant pathways on proximal surgical field.
- Place tourniquet on proximal thigh so that distal femur can be easily manipulated during case for adequate imaging and reduction techniques.

References

1. Evans AR, Henley MB. Tibial Shaft Fractures. In: Gardner MJ and Henley MB, eds. *Harborview Illustrated Tips and Tricks in Fracture Surgery.* Philadelphia, PA: Lippincott Williams and Wilkins; 2011:277–304.
2. Boraiah S, Gardner MJ, Heflet DL, et al. High association of posterior malleolus fractures with spiral distal tibial fractures. *Clin Orthop Relat Res.* 2008;466(7):1692–1698.

Chapter 25
Ankle/Pilon Fractures

W. MICHAEL PULLEN*
CHRISTOPHER S. SMITH*
MICHAEL J. GARDNER
CHRISTIAAN N. MAMCZAK

Bony Anatomy

- The ankle joint is a complex hinge joint consisting of two articulations, the talocrural joint and the distal tibiofibular joint, with bony contributions from the distal tibia, distal fibula, and the talus.
- The distal tibia is subcutaneous on its anteromedial aspect contributing the medial malleolus and medial articular surface, the distal articular surface or plafond, and the tibial incisura. The articular surface is concave with distal extensions anteriorly and posteriorly.
- The distal fibula is subcutaneous laterally at its distal aspect and sits within the tibial incisura contributing the lateral malleolus with an irregular convex articular surface.
- The talus contributes a more uniform convex articular surface, which is wider at its anterior portion when contrasted with the posterior portion.
- Ankle stability is provided by ligamentous structures, with the deep deltoid ligament being the primary medial stabilizer, the syndesmotic complex being the primary stabilizer of the tibiofibular joint, and the lateral collateral ligament complex being the primary lateral stabilizer.[1]

Radiographic Anatomy

Anteroposterior (AP) View

- The AP view, in the intact ankle, demonstrates congruent articular surfaces with overlap of the distal tibia and fibula within the incisural notch (Fig. 25-1).
- With ankle fractures, there can be incongruent articular surfaces, decreased distal tibia and fibular overlap, and/or loss of fibular length. Note the double density of the displaced posterior malleolus, fibular shortening, and loss of tibiotalar joint space associated with this AP image of a trimalleolar fracture with posterior dislocation (Fig. 25-2).
- Postreduction AP imaging should demonstrate restoration of the articular congruity, fibular length, and distal tibiofibular overlap. Shortening of the fibula in relationship to the talocrural joint or the talus as well as decreased tibiofibular overlap may be concerning for malreduction.
- Tibial plafond, or pilon, fractures involve various degrees of articular involvement and may be associated with substantial comminution and shortening as depicted below (Fig. 25-3):

Mortise View

- The mortise view is performed with the ankle in dorsiflexion to neutral, to place the widest portion of the talus within the joint, and with the tibia internally rotated 10 to 15 degrees (Fig. 25-4).
- This view is utilized to evaluate the medial clear space and distal tibiofibular joint relationship as surrogates of (deltoid and/or syndesmotic) ligamentous integrity to evaluate for the

*The views expressed in this chapter are those of the author(s) and do not necessarily reflect the official policy or position of the Department of the Navy, Department of Defense or the United States Government. W. Michael Pullen and Christopher S. Smith are military service members and this work was prepared as part of their official duties. Title 17 U.S.C. 105 provides that 'Copyright protection under this title is not available for any work of the United States Government.' Title 17 U.S.C. 101 defines a United States Government work as a work prepared by a military service member or employee of the United States Government as part of that person's official duties.

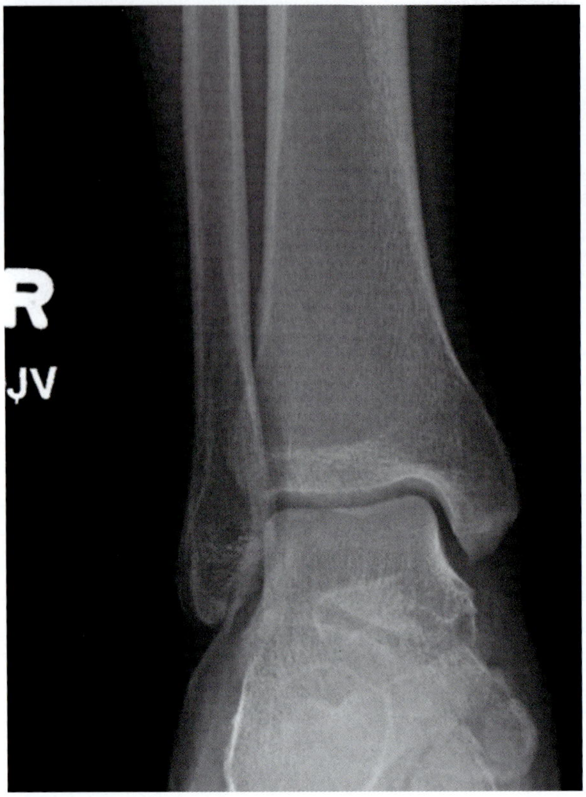

Figure 25-1 | Normal AP projection of a right ankle.

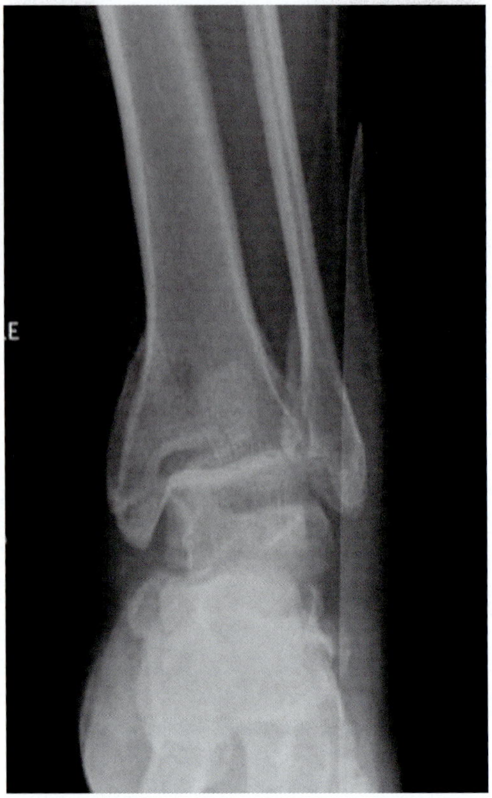

Figure 25-2 | AP projection with a trimalleolar ankle fracture. Note the double density due to the posterior malleolus fracture, overlap in the joint space due joint dislocation, and fibular shortening.

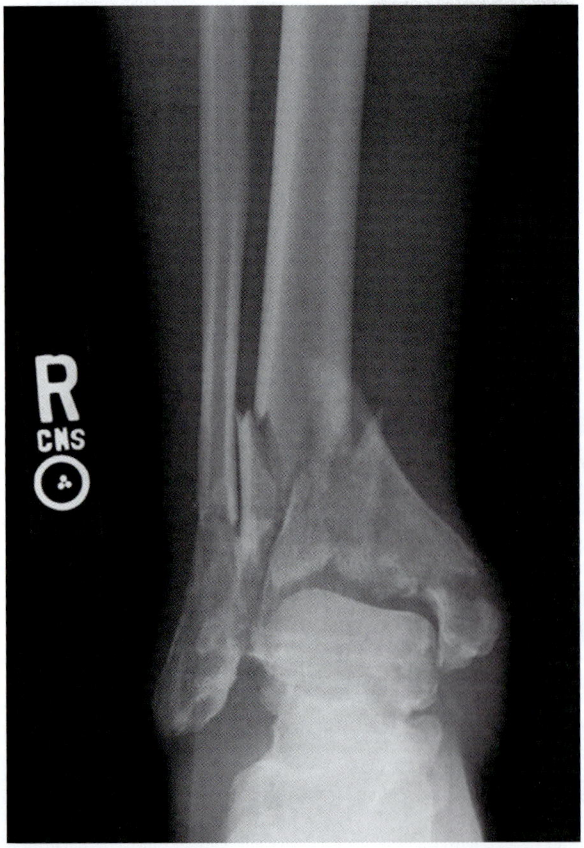

Figure 25-3 | AP projection of a comminuted pilon fracture.

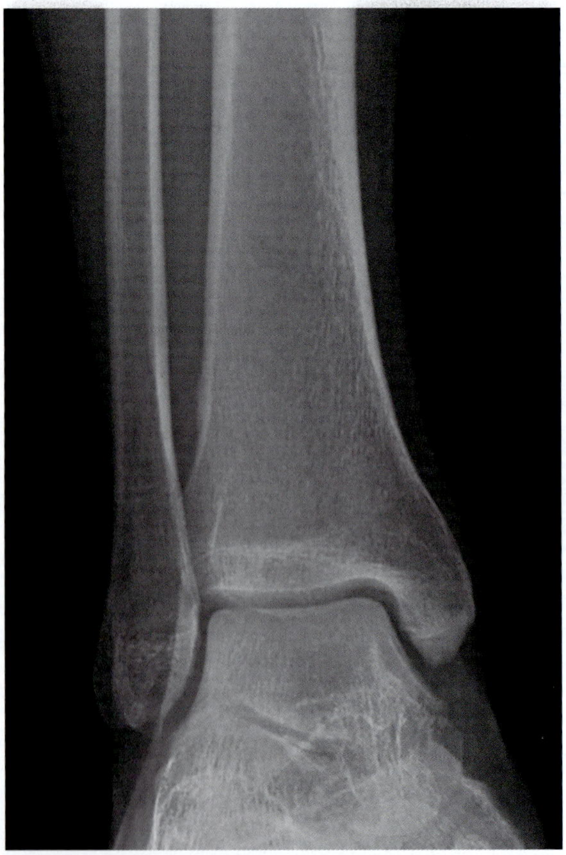

Figure 25-4 | Normal mortise view of a right ankle.

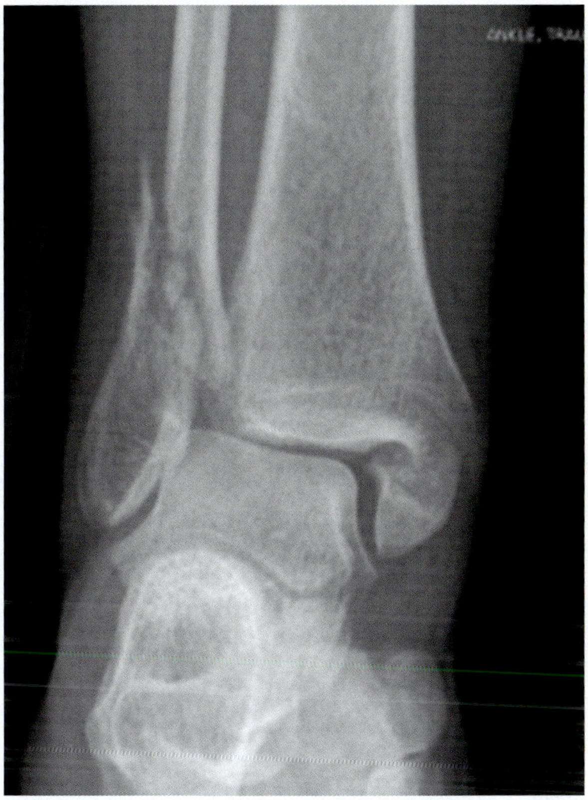

Figure 25-5 I Mortise view of a bimalleolar ankle fracture. Note the lateral subluxation of the talus and fibular shortening. An increase in the medial clear space can be seen when comparing the distance between the superior tibiotalar distance to the distance between the medial border of the talus and the medial shoulder of the tibia.

stability of the ankle fracture either preoperatively or intraoperatively. This mortise view demonstrates a bimalleolar ankle fracture with lateral talar subluxation and fibular shortening (Fig. 25-5).

- Normal medial clear space is typically <4 mm measured at the proximal and medial aspect of the talus; however, in the absence of a scaled image to account for image magnification, this measurement should be symmetric to the superior tibiotalar distance. This asymmetry can be seen on static images or on stress radiographs.
- Postreduction mortise images should demonstrate restoration of the articular congruity, reduction of the medial clear space, and restoration of fibular length.
- The "dime sign" is a radiographic marker best visualized on the ankle mortise view where a dime placed laterally should uniformly touch the peroneal groove of the distal fibula and the lateral talar process. Asymmetry is usually associated with fibular fracture shortening that must be reconstructed intraoperatively. Even a few millimeters of fibular shortening will have a profound effect on ankle mortise congruity and ligamentous stability (as depicted below) (Fig. 25-6A and B).

Lateral View

- The lateral view is performed with the ankle in neutral dorsiflexion and directed perpendicular to the AP projection, with the medial and lateral dome of the talus superimposed, which typically requires slight adduction and internal rotation.
- On a perfect "dome" lateral, three distinct anatomic ankle projections should always be evaluated: (1) the medial malleolus with anterior and posterior colliculi (blue), (2) the posterior malleolar congruity or fracture reduction (yellow), and (3) the posterior syndesmotic tibiofibular overlap (orange), which should be matched to a saved image of the patient's contralateral, uninjured ankle (Fig. 25-7).
- In ankle fractures, the lateral view is also utilized to determine the obliquity of the fracture to determine fracture classification as well as guide proper lag screw placement and plate position. The presence or absence of a posterior malleolar fragment can also be appreciated (Fig. 25-8).
- The degree of articular impaction is greatly appreciated on the lateral view of pilon injuries (Fig. 25-9).

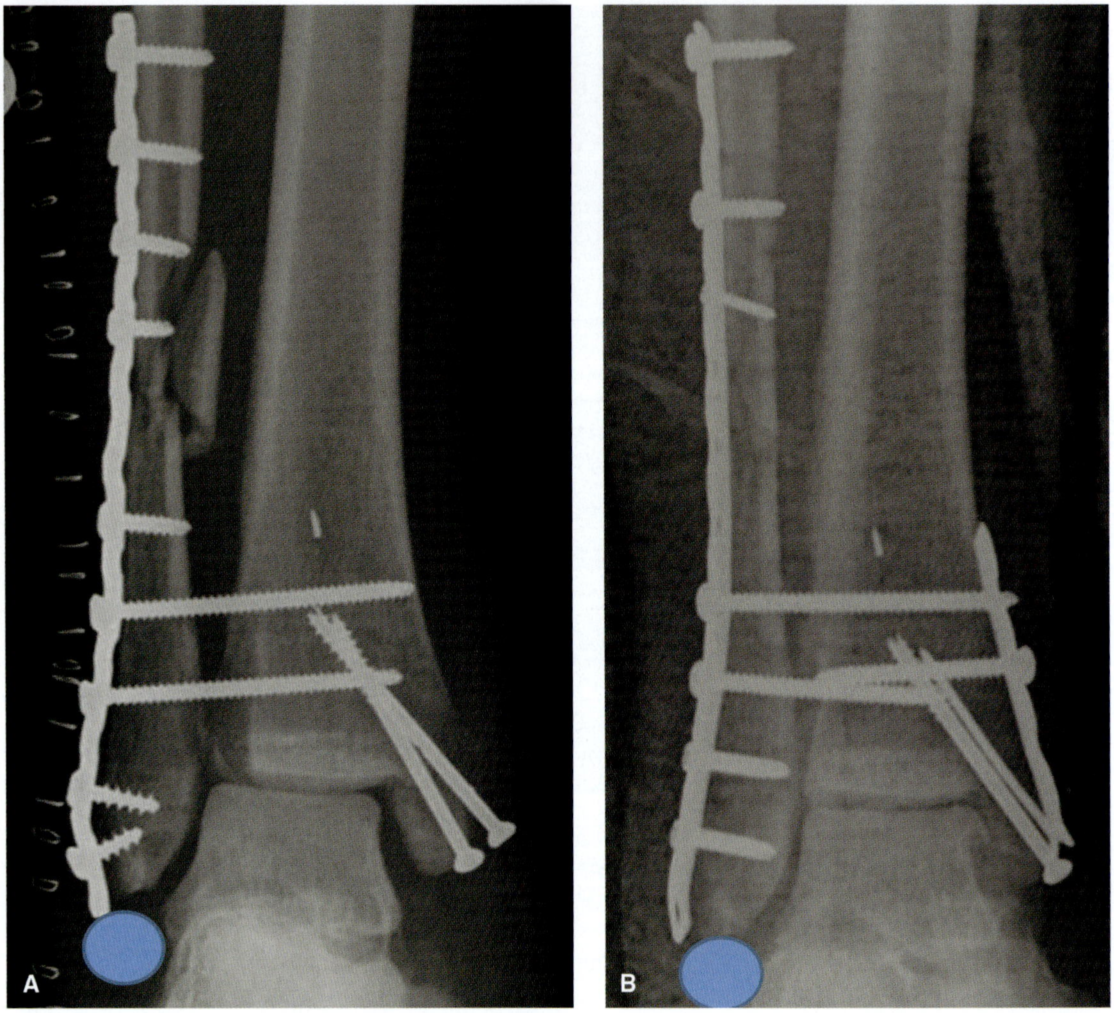

Figure 25-6 | A: Ankle fracture malreduction which can be confirmed by inadequate dime sign. Note the persistent fibular shortening and mortise malreduction. **B:** After revision, the dime sign is appropriately in contact with the peroneal groove and lateral process of the talus. Note improved reduction of the ankle and restoration of fibular length.

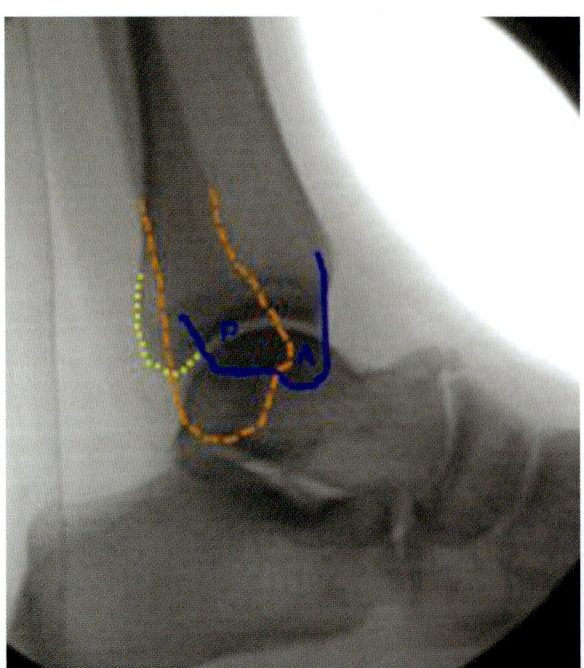

Figure 25-7 | Lateral fluoroscopic projection demonstrating the medial malleolus (*blue*), posterior malleolus (*yellow*), and posterior tibiofibular overlap (*orange*).

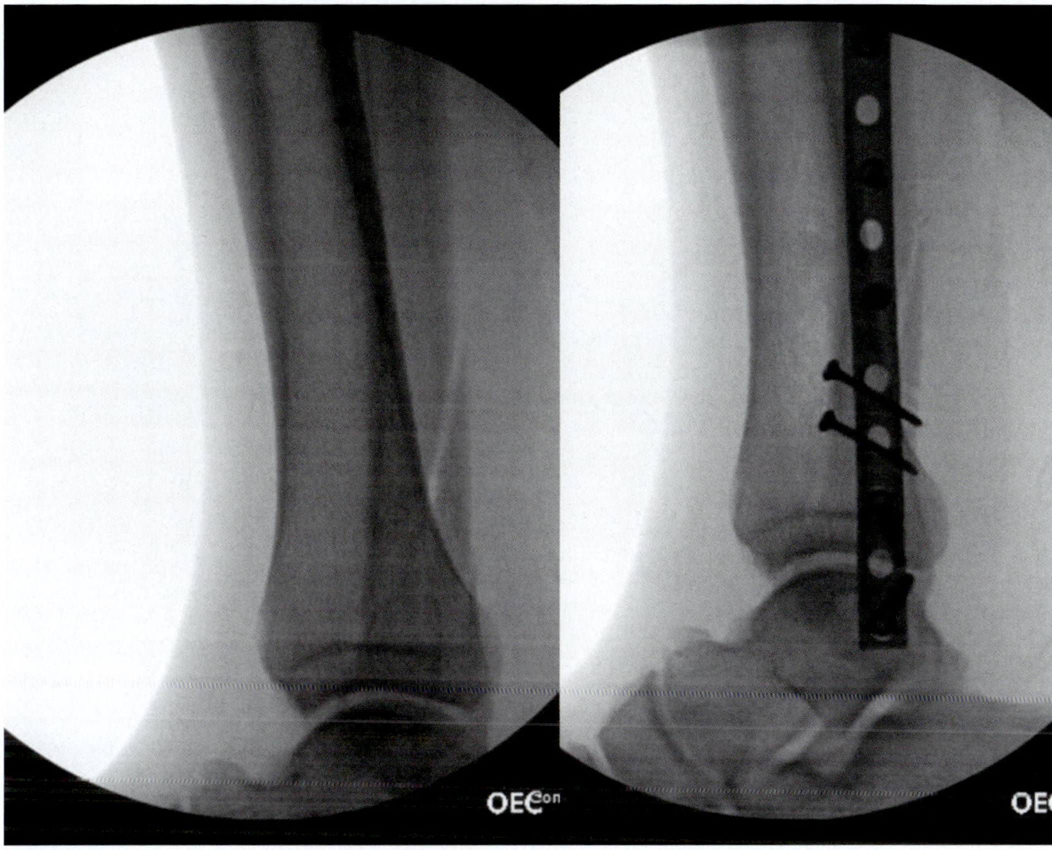

Figure 25-8 | A: Lateral fluoroscopic imaging demonstrates an oblique fracture from proximal posterior to distal anterior. No posterior malleolus fracture is seen on this projection. This can help guide lag-screw fixation trajectory as seen in the post-fixation image **(B)**.

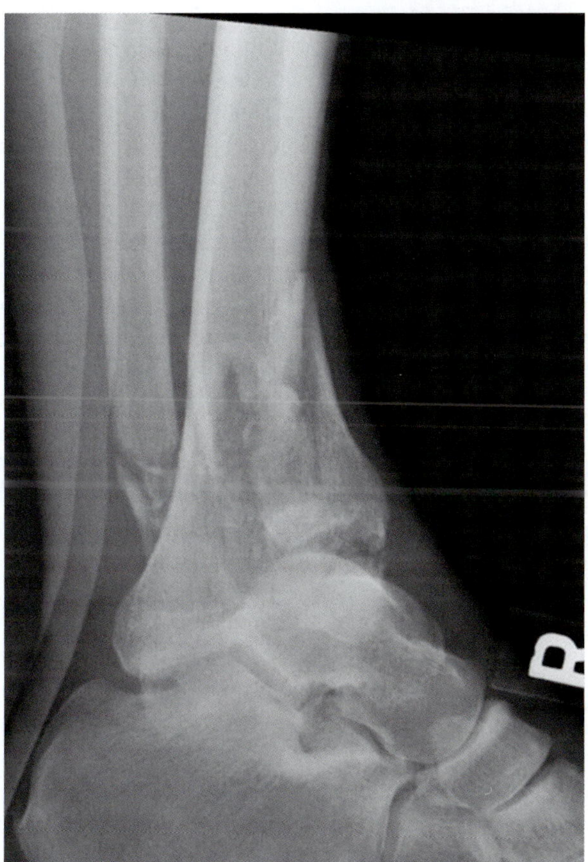

Figure 25-9 | Lateral projection of a comminuted pilon fracture demonstrated significant articular impaction.

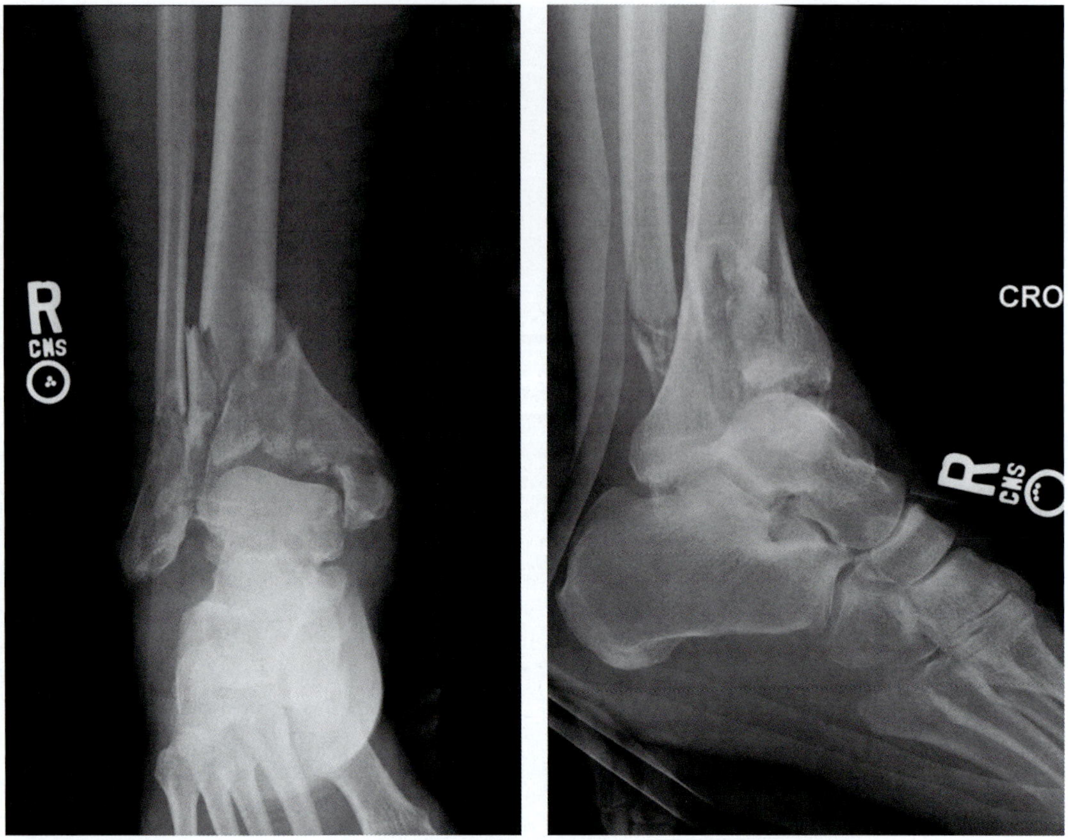

Figure 25-10 | AP and Lateral projections of a comminuted and shortened pilon fracture. The fracture pattern and articular surface is difficult to assess due to the shortening and comminution.

Preoperative Imaging

- The radiographic indication for operative treatment of an ankle fracture is articular impaction or incongruity and mortise instability secondary to fractures of two or more malleoli, a combination of osseous injury with ligamentous injury, or severe ligamentous injury. By the nature of their articular disruption, most pilon fractures are treated surgically to restore joint congruity.
- Standard radiographic views including an AP, mortise, and lateral are good screening tools for ankle fractures; however, bony overlap may obscure posterior malleolus fractures. Advanced imaging such at CT scans may be necessary to elicit the extent of articular involvement (see above).
- Stress radiographs, performed via a manual external rotation or gravity rotation, can demonstrate ligamentous instability.[2] A stress mortise view may show medial clear space widening and lateral displacement of the fibular fracture indicating deltoid ligament injury and/or syndesmotic sprain. Intraoperatively, these maneuvers, or a Cotton test, are performed following osseous fixation to evaluate for persistent ligamentous instability that may require further fixation.
- A staged protocol of treating pilon fractures with an index closed reduction and ankle spanning external fixation is a widely accepted method for allowing the soft tissue swelling to subside before definitive fracture fixation. CT scans should be performed after the external fixation frame when the tibial length has been restored noting that slight overdistraction plays favorably into achieving subsequent fracture reduction when several weeks of soft tissue rest are necessary to achieve a positive wrinkle sign (Figs. 25-10 and 25-11).

Intraoperative Imaging Pearls

- Postreduction lateral images should demonstrate restoration and congruency of the articular surface and restoration of the distal tibiofibular relationship. Note the small superiorly displaced posterior malleolar fragment (yellow bracket) is realigned at the joint surface (yellow arrow) via ligamentotaxis after surgical restoration of the fibular length and alignment utilizing a push-pull screw plating technique (blue arrow) (Fig. 25-12).

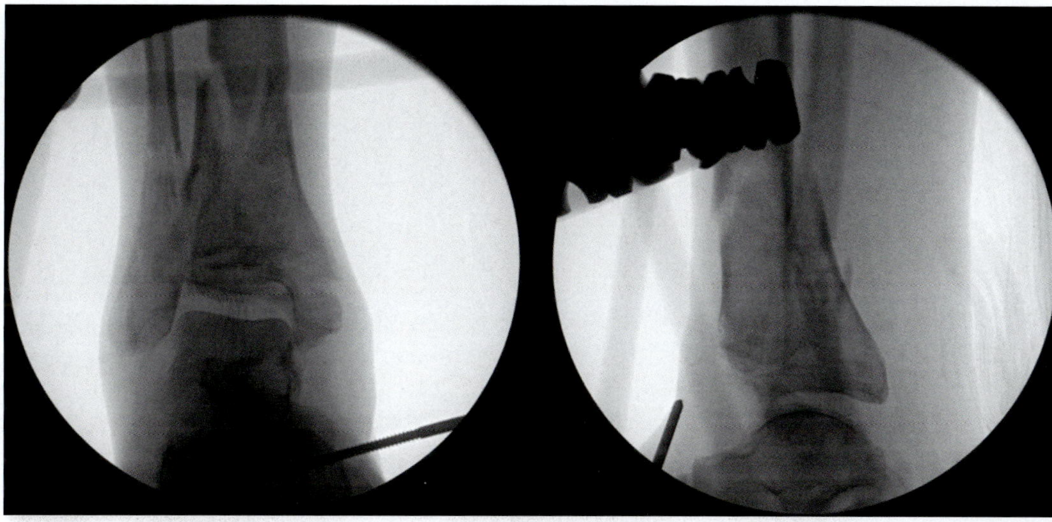

Figure 25-11 | Pilon fracture after spanning external fixator. Note slight over-distraction of the joint and improved ability to assess the fracture pattern and identify bony fragments.

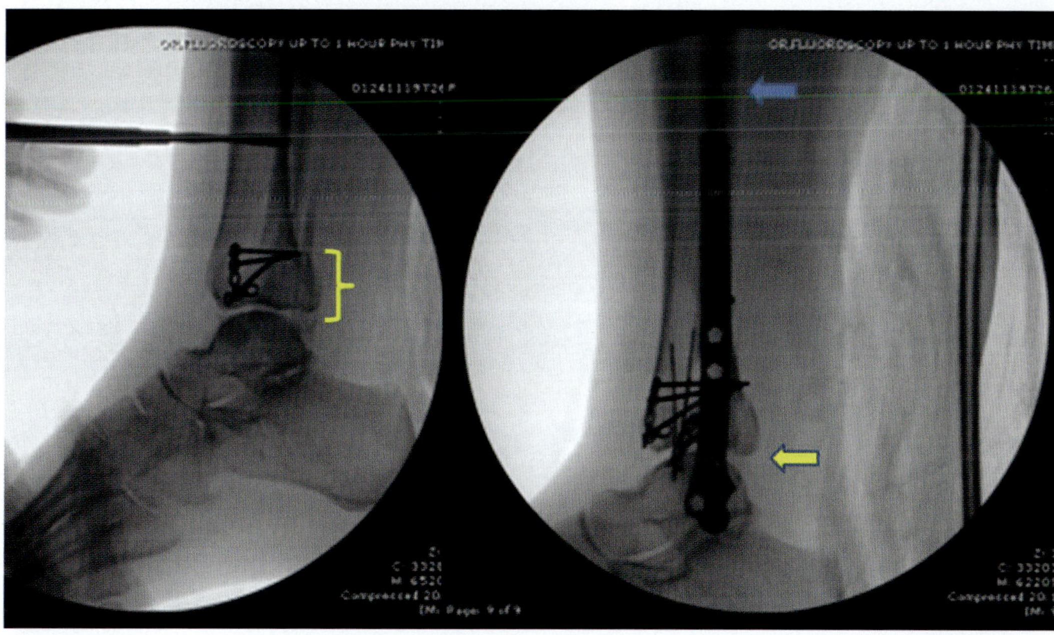

Figure 25-12 | Posterior malleolus fracture (*yellow bracket*) which is seen to reduce (*yellow arrow*) utilizing ligamentotaxis and a push-pull technique (*blue arrow*).

- Larger or comminuted posterior malleolar fractures, especially those associated with articular die-punch fragments blocking the reduction, may require a formal open reduction (Fig. 25-13).
- A modified lateral with slight external rotation may better delineate the obliquity of the posterior malleolar fracture and reduction (Fig. 25-14).
- Note that posterior malleolar fixation should precede lateral malleolar fixation in order to accurately determine adequate tibial articular reduction without impairment from lateral hardware (Fig. 25-15).
- Lateral imaging of pilon fractures should confirm both articular congruity and correct sagittal plane alignment of the joint surface relative to the tibial shaft. The fluoro sequence below depicts cortical fracture lines at the metadiaphyseal and metaphyseal junctions (Fig. 25-16A yellow lines). Note the highlighted circle of posterior metaphyseal step-off corresponding to a subtle but important sagittal plane fracture of the articular surface. Anterior metadiaphyseal reduction with a reference wire parallel to the joint surface makes the lateral plantar flexion deformity more noticeable (Fig. 25-16B). Stout wires can be used to reduce the joint surface into a more plantigrade alignment for definitive fixation (Fig. 25-16C). The posterior metaphyseal reduction is highlighted with a rotational view to move the fibular plate out of the way (Fig. 25-16D).

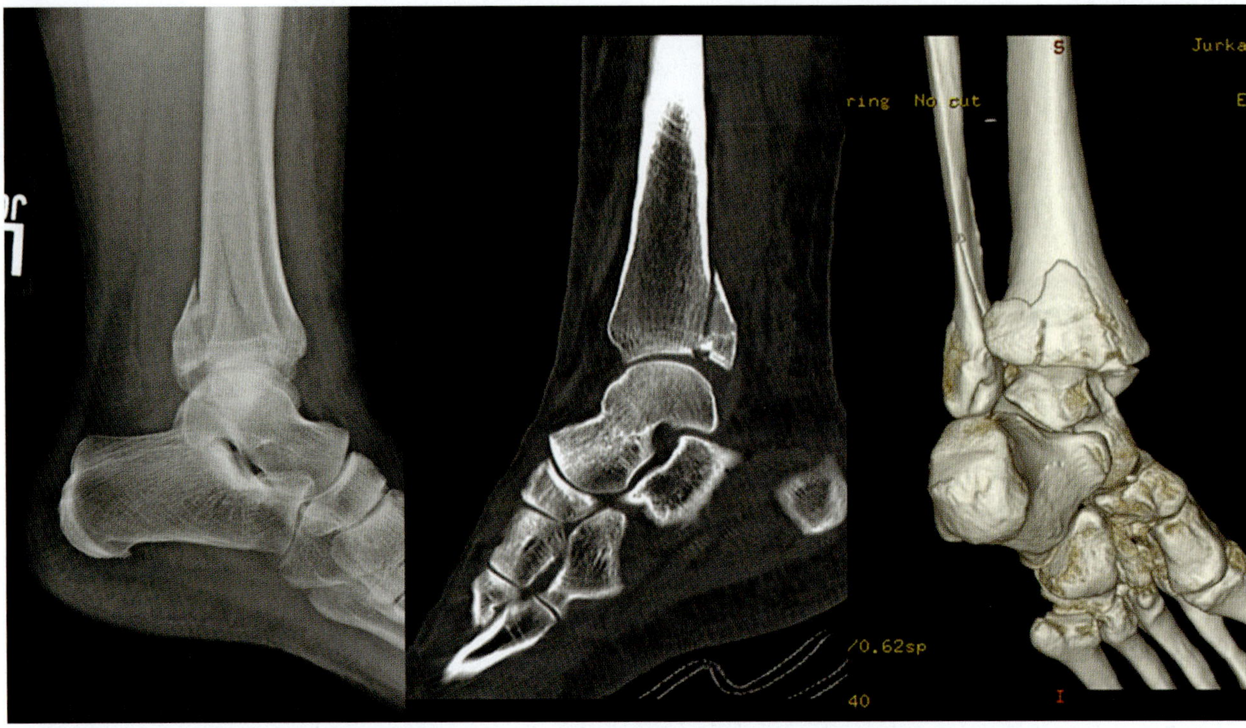

Figure 25-13 | Lateral radiographs and selective CT and reconstructive images demonstrating a large posterior malleolus fracture involving a large portion of the articular surface with an impacted, die-punch articular segment.

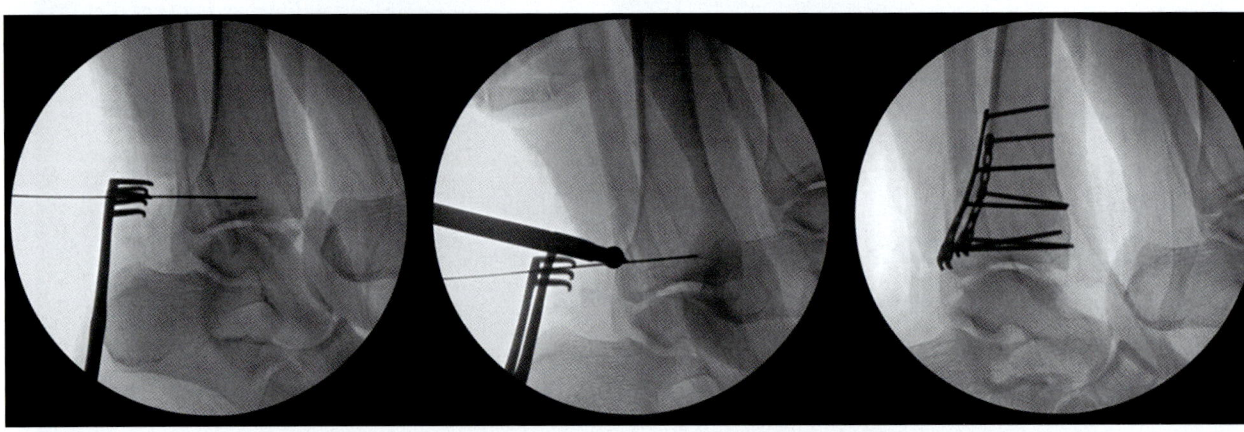

Figure 25-14 | Intraoperative fluoroscopic image demonstrating a modified, semi-oblique lateral in the plane of the posterior malleolus fracture which allows for easy visualization of reduction and fixation.

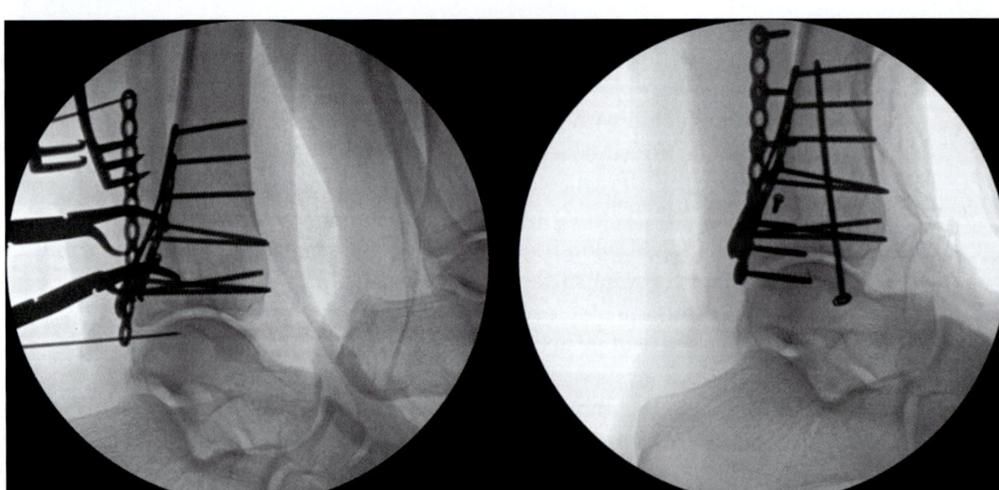

Figure 25-15 | Lateral projection demonstrating suggested order of fixation. Note the potential image obstruction if lateral malleolus fixation is performed first as the screws and plate will often obstruct the articular surface.

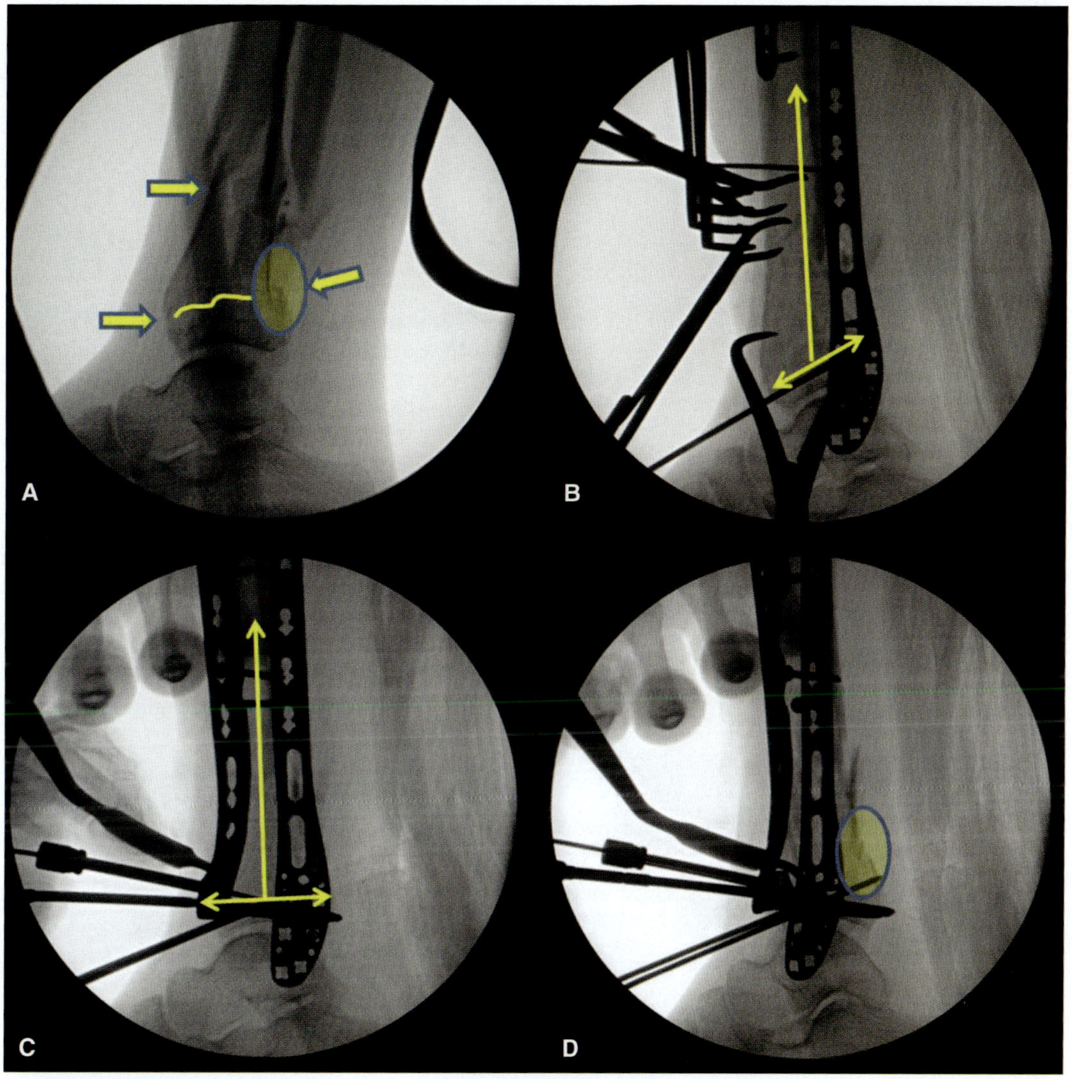

Figure 25-16 | Lateral imaging of a pilon fracture. **A:** Cortical fracture lines of both the diaphyseal and metadiaphyseal portion of the distal tibia (*yellow arrows*) with posterior metaphyseal displacement (*circle*). **B:** after anterior metaphyseal reduction the articular surface has a plantarflexion deformity (*yellow arrows*). **C:** K-wires placed parallel to the joint are used to reduce the articular surface. **D:** reduction of the posterior metaphyseal displacement can be observed (*circle*).

- An intraoperative Cotton Test (lateral-based clamp distraction of fibula) may demonstrate persistent syndesmotic instability and medial clear space widening following anatomic fixation of the lateral malleolus (Fig. 25-17A). This requires ankle mortise reduction with a clamp (Fig. 25-17B), and fixation is achieved via transsyndesmotic screws (Fig. 25-17C). The lateral view (Fig. 25-17D) demonstrates the screw trajectory from posterior to anterior traveling from lateral to medial.
- Syndesmotic malreduction remains a challenging aspect of ankle fracture surgery with malreduction rates approaching 30+% (Fig. 25-18). Injury patterns, as well as clamp and screw vectors, can lead to malreduction or even overcompression. Saved perfect "dome" lateral images of the uninjured ankle offer a reference for sagittal plane reduction. Note in this fluoro sequence the normal location of where the posterior cortex of the fibula crosses the tibial plafond on the contralateral ankle (orange) and the posterior (blue arrow) and anterior (yellow arrow) instability of the syndesmosis depicted in this pronation-external rotation fracture pattern (Fig. 25-19).
- Sagittal reduction and final syndesmotic screw dome lateral images should be meticulously compared to saved, preoperative images of the uninjured ankle to assure adequate reduction (Fig. 25-20).
- Pre- and postdynamic stress images (i.e., Cotton Test) should also be saved to document the presence and fixation of ankle instability (Fig. 25-21).
- Again, images of the uninjured ankle serve as a reference for restoring the fibular length and alignment (i.e., fibular dime sign). Note that the articular facet orientation of the fibula is comparable to the uninjured ankle denoting proper rotational alignment (Fig. 25-22).

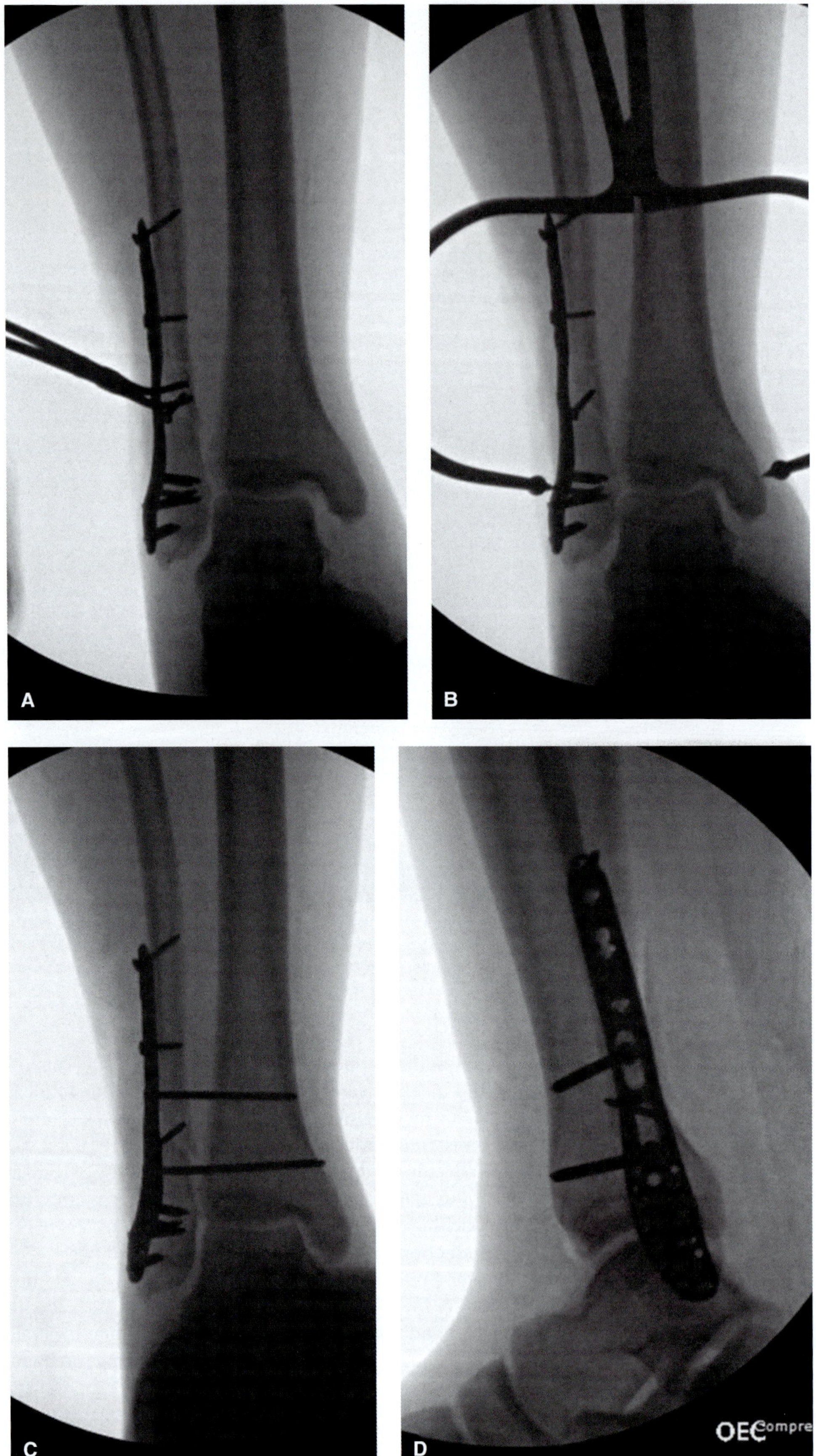

Figure 25-17 | A: intraoperative cotton test demonstrating medial clear space widening. **B:** Reduction was achieved with a clamp and transsyndesmotic screws were placed **(C)**. Lateral projection demonstrates posterior to anterior trajectory of syndesmotic screws **(D)**.

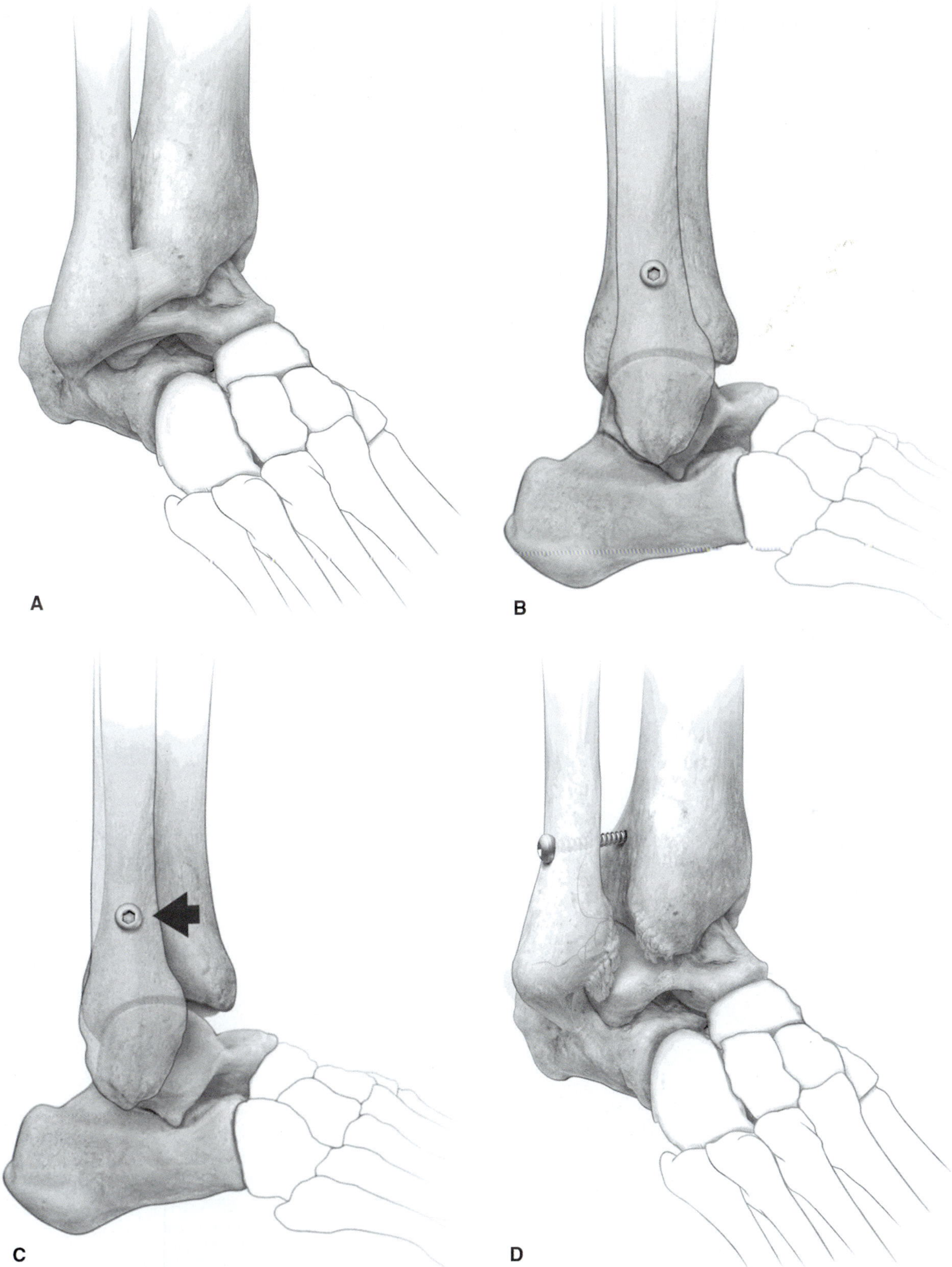

Figure 25-18 | Intraoperative recognition of syndesmotic disruption is an important part of treating ankle fractures. Multiple studies have shown that syndesmotic malreduction remains a common occurrence; contributing factors include a shallow tibial incisura, improper clamp vectors, translation or rotation during screw placement, and poor fibular reduction. These illustrations depict syndesmotic malreduction with posterior translation of the fibula leading to persistent gap of the anterior ligaments and resulting changes in joint congruity. The normal ligamentous relationships can be appreciated anterolaterally **(A)**. Anatomic reduction **(B)** can be seen in contrast with posterior malreduction **(C)**. In the case of malreduction, persistent anterolateral gapping can be seen resulting in ligament gapping and joint incongruity **(D)**.

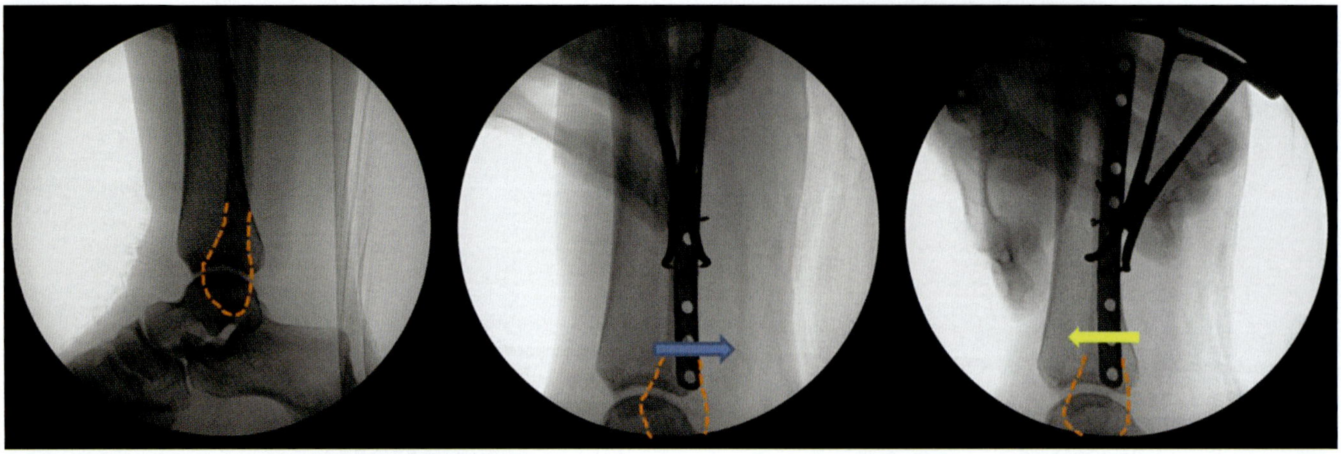

Figure 25-19 | Normal contralateral ankle demonstrates the patients tibiofibular relationship (*orange*). Syndesmotic instability can allow for posterior (*blue arrow*) or anterior (*yellow arrow*) tralsnation of the fibula.

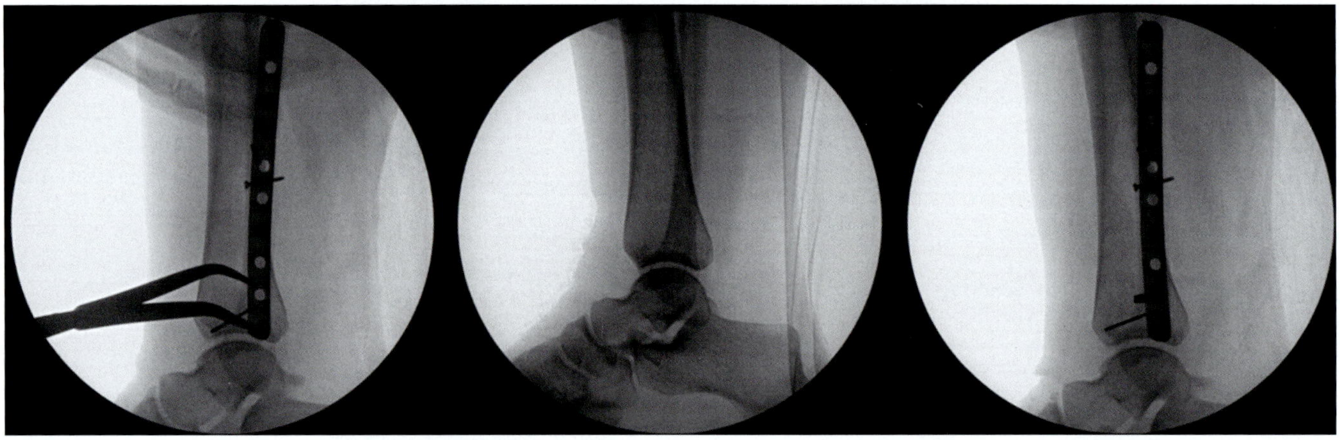

Figure 25-20 | Fluoroscpoic images demonstrating reduction images (*left*) and after fixation images (*right*) compared with the uninjured contralateral side (*center*).

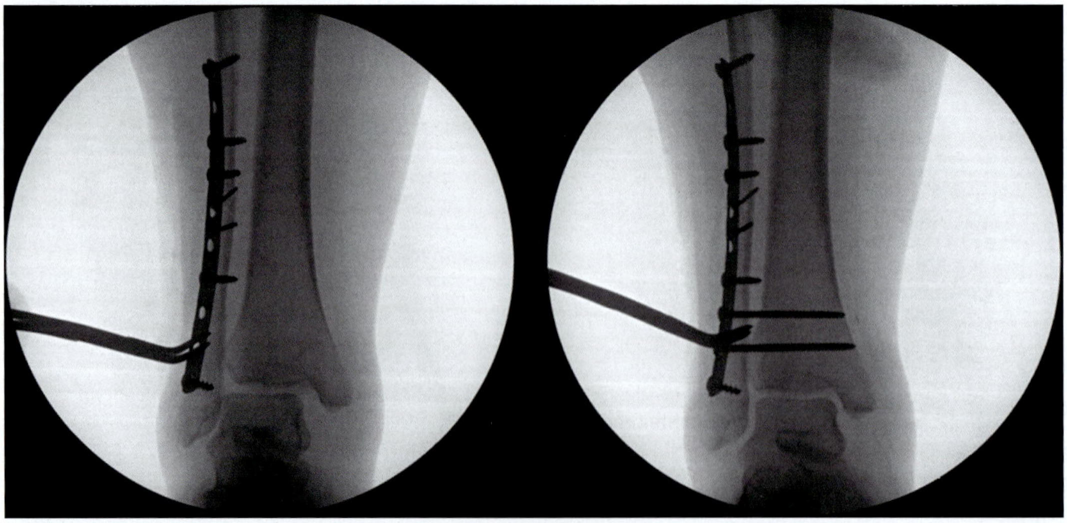

Figure 25-21 | Intraoperative cotton test before and after syndesmotic fixation. Note increased medial clear space and lateral talar subluxation on the stress images which is stabilized with 2 transsyndesmotic screws.

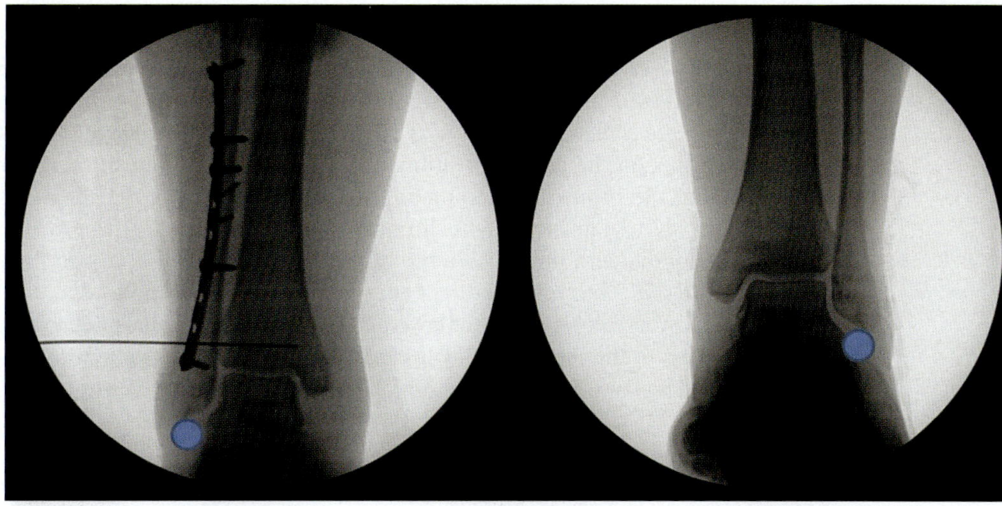

Figure 25-22 | Post reduction fixation compared with the uninjured contralateral side. Note restoration of length and rotation by symmetry of the dime sign.

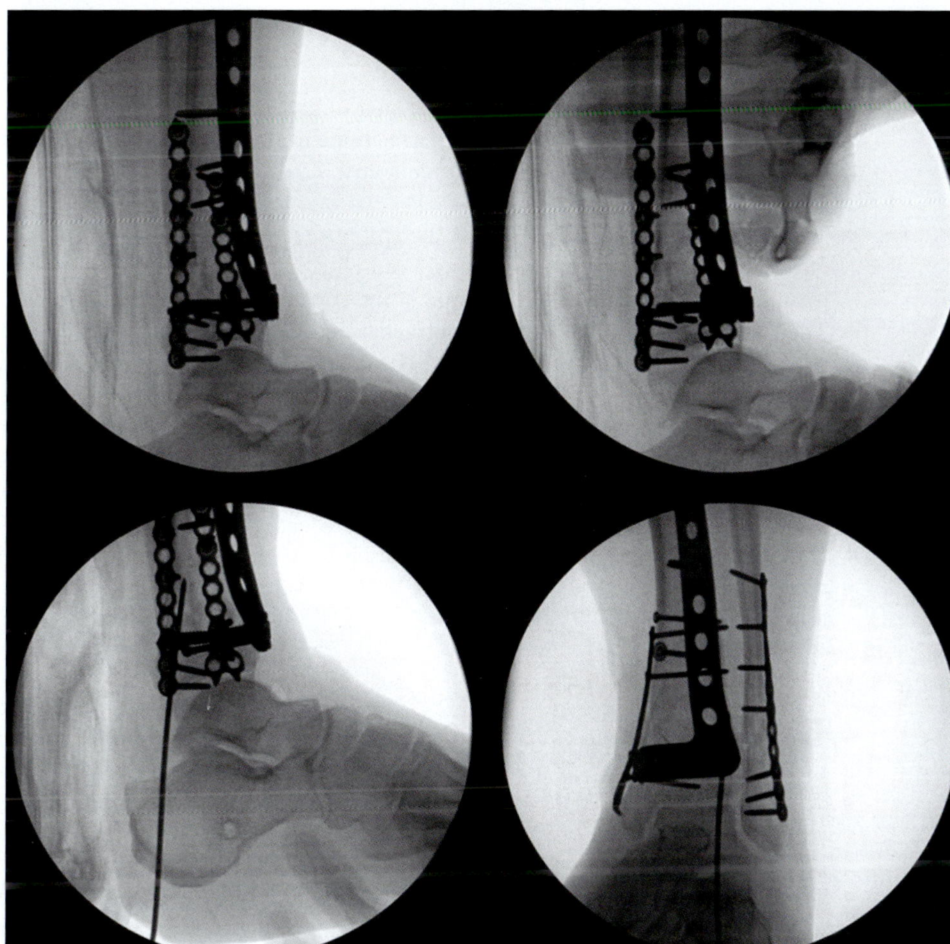

Figure 25-23 | Intraoperative imaging following pilon fixation demonstrating the need for anterior and posterior stress testing in complex ankle fracture-dislocations. Note the persistent instability after osseous stabilization with anterior talar subluxation with an intraoperative anterior drawer. This was managed with closed reduction and joint-sparing percutaneous fixation.

Medial and lateral ligamentous injuries are also possible, especially in complex fracture patterns and dislocations. Failure to perform intraoperative stress examinations may lead to missing these injuries. Note the anterior drawer laxity seen after fixation of this pilon fracture and the closed reduction and joint-sparing percutaneous pinning (Fig. 25-23).

Intraoperative Positioning

- Surgical fixation of ankle fractures depend on the fracture pattern, portions of the ankle to be surgically addressed, and the planned surgical approach.
- There are unique challenges, both surgical and anesthetic, and varying access around the ankle depending on the patient positioning, with the common positions being supine, lateral or semilateral, and prone. Depending on the fracture pattern, it may be necessary to use a combination of these positioning techniques during a single surgical procedure.
- Supine positioning with the use of a hip bump allows excellent access to the medial and lateral malleoli; however, it has limited direct access to the posterior malleolus.
- Lateral positioning allows excellent access to the lateral malleolus and posterior malleolus; however, access to the medial malleolus may be limited, requiring external rotation through the hip or require repositioning. It offers greater airway access for anesthesia when contrasted with the prone position.
- Prone positioning allows direct access to the posterior malleolus and lateral malleolus, with access to the medial malleolus available through internal rotation of the limb. A small sheet bump under the contralateral hip facilitates this access.
- Ideally, a radiolucent extension on the foot of the table is used as it facilitates the most degrees of freedom with fluoroscopic imaging.

1. Supine Positioning

- The supine position offers access to the lateral malleolus and medial malleolus. Adding a bump under the ipsilateral operative hip may facilitate improved access to the distal fibula without compromising access to the medial malleolus. Access to the posterior malleolus may be difficult from this position.
- The patient should be positioned at the end of the bed to facilitate surgical access as well as facilitate fluoroscopic imaging. Using a radiolucent leg ramp or elevator will help facilitate lateral imaging by moving it out of the plane of the contralateral extremity.
- The C-arm should enter from the contralateral side to the operative extremity to facilitate imaging without compromising surgical access. The C-arm should enter perpendicular to the table to facilitate transition from the AP, mortise, and lateral projections without having to move the C-arm base.
- AP imaging is taken with the C-arm in the upright position. Adjustments in rotation can be made by the surgeon through internal or external rotation of the tibia. The mortise view is typically performed with 10 to 15 degrees of internal rotation of the tibia without needing repositioning of the C-arm.
- Lateral imaging is performed through rotating the C-arm through its arc. Use of a half-sheet drape or C-armor permits movement of the C-arm through its arc without compromising sterility (Fig. 25-24).

2. Lateral Positioning

- This position allows access to the posterior and lateral malleoli; however, there is limited access to the medial malleolus.
- The patient is placed in the lateral decubitus position or the semilateral position and stabilized using either a beanbag or chest rolls. An axillary roll or thoracic wedge should be used for the down upper extremity.
- The down extremity is placed in a down leg holder with the operative extremity placed on the working surface. Alternatively, in the semilateral position, the radiolucent leg ramp is utilized to position the operative extremity. Subsequently, for improved access to the medial malleolus, the beanbag can be deflated or the posterior chest roll can be removed.
- The C-arm should enter from the front of the patient orientated perpendicular to the table to facilitate AP, mortise, and lateral imaging without need to move the C-arm base (Fig. 25-25).

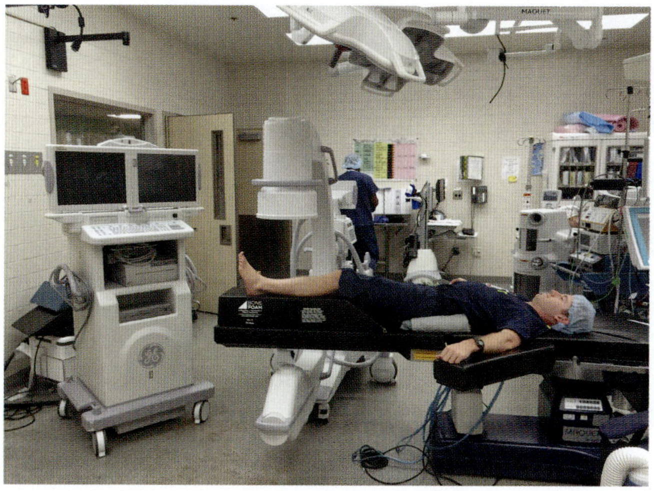

Figure 25-24 | Patient position and C-arm position for supine positioning. The ipsilateral upper extremity is taken across the body and secured to increase space for the surgeon and assistants. A size appropriate hip bump is utilized to internally rotate the lower extremity to ease lateral access. Note the use of a leg ramp to facilitate lateral imaging utilizing the arc of the C-arm without need for repositioning the leg or the fluoroscopy machine. The C-arm enters from the contralateral side of the patient to allow the surgeon un-obstructed access to the lateral ankle.

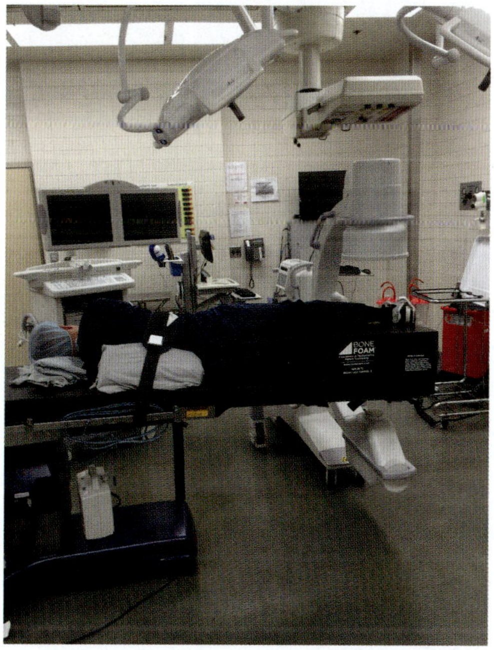

Figure 25-25 | Patient position and C-arm position for lateral positioning. The upper trunk is supported in a lateral decubitus or semi-lateral position utilizing chest rolls or a beanbag. The up arm is supported either on pillows or a specific arm board. An axillary roll or thoracic wedge is needed for the down extremity (not pictured). The down leg is placed on the table with care taken to ensure the peroneal nerve is appropriately protected. In this example, the operative extremity is placed on the working surface of a down-leg holder. Medial malleolus access can be limited in this position, but improved by deflating the beanbag or removing the posterior chest roll allowing the body and lower extremity to externally rotate.

3. Prone Positioning

- This positioning provides direct access to the posterior malleolus, access to the posterior or lateral surfaces of the distal fibula, and access to the medial malleolus.
- The patient is positioned prone utilizing chest rolls to free the abdomen and facilitate anesthesia. Padding is applied to the bilateral patella. The nonoperative leg is elevated slightly to flex the knee on blankets or pillows with the operative leg elevated further on either foam pads or blankets to facilitate fluoroscopic imaging without overlap.
- The contralateral iliac crest is bumped to allow access to the medial malleolus and facilitates the lateral view.
- The C-arm enters from the nonoperative side of the patient. Lateral imaging is obtained similarly to supine positioning; however, AP and mortise views require cranial to caudal (inlet) tilt to match the elevated positioning of the ankle (Figs. 25-26 and 25-27).

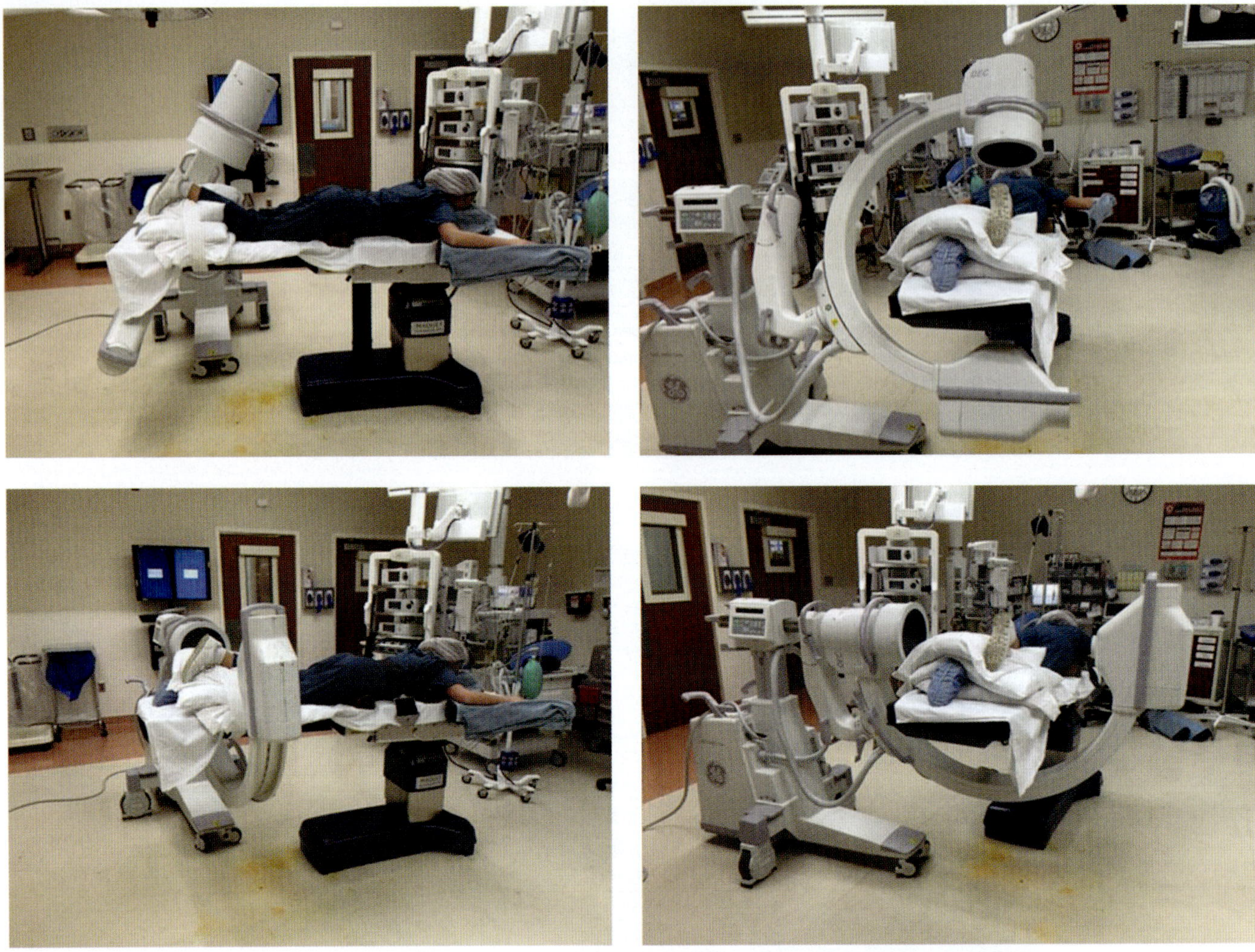

Figure 25-26 | Patient position and C-arm position for prone positioning. The patient is placed on chest rolls to allow the abdomen to be free. Padding is required for all down bony prominences, namely the patella and anterior superior iliac spine. The nonoperative extremity is slightly flexed and well padded. The operative extremity is elevated with either a radiolucent leg ramp or pillows. C-arm enters from the nonoperative side. Note that to obtain accurate AP and mortise views cranial to caudal tilt of the C-arm is required. Lateral imaging is obtained similar to supine positioning.

Additional Positioning Tips

- Discuss positioning need with anesthesia, specifically when prone positioning is expected as this may represent specific anesthesia concerns.
- When using lateral or semilateral positioning, it is important to ensure adequate padding and elevation of the nonoperative fibular head to protect the peroneal nerve.
- If utilizing a tourniquet and using the prone position, placing the tourniquet on the thigh prior to final positioning facilitates easier tourniquet placement.
- Use of a radiolucent table and radiolucent foam ramps allows freedom of fluoroscopic imaging.
- Obtaining contralateral ankle films prior to prepping and draping provides a reference for accurate restoration of the anteroposterior relationship of the distal fibula to the tibia.
- Taking a preoperative radiograph superimposing the planned implant can facilitate the length of incision needed (Fig. 25-28).

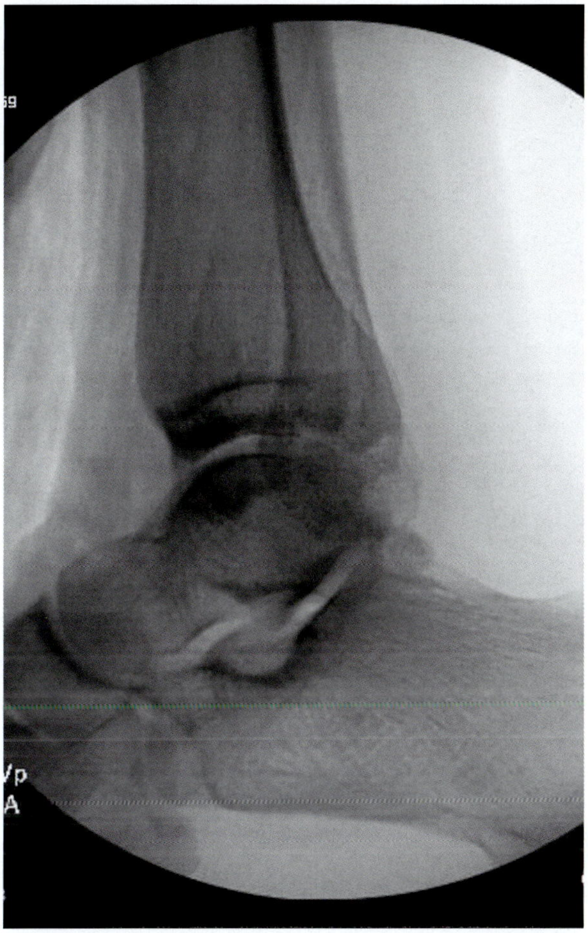

Figure 25-27 | Lateral radiograph obtained in the prone position demonstrating a posterior malleolus fracture.

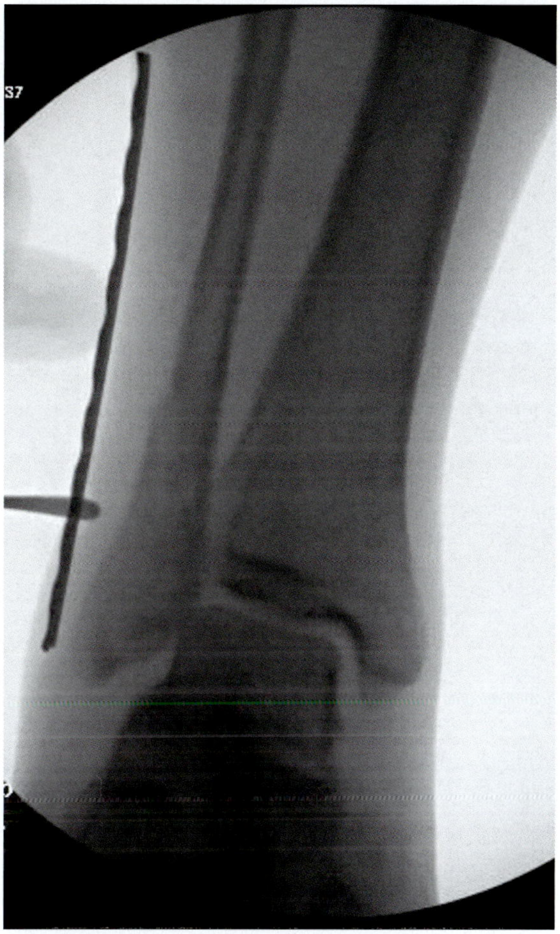

Figure 25-28 | Preoperative radiograph with superimposed implant can assist in predicting the needed length of incision.

References

1. Michelson JD. Ankle fractures resulting from rotational injuries. *J Am Acad Orthop Surg*. 2003;11(6):403–412.
2. Schock HJ, Pinzur M, Manion L, et al. The use of gravity or manual-stress radiographs in the assessment of supination-external rotation fractures of the ankle. *J Bone Joint Surg Br*. 2007;89(8):1055–1059.

Chapter 26
Lisfranc Injuries

JOHN W. MUNZ
RYAN TAYLOR

- Lisfranc Injury
  - A Lisfranc injury is any osseous or ligamentous pathology involving the tarsometatarsal (TMT) joint complex of the midfoot ranging from subtle instability to frank dislocations.
  - May involve the medial or lateral columns, or both, depending on the mechanism of injury.
  - Lower-energy Lisfranc injuries are often misdiagnosed as foot sprains and may be missed altogether with a delayed posttraumatic diagnosis.
  - Missed Lisfranc injuries can lead to chronic midfoot instability and degeneration.
- Anatomy
  - The Lisfranc joint articulations include the base of the metatarsals with the three cuneiforms (1st through 3rd) and the cuboid (4th and 5th).
  - The first three metatarsal bases are configured in a Roman arch–style pattern with the 2nd metatarsal head residing the most dorsally and proximally.
  - In general, the 1st through 3rd tarsometatarsal articulations are relatively immobile and firmly fixed, while the 4th and 5th TMT articulations are more mobile.
  - The depth from dorsal to plantar of the metatarsal bases varies with the 1st metatarsal head being the largest with an average dorsal to plantar depth of approximately 30 mm. The 2nd metatarsal has the shortest dorsal to plantar depth being approximately 22 mm. The 3rd metatarsal base is approximately 26 mm from dorsal to plantar.
  - The Lisfranc ligament originates from the plantar aspect of the medial cuneiform and inserts on the plantar aspect of the base of the 2nd metatarsal. On occasion, an avulsion of the Lisfranc ligament from the base of the 2nd metatarsal (a.k.a. "fleck sign") may be the only radiographic marker of this injury.
  - Interosseous ligaments link the 2nd through 5th metatarsals. There is no intermetatarsal ligament that connects the 1st metatarsal base to the 2nd metatarsal base.
  - Secondary stabilizers of the Lisfranc articulation include the plantar fascia, the peroneus longus, and the foot intrinsics.

Preoperative Imaging

- Radiographs
  - Three views of the foot are necessary to fully evaluate the tarsometatarsal joints. The most common views are the AP, the internal rotation oblique, and the lateral.
  - Each view has characteristic relationships that must be evaluated to properly assess for the presence or extent of an injury (Fig. 26-1).
  - Oftentimes, injuries are not so obvious, and comparison views of the uninjured side are helpful for diagnosing subtle injuries.
  - Bilateral weight-bearing views are also helpful in identifying subtle instability.
- Relationships
  - On the AP view, the medial border of the 2nd metatarsal base should be in line with the medial border of the middle cuneiform (red arrow Case A below). Note the two extremes of Lisfranc injuries depicted below with Case B showing a divergent TMT dislocation of the medial column (navicular-cuneiform, intercuneiform, and TMT joints) and lateral dislocation of the 2nd to 5th TMT articulations (Fig. 26-2).

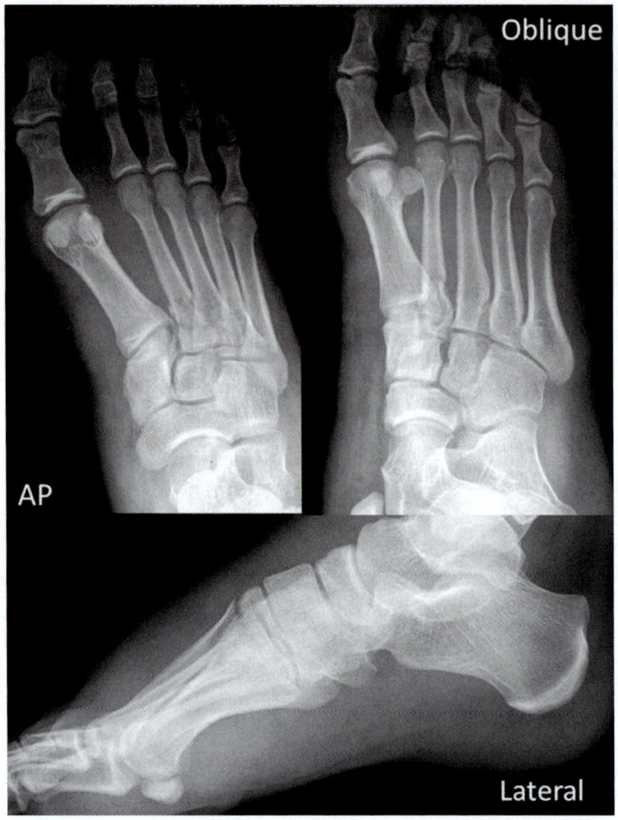

Figure 26-1 |

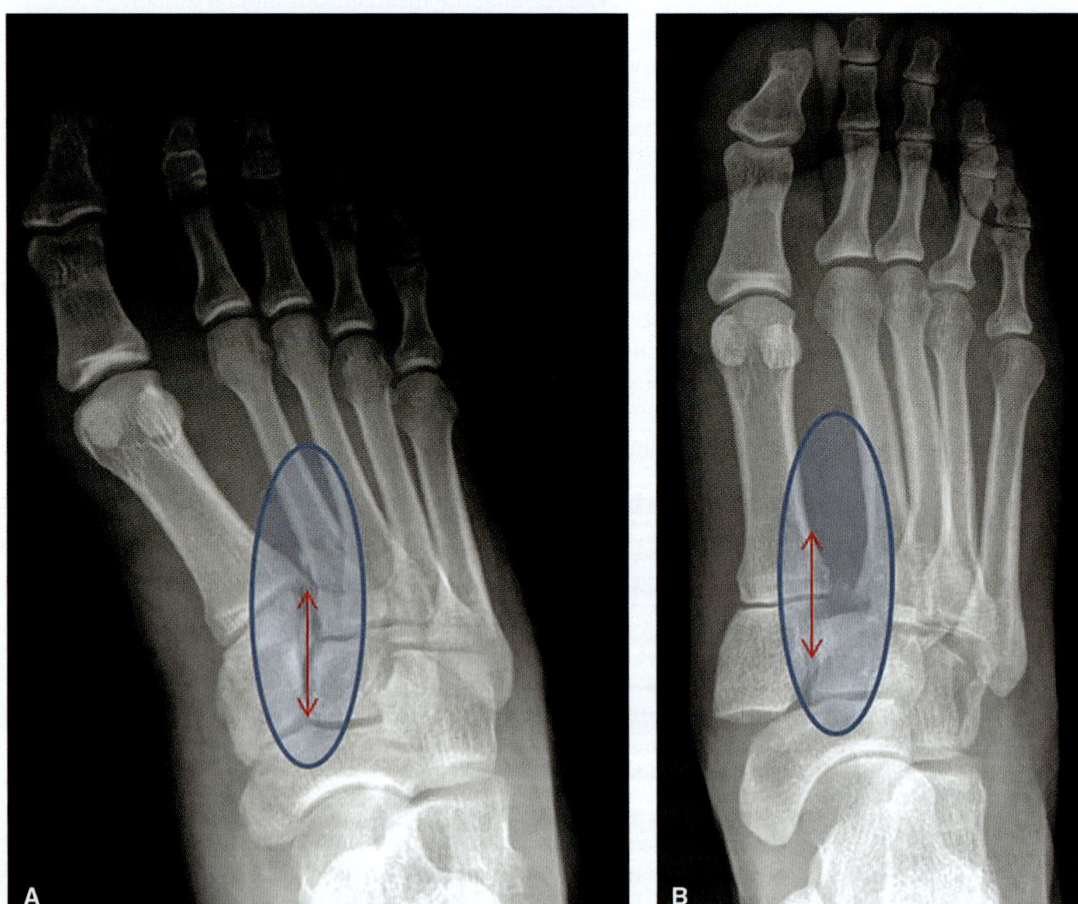

Figure 26-2 |

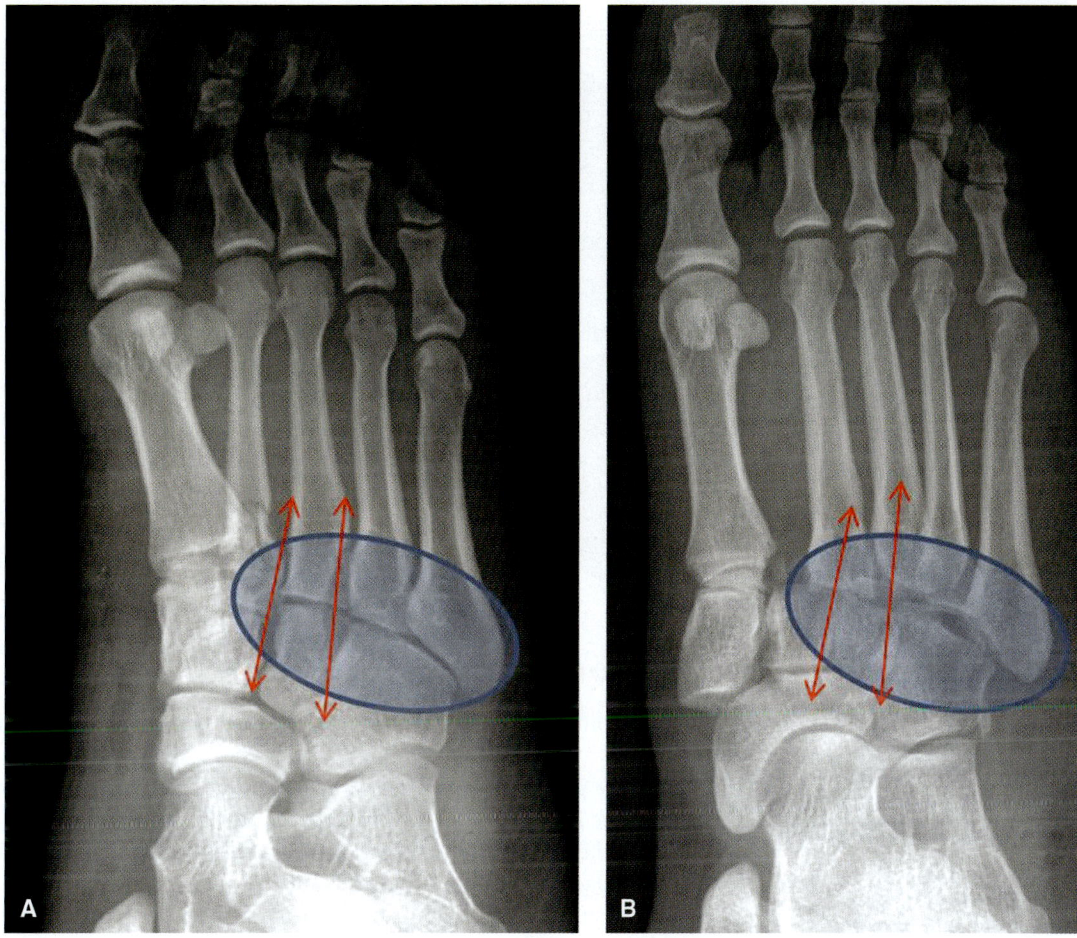

Figure 26-3 |

- On the oblique view, the medial border of the 3rd metatarsal base should be in line with the medial border of the lateral cuneiform (left red arrow Case A above), the medial border of the 4th metatarsal base should be in line with the medial border of the cuboid (right red arrow Case A above), and the 5th metatarsal base should articulate with the lateral cuboid. Again, note the two extremes of Lisfranc injuries depicted above with Case B showing a divergent TMT dislocation with lateral dislocation of the 2nd to 5th TMT articulations disrupting the radiographic lines (Fig. 26-3).
- On the lateral view, the dorsal surface of the 1st metatarsal base should be in line with the dorsal surface of the navicular (thin solid red arrow below). In addition, a straight and parallel line (dashed arrow below) should traverse from the midportion of the talus through the middle of the navicular, medial cuneiform, and 1st metatarsal (a.k.a. Meary's line). The 2nd metatarsal base is more proximal and can be seen through the midportion of the medial cuneiform. Note, on this lateral view, the dorsal subluxation of the base of the 2nd metatarsal associated with a Lisfranc injury (blue arrow) (Fig. 26-4).

Advanced Imaging

- After the diagnosis is made, advanced imaging in the form of computed tomography (CT) is often helpful in delineating the extent of the injury. Minimally displaced fractures, mildly subluxated joints, and midfoot comminution are often not apparent on plain radiographs.
- Magnetic resonance imaging (MRI) is usually only indicated if there is high suspicion of ligamentous injury and all other imaging modalities are negative.

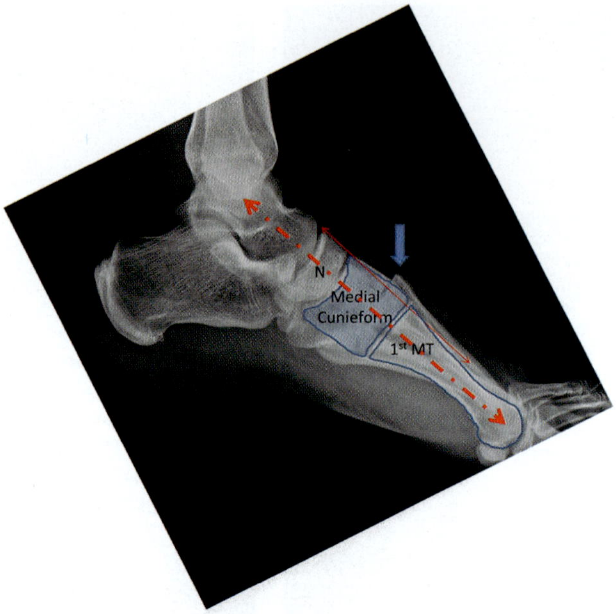

Figure 26-4 |

Intraoperative Positioning

- Intraoperative positioning is crucial to obtaining and maintaining adequate fluoroscopic views of the Lisfranc joint.
- The patient should be positioned supine on a radiolucent table with or without an extension. A small bump under the ipsilateral hip prevents the lower extremity from externally rotating.
- Prior to prepping and draping, ensure that adequate imaging can be obtained without the interference of radiopaque components of the table or the contralateral limb (lateral images).
- Once prepped and draped, a radiolucent triangle can be used to bring the plantar aspect of the foot parallel to the bed with a stack of towels under the foot providing a stable base to work on. This position also facilitates imaging without having to manipulate the foot (Figs. 26-5 and 26-6).

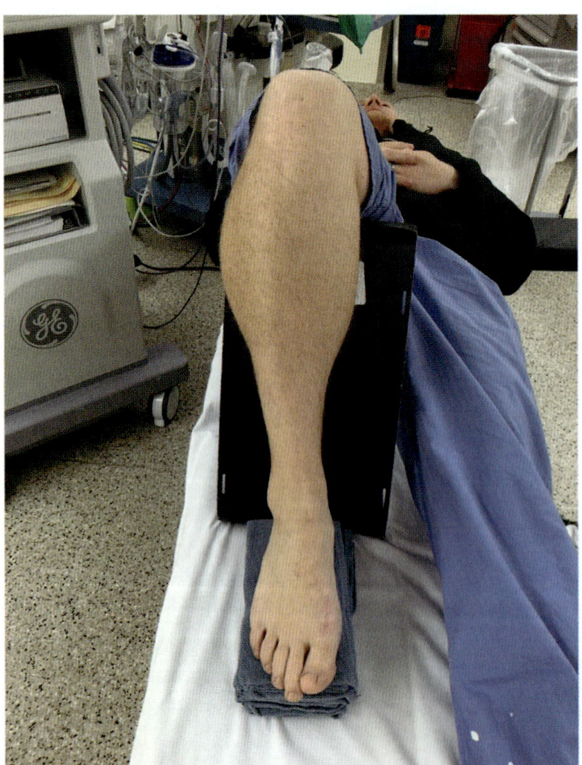

Figure 26-5 |

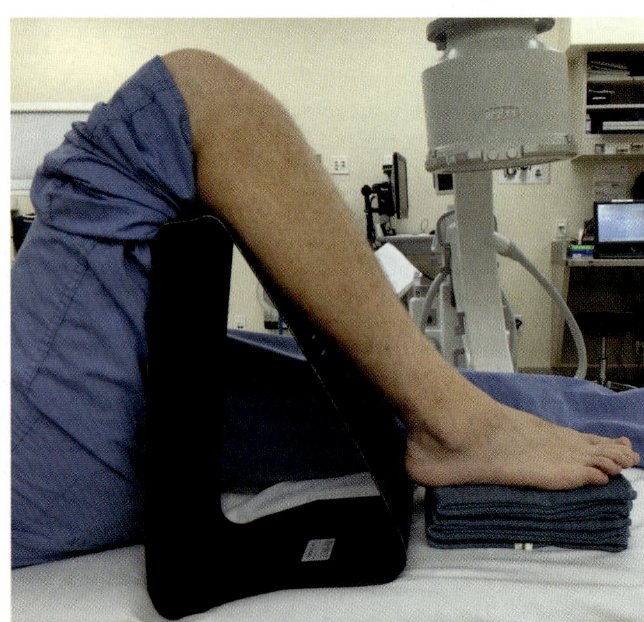

Figure 26-6 |

Fluoroscopy Pearls

- Position the C-arm to come in from the contralateral side with the monitor at the head of the bed on the ipsilateral side, as the surgeon will stand at the foot of the bed facing the patient's head (Fig. 26-7).
- Once the foot is in an appropriate position and an adequate AP foot view is obtained, do not move the root; rather have the C-arm operator maneuver the C-arm for oblique (partial rollover) and lateral views (complete rollback). A radiolucent triangle helps position the foot in space to bring the AP and lateral views orthogonal and parallel to the floor for ease of imaging (Fig. 26-8).

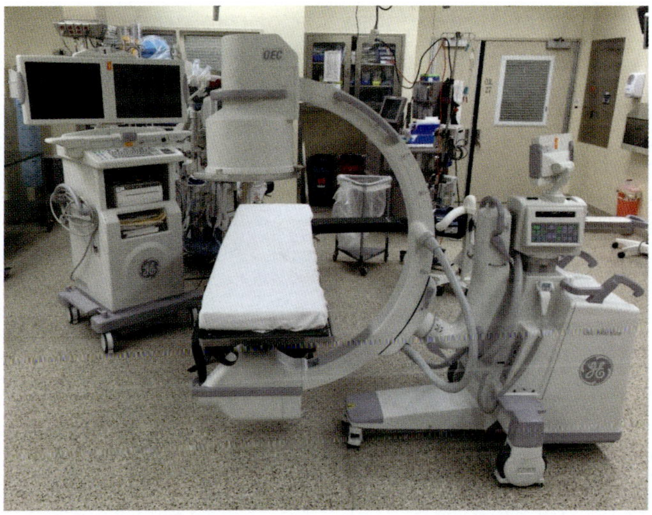

Figure 26-7 |

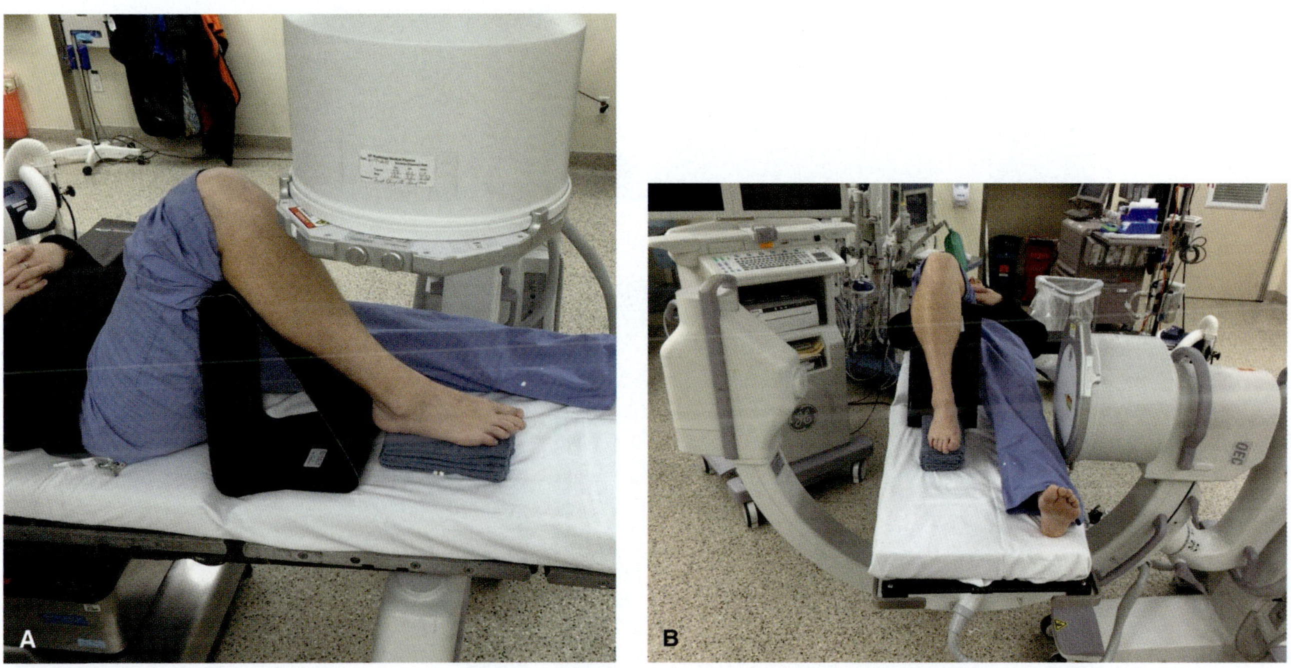

Figure 26-8 |

Stress Examination

- Due to the subtle nature of some injuries, a stress examination is necessary to identify occult instability. A stress examination is also helpful to identify which of the tarsometatarsal articulations are involved in the injury leading to instability.
- The stress examination should begin on an AP view sighting directly down the 1st tarsometatarsal joint (Fig. 26-9).
- The hindfoot is then stabilized with pressure exerted over the lateral midfoot. The forefoot is then abducted, and a repeat AP image is obtained. Fluoroscopic stress examination is useful for both identifying occult unstable injuries at the 1st tarsometatarsal articulations as well as uncovering instability at the 2nd through 5th tarsometatarsal articulations with known 1st tarsometatarsal instability (Fig. 26-10).

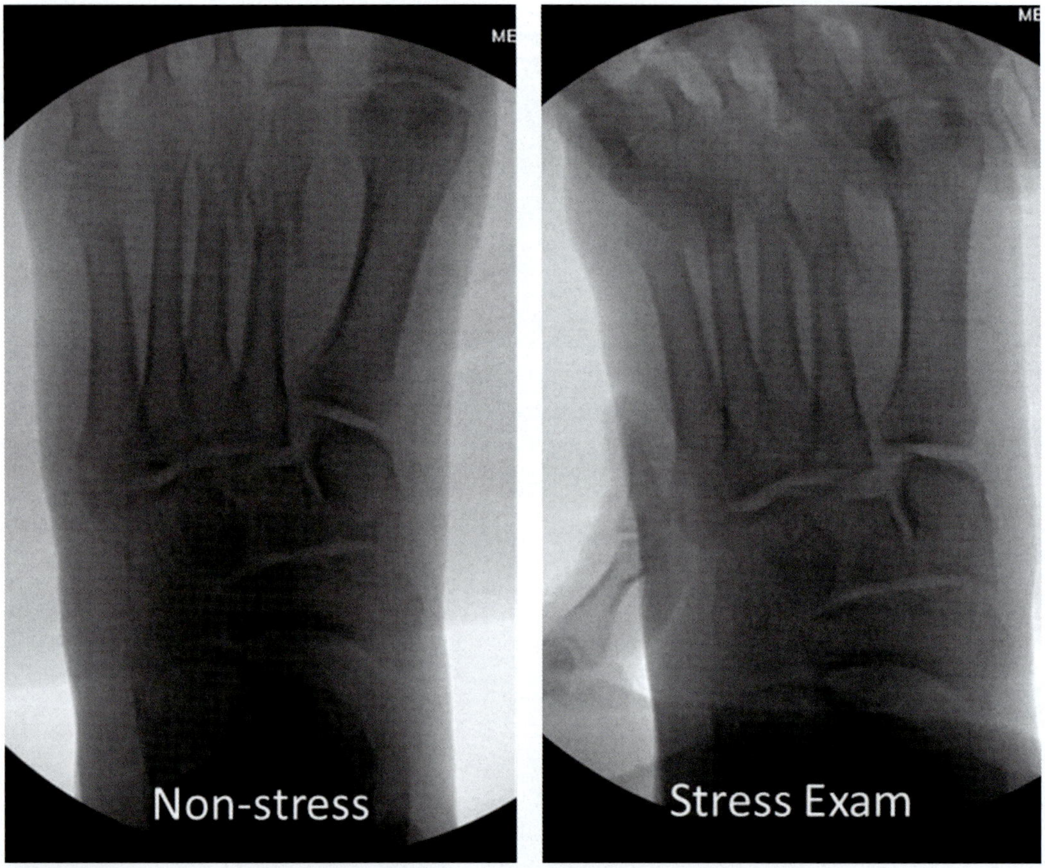

Figure 26-9 |

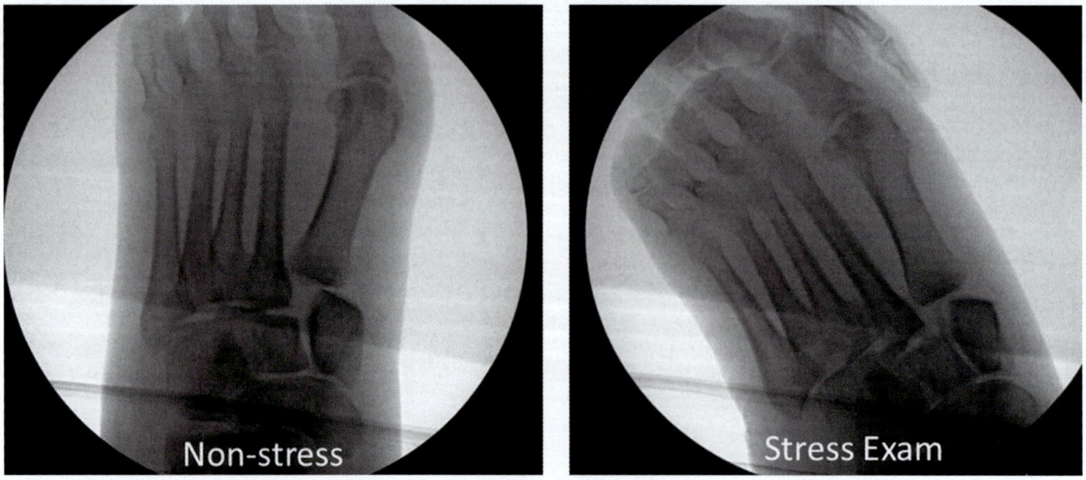

Figure 26-10 |

Fixation

- For both provisional and definitive stabilization of the 1st tarsometatarsal joint, the AP view profiling the 1st tarsometatarsal joint is ideal. A lateral view is also necessary to confirm reduction in the sagittal plane with no residual displacement of the base of the 1st metatarsal base relative to the medial cuneiform. To best visualize the plantar extent of the 1st metatarsal base and the medial cuneiform, the foot must be pronated. This helps evaluate both reduction and screw lengths (Fig. 26-11).
- The more plantar screw often appears to violate the navicular-cuneiform joint on the AP or oblique views; however, this is due to the concavity of the proximal aspect of the medial cuneiform. An adequate lateral view will show that the screw is actually positioned in the most plantar and proximal aspect of the medial cuneiform and does not violate the joint (Fig. 26-12).
- Reduction of the 2nd tarsometatarsal can be done in the AP view with reconstitution of line between the medial border of the base of the 2nd metatarsal and the medial border of the middle cuneiform (Fig. 26-13).

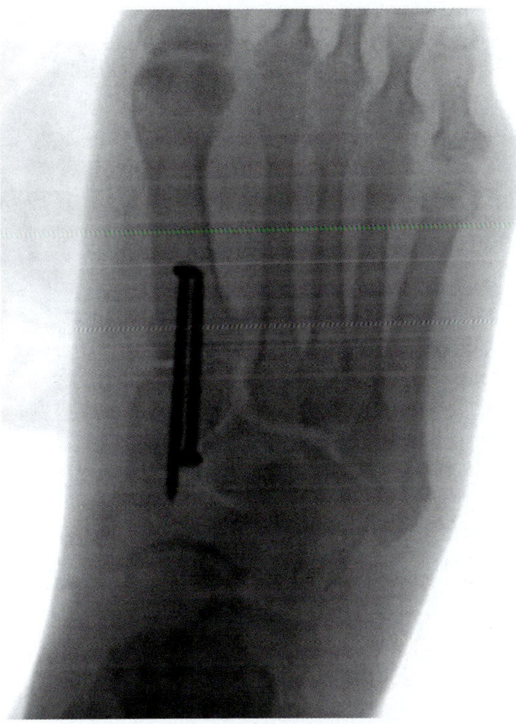

Figure 26-11 |

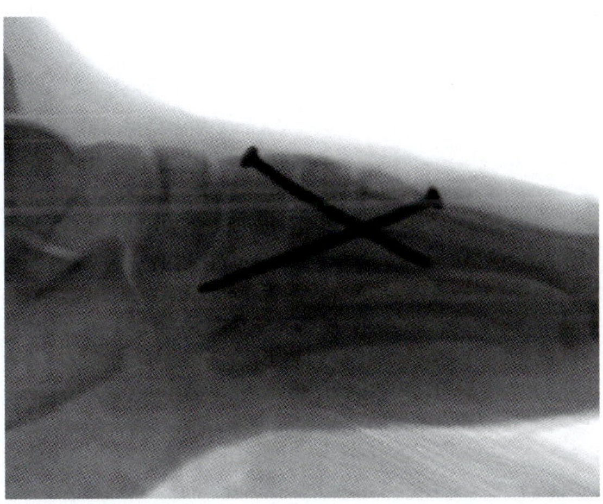

Figure 26-12 |

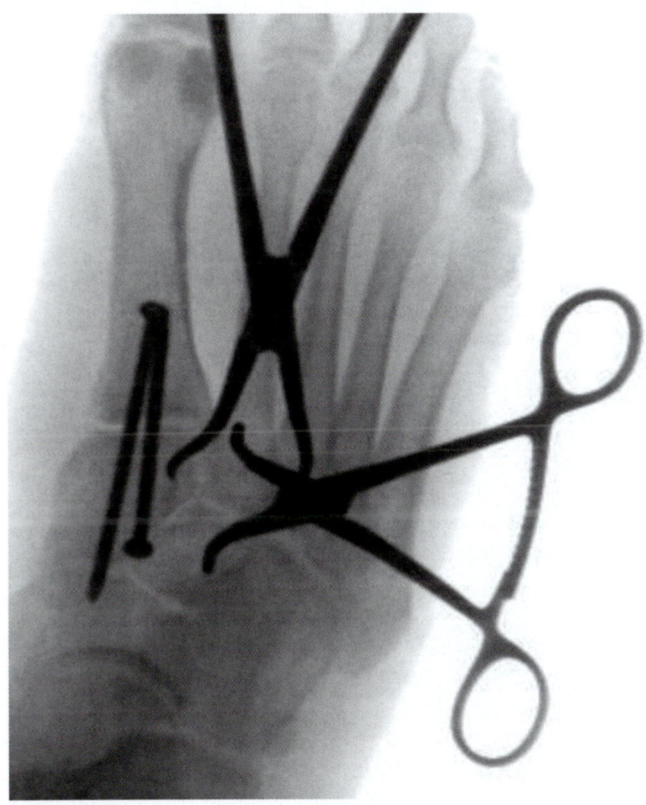

Figure 26-13 |

- After sequential reduction of each tarsometatarsal articulation, AP, oblique, and lateral views should be checked to insure that normal radiographic relationships are restored. On the lateral view, the plantar extent of the lesser metatarsal bases can be accentuated by varying degrees of pronation and supination of the foot. The dorsal articulation can also be evaluated (Fig. 26-14).
- Restoration of the 4th and 5th tarsometatarsal articulation with the cuboid should be done in the oblique and lateral view (Fig. 26-15).
- For fractures with significant articular involvement or that are length unstable, dorsal plates can be used to span the joint.

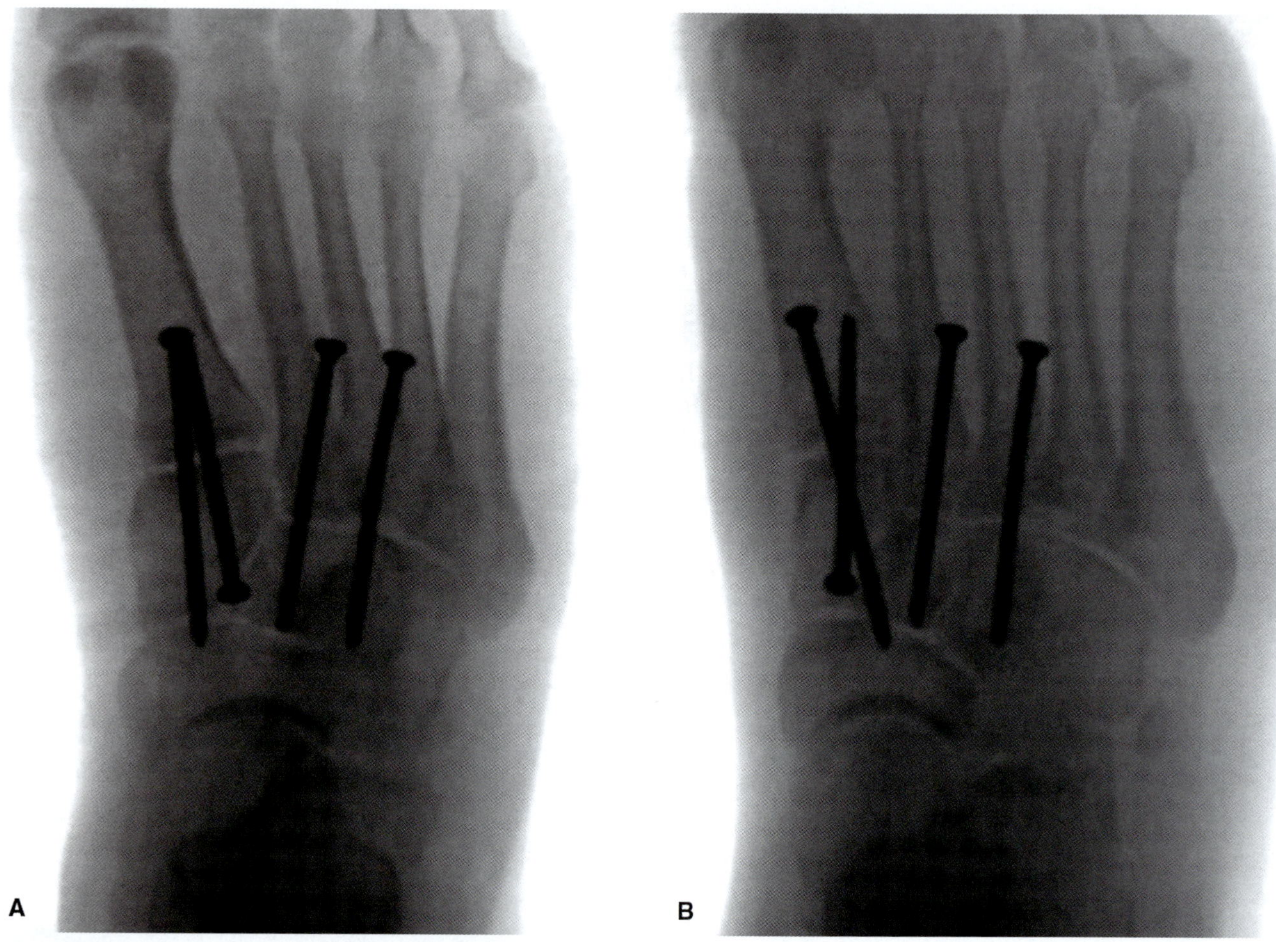

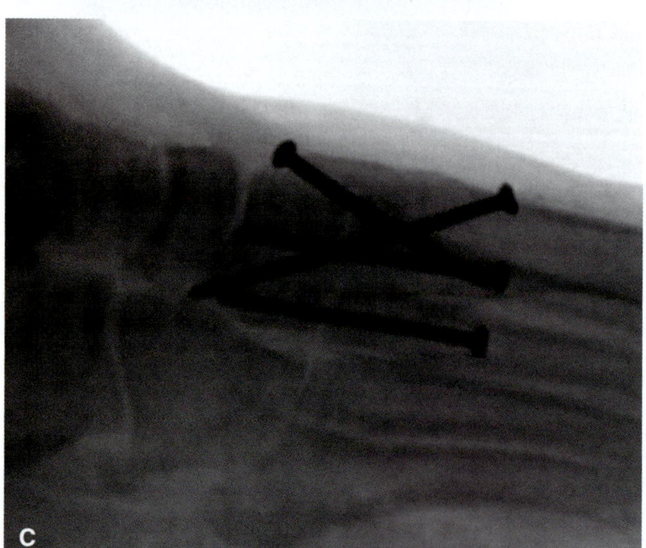

Figure 26-14 |

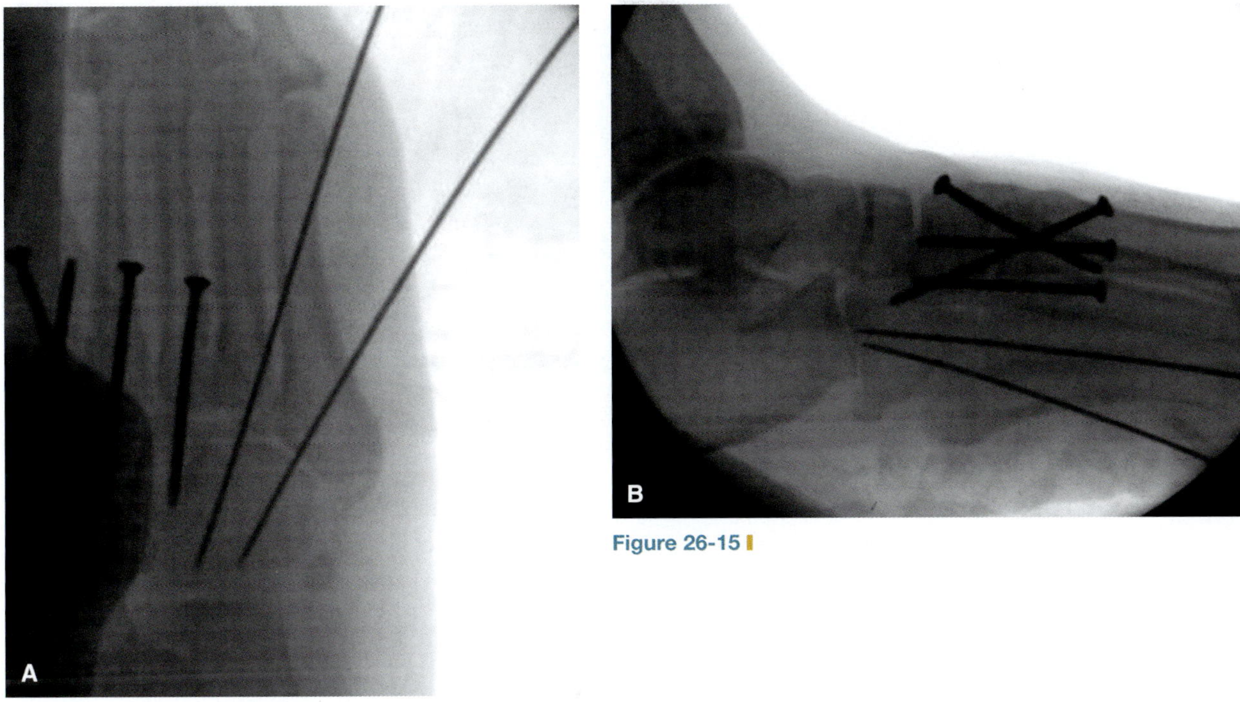

Figure 26-15

- When applying a plate to the 1st tarsometatarsal articulation, the AP and oblique views can be used. Due to soft tissue and anatomic restrictions, the plate usually sits on the dorsal and medial side of the articulation. On the AP view, the plate will appear to be medialized (Fig. 26-16).
- The pronated lateral view is used to visualize screw length on a spanning plate and assess reduction of the dorsal surfaces (Fig. 26-17).

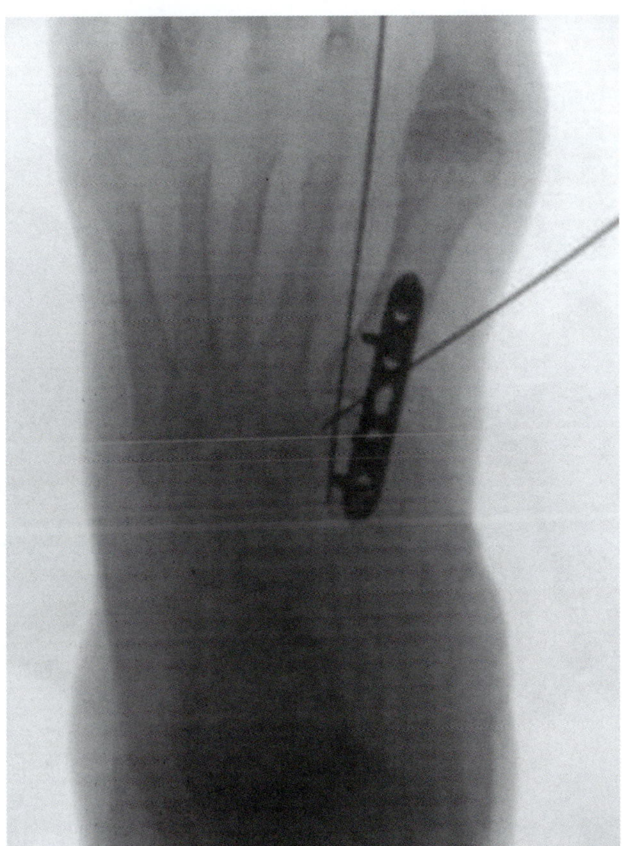

Figure 26-16

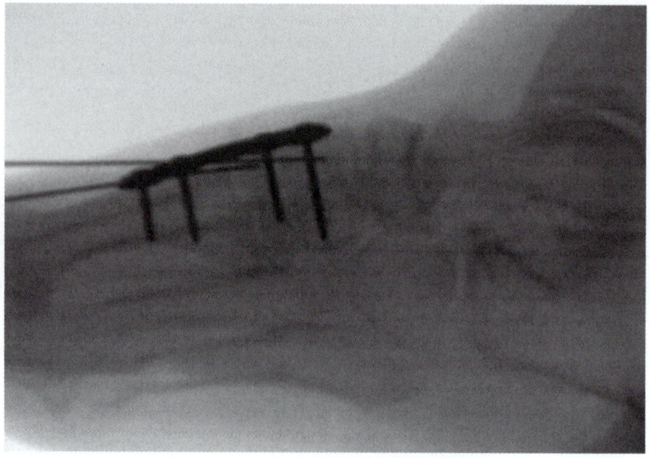

Figure 26-17 |

- AP and oblique views can be useful to assess reduction at the 2nd and 3rd tarsometatarsal joint as well as to verify there is no screw penetration into the intercuneiform joint (Fig. 26-18).
- Varying degrees of pronation and supination can be utilized to assess the screw lengths at different metatarsal and cuneiform articulations (Figs. 26-19 and 26-20).
- A dorsal plate can be applied to the 3rd tarsometatarsal joint in similar fashion (Figs. 26-21 and 26-22).
- For injuries that involve both the tarsometatarsal joints and the midtarsal joints, additional fixation is needed in the midfoot.
- Intercuneiform screws must be placed in the dorsal aspect of the medial cuneiform in order to traverse the middle cuneiform. Relative to the medial and lateral cuneiforms, the middle cuneiform has a shallow dorsal to plantar depth (Figs. 26-23–26-25).
- For injuries that involve the navicular-cuneiform joint, screws can be targeted from distal medial to proximal lateral in the AP and from dorsal to plantar in the lateral (Fig. 26-26).

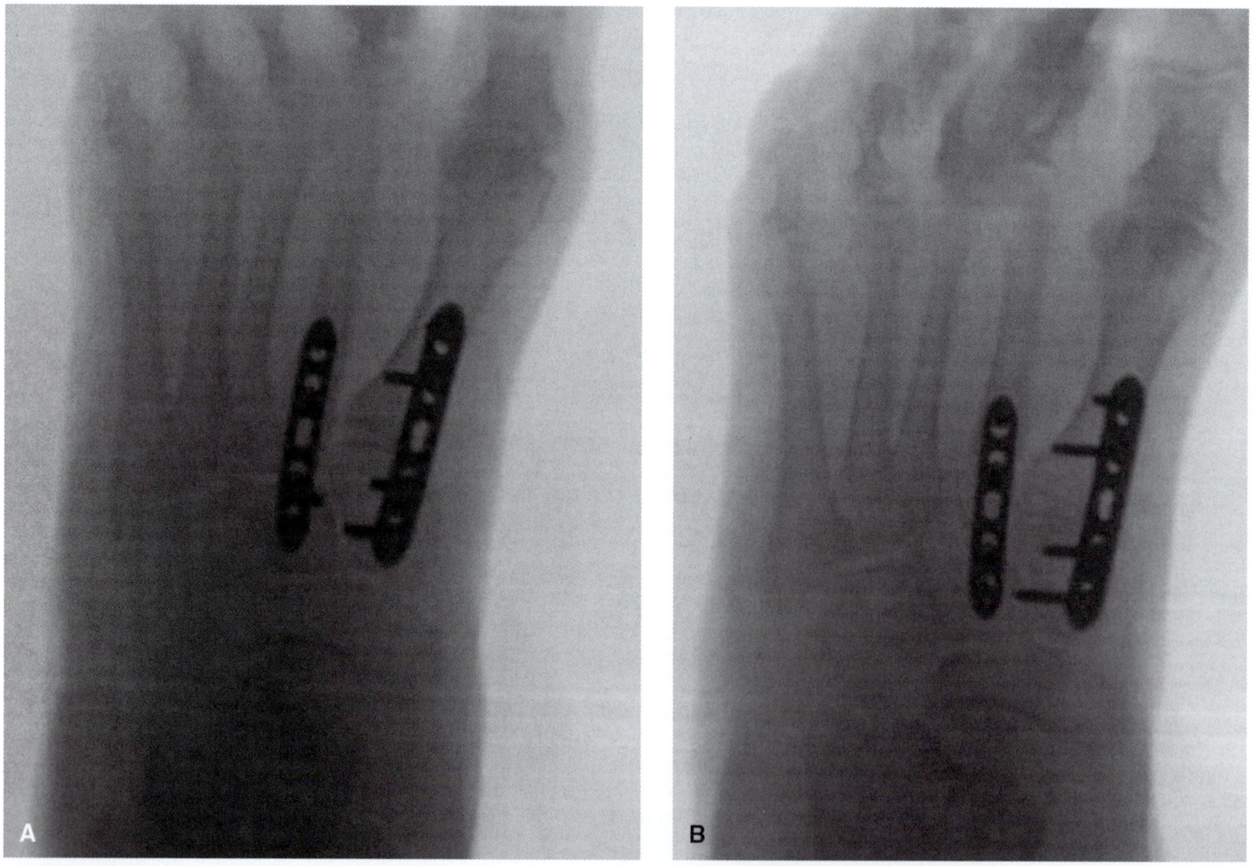

Figure 26-18 |

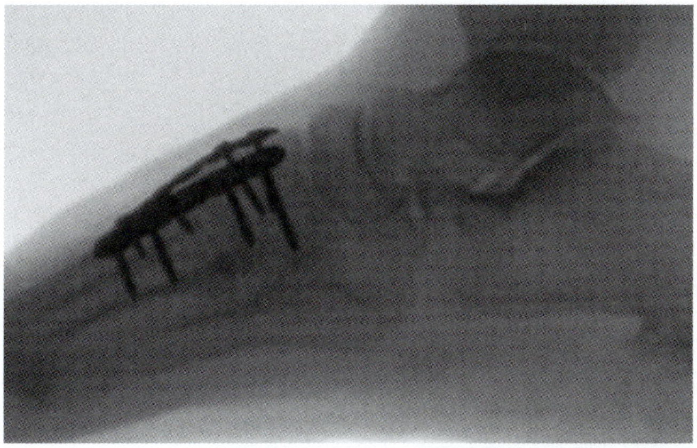

Figure 26-19 |

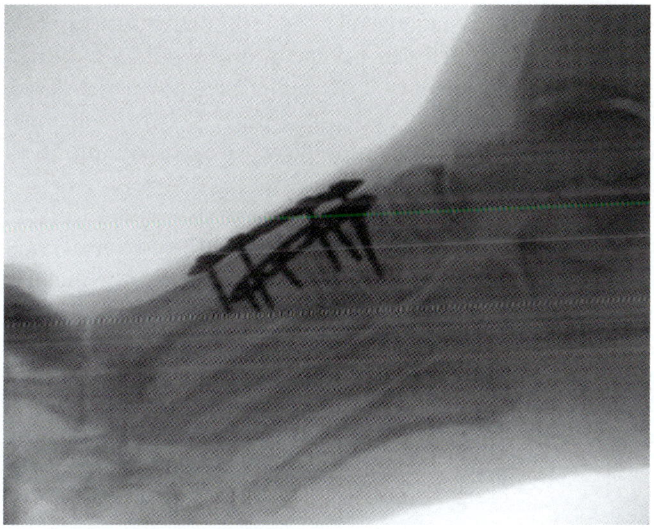

Figure 26-20 |

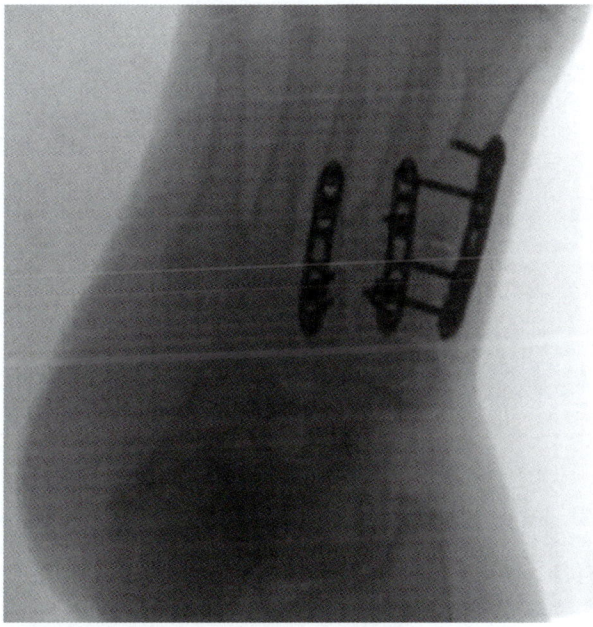

Figure 26-21 |

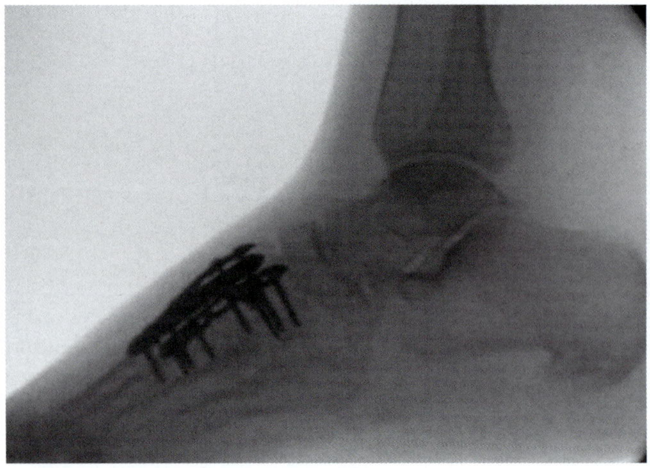

Figure 26-22

- An AP view is used to evaluate the metatarsal cuneiform line as well as the reduction of the cuneiform-navicular joint. The cuneiform-navicular joint should also be concentric on the lateral with no dorsal or plantar displacement of the cuneiform. Screw penetration into the talonavicular joint should be avoided (Fig. 26-27).
- Again, the oblique and lateral views are used to place wire fixation into the 4th and 5th tarsometatarsal articulations.
- The oblique view allows visualization of the reduction to the cuboid while the lateral is used to ensure wires are placed into the cuboid but do not violate the calcaneal cuboid joint.
- The trajectory of these wires is from distal lateral and plantar on the metatarsal base to proximal medial and dorsal into the cuboid (Fig. 26-28).

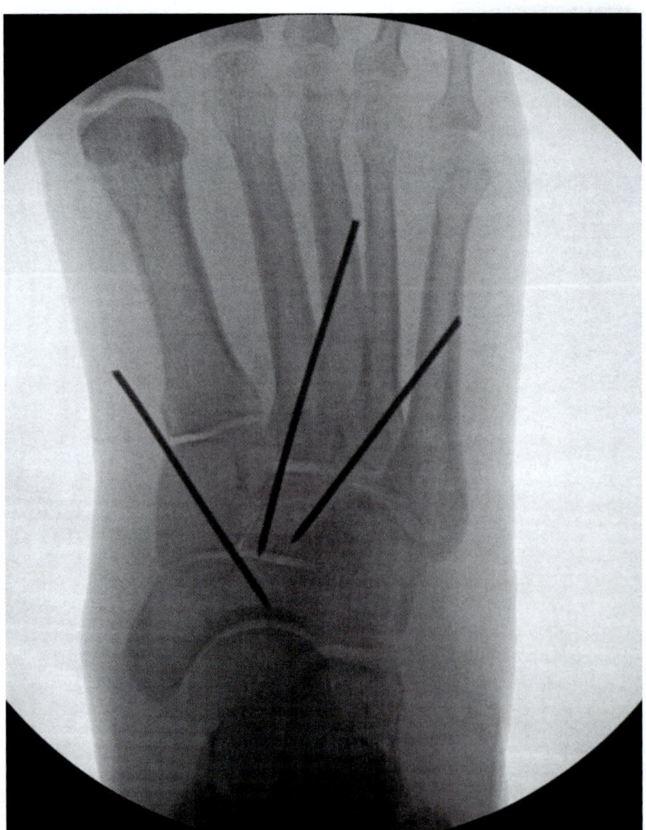

Figure 26-23

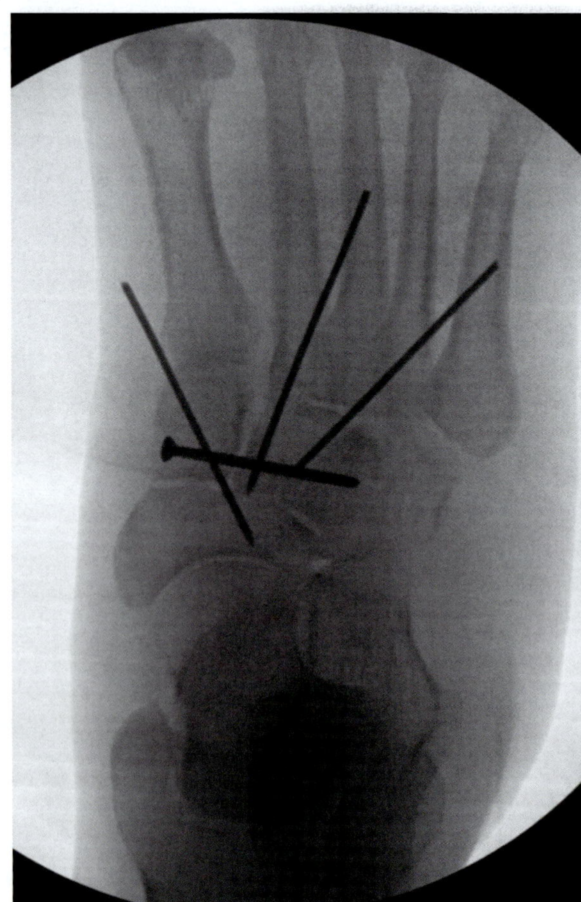

Figure 26-24

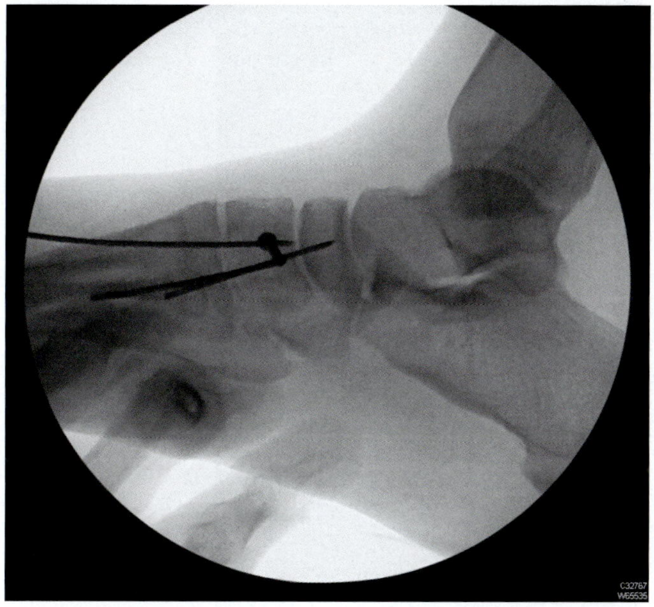

Figure 26-25 |

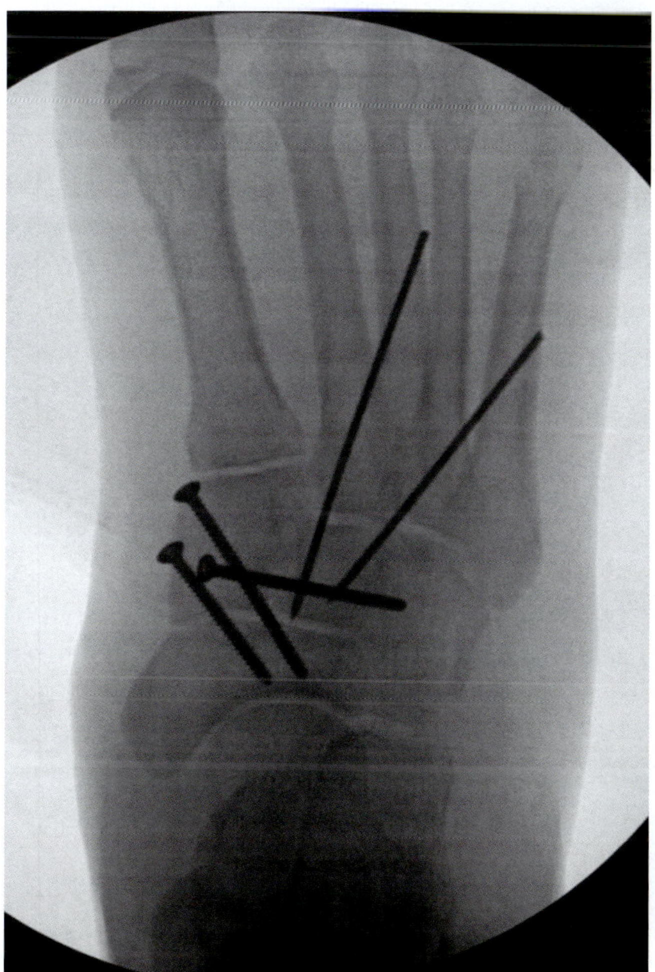

Figure 26-26 |

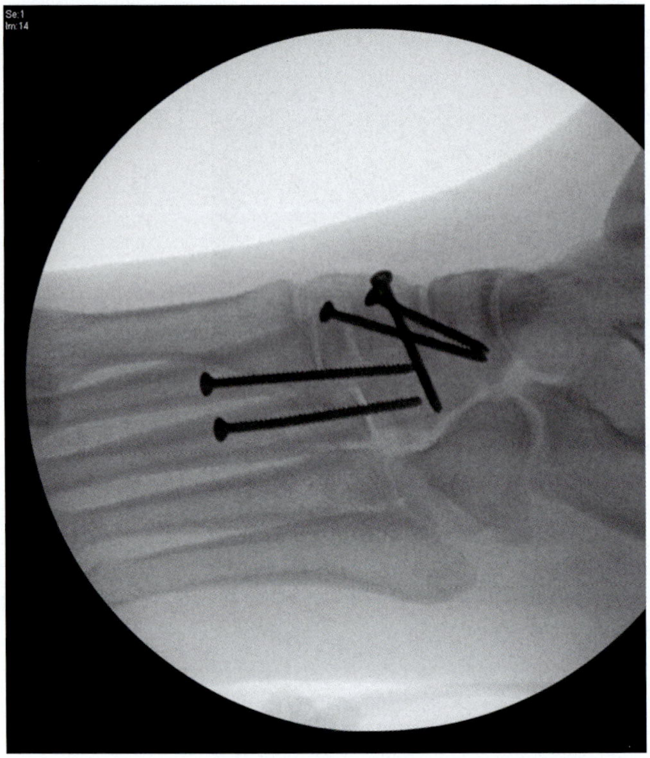

Figure 26-27 |

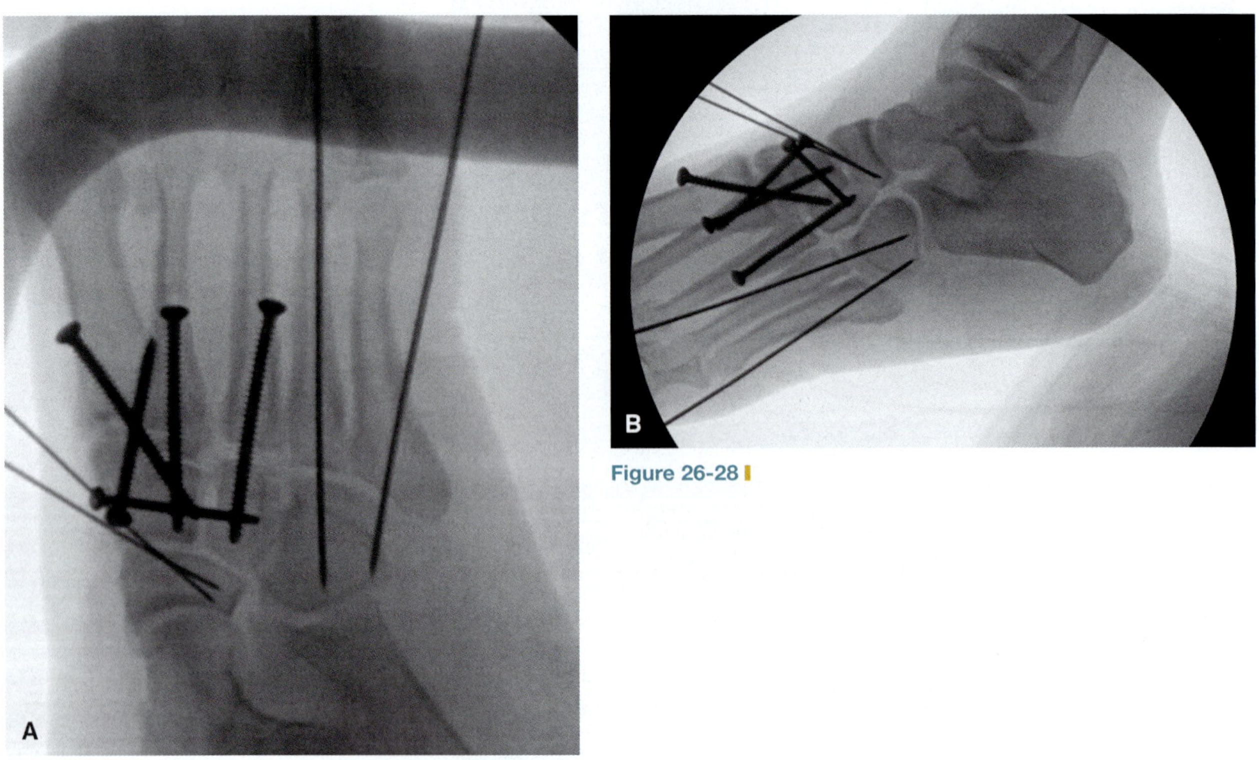

Figure 26-28 |

Chapter 27
Talus Fractures

TYLER SNOAP
ROBERT R. GORMAN III
JASON W. ROBERTS

Bony Anatomy

- The talus has complex anatomy; over 60% of the bone is covered with articular cartilage.
- The talus articulates superiorly with the tibia and fibula at the ankle joint, inferiorly with the calcaneus at the subtalar joint and anteriorly with the navicular at the talonavicular joint.
- The inferior portion of the talus has anterior, middle, and posterior facets, which articulate with their respective calcaneal facets.
- Between the posterior and middle facets is a groove, which exits laterally to form the sinus tarsi.
- Fractures of the talus are often classified into the body, neck, head, and processes.
- The talar neck, in relation to the talar body, is oriented 10 to 44 degrees medial and 5 to 50 degrees plantar.
- Different radiographic views are required to accurately assess each of the anatomic segments and their articulations.

Radiographic Anatomy

AP/Mortise View Ankle

- Assess involvement and fracture displacement of the talar body.
- Assess congruence of the tibiotalar articulation.
- Visualize the lateral process (Figs. 27-1–27-3).

Lateral View Ankle/Foot

- Assess congruence of the subtalar articulation.
- Assess sagittal plane alignment of the tibiotalar, talonavicular, and midfoot articulations (Figs. 27-4–27-6).

Canale View

- Oblique imaging of the talar neck that removes the overlap of the calcaneus to more accurately assess the talar neck.
- Taken with 75 degrees cephalad tilt with foot in 15 degrees eversion and plantar flexion.
- Allows visualization of the lateral shoulder and medial cortex.
- This is not a standard injury film; it is more widely used intraoperatively to assess the reduction of the talar neck.
- AP view of the foot can also assist in evaluating the reduction of the talar neck; however, the Canale view provides more valuable information by assessing the neck in profile while removing the overlap of the talus and calcaneus (Fig. 27-7).

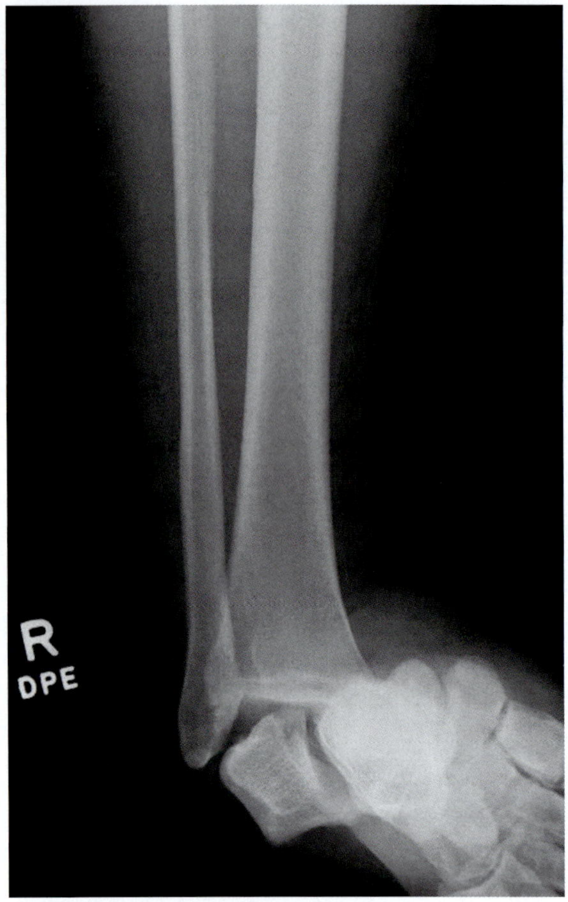

Figure 27-1 | AP view of the ankle: tibiotalar dislocation with evidence of talar neck fracture. Note the talonavicular articulation appears to be intact on this view.

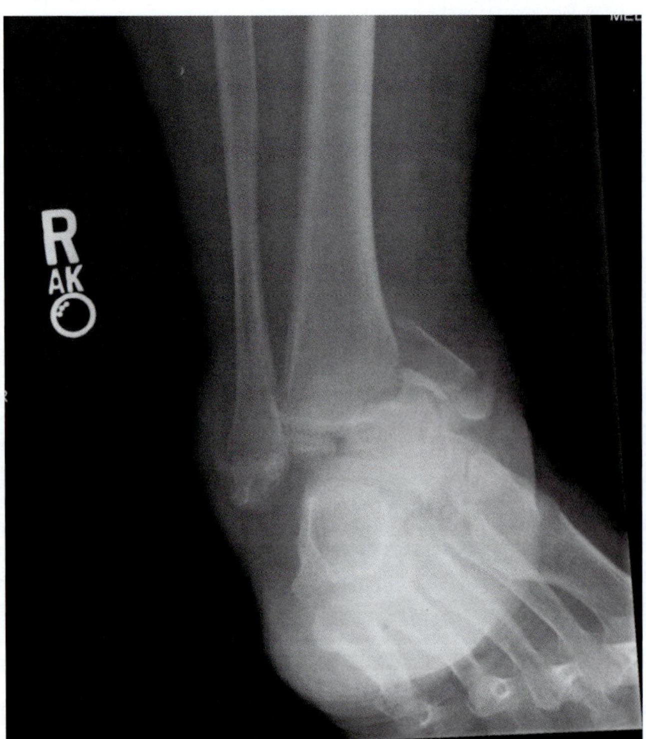

Figure 27-2 | Mortise view of the ankle: there is a talar body fracture with an associated vertical medial malleolus fracture.

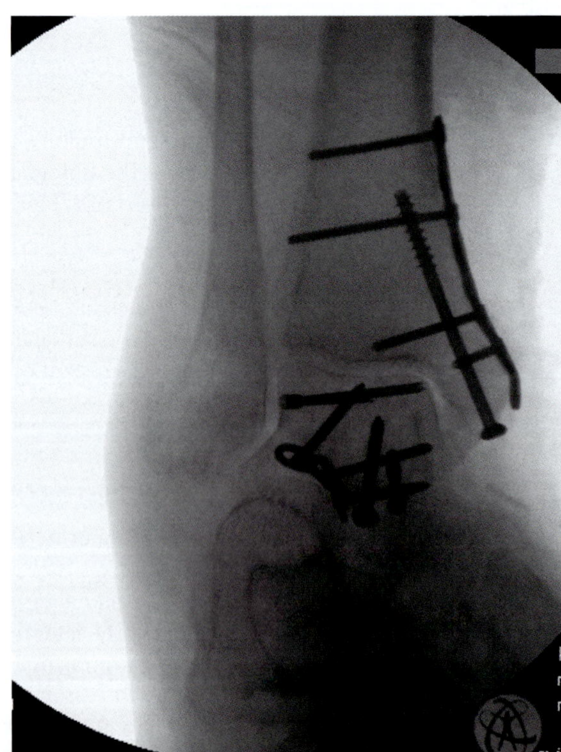

Figure 27-3 | Intraoperative mortise view with definitive fixation of the medial malleolus, talar body, and talar neck.

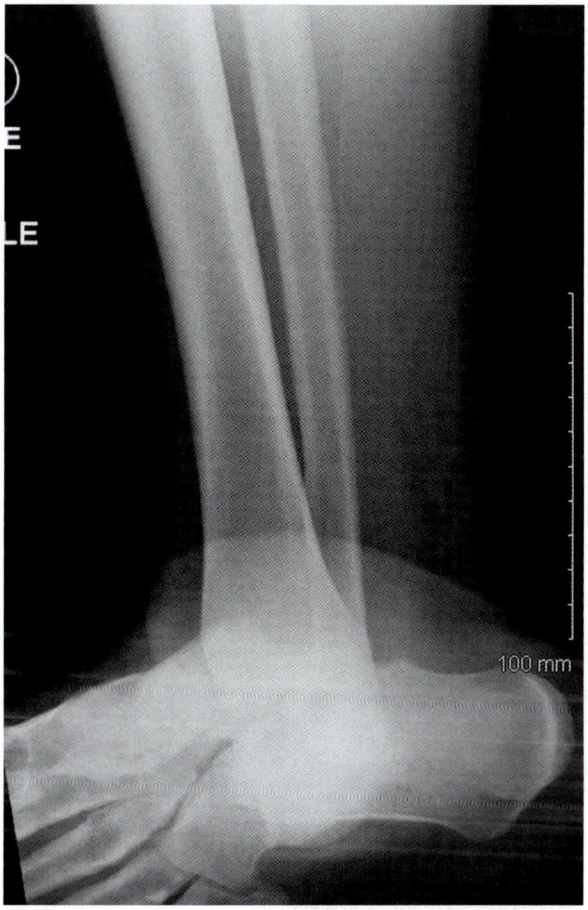

Figure 27-4 | Lateral view of the ankle: there is loss of normal contour of the tibiotalar joint with evidence of a talar neck fracture. The talonavicular joint appears congruent on this view.

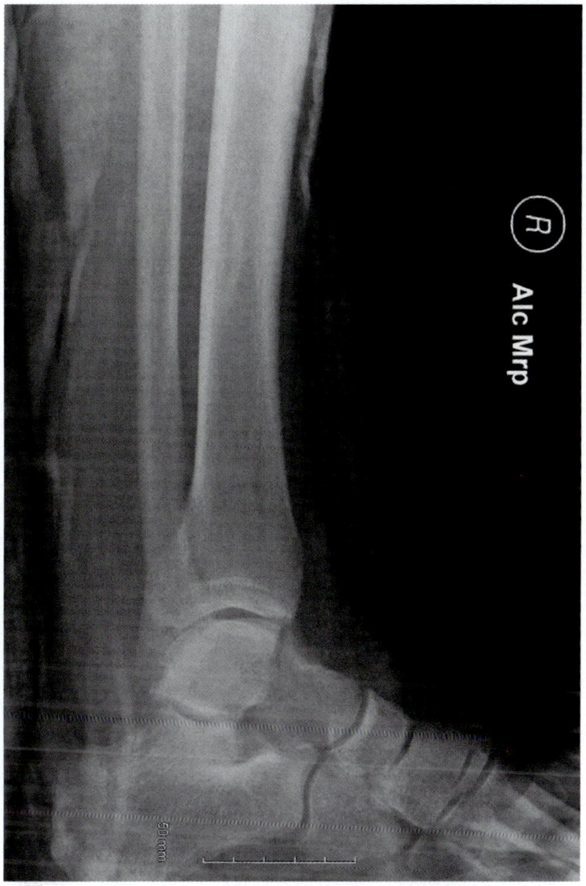

Figure 27-5 | Postreduction lateral view of the ankle: there is a minimally displaced talar neck fracture with intact articulations at the tibiotalar and talonavicular joints. A CT would help assess the subtalar articular congruency and fracture morphology in more detail.

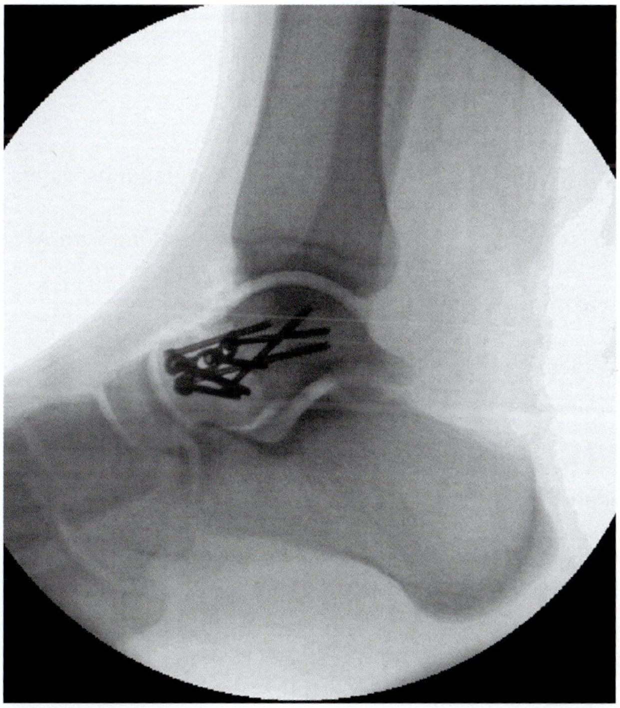

Figure 27-6 | Intraoperative lateral view after definitive fixation of a talar neck fracture.

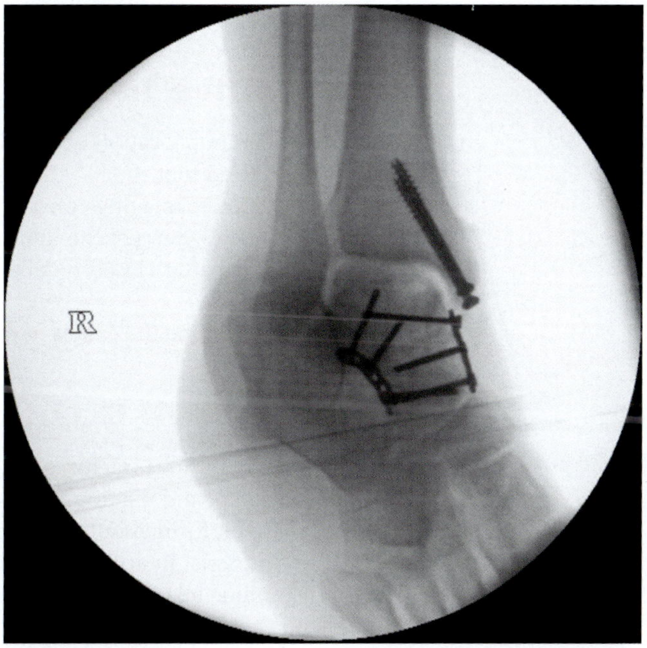

Figure 27-7 | Intraoperative Canale view demonstrating reduction and fixation of a comminuted talar neck fracture with dual plating and screw fixation of an associated medial malleolus fracture.

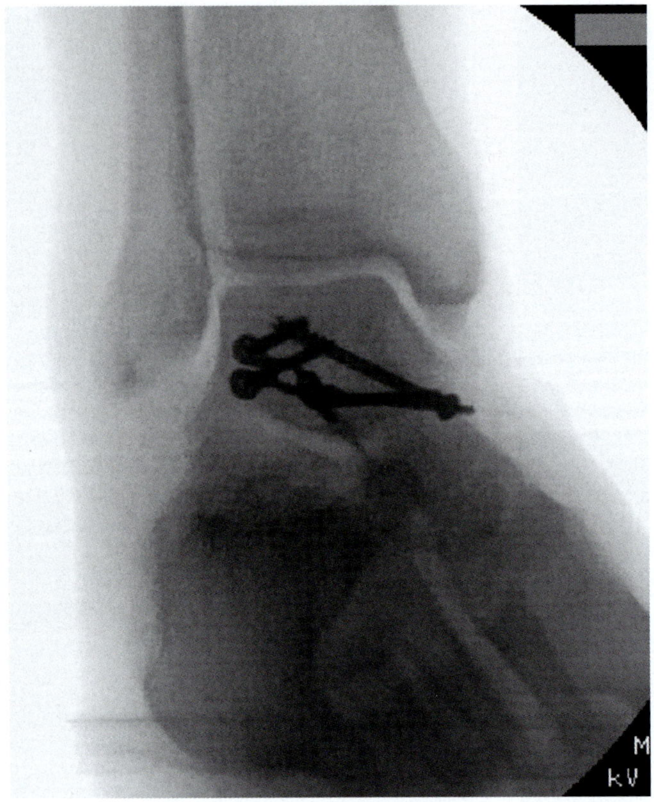

Figure 27-8 | Intraoperative Broden's view after definitive fixation. This construct consists of a lateral plate and screws along with a medial retrograde screw.

Broden's View

- Classically described for calcaneus fractures because it provides radiographic assessment of the posterior facet of the subtalar joint; it can be helpful with talus fractures as well
- Taken with 45 degrees internal rotation, angling image 10 to 40 degrees, and varying foot position until the posterior facet is seen in profile
- Similar to a Canale view; this is not a standard injury radiograph but more of an intraoperative tool that can assist in gauging the accuracy of the reduction (Fig. 27-8)

Preoperative Imaging

- Due to the anatomic location of the talus and its complex articulations, initial imaging must assess both the ankle and foot.
- Typical preoperative imaging consists of AP, lateral, and mortise views of the ankle along with AP, oblique, and lateral views of the foot.
- Imaging obtained after closed reduction gives improved understanding of the fracture morphology.
- CT is helpful to define the extent of displacement and aid in preoperative planning.

Intraoperative Positioning

- Surgical fixation of talus fractures is dependent upon the fracture pattern, approach (one incision vs. dual incisions), and fixation preference (screw vs. plate fixation).
- Most cases are performed in the supine position; various positioning strategies and surgical accessories can assist in accurate imaging.
- Due to the unique talar anatomy, there is not one view that can ensure safe hardware placement; multiple images must be obtained to confirm accurate hardware placement.
- A radiolucent table is required, preferably one in which the end toward the foot of the table is free and does not have a floor attachment. This allows the fluoroscopy to move unimpeded and the surgeon to work at the foot of the table more easily.

Supine Position

- A supine position on a radiolucent table allows for a dual-incision approach with easy access to the medial and lateral aspects of the talus.
- A bump can be placed under the patient's hip to assist with foot positioning.
- An extremity pad can be placed beneath the operative leg; this allows for easier access and more degrees of freedom when obtaining intraoperative fluoroscopy.
- The contralateral extremity is taped down along with the extremity pad for stability during the procedure.
- The room should be positioned to allow image to come in at a 90-degree angle to the longitudinal axis of the patient's extremity; image typically is positioned on the side opposite the operative extremity (Figs. 27-9–27-11).

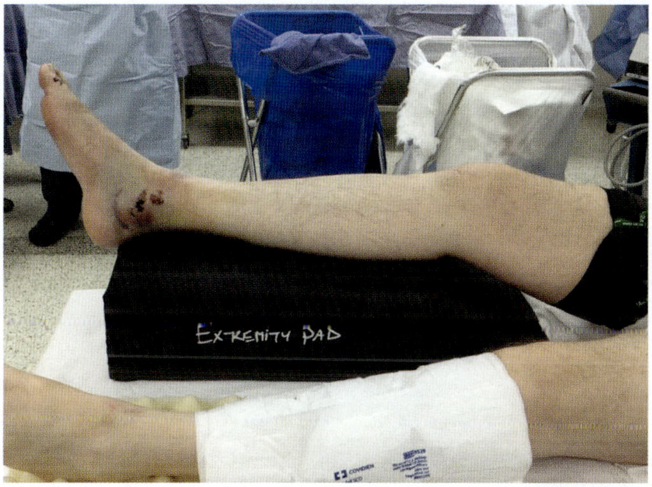

Figure 27-9 I An extremity pad placed under the operative leg with tourniquet applied to the thigh. This position allows multiple views while moving only the C-arm, not the operative limb.

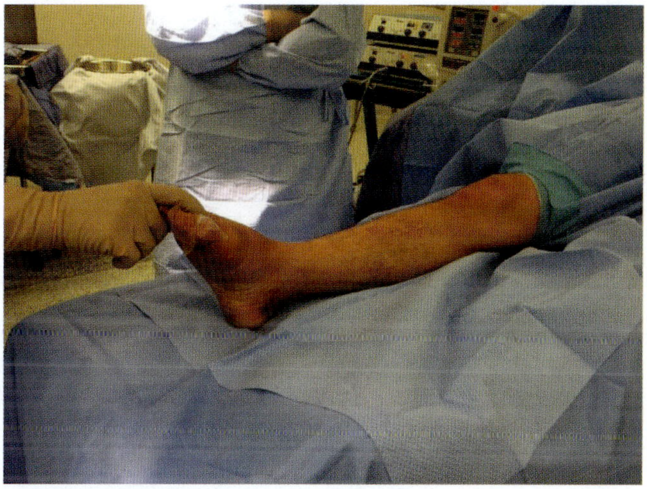

Figure 27-10 I Intraoperative positioning with a bump placed under the ipsilateral hip. A thigh tourniquet was placed and the prep was applied to the level above the knee allowing for ease of manipulation of the operative limb.

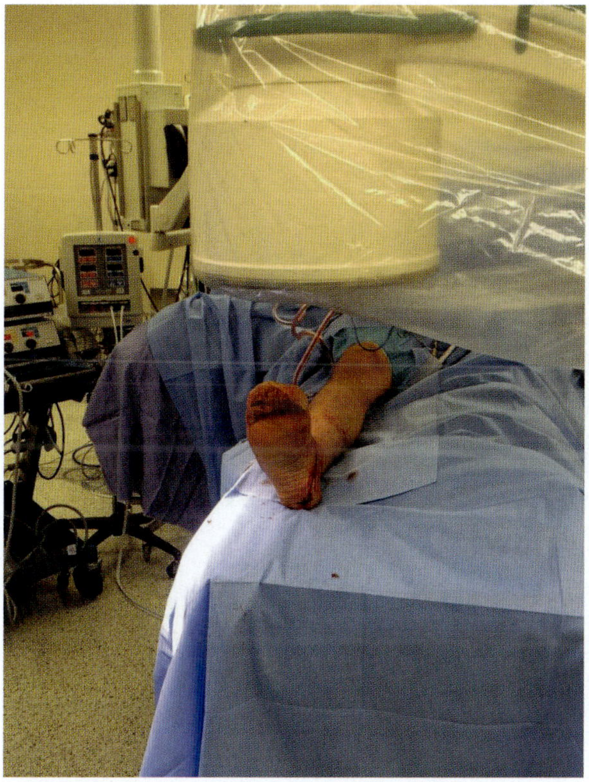

Figure 27-11 I C-arm comes in perpendicular to the longitudinal axis of the patient. This allows for imaging in the AP plane. Swinging the C-arm under the bed from this angle allows easy positioning to obtain a lateral view without moving the base of the C-arm as well.

Additional Imaging Tips

- Prep operative extremity above the knee to allow freedom of manipulation and positioning.
- AP, mortise, and lateral views of the ankle are obtained in a similar fashion to those achieved during standard ankle fracture fixation.
- An army/navy retractor, a mallet, or a metal plate covering from a set tray can assist in obtaining accurate radiographs while minimizing radiation to the surgeon's hands.
- The Canale view can be difficult to obtain intraoperatively. To assist the surgeon, a triangle can be placed under the knee to improve visualization of the talar neck in profile.
- Rotation through the patient's hip can create the internal rotation component of the image. An army/navy retractor can allow for the eversion component while minimizing exposure to fluoroscopic radiation.
- Canting the C-arm can be useful for to achieve the cephalad tilt required to see the entire axis of the talus.
- Broden's view can also be difficult to obtain intraoperatively. The C-arm can generally remain stationary above the patient's foot and ankle. The surgeon internally rotates the operative limb varying degrees until the posterior facet is visible. Eversion at the subtalar joint and plantarflexion at the tibiotalar joint can assist in bringing the posterior facet into profile (Figs. 27-12–27-20).

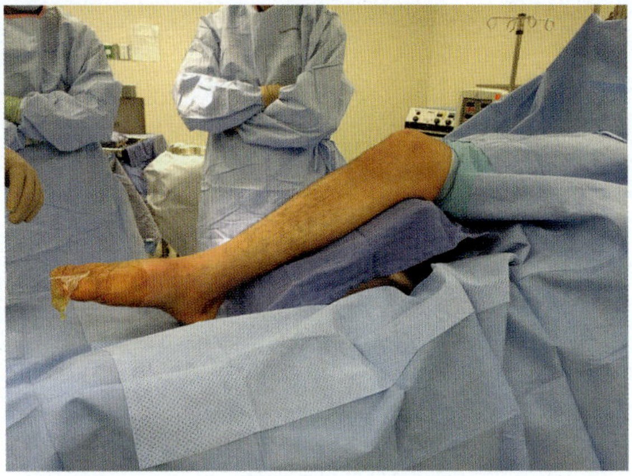

Figure 27-12 | Intraoperative positioning utilizing a triangle. This position allows the foot to be imaged in profile and is especially beneficial for AP and Canale views of the foot.

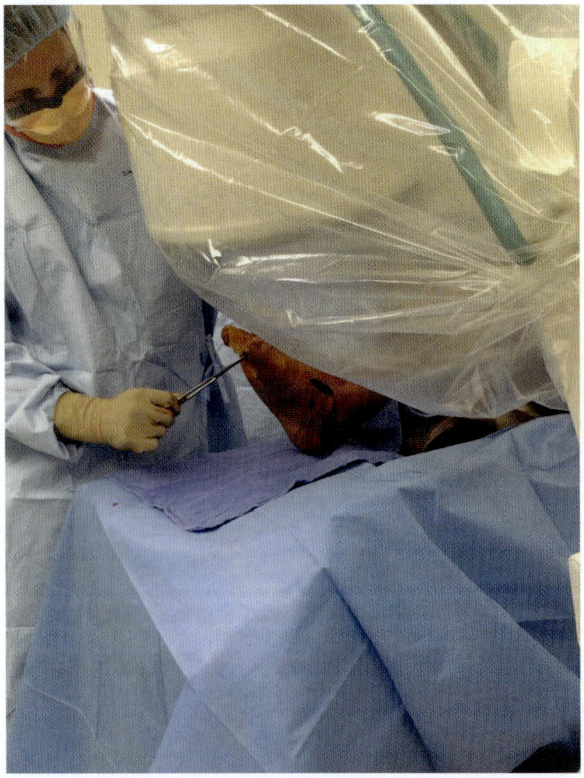

Figure 27-13 | Intraoperative mortise view of the ankle. Note the position of the C-arm as well as the army/navy retractor that can assist in obtaining accurate radiographs while minimizing direct radiation to the surgeon's hands.

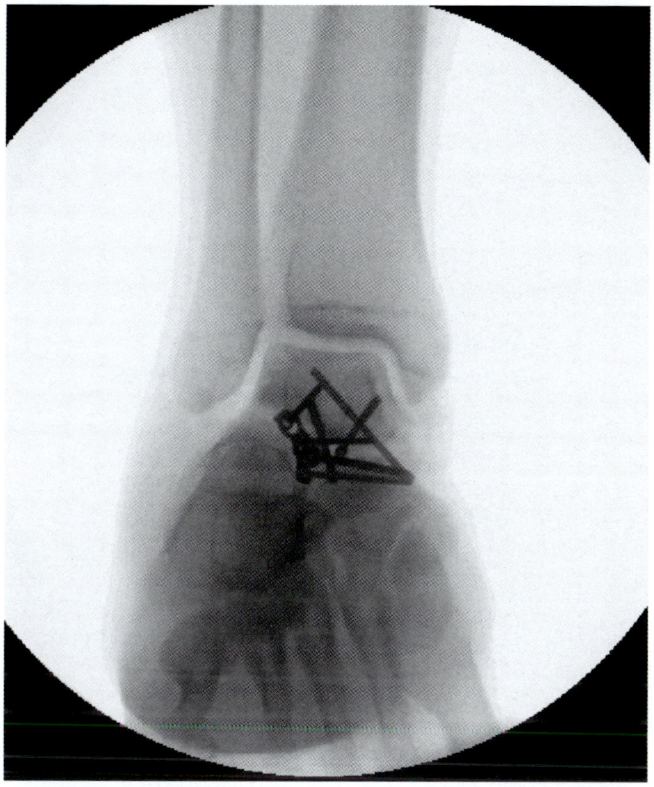

Figure 27-14 | Intraoperative mortise view of the ankle confirming safe hardware placement and congruence of the tibiotalar joint.

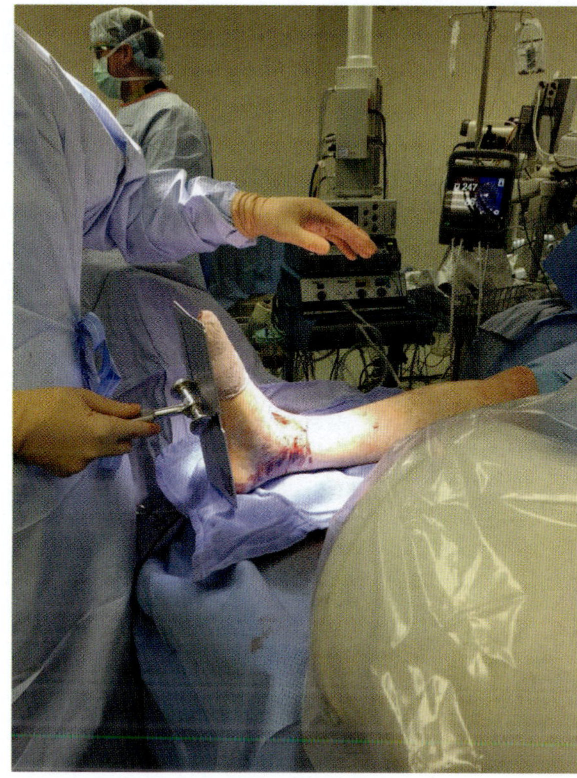

Figure 27-15 | Lateral view of the foot/ankle using a metal plate from a set tray for positioning.

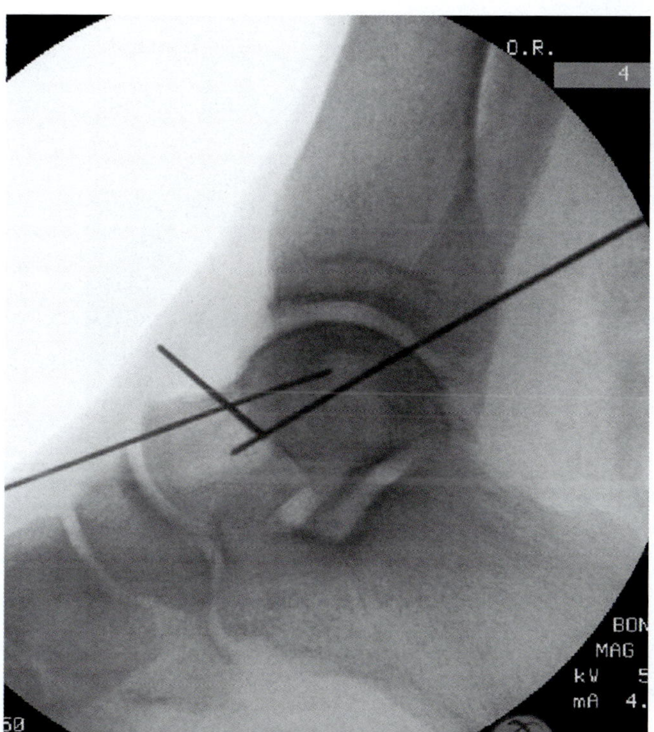

Figure 27-16 | Lateral view of the ankle demonstrating anatomic reduction after provisional fixation of a talar neck fracture.

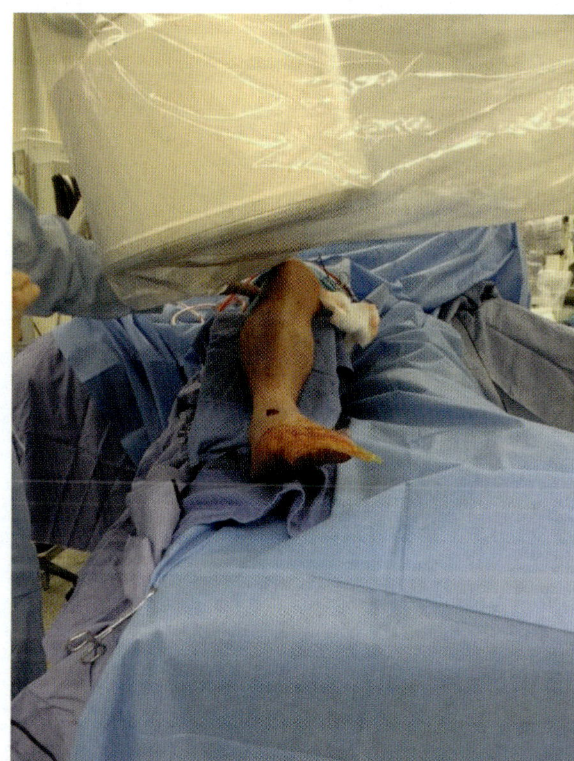

Figure 27-17 | Intraoperative Canale view. There is a bump under the ipsilateral hip. A triangle is placed beneath the operative knee to align the foot for better visualization of the talar neck in profile. The C-arm is canted caudad.

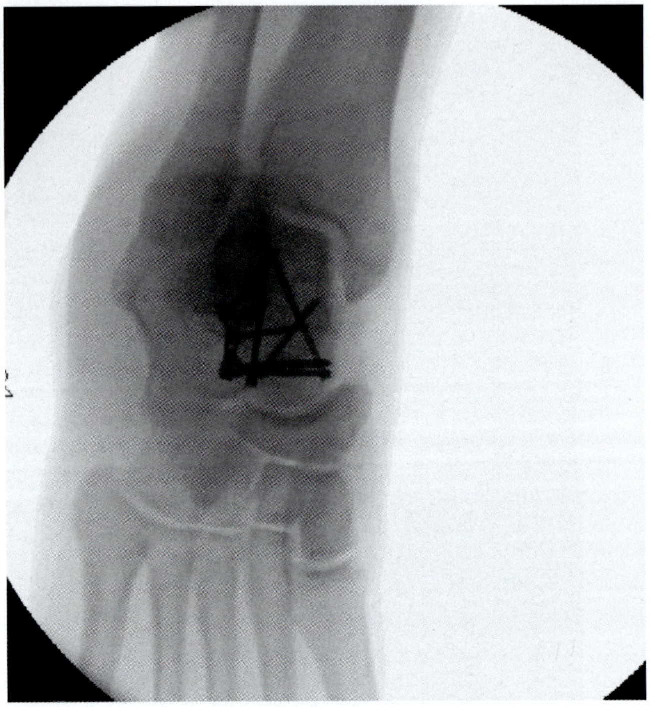

Figure 27-18 | Intraoperative Canale view confirming reduction of the talar neck and hardware position.

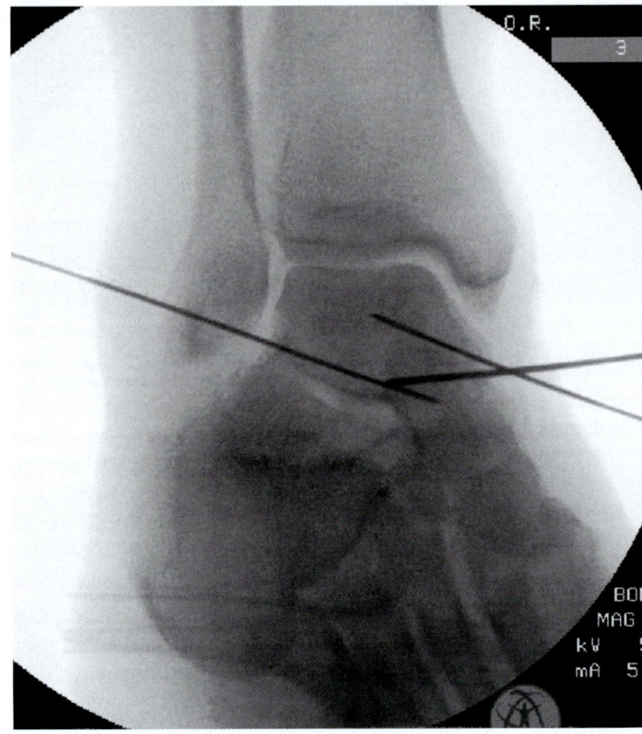

Figure 27-20 | Intraoperative Broden's view with provisional K-wire fixation. Note the subtalar joint congruency, specifically at the posterior facet articulation.

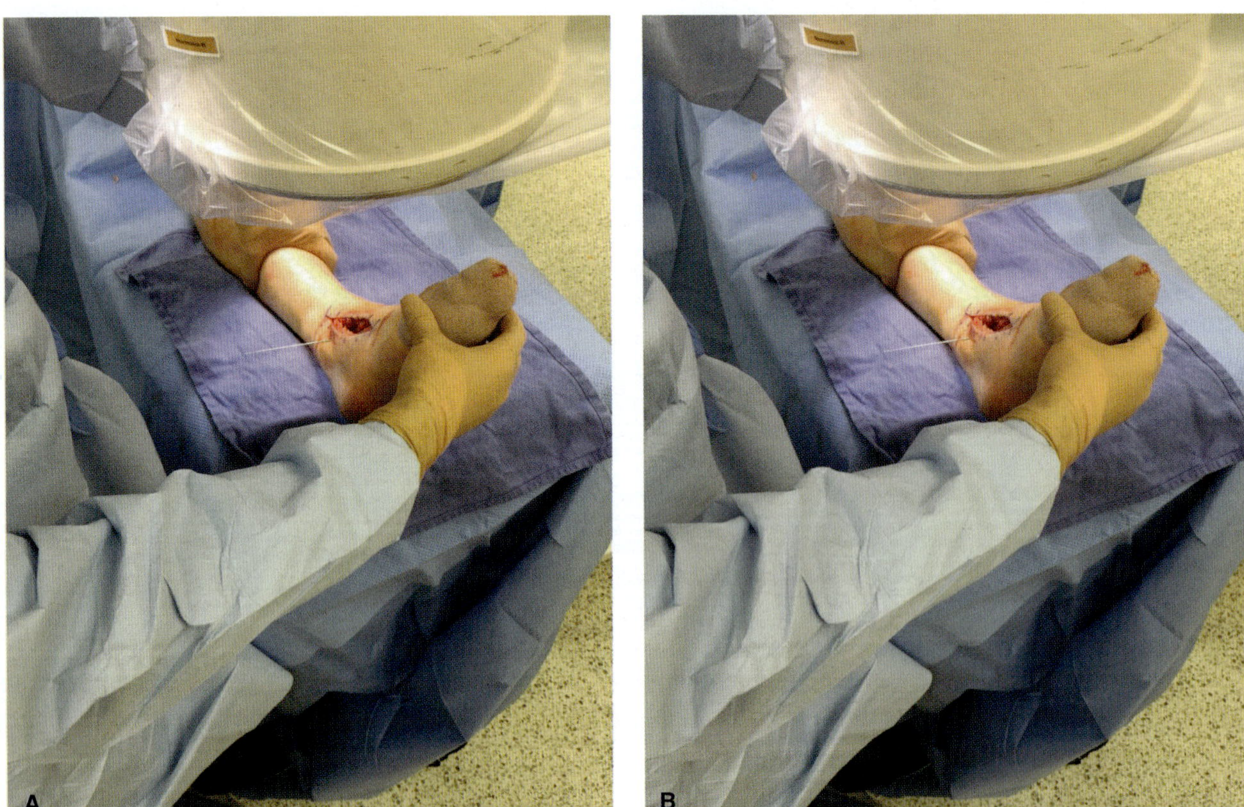

Figure 27-19 | Intraoperative positioning for Broden's view. Note the surgeon plantar flexing the ankle, internally rotating the foot, and also applying an eversion force to get the posterior facet in profile.

Chapter 28
Calcaneus Fractures

BRAD J. YOO
JAMES E. MEEKER

Bony Anatomy

- The calcaneus is asymmetrically shaped, with multiple osseous prominences: the calcaneal tuberosity posteriorly, the sustentaculum tali medially, the anterior process anteriorly, and the peroneal tubercle laterally (Fig. 28-1).
- There are four articular facets: the planar calcaneocuboid; the talar articulations: the anterior facet and middle facets; and the convex posterior facet.
- Calcaneal fractures most commonly occur following a severe axial load.
- Axial force and subtalar eversion result in the lateral talar process striking the superior margin of the critical angle of Gissane as a fulcrum, resulting in primary and secondary fracture lines.
- Primary fracture line: Originates superolaterally, distal to posterior facet articular cartilage margin, and exits medially, caudal to the sustentaculum tali. Two fragments are created: the tuberosity/posterior facet[1] and the anterior process/medial facet[2] (Fig. 28-2).
- Secondary fracture lines created depending upon the energy absorbed and the foot position at time of impact. Distally, stellate fractures in the sagittal plane are common extending into the calcaneocuboid articulation or middle facet. Proximally, fracture lines may occur in the sagittal plane or the axial plane. If a sagittal plane fracture occurs proximally from fracture origination, a separate osteochondral fragment of the posterior facet is created (Essex-Lopresti joint depression fracture). If an axial plane fracture occurs proximally from fracture origination, the tuberosity is detached as a separate fragment with or without a variable portion of the posterior facet (Essex-Lopresti tongue-type fracture) (Fig. 28-3).
- Common deformities visualized on a lateral x-ray include (1) calcaneal height loss, (2) calcaneal length loss, and (3) incongruity of the posterior talocalcaneal facet (Fig. 28-4).[3]
- Common deformities visualized on a Harris axial x-ray include (1) the primary fracture line; (2) varus tuberosity malpositioning; (3) calcaneal width increase, with pathologic lateral translation of the lateral calcaneal wall; and (4) involvement of the posterior facet (Fig. 28-5).
- Soft tissue injuries are almost as important to determining treatment if not more than the fracture pattern.[3] They are not well visualized radiographically, but require close physical examination for proper assessment and optimal outcomes.
- The affected foot and ankle should not demonstrate significant swelling prior to operative intervention. Soft tissue readiness is heralded by the appearance of fine soft tissue wrinkles and the mobility of the skin over the underlying connective tissue. Failure to wait for soft tissue quiescence increases the risk of soft tissue wound complications and infection (Fig. 28-6).

Radiographic Anatomy

- Orthogonal x-rays for calcaneus evaluation include a lateral heel view, a Harris-Beath axial view, and an AP view of the foot.
- Lateral heel view identifies posterior facet involvement, Bohler's angle, (critical) angle of Gissane, and tuberosity position (cranial migration) (Fig. 28-7).

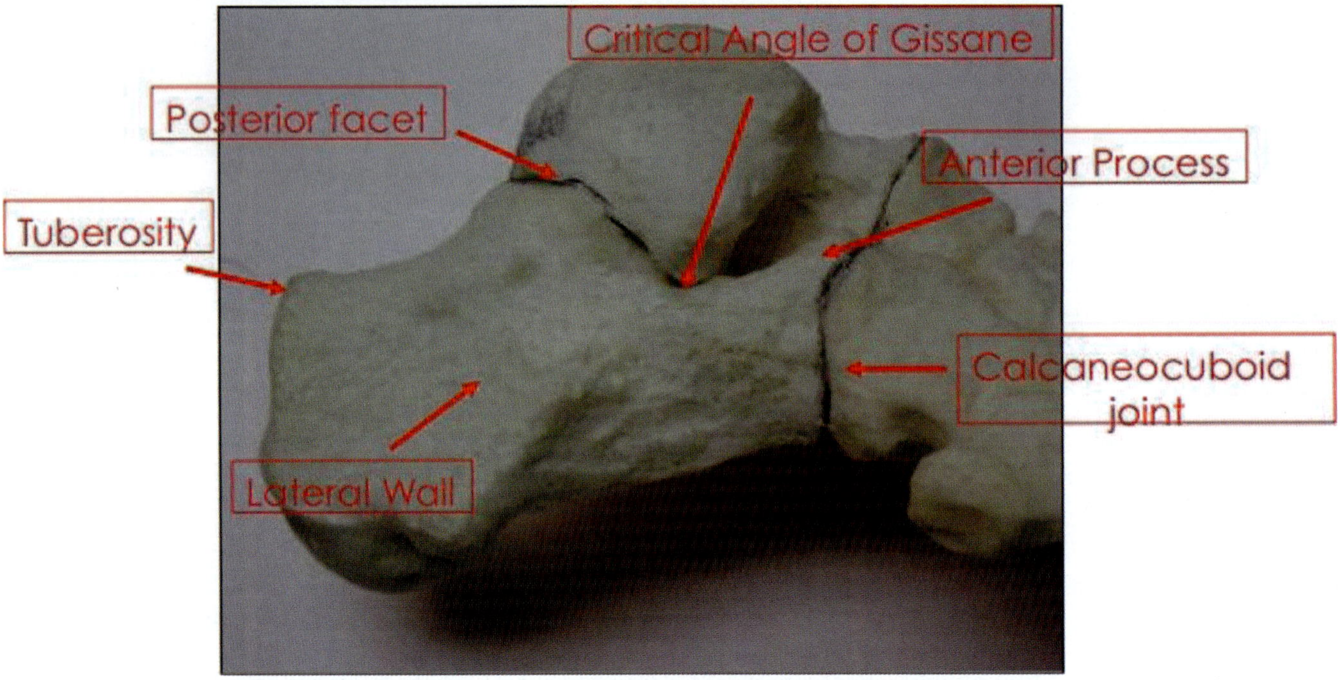

Figure 28-1 I Lateral calcaneus normal anatomy.

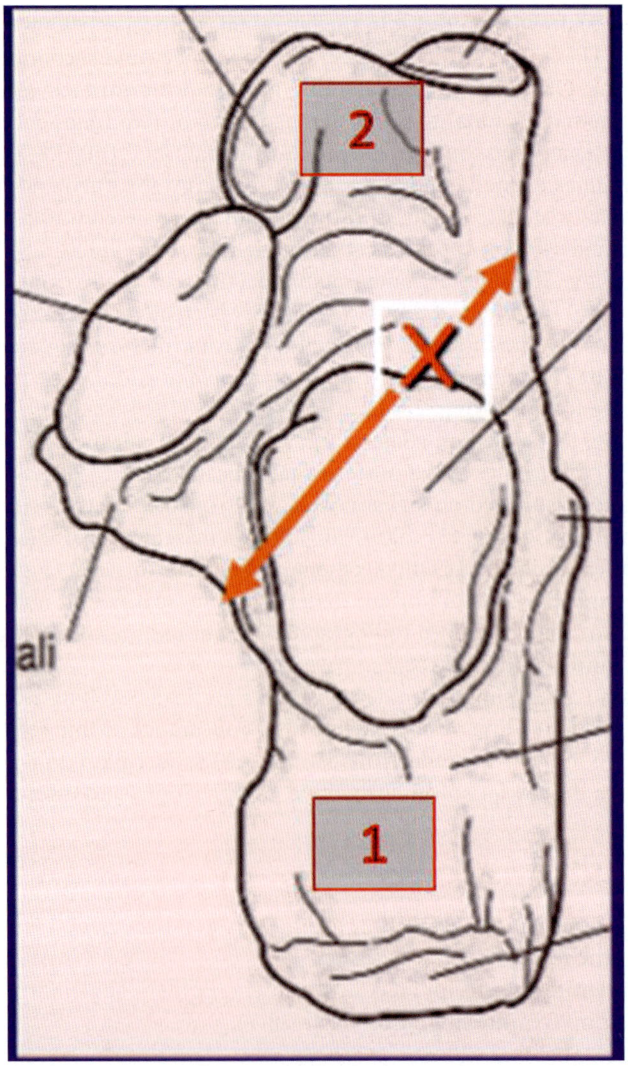

Figure 28-2 I The primary fracture line with the creation of two major fragments, the tuberosity and posterior facet segment (1) and the anterior process and sustentacular segment (2).

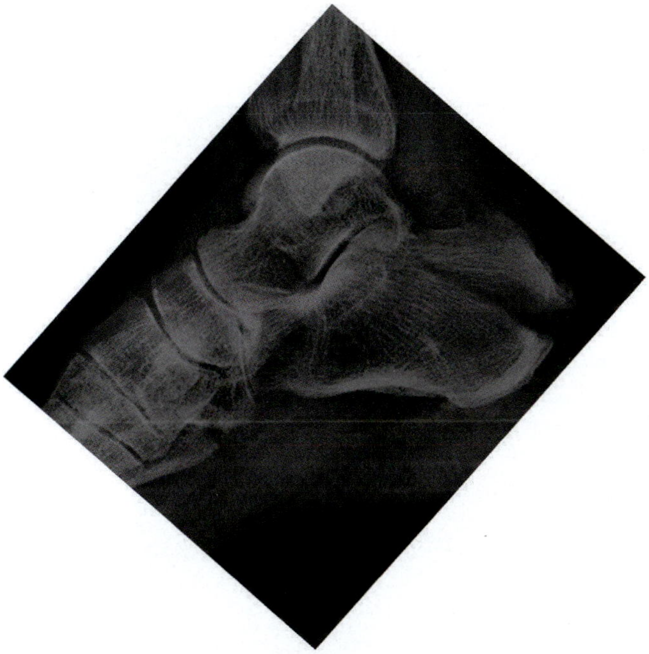

Figure 28-3 | Tongue-type calcaneus fracture.

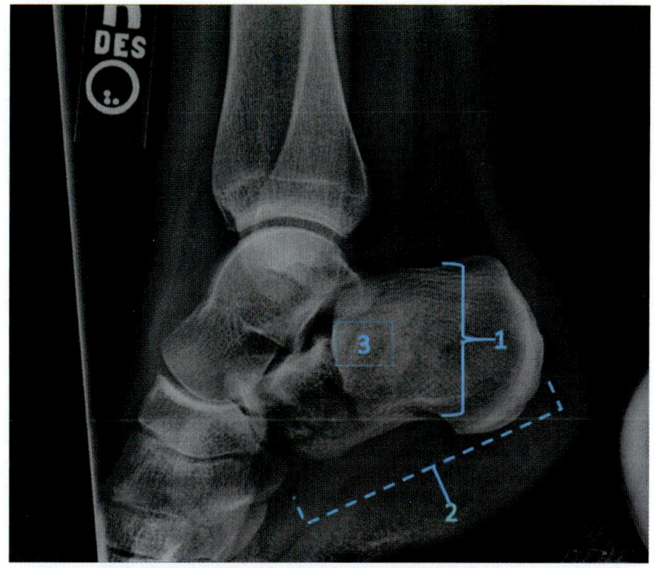

Figure 28-4 | Joint depression calcaneus fracture.

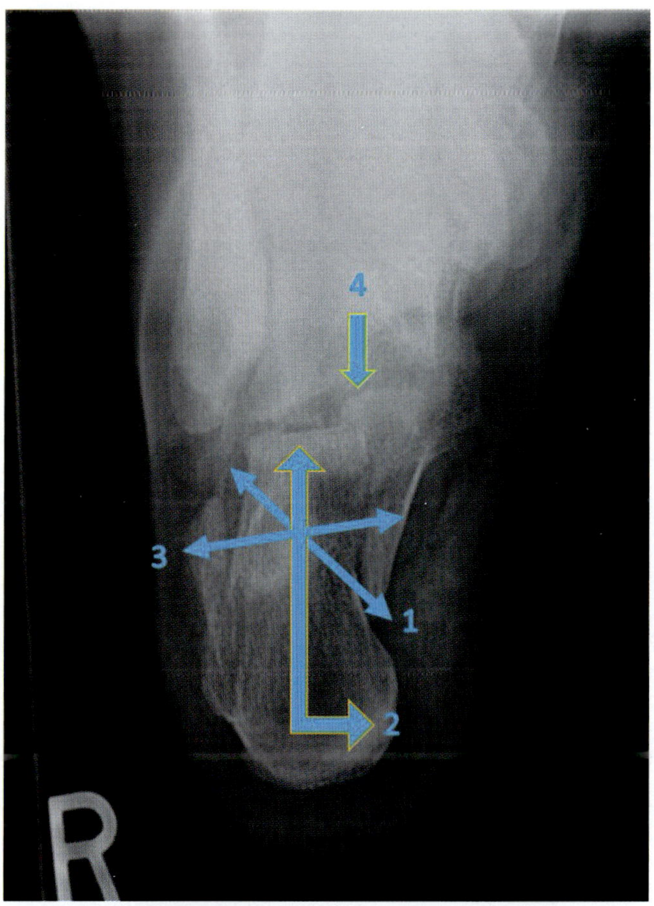

Figure 28-5 | Fracture preoperative calcaneus Harris axial.

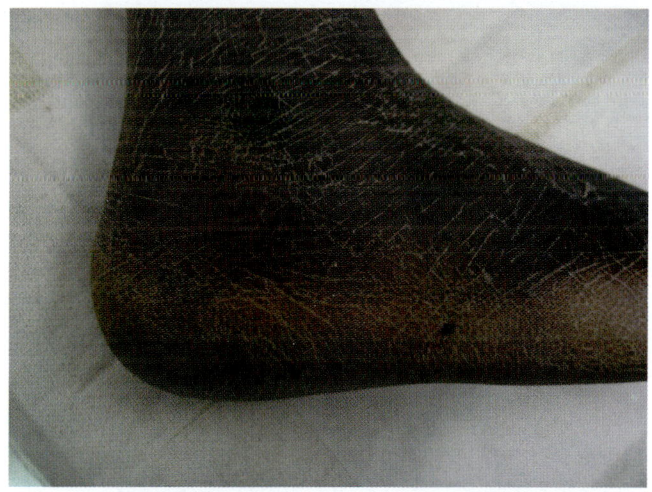

Figure 28-6 | Wrinkled foot.

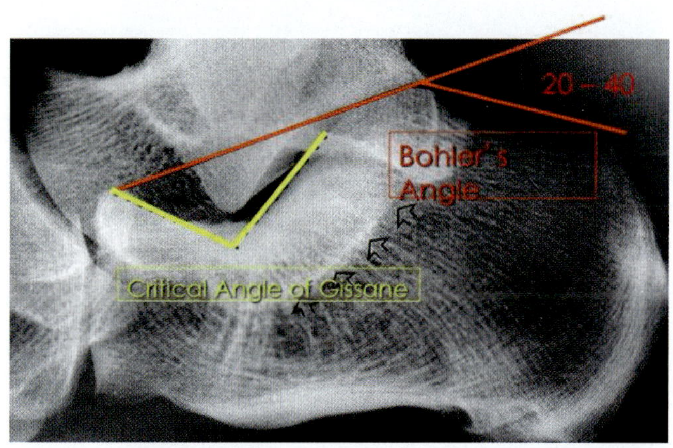

Figure 28-7 | Calcaneus lateral x-ray.

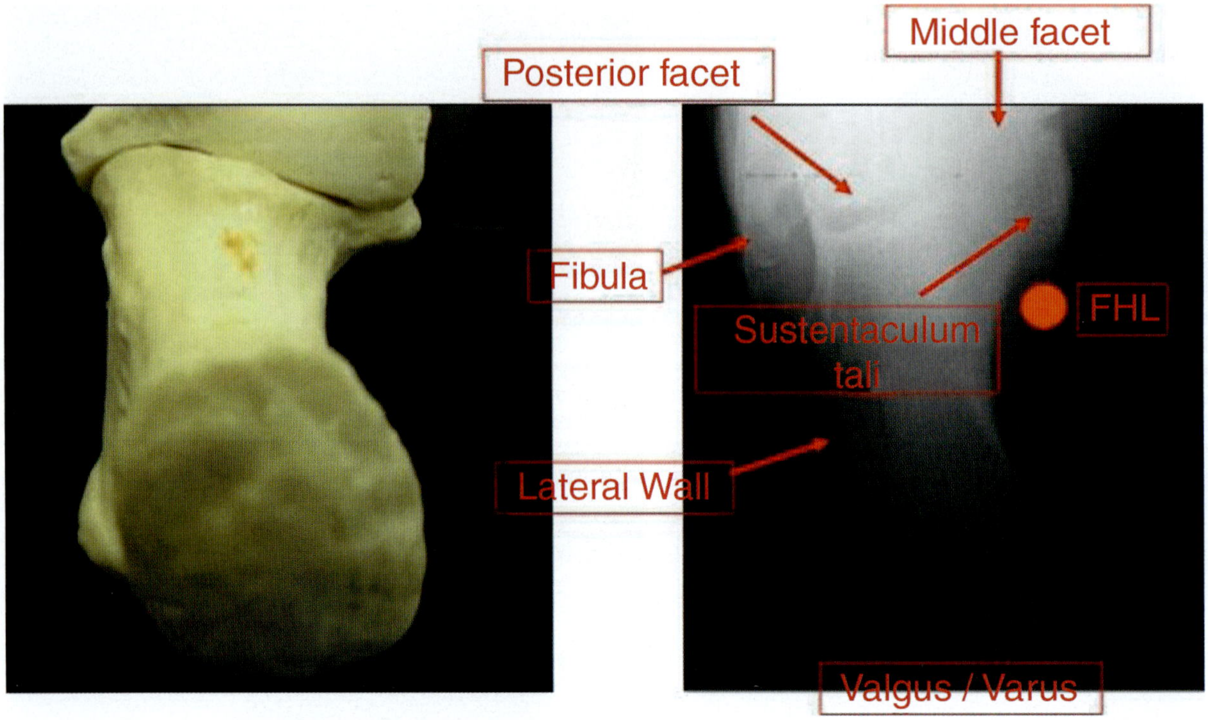

Figure 28-8 | Harris-Beath calcaneus intact.

- Axial view (Harris-Beath) visualizes tuberosity position (varus-valgus), primary fracture line, calcaneal height loss, calcaneal widening, and a portion of the posterior facet (Fig. 28-8).
- AP view of the foot exhibits secondary fracture lines into the anterior process and incongruity of the calcaneocuboid joint (Fig. 28-9).

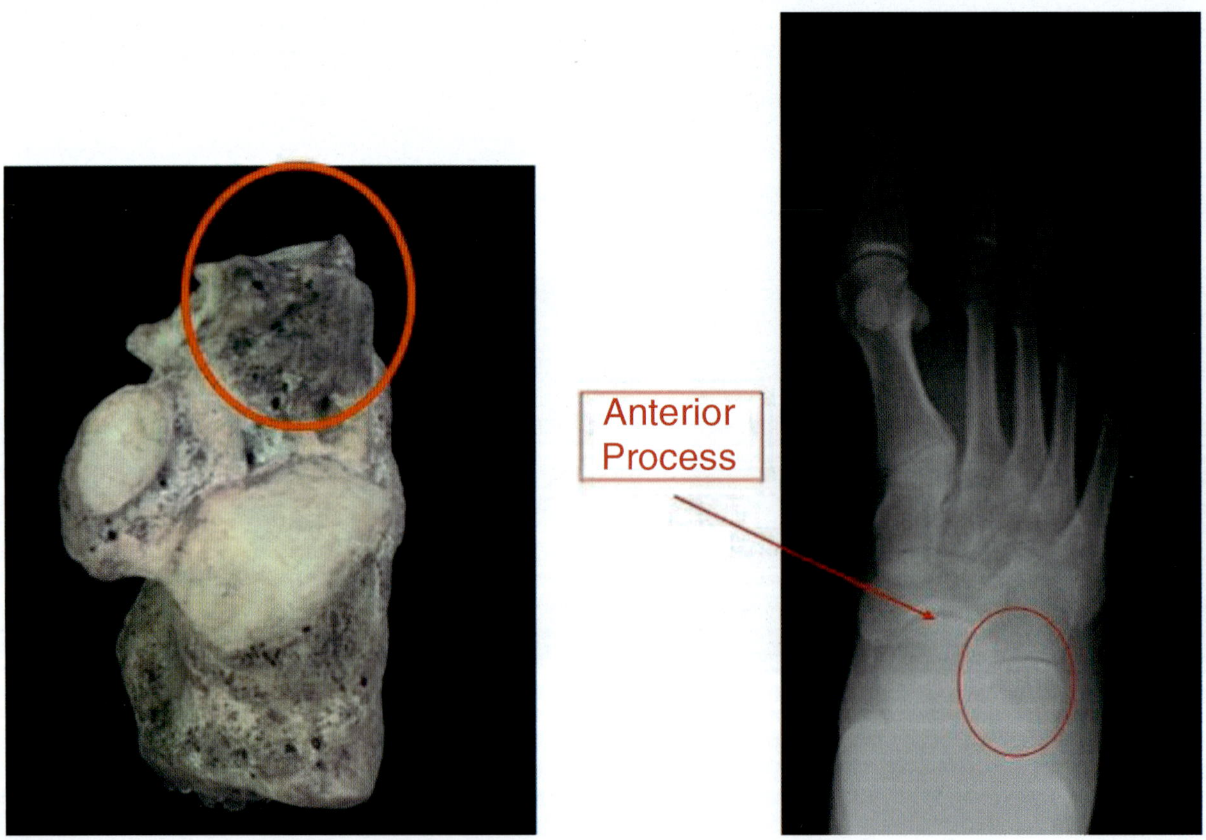

Figure 28-9 | AP foot normal anatomy.

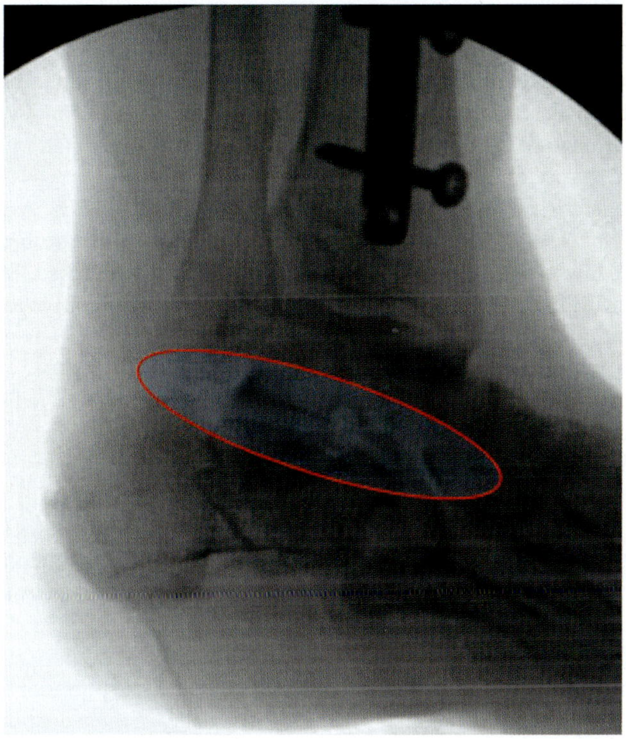

Figure 28-10 | Broden's view.

- Radiographs can be obtained from multiple perspectives to obtain a comprehensive assessment of the posterior facet (Broden x-ray views) (Fig. 28-10).[4]
- Computed tomography clarifies fracture line configuration. Sagittal and coronal reconstructed images may further help understanding of fracture patterns. Axial, coronal, and sagittal CT images below depict a significantly comminuted, intra-articular calcaneal fracture with joint depression, lateral wall blowout, widening, shortening, and ankle subluxation (Fig. 28-11).

Surgical Positioning and Imaging

- The extensile lateral approach (Letournel) requires positioning the patient in the lateral position. The patient is positioned with the uninjured side down. Note that a prone position on padded jelly rolls may be considered in cases of bilateral calcaneal fractures undergoing ORIF.

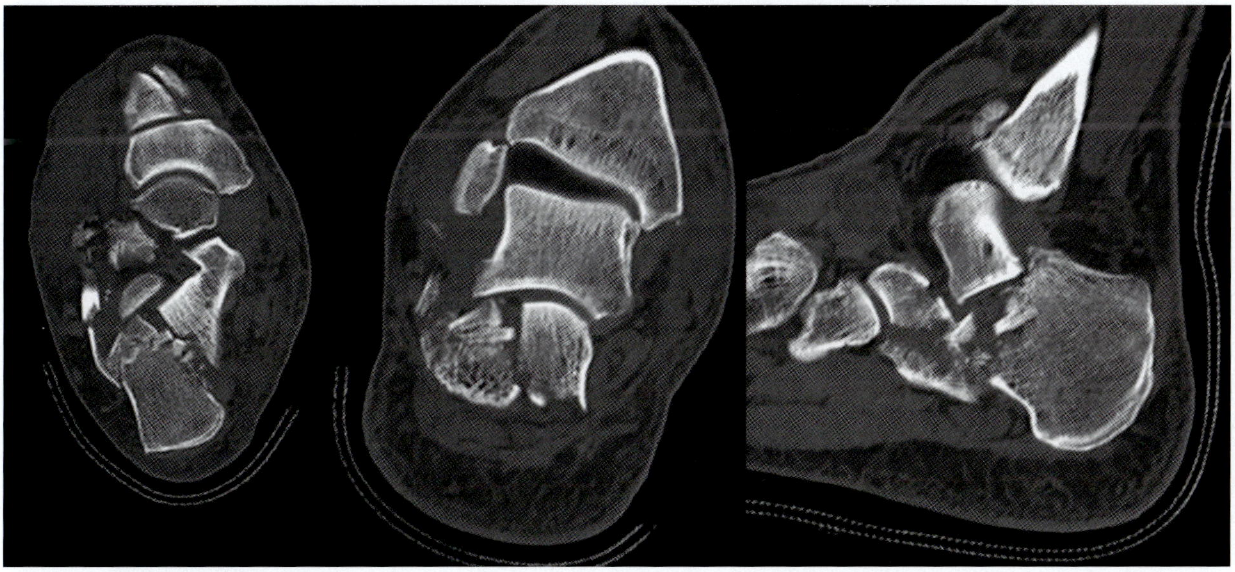

Figure 28-11 | CT images.

- A tourniquet is placed around the operative thigh prior to lateral positioning to facilitate ease of application and proper application.
- An axillary roll is used to facilitate lung ventilation and release pressure upon the down side brachial plexus. The ipsilateral arm may be suspended with a well-padded arm holder.
- Preoperative saved images of the contralateral Harris axial and lateral radiographs will serve as an invaluable template to model fracture reduction upon.
- A radiolucent table is critical for proper intraoperative imaging.
- Folded blankets or speciality pillows are used to support the operative limb at an elevated position compared with the down, nonoperative limb. The operative limb is flexed, while the nonoperative limb is positioned with knee extension. This permits lateral intraoperative radiographs without overlap with the nonoperative limb. With knee flexion, the tendoachilles is more relaxed, which helps with tuberosity reduction (Fig. 28-12).
- Intraoperative calcaneus radiography is facilitated by placing the operative limb in the distal posterior corner of the radiolucent operative table.
- In this position, the C-arm may be introduced into the surgical field from the foot of the bed. Lateral radiographs may be readily obtained (Fig. 28-13).
- Positioning the C-arm parallel with the floor will allow a Harris axial view (Fig. 28-14).
- The C-arm may be kept parallel with the floor but repositioned perpendicular to the Harris axial view to obtain an AP view of the foot. Another option is to utilize the lateral C-arm position and rotate the limb (via the hip) to obtain an AP foot view (Fig. 28-15).
- Broden views permit subtalar articular assessment.
- Broden described an imaging series to show the articular surface of the posterior facet. This can be helpful in evaluating fracture displacement preoperatively and also quality of the reduction during surgery.
  - Broden views can be obtained with the patient in the lateral position. The ankle is held in neutral position with respect to dorsiflexion and plantar flexion.
  - The fluoro beam is directed through the subtalar joint at an angle that is 45 degrees from true lateral (i.e., positioned half way between AP ankle and true lateral ankle).
  - The four Broden projections are obtained with the beam tilted 10, 20, 30, and 40 degrees cephalad. This permits evaluation of fracture lines and displacement along the majority of the posterior facet.
    - The 10-degree tilt images the posterior aspect of the joint while the 40-degree view images the anterior aspect.
    - The 20- and 30-degree views show the midportion of the posterior facet and are best at demonstrating the sustentaculotalar articulation (Fig. 28-16).

Intraoperative Technique

- Incisions are marked prior to incision to ensure proper location. The descending limb is posterior to the midpoint between the posterior fibular border and the Achilles tendon.[5] The transverse limb is along or slightly cranial to the glabrous and nonglabrous skin junction. Marking out the anticipated course of the superficial peroneal nerve, the sural nerve, the peroneal tendons, and the base of the 5th metatarsal is helpful (Fig. 28-17).

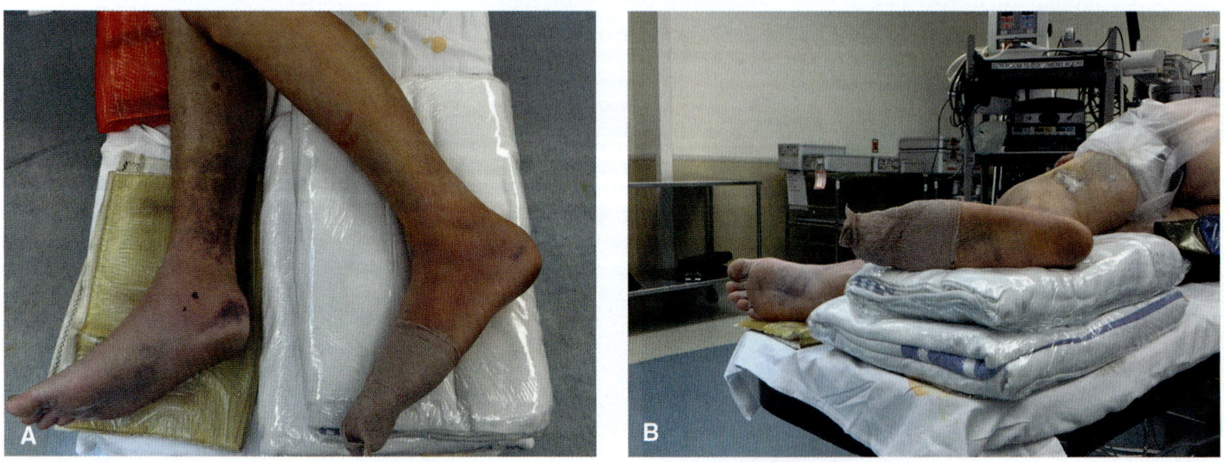

Figure 28-12 | Lateral calcaneus positioning **(A)** and lateral calcaneus positioning **(B)**.

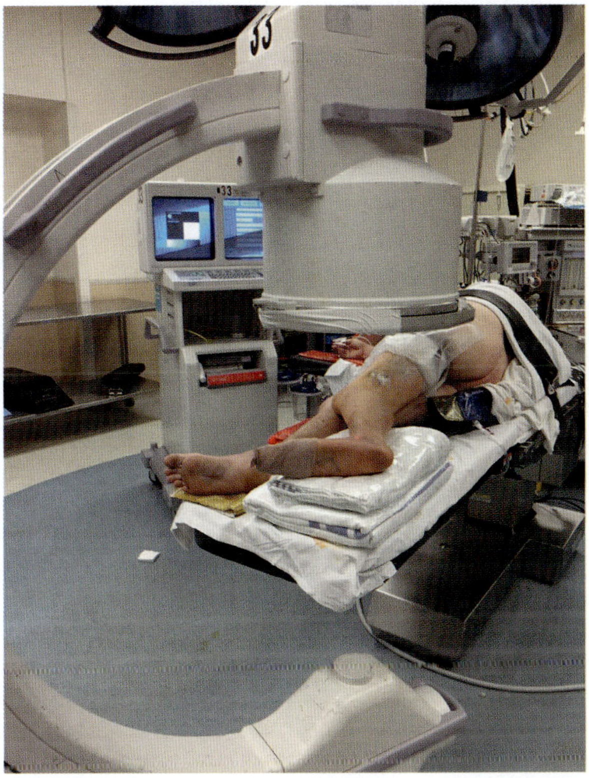

Figure 28-13 | Lateral x-ray C-arm positioning.

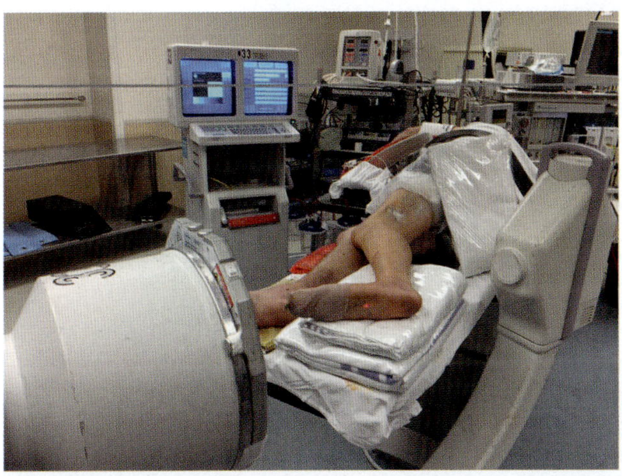

Figure 28-14 | Harris axial x-ray C-arm positioning.

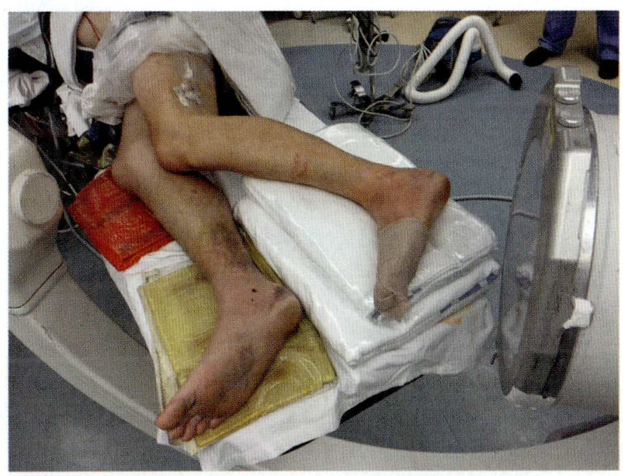

Figure 28-15 | AP x-ray C-arm positioning.

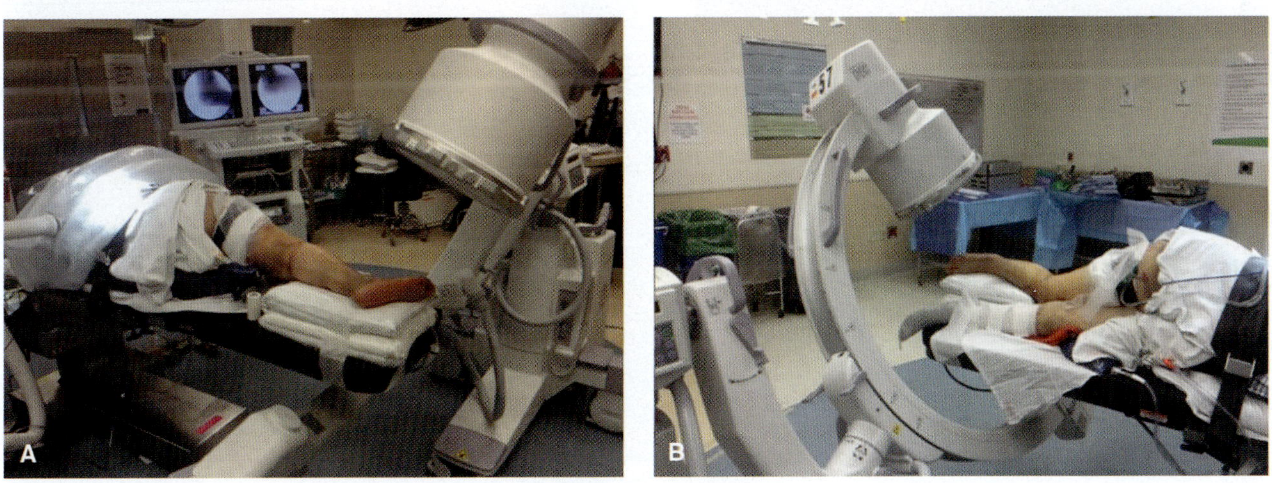

Figure 28-16 | Broden's fluoro positioning. **A:** Posterior view. **B:** Anterior view.

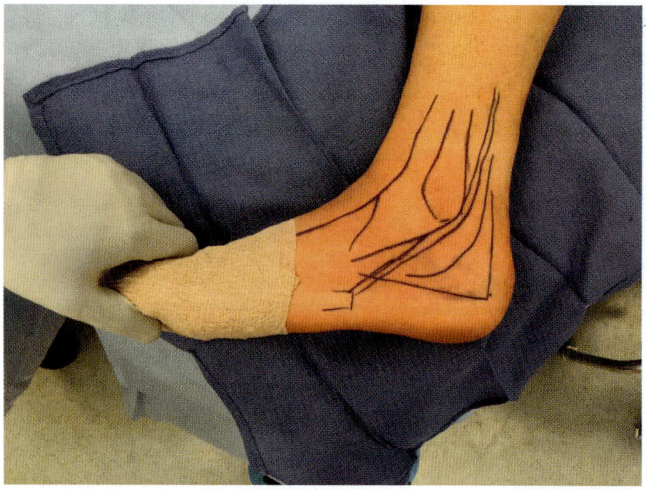

Figure 28-17 | Lateral foot incisions.

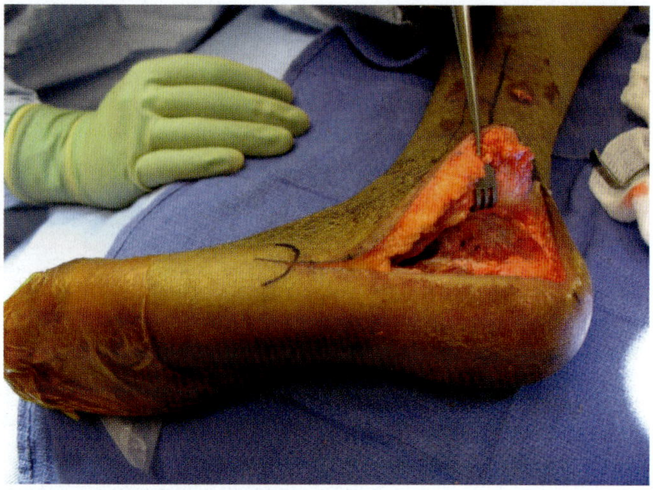

Figure 28-18 | Periosteal flap elevation.

- The limb is exsanguinated, and the tourniquet is elevated.
- The goal is to raise a full-thickness periosteal-cutaneous flap, with all neurovascular and tendinous structures protected within the flap.
- The cranial extent of the dissection occurs to the superior aspect of the calcaneal tuberosity. The distal extent of the dissection occurs to the calcaneocuboid joint. If desired, Kirschner wires may be placed into the talar neck and cuboid to serve as soft tissue retractors (Fig. 28-18).
- Place retractors upon the periosteum only. Avoid retractors on the skin or subcutaneous flap tissue.
- Towel bumps under the ankle will permit foot inversion and facilitate subtalar joint visualization (Fig. 28-19).
- In general, reduction occurs from anteromedial to posterolateral. Thus, the sagittal fractures in the anterior process or articular impaction of the calcaneocuboid joint are addressed first. Occasionally, joint reduction may be performed indirectly by reducing the cranial cortex of the anterior process. Reduction may be provisionally stabilized with small-caliber Kirschner wires and confirmed with an AP radiograph of the foot.
- Lateral wall and depressed posterior facet fragments may be extricated from the surgical field and held on the back table for later handling. In this extracorporeal setting, multiple posterior facet fragments may be reduced and held in place with small caliber fixation (Fig. 28-20).

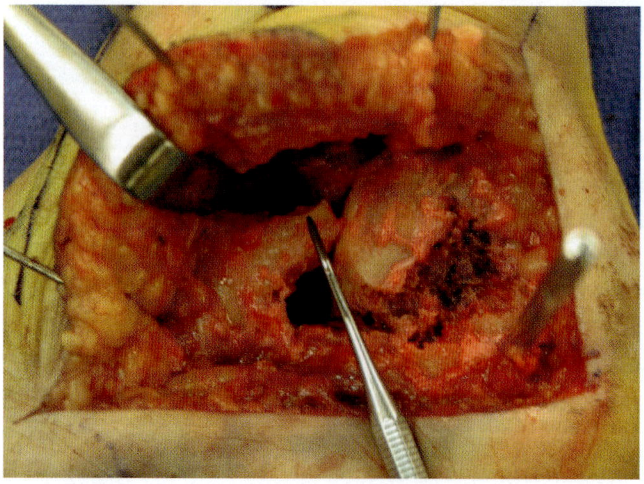

Figure 28-19 | Gross fractured calcaneus.

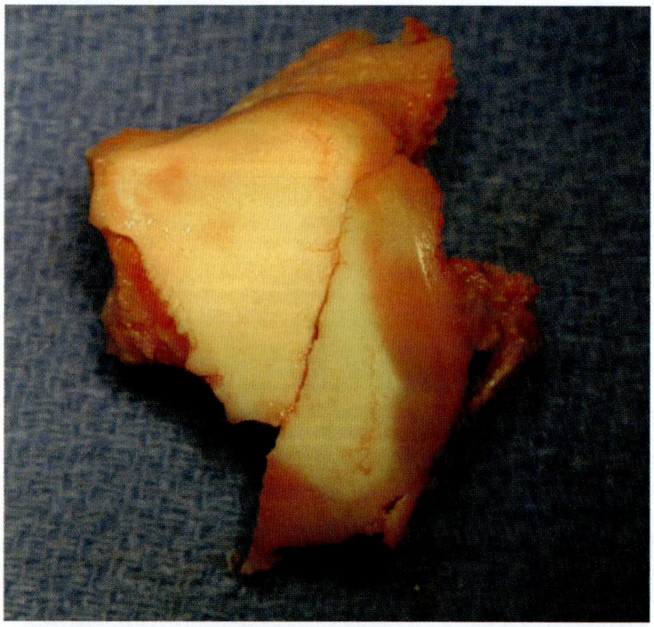

Figure 28-20 | Posterior facet.

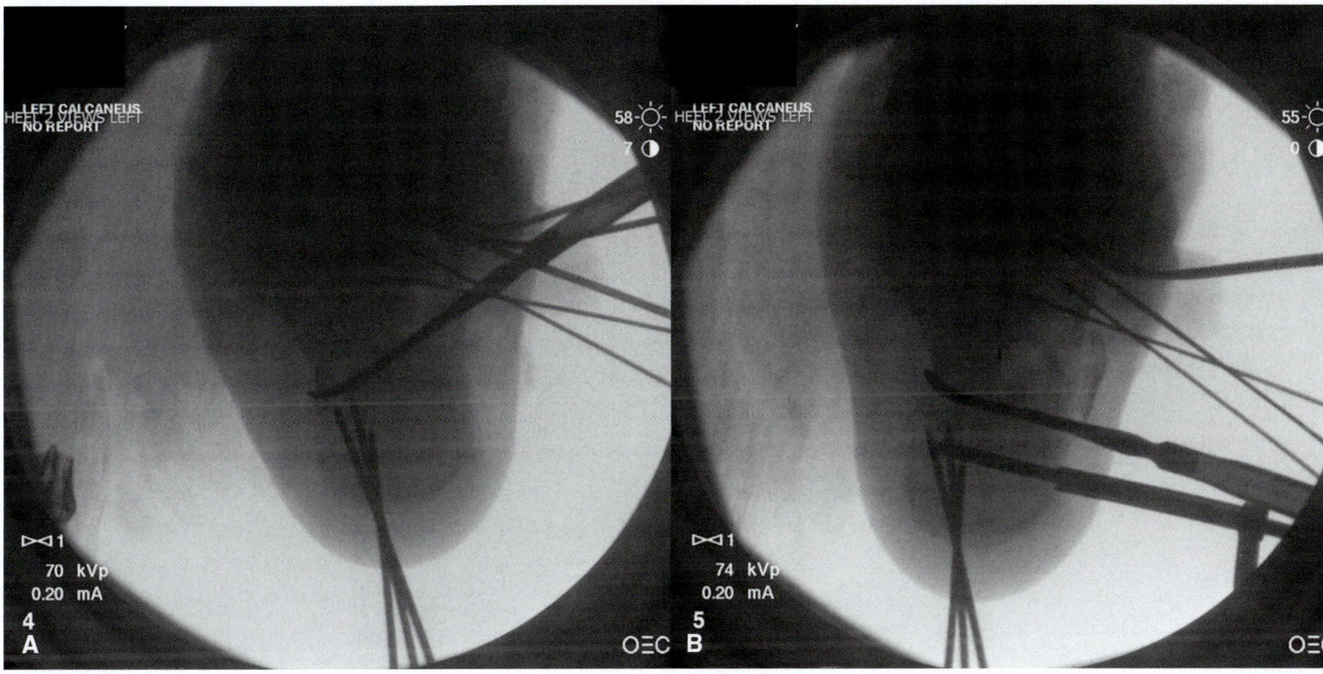

Figure 28-21 | Primary fracture line reduction prior to reduction manuovor **(A)** and after reduction manuever **(B)**.

- The primary fracture line may be found with an elevator instrument and used as a lever to reduce the lateral tuberosity translation and height loss. A Schanz pin inserted into the tuberosity laterally or posteriorly will aid in tuberosity and primary fracture line reduction. Axially placed Kirschner wires will maintain the reduction once accomplished (Fig. 28-21).
- Anatomic primary fracture line and tuberosity reduction will create space to reinsert the posterior facet back into the surgical field. The critical angle of Gissane, if well corticated, can be reduced, which can aid with posterior facet reduction. Posterior facet articular reduction is then performed both with direct visualization and with intraoperative imaging (Figs. 28-22 and 28-23).
- A lateral plate is applied. Although grossly reduced at this point, the calcaneus still remains wide in its medial to lateral dimensions. Through the plate, a "working" lag screw is introduced into the sustentaculum to enable horizontal fracture compression. This screw will ultimately be longer than the width of the calcaneus and will need to be revised to a shorter screw after subsequent points of fixation are in place (Fig. 28-24).

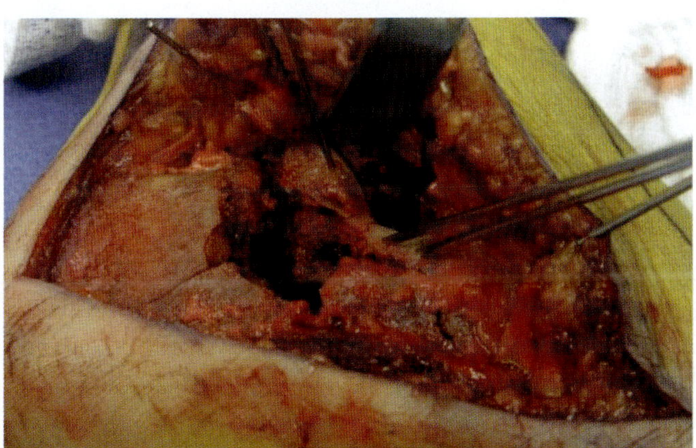

Figure 28-22 | Intraoperative temporary fracture reduction.

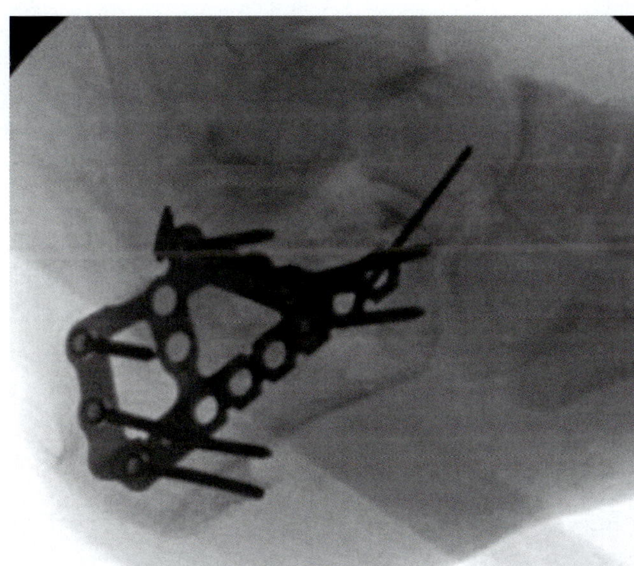

Figure 28-23 | Broden's intraoperative fluoro.

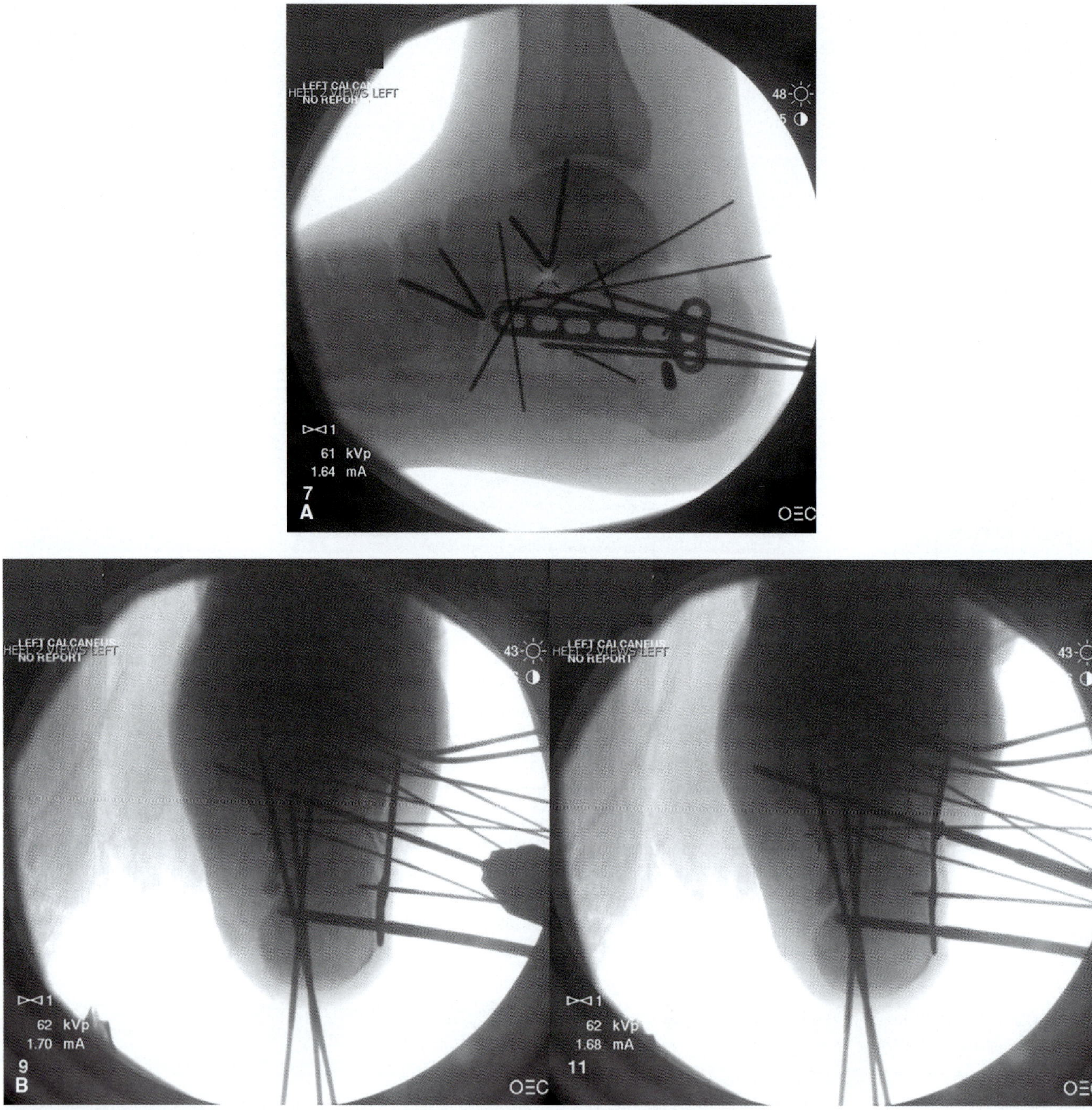

Figure 28-24 | Plate positioning calcaneus lateral, plate positioning calcaneus axial **(A)**, and plate positioning calcaneus **(B)**.

- Screw fixation, with or without lag screw by technique, is performed in the anterior process, the posterior facet, and the tuberosity to secure the calcaneal fracture components. Confirmation of proper implants and screw lengths is performed with Harris axial, lateral, and AP foot intraoperative views (Figs. 28-25–28-30).

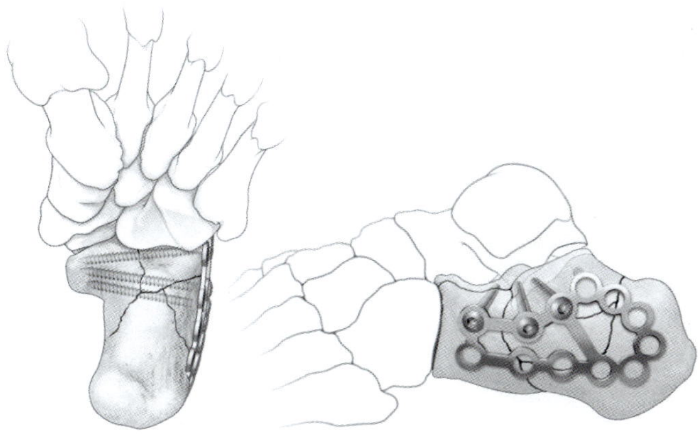

Figure 28-25 | The sustentaculum often remains the "constant (medial) fragment" to which complex intra-articular calcaneal fractures are reconstructed. When sustentacular comminution is present, this dense condensation of bone offers an excellent point of fixation, but proper screw trajectory is critical to accurately capture this fragment without injuring the FHL tendon and neurovascular structures. The more anteriorly based sustentaculum is usually only amenable to more anterior screw options in conventional calcaneal plates. These lateral and Harris view perspective illustrations demonstrate the appropriate vectors for superior-anterior screw holes. Note that the screw angles change in the anterior to posterior direction depending on the hole location but remain fairly transverse and directed under the subtalar joint surface.

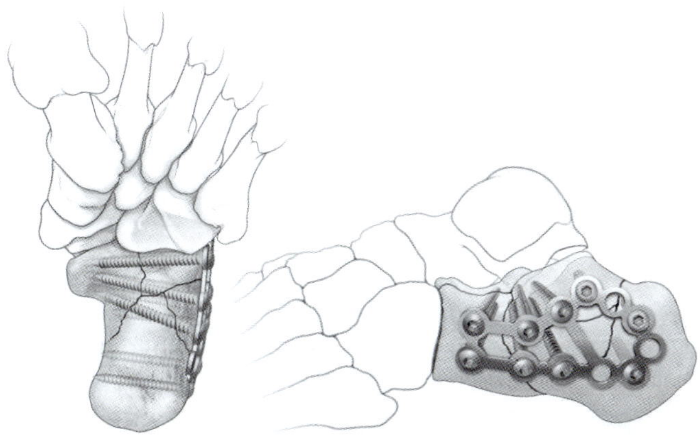

Figure 28-26 | In contrast, anteroinferior plate holes often require a more cranial screw trajectory in order to engage the sustentaculum. This can result in an oblique screw purchase in the medial cortex and irritation of the FHL tendon if too long of a screw length is selected or if the screw length "grows" with compression of the fracture or plate against the lateral cortex.

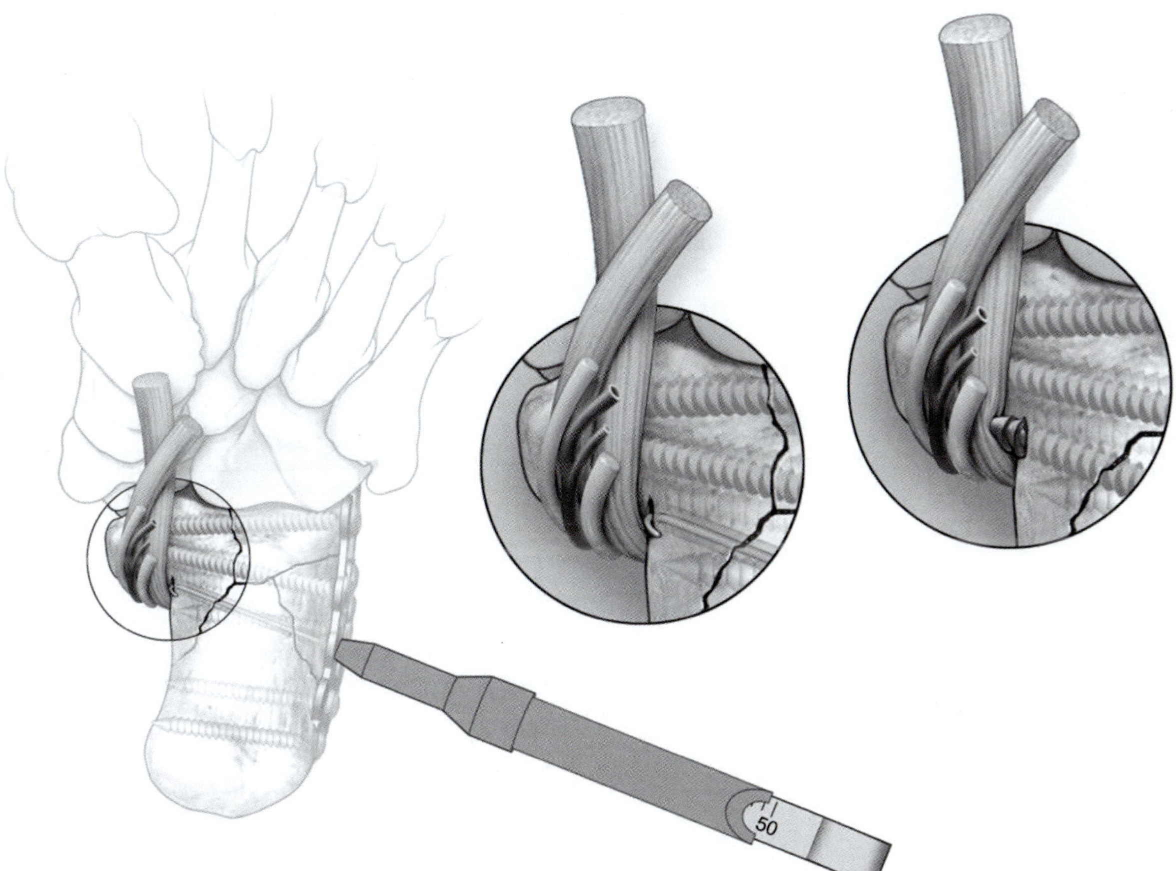

Figure 28-27 | Screw length measurements near the sustentaculum can be difficult to accurately assess based on the irregular cortical topography and screw vector obliquity. Numerous measurements should be performed noting that excessively long screw selection with conflicting shorter measurements put the medial FHL tendon and neurovascular structures at risk of iatrogenic injury as depicted in these illustrations.

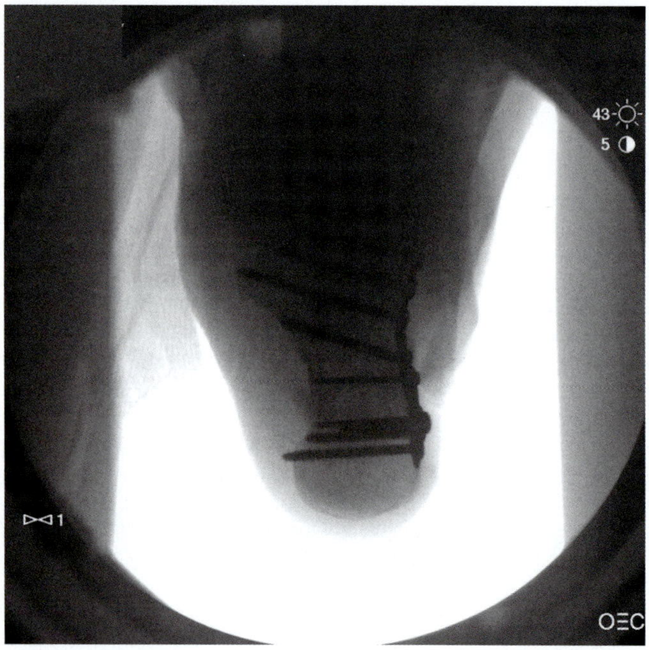

Figure 28-28 | Final Harris axial.

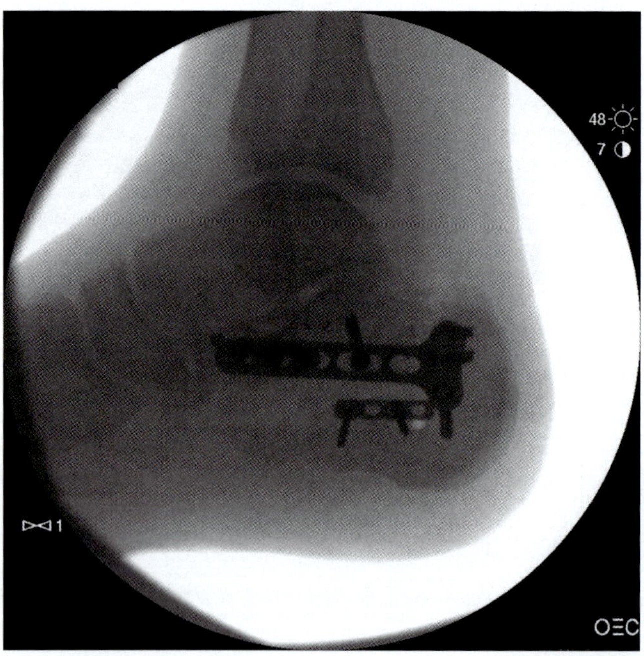

Figure 28-29 | Final lateral.

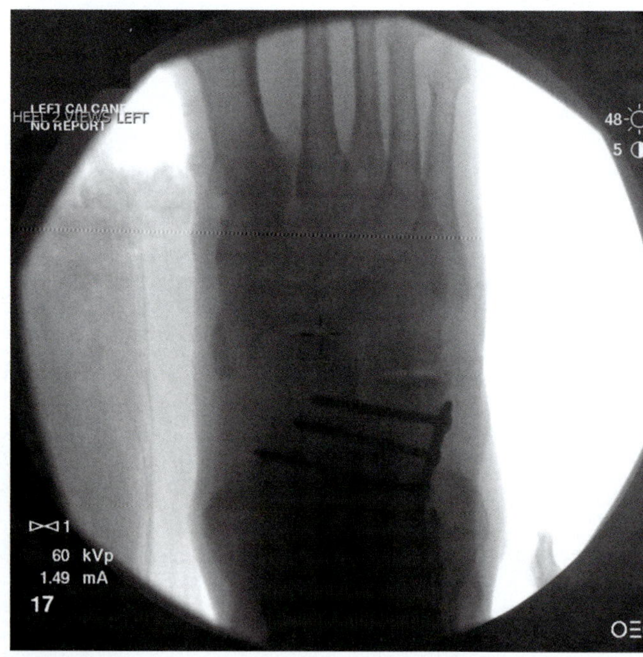

Figure 28-30 | Final AP foot.

References

1. Letournel E. Open treatment of acute calcaneal fractures. *Clin Orthop Relat Res.* 1993;290:60–67.
2. Bernischke SK, Sangeorzan BJ. Extensive intraarticular fractures of the foot. Surgical management of calcaneal fractures. *Clin Orthop Relat Res.* 1993;292:128–134.
3. Sanders R. Displaced intraarticular fractures of the calcaneus. *J Bone Joint Surg Am.* 2000;82:225–250.
4. Broden B. Roentgen examination of the subtaloid joint in fractures of the calcaneus. *Acta Radiol.* 1949;31(1):85–91.
5. Borrelli J, Lashgari C. Vascularity of the lateral calcaneal flap: a cadaveric injection study. *J Orthop Trauma.* 1999;13:73–77.

Appendix 1
Fluoroscope Movements

A modern fluoroscopy machine can be a versatile addition to fracture fixation. Orthopaedic surgeons should be well versed in its movements, basic settings, and terms for communicating intraoperative views to the x-ray technician.

Customary C-Arm Levers and Movements

This figure highlights the numerous levers available to control C-arm movements within uniplanar vectors. These motions are discussed in detail below.

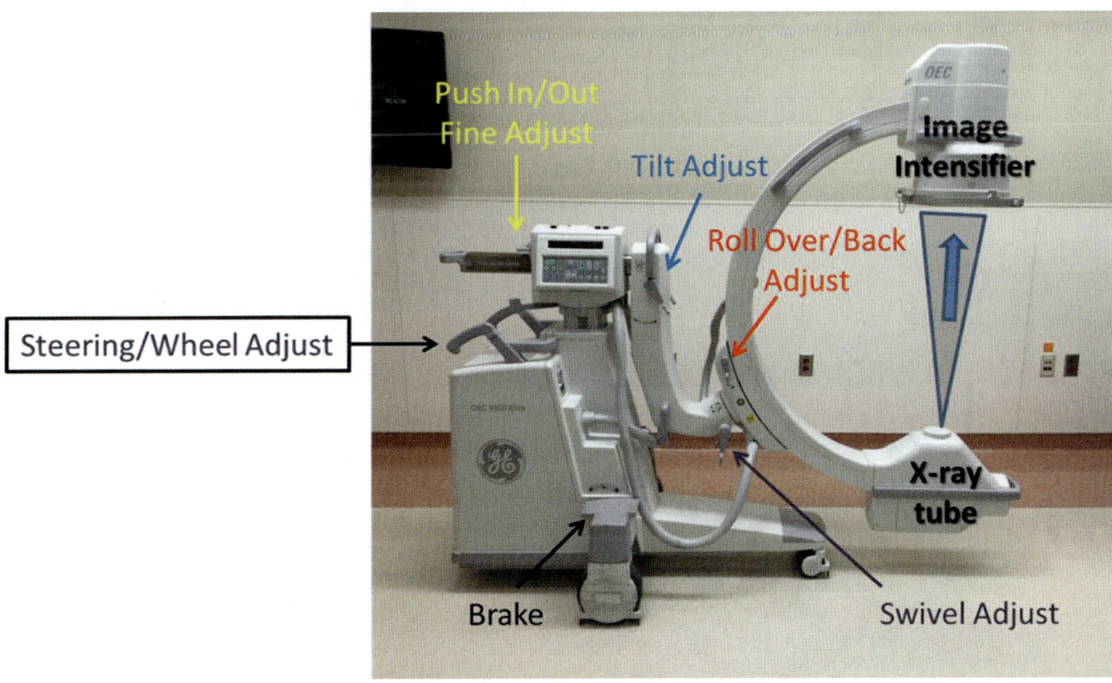

Figure A1-1

C-Arm Base Controls

The control panel on a C-arm base allows movement of the machine up and down along with image capture and fine-tuned image control (i.e., kVP and mA generator adjustment, collimation, contrast adjustment, and image orientation).

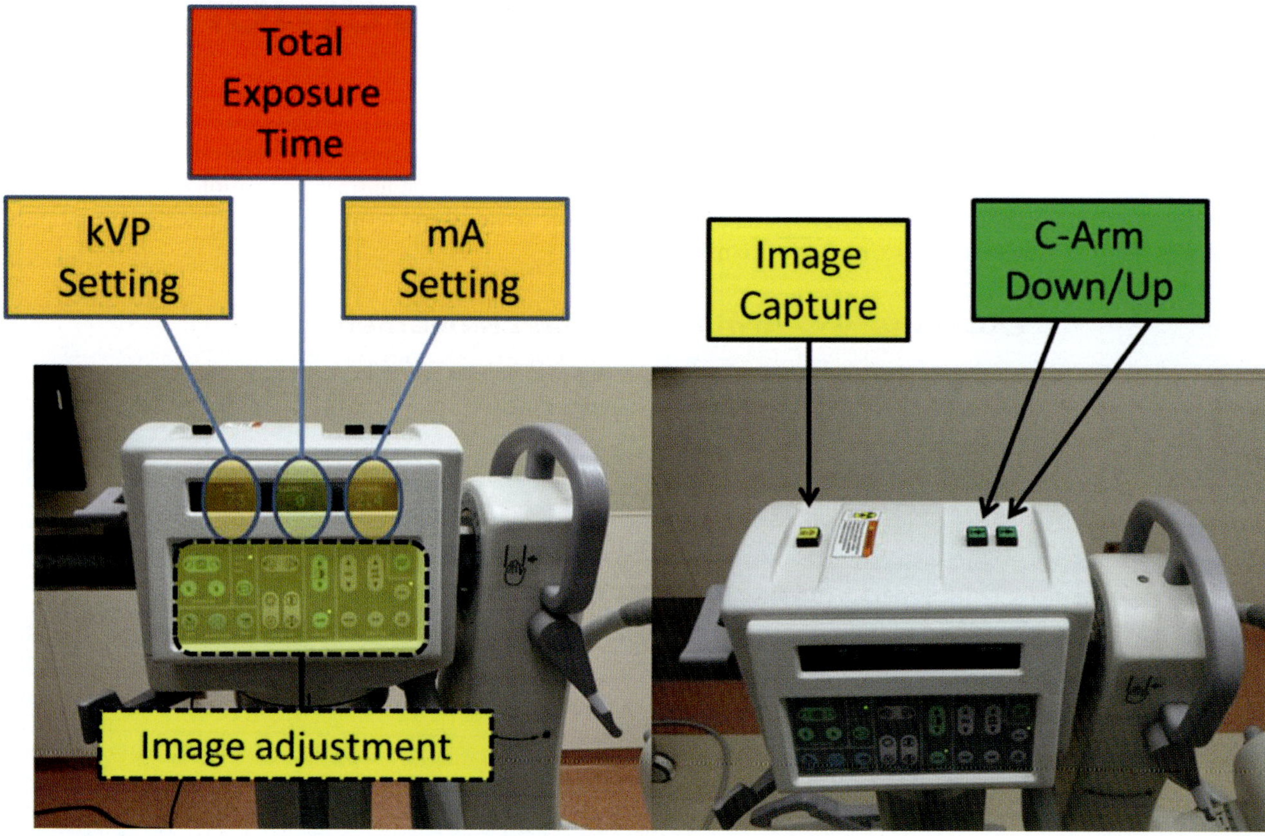

Figure A1-2 |

C-Arm Monitor Controls

The control panel on a C-arm monitor is used to enter patient information and offers an image directory function to review the images captured during the case. Advanced contrast adjustments are available to enhance the image, filter noise, create a negative image, and zoom.

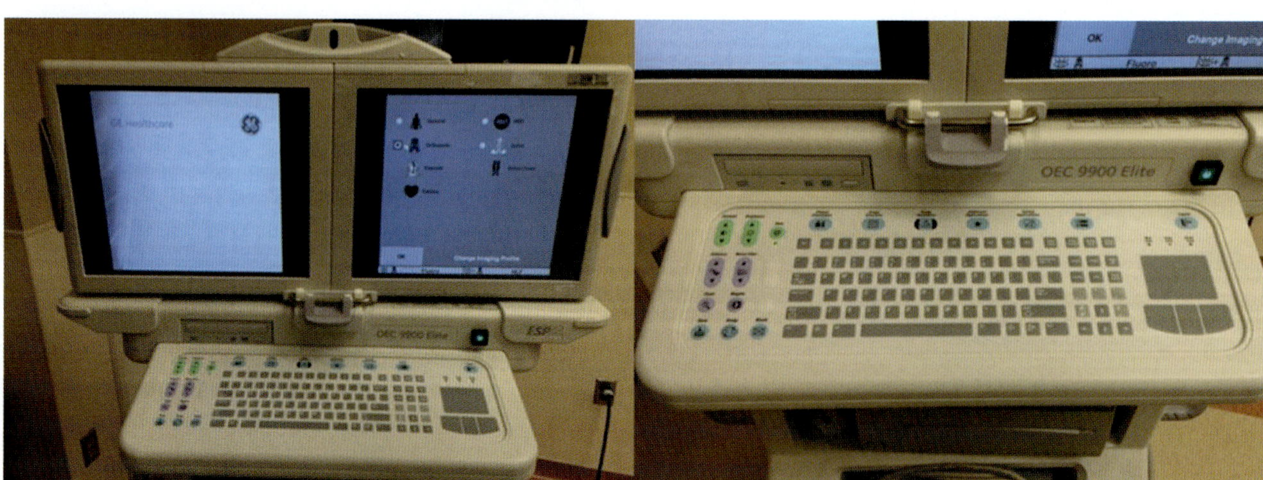

Figure A1-3 |

C-Arm Movements

(Micro) Push In/Out—Uniplanar micro adjust movement limited to length of the C-arm boom (as the base remains in a fixed position).

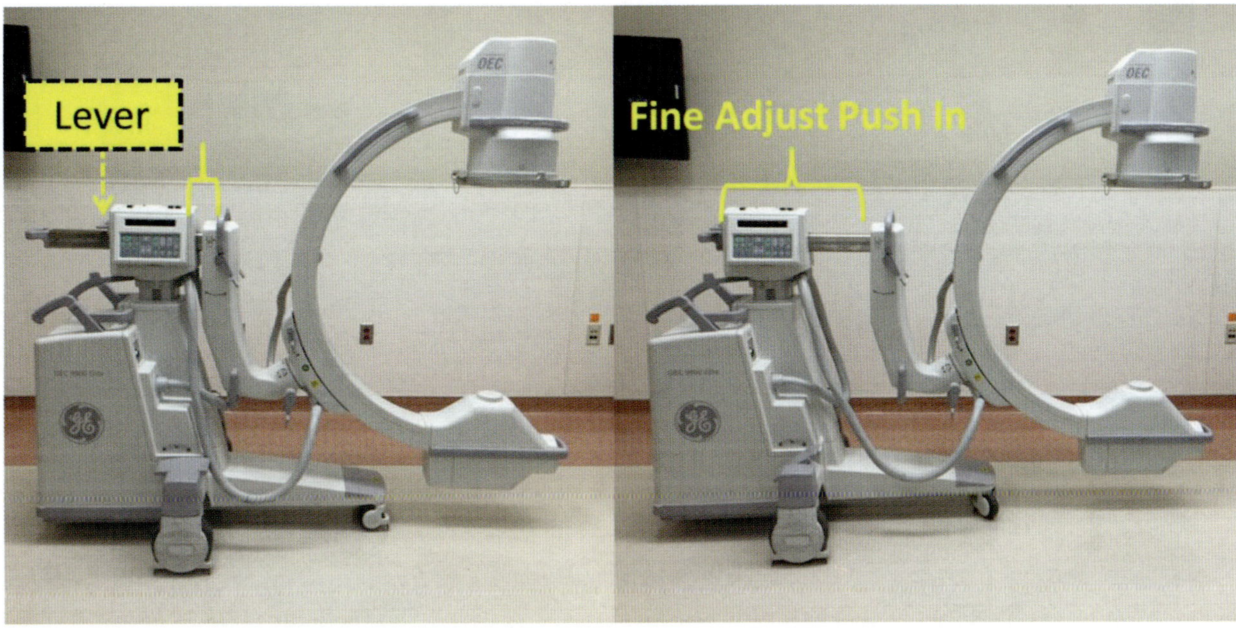

Figure A1-4 |

Raise Up/Down—Uniplanar movement limited to maximum height C-arm elevation and interference with operating table.

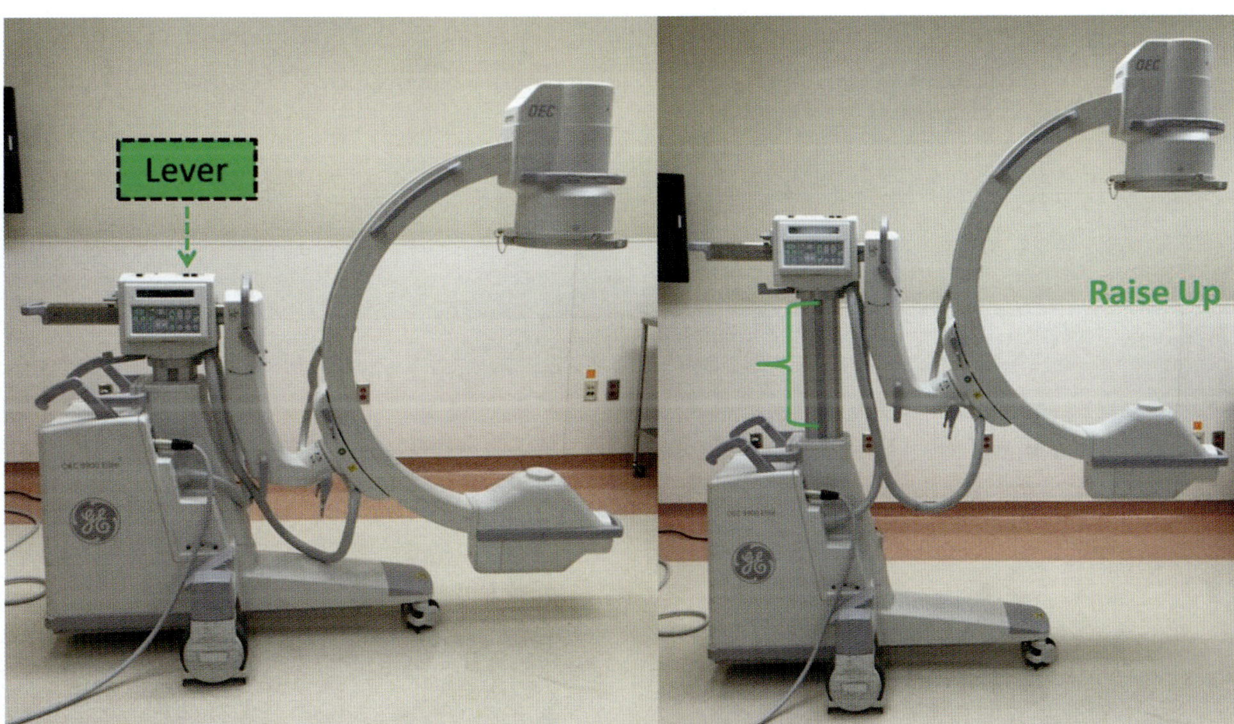

Figure A1-5 |

(Macro) Push In/Out, Move Right/Left and Wag—Uniplanar macro movements to adjust the position of the C-arm base in the plane of the floor (*around the patient and/or operating table*). Make sure C-arm approaches the OR table at a 90 degree angle and the intensifier is parallel to the floor.

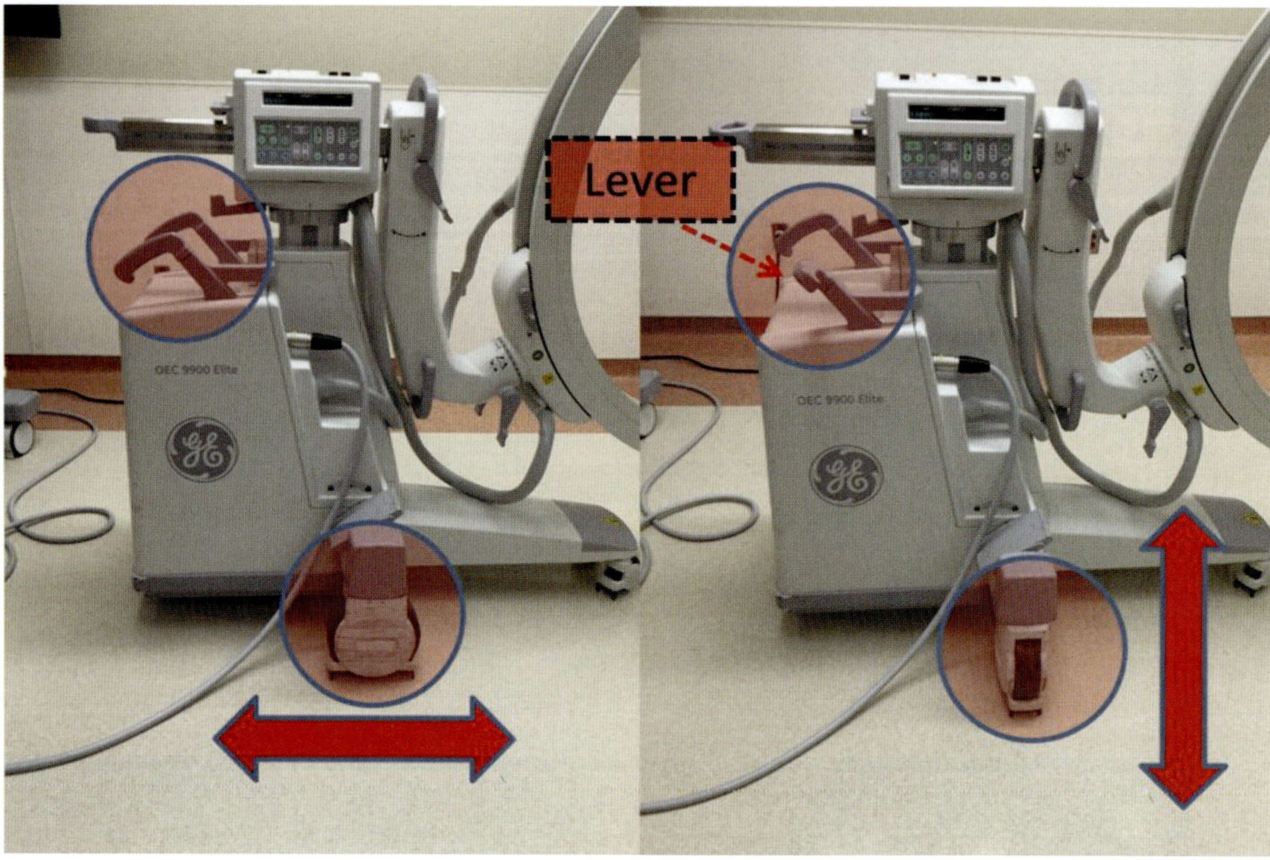

Figure A1-6 |

(Micro) Wag—Uniplanar micro adjust limited to approximately 15 degrees in each direction (as the base remains in a fixed position).

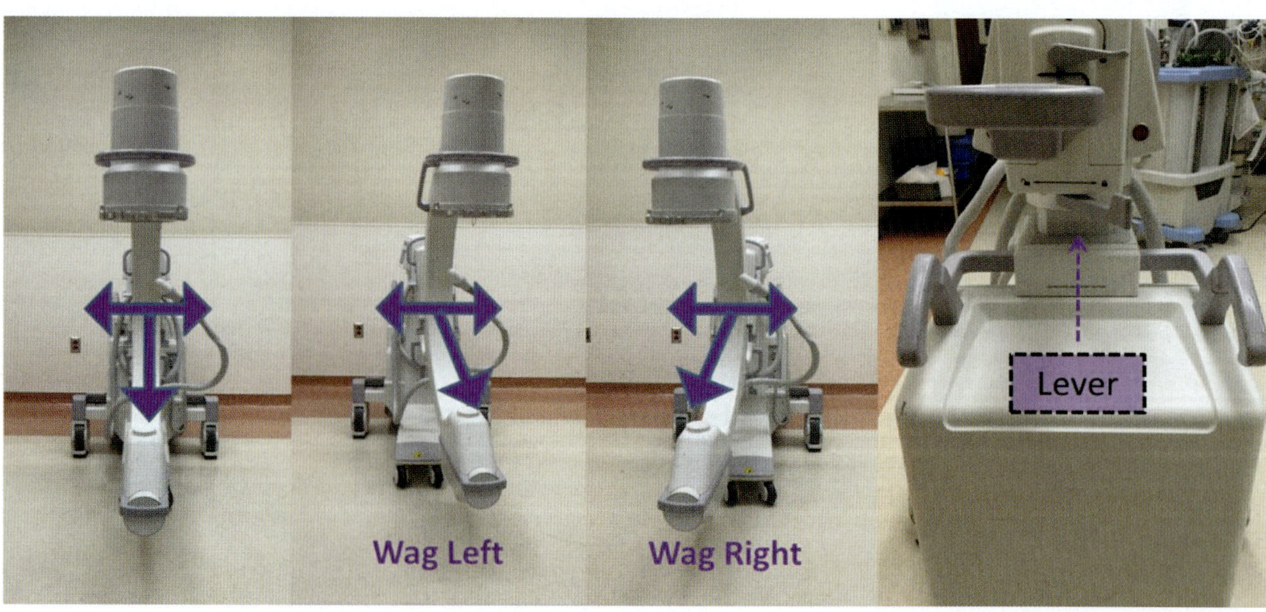

Figure A1-7 |

Inverted C-Arm—Allows the C-Arm Image Intensifier to function as operating table, which maximally enhances image detail and focus (i.e., hand and pediatric supracondylar fractures).

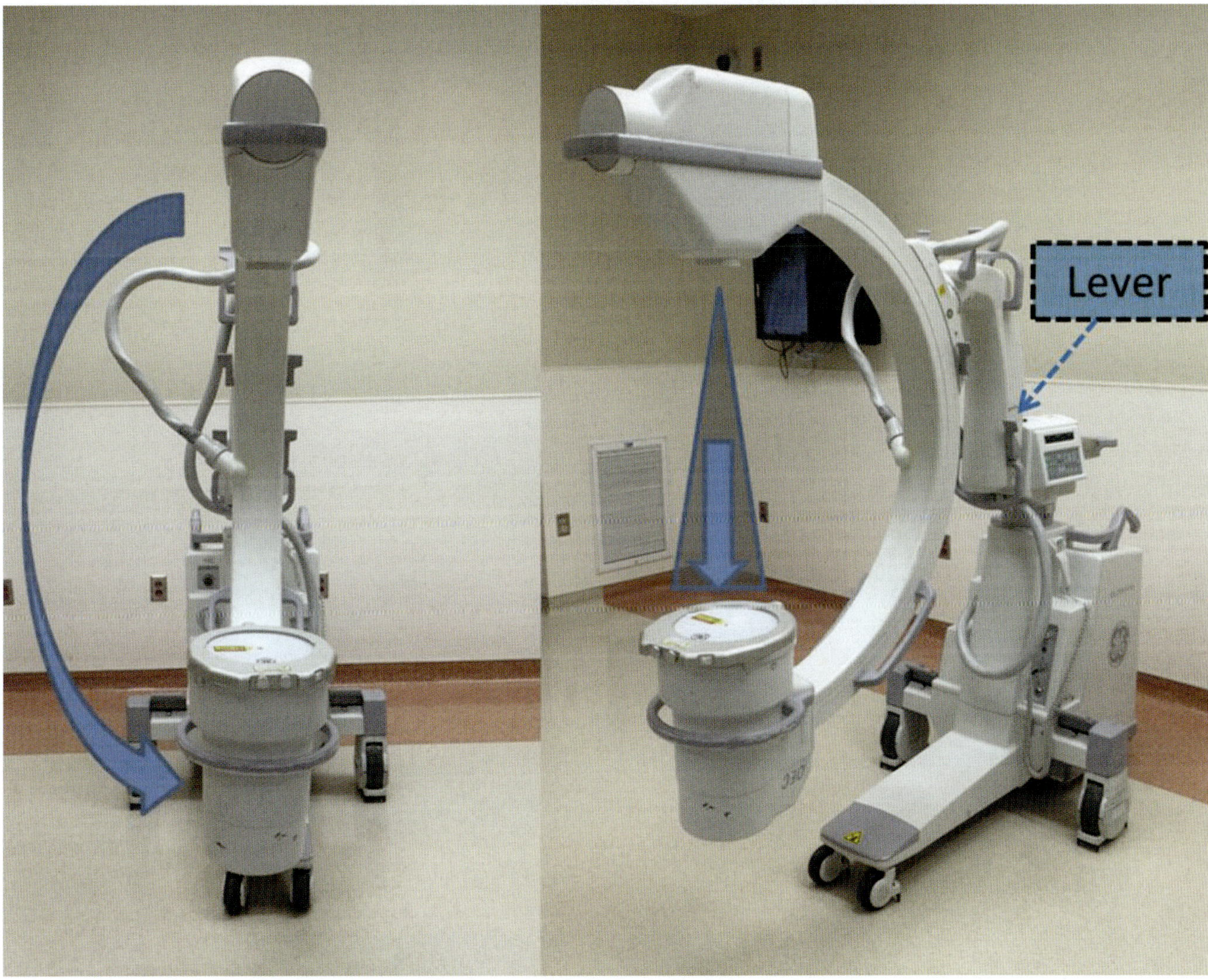

Figure A1-8 |

Roll Over/Back (a.k.a Rainbow Over/Back or "C" Over/Back)—Uniplanar movement limited to approximately 35 degrees roll over and 90 degrees roll back. Most commonly used for obtaining AP, lateral, and oblique views.

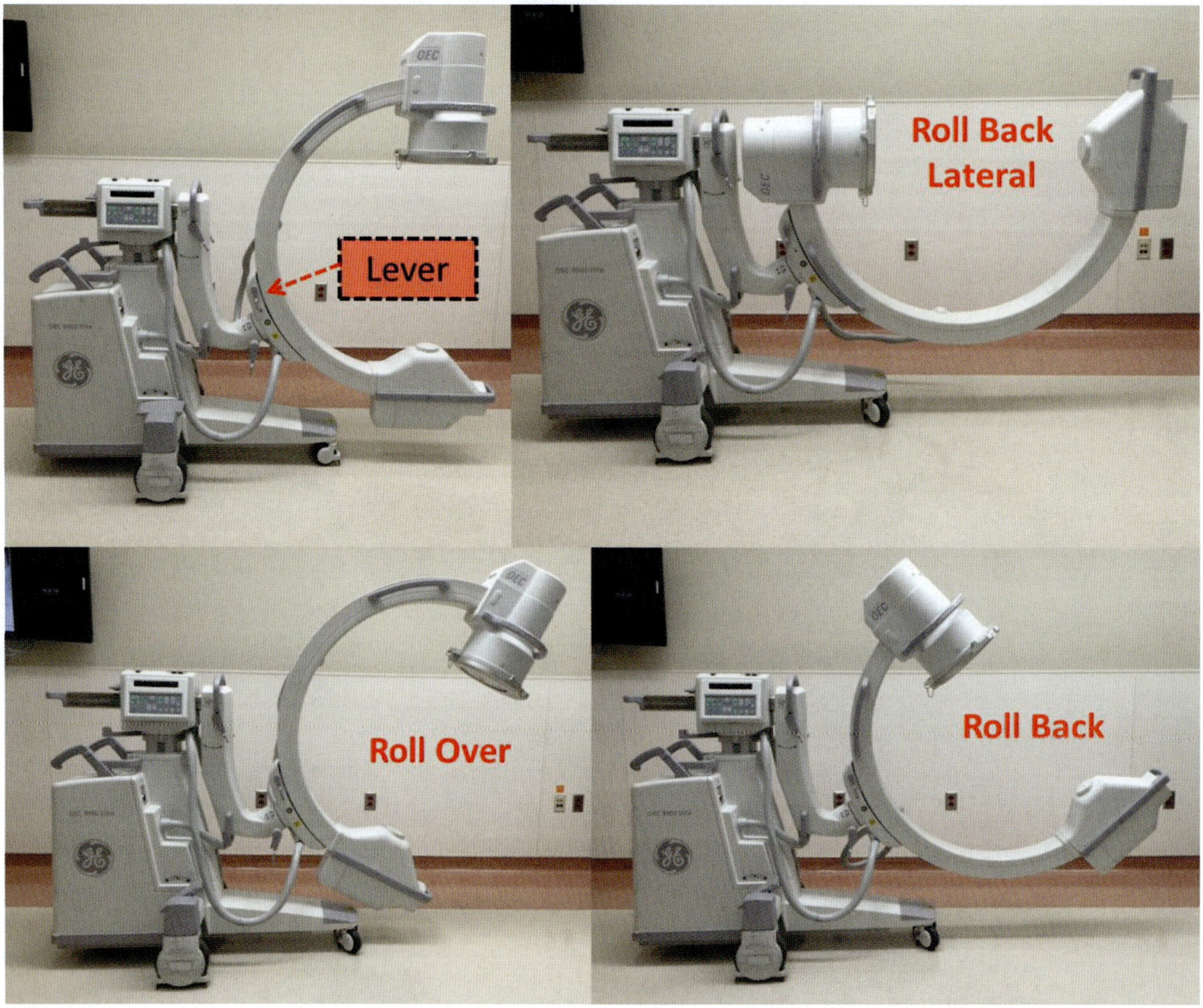

Figure A1-9 |

Tilt or Cant—Uniplanar movement typically limited by desired image and the patient's body habitus or operating table. Enables one to angle the base cephadad or caudad.

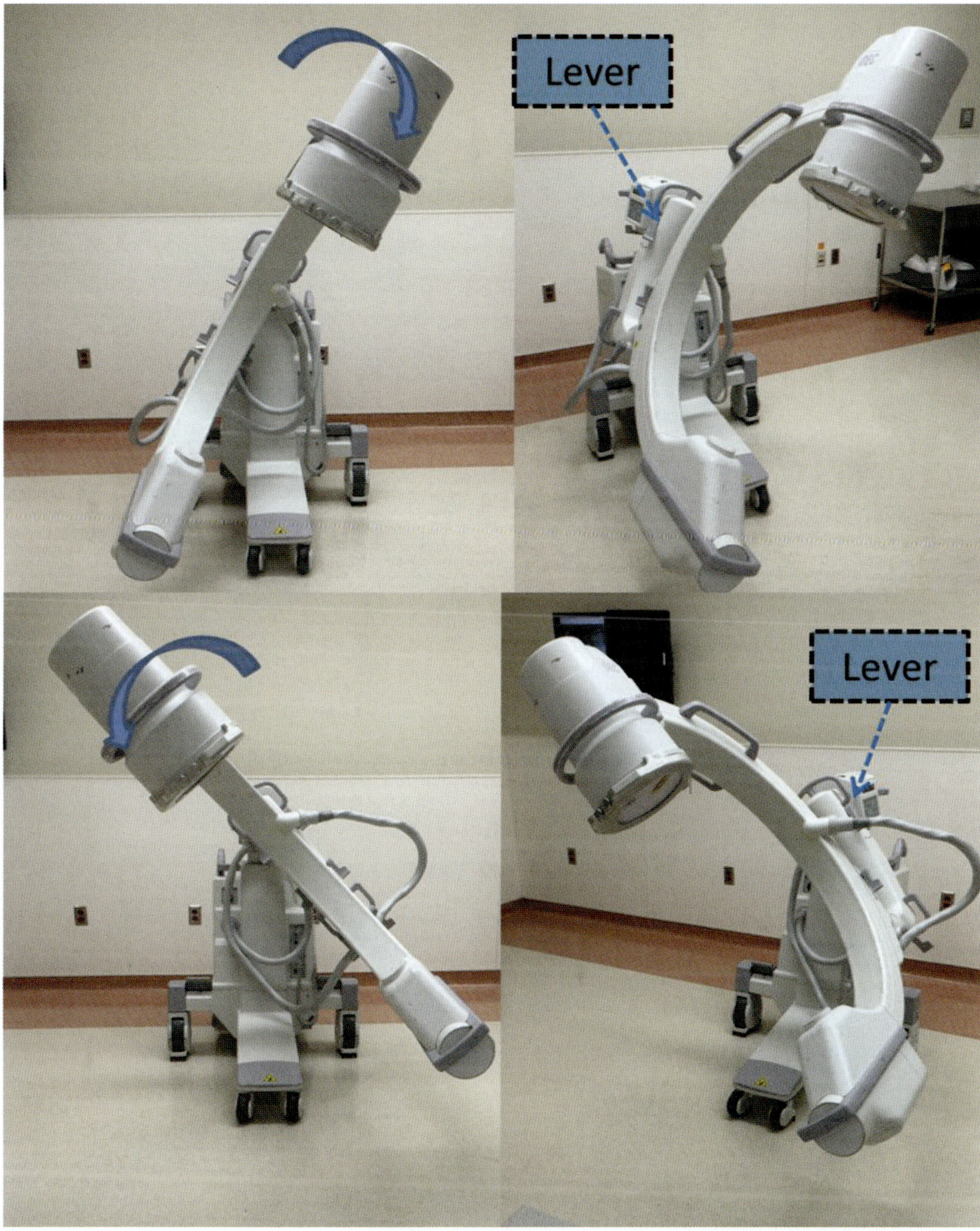

Figure A1-10 |

Multiplanar Movements—Movement in numerous planes can be accomplished by a combination of uniplanar levers (i.e., obturator-outlet view = outlet + roll over and smart view).

1. **Example: Swivel Movement**—can be used alone or with roll over/back as depicted.

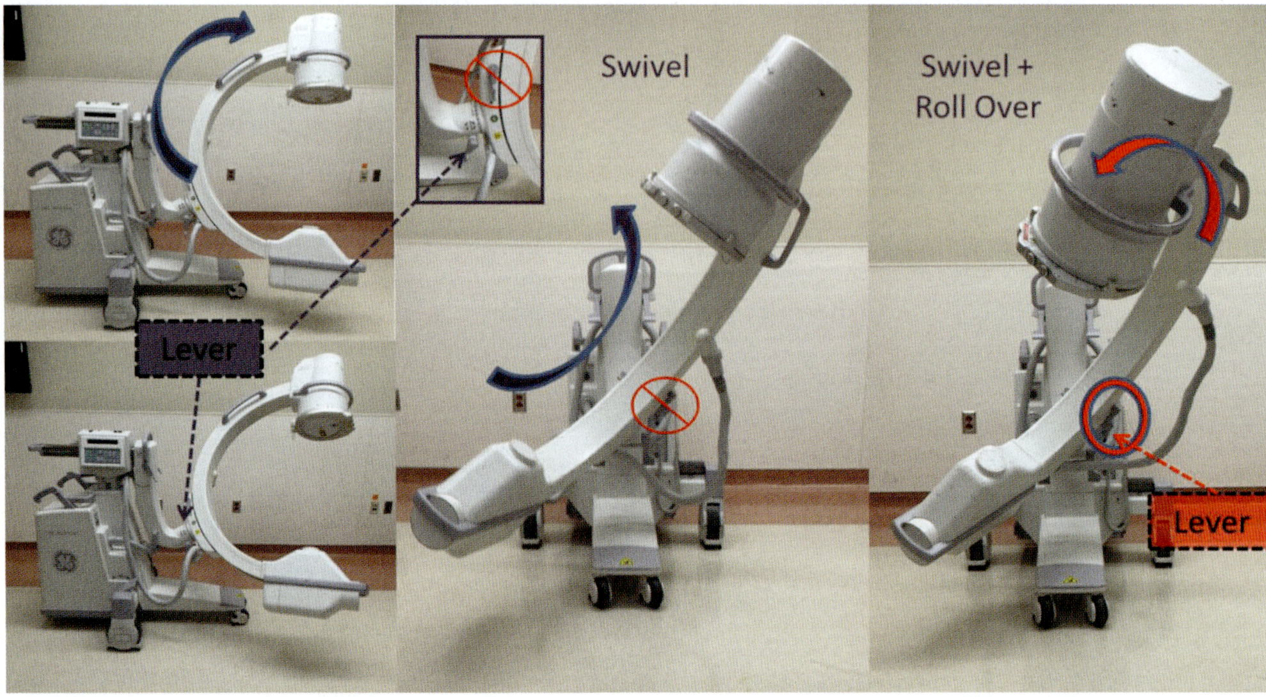

Figure A1-11 |

2. **Example: Obturator Outlet**—Combination of uniplanar movements commonly used for pelvic and acetabular surgery.

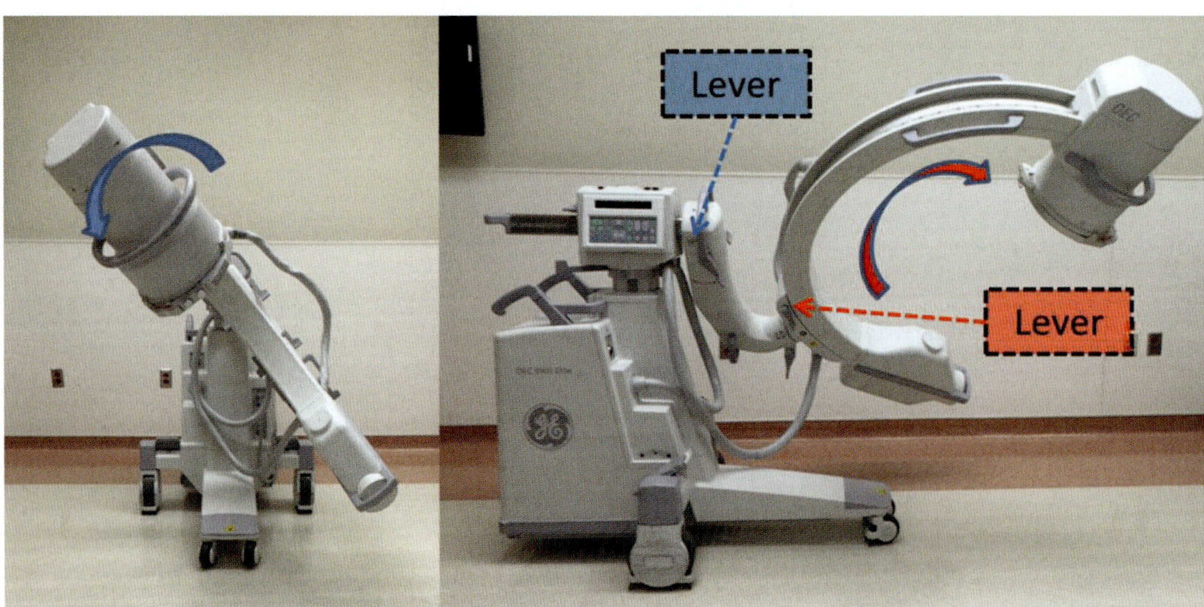

Figure A1-12 |

3. **Example: Smart View**—Combination of uniplanar movements (inlet/outlet 1st, swivel 2nd) to create an altered C-arm base having greater roll over/back than uniplanar roll alone (an adjunctive option for pelvic and acetabular surgery).

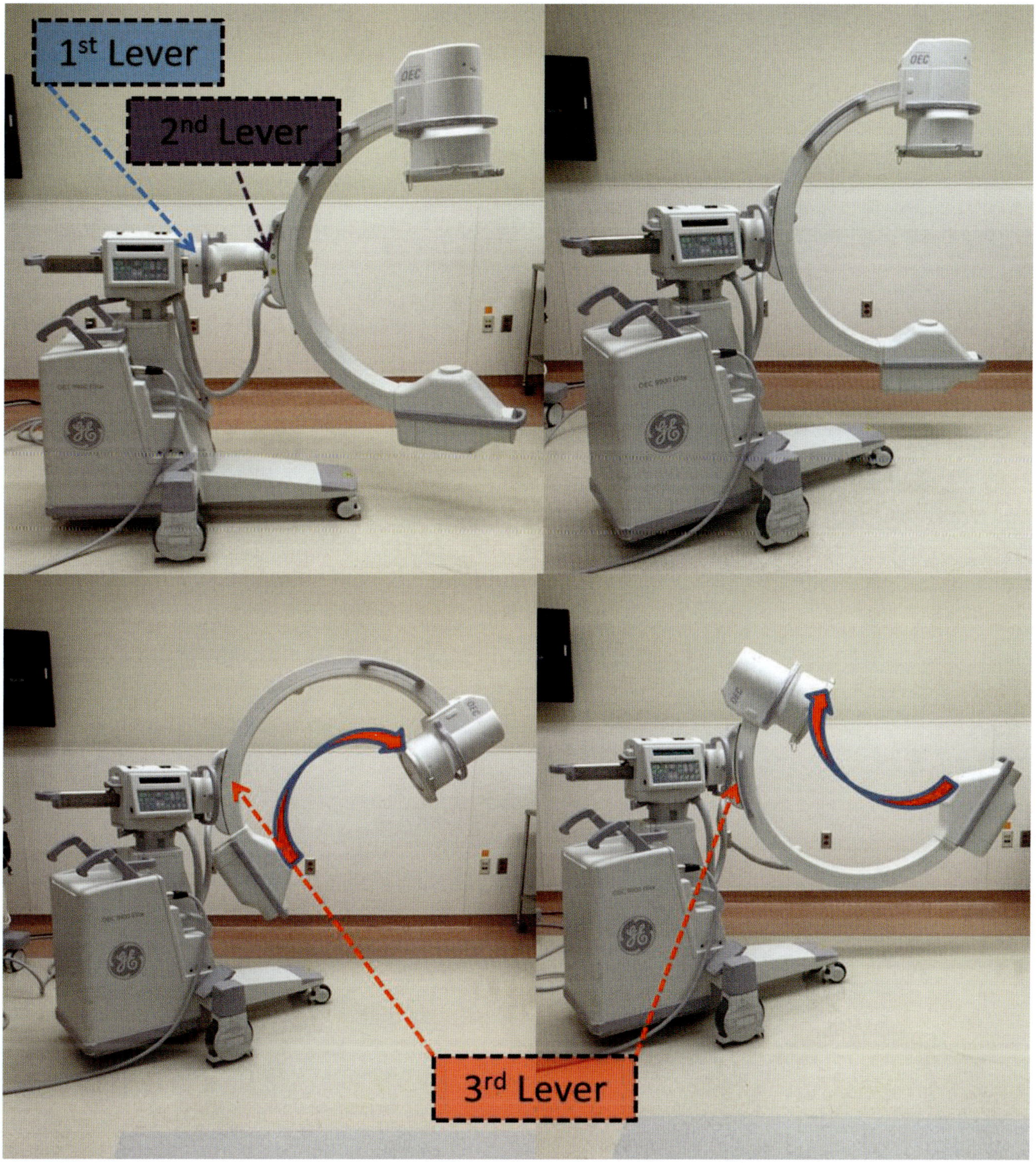

Figure A1-13

Index

Note: Page numbers in *italics* refer to figures.